Clinical echocardiography

Clinical echocardiography

NAVIN C. NANDA, M.D.

Director, Noninvasive Cardiology Laboratory (Graphics-Echo),
Assistant Professor of Medicine and Radiology,
University of Rochester School of Medicine
and Dentistry; Associate Physician and Cardiologist,
Strong Memorial Hospital;
Consultant in Cardiology,
Genesee Hospital, Rochester, New York

RAYMOND GRAMIAK, M.D.

Professor, Department of Radiology,
Chief, Ultrasound Division, Division of Diagnostic Radiology,
University of Rochester School of Medicine
and Dentistry, Rochester, New York

with 695 illustrations

The C. V. Mosby Company

Saint Louis   1978

The C. V. Mosby Company
11830 Westline Industrial Drive, St. Louis, Missouri 63141

Library of Congress Cataloging in Publication Data

Nanda, Navin C   1937-
    Clinical echocardiography.

    Bibliography: p.
    Includes index.
    1. Heart—Diseases—Diagnosis. 2. Ultra-
sonic cardiography. I. Gramiak, Raymond,
1924-   joint author. II. Title.
[DNLM: 1. Echocardiography. WG141.5.E2 N176c]
RC683.5.U5N36   616.1′2′0754   78-4116
ISBN 0-8016-3622-1

GW/CB/B   9 8 7 6 5 4 3 2 1

To our parents
Maya Vati and Dr. Balwant Rai Nanda
and
Tekla and Peter Gramiak

Foreword

Ultrasonic cardiography, or echocardiography, has grown considerably in just a little over ten years. Within this relatively short period of time, echocardiography has become one of the most useful noninvasive techniques in the diagnosis of cardiovascular disease throughout the world.

Drs. Nanda and Gramiak have written an excellent book for the use of cardiologists, trainees, and technologists in cardiology who desire to learn clinical echocardiography. This book covers the basic principles, instrumentation, and techniques of echocardiography and, in addition, details the echocardiographic findings present in various types of acquired and congenital cardiovascular diseases. The authors have compiled an enormous store of clinical findings, based upon their own personal collections, and have organized and presented the data in a remarkably lucid manner. They have been able to link beautifully the results of their experience in research and their day-to-day clinical observations. The inclusion of a comprehensive chapter on real-time, two-dimensional cardiac imaging is most welcome and emphasizes this system as a major and important direction in the field of current and future echocardiography. The illustrations in this book are abundant and of good quality, and the bibliography is up-to-date and extensive.

It has been my privilege to witness the formation, growth, and expansion of the echocardiographic laboratory in this medical center, from which many publications of original work emanated and in which an active investigational and educational program is in progress. I wish to compliment the authors for the completion of this fine book, which I am sure will provide important and pertinent information concerning clinical echocardiography for many interested readers.

Paul N. Yu, M.D.

Sarah McCort Ward Professor of Medicine
Head, Cardiology Unit
University of Rochester
School of Medicine and Dentistry

Preface

The recent enormous growth and wide acceptance of echocardiography have emphasized the need for a textbook directed at the trainee enrolled in a structured program or learning the technique independently. The available textbooks are excellent reference sources containing comprehensive descriptions of clinical echocardiography, but they do not cater to the special needs of a beginner who must first master the everyday aspects of the echocardiographic examination, quickly grasp the salient diagnostic findings in various conditions, and understand the value of echocardiography in clinical diagnosis and patient management. With progressive development, greater depth in the fine points of diagnosis, embellishment of technique, and the avoidance of pitfalls assume major importance.

We have attempted to compile a simplified learning or teaching textbook that is expected to fulfill the needs of the beginning echocardiographer and at the same time provide a comprehensive overview of the field that encompasses acquired and congenital heart disease. Although this book is mainly directed to trainees in cardiology and other medical specialties, the simple and direct approach employed should make it equally useful to technologists. The experienced echocardiographer may also benefit from the unique organization of our text as a ready reference or review, from the detail offered in the interpretation of echocardio-

graphic findings, as well as the analysis of pitfalls in interpretation. This text offers a review of our long experience, which encompasses several years and more than 11,000 clinical examinations performed by us or by trainees under our close supervision. In almost all instances, continuous records in a strip chart format have been obtained using a 35-mm camera with continuously moving film.

Some features of this text are directed at the special needs of a beginning echocardiographer. The style is straightforward and concise, with fundamental concepts heavily illustrated by sketches. Numerous echocardiographic illustrations have been used to exemplify findings in normal and diseased states as well as examination pitfalls and artifacts. They have mostly been selected from our files to maintain uniformity of presentation. Generally, high-speed recordings have been employed to present details in motion patterns in individual cardiac cycles. Judicious cropping minimizes distraction and provides emphasis for elucidation of specific diagnostic findings or concepts. The accompanying legends are detailed and comprehensive to make each illustration self-explanatory.

Literature citations at the ends of chapters provide background reading material and acknowledge the work of the numerous investigators who have contributed to the advancement of echocardiography. Simplicity of presentation precludes mention of individual authors by name in the text, and for this we apologize.

At the suggestion of trainees and technical staff in our laboratory, the text begins with a short summary of the important concepts in clinical cardiology that is oriented toward the special needs of an echocardiography technologist. The section describes normal cardiac anatomy and function, changes in structure and function produced by disease, and the clinical investigations commonly employed to detect disease or to obtain proof of the fundamental pathology present. We expect that the physicians supervising the training of technologists will find this section particularly useful as a supplement to their efforts.

The second chapter explains the basic principles of ultrasound as they apply to echocardiography. The material is presented in a narrative form, minimizing mathematical formulas not of practical value. Physical factors as they pertain to image formation, operational concepts of clinical devices, the function of instrument controls, signal processing as it affects the images, potential biologic effects, and recording techniques are included. The section on echocardiographic examination technique explains in-depth aspects of patient interaction, the recording of auxiliary information such as the ECG and phonocardiogram, transducer manipulation, and instrument control settings. Cardiac target characteristics are described by their position, motion, and echo amplitude. The anatomy of cardiac structure presentation is explained and illustrated for all common beam positions and is followed by a discussion of recording philosophy, the use of interventions, and a series of comments emphasizing techniques used to produce an ideal examination.

The major portion of this book deals with clinical echocardiography and is generally organized according to a structure of interest such as the mitral valve. Each section begins with a review of the structures in the beam, followed by a description of a normal tracing and technical comments. In disease descriptions, anatomic and pathologic changes as well as clinical findings pertinent to the echocardiographic examination are summarized and are followed by a listing of the salient echocardiographic features. Brief, individual comments describe variations in findings, differential diagnosis, alert the examiner to other areas in which the disease process may produce changes in the echocardiogram, and highlight subtle technical details that enhance the quality of the examination. They also emphasize pitfalls in the echocardiographic assessment, with special reference to improper technique and misinterpretation of echocardiographic findings. The beginner may choose to postpone in-depth perusal of the comments sections until some familiarity with the basic examination techniques and salient diagnostic findings has been attained. Each disease process description concludes with a statement that evaluates the role of echocardiography in patient management.

Congenital lesions, when they involve a single structure, are incorporated into the sections dealing with specific valves or cavities. A separate chapter on complex malformations begins with a brief summary of relevant embryology for the understanding of the development of various congenital anomalies. Individual lesions are presented in the same format as other clinical chapters.

The final chapter discusses the emerging technique of real-time, two-dimensional echocardiography and highlights the features of current systems. We have attempted to present a comprehensive and systematic approach to the demonstration of cardiac anatomy for single structures as well as for regional examination by describing a series of planes usually designated by contained heart valves or by their relationship to valve-based landmarks. Numerous drawings show the orientation of these examining planes in the heart and include the disposition of anatomic structures encountered. Images obtained from a mechanical sector scanner illustrate the anatomy and the changes produced by disease.

The appendix contains tables of normal values measured from echocardiograms and outlines of the differential diagnosis of various common echocardiographic findings.

It is our hope and expectation that this book provides a valuable fundamental reference source for the beginning echocardiographer to speed the understanding of funda-mental concepts and to accelerate the development of technical expertise in echocardiography.

Navin C. Nanda
Raymond Gramiak

Acknowledgments

The writing of this textbook has revealed to us the complexity of our activities and has emphasized the enormous support and help that we enjoy in our work at the University of Rochester. We have attempted to identify those individuals who have made a direct contribution to the preparation of this book but suspect that our review is not all-inclusive. We therefore apologize to all who have been helpful and who have been inadvertently omitted.

We must first thank those individuals who have been instrumental in the growth and development of our echocardiographic laboratory through the provision of support and by their active cooperation in our activities. Dr. Harry W. Fischer, Chairman of the Department of Radiology, has generously provided space and facilities as well as encouragement in our activities. Dr. Paul N. Yu, Chief of Cardiology Unit, has given us strong clinical support and has enthusiastically encouraged us in all our activities, including working in the cardiac catheterization laboratory. Dr. James Manning, Chief of Pediatric Cardiology, has provided us a rich clinical environment, warm support, and the opportunity to perform echocardiographic studies in the pediatric catheterization laboratory. Most important, all have encouraged trainees to enter our training program and to engage in the investigative activities of our group. We owe special thanks to Dr. Pravin M. Shah, whose contribution during our early development is sincerely appreciated. Dr. Chloe Alexson and Dr. Peter Harris, of pediatric cardiology, have offered continued stimulation and valuable suggestions in our clinical activities. We also thank Drs. James DeWeese and Scott Stewart for providing surgical correlations important in our work. Dr. DeWeese kindly supplied us specimens of the diseased mitral and aortic valves illustrated in this book.

Our major vote of thanks is to the trainees who have been part of our training program. It is their need for answers to questions that indicated a need for a textbook of this type. Their progression through stages of development helped us conceive the organization of the text. Their clinical examinations and investigations supplied valued data and demonstrations of clinical findings, pitfalls, and artifacts. For this experience we are grateful to Drs. Trevor Robinson, Charles Gross, William Reeves, Ullrich Ettinger, Harry Lever, Anthony Lombardi, James Scovil, Paul Hess, Andrew Ross, Robert Combs, Karl Sze, John Zesk, David Schwenker, David Pocoski, and William Epps (all cardiology trainees); Seth Borg and Kenneth Thomson (radiology trainees); and Kyung Chung (pediatric cardiology trainee).

Medical students Ronald Schwartz and James Powers also carried out investigations and have allowed us to refer to their work in our text. Dr. Angel Dela Torre, Chief of Cardiology, St. Vincent's Medical Center,

Jacksonville, Florida, kindly supplied the photograph of a myxomatous mitral valve.

Many persons aided us in the preparation of the manuscript and illustrations. We acknowledge the generous help of Dr. William Reeves in preparing references; Ben Emerson and Nicholas Graver for their expert photographic efforts; Robert Wabnitz, Laura Hayward, Richard Howe, Anita Matthews, and William Coons for their artistic contributions; Michelle Berdych, Julie Warner, Colleen Krebbeks, and Karen Wickman for help in assembling illustrations; Ginny Bleier and Erna Larusdottir for library assistance; Adele Khuzami for manuscript typing and general organization of multiple aspects of our effort; and Beth Nestorowycz, Judy Olevnik, and Bonnie Hadden for assistance in manuscript preparation.

The evaluation of manuscript content was aided by Drs. Paul Hess and James Scovil, who were trainees in our department at the time of manuscript writing and by Dr. Serge Barold, Chief of Cardiology Division, The Genesee Hospital. Their reviews are gratefully acknowledged. Donna Bowles, a special project nurse in the cardiology unit, was extremely helpful and provided excellent suggestions that were used to formulate the section on the fundamentals of clinical cardiology. We are grateful to Drs. Serge Barold, Ling Ong, Robert Heinle, and Michael Falcoff of the cardiology division of The Genesee Hospital for helpful advice and for permitting us to use some of the work done in the Louis and Molly Wolk Ultrasound Laboratory of the Department of Medicine.

We extend our gratitude to Drs. Paul Hess, Williams Reeves, Andrew Ross, Karl Sze, Robert Combs, John Zesk, and David Schwenker for their helpful suggestions and advice as well as for their patient examination efforts, which provided us with additional hours that could be devoted to the many tasks required for completion of our book. We are grateful to Drs. David Pocoski and William Epps for their help in carrying out two-dimensional contrast studies.

Our engineering colleagues, Dr. Robert C. Waag, Paul P. K. Lee, and Peter Helmers, were kind enough to support our efforts in describing the physical aspects of ultrasound and to offer guidelines in reducing complex concepts to easily understood narrative description.

The chapter on two-dimensional imaging could not have been written without the strong support of the Picker Corporation, which supplied the clinical imager from which illustrations of normal and abnormal anatomy were made.

Finally, we would like to acknowledge the warm support and understanding of our wives and families, who tolerated our absence from home during long and irregular working hours.

Contents

PART ONE
Fundamentals of echocardiography

1 Clinical cardiology, 3

2 Basic principles of ultrasound, 28

3 Echocardiographic examination technique, 54

PART TWO
Clinical echocardiography

4 Mitral valve, 87

5 Aortic valve, 160

6 Tricuspid valve, 192

7 Pulmonary valve, 222

8 Left ventricle, 244

9 Pericardial effusion, 268

10 Prosthetic valves, 293

11 Complex malformations, 312

12 Two-dimensional echocardiography, 369

Appendix, 432

General review articles, 437

PART ONE

Fundamentals of echocardiography

1 Clinical cardiology

NORMAL CARDIAC ANATOMY AND FUNCTION

The structures surrounding the heart influence the quality and completeness of an echocardiogram. Bone and lung are barriers that are essentially impenetrable to ultrasound and obscure portions of the heart.

Cardiac relationships

The heart lies in a midline position with the apex or lowermost point extending to the left (Fig. 1-1). It is contained in a fibrous sac, the pericardium, which isolates and protects it from invasion by adjacent disease processes. The pericardium secretes a small amount of fluid (normally less than 25 ml), which lubricates the moving surface of the heart walls. The outer surface of the heart consists of a thin, smooth lining, the epicardium, which contains variable amounts of fat between it and the muscular walls, the myocardium. Internally, the cavities of the heart are lined by a similar thin membrane, the endocardium, which separates the muscle from the contained blood.

The heart and pericardium lie immediately below the chest wall, which includes the sternum (breastbone), ribs, and costal cartilages, which are semiflexible and connect the ribs to the sternum. In children the sternum is comprised mainly of cartilage and, like the costal cartilages, transmits sound easily and does not limit examination of the heart with ultrasound. In adults the sternum is regularly calcified and blocks passage of the beam.

With increasing age the costal cartilages also calcify and may make examination difficult.

In the chest the right heart structures occupy an anterior location somewhat more to the right (closer to midline) than are the more deeply situated posterior left heart structures. Their relative positions during echocardiographic examination are discussed in more detail when the examination of specific valves is discussed.

The left lung lies laterally and surrounds the apex and posterior wall to a variable degree. Anteriorly, there is usually enough lung-free space to provide a window through which the heart can be examined (Fig. 1-2). Posteriorly, the lung extends to the margin of the mediastinum, a central compartment containing the heart, esophagus, thymus gland, trachea, aorta, and other structures. The mediastinum separates the two lungs and lies in contact with the central posterior portion of the pericardium. It extends from the diaphragm inferiorly to the base of the neck superiorly. It provides another lung-free path through which the heart and great vessels may be examined ultrasonically by placing the probe in the notch at the upper end of the sternum, the suprasternal notch, or at the lower end of the sternum, the xiphoid process.

The lung is contained in a fibrous sac, the pleura, which is similar to the pericardium in structure and function. The pleura, like the lung, does not extend completely around the heart posteriorly into the midline.

3

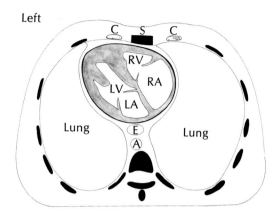

Fig. 1-1. Normal anatomic relationships. This cross section of the thorax shows position of heart relative to lung, bony structures, mediastinal contents, and costal cartilages. Apex of heart is directed toward the left, and right heart chambers are located medially and anteriorly in respect to the left heart. S, sternum; C, costal cartilage; RV, right ventricle; RA, right atrium; LV, left ventricle; LA, left atrium; E, esophagus; A, descending aorta.

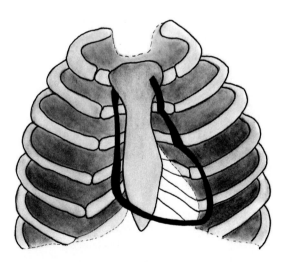

Fig. 1-2. Cardiac window. This schematic frontal view of the chest shows the heart partially covered by the centrally placed sternum and by the lung, which is shown in gray. The clear area over the lower portion of the heart is the cardiac window, through which ultrasonic examinations are carried out. The costal cartilages that pass across the window are generally sonolucent and do not impede the ultrasonic examination. The window varies widely, depending on the size of the heart, the shape of the chest, and body position. Since the window does not permit direct access to all portions of heart, beam angulation techniques are important to look under barriers such as bone and lung for structure detection.

Position and function of chambers

Functionally, the heart is divided into right and left or pulmonary and systemic circuits (Fig. 1-3). The function of the right heart is to accept nonoxygenated blood, which flows into the heart from the superior vena cava, which drains the upper half of the body, and the inferior vena cava, which drains the abdomen and lower extremities. The right heart pumps blood through the pulmonary artery into the lungs for oxygenation. The left side receives oxygenated blood via the pulmonary veins and delivers it to the body through the aorta and systemic arteries.

The heart chambers in each circuit consist of a receiving portion, the atrium, and a muscular pump, the ventricle. Valves are present between these chambers as well as between the ventricles and outflow vessels to prevent backflow within the heart during ventricular contraction (systole) or from the great vessels during ventricular relaxation and filling (diastole). The right and left atria lie adjacent to each other and are separated by a common partition, the atrial septum. Similarly, the left and right ventricles are isolated from each other by the ventricular septum. This division assures that mixing of the oxygenated and nonoxygenated blood does not occur. Cardiac valves are composed of thin sheets of fibrous tissue covered by a smooth lining called the endocardium. The areas of their attachment are circular and are called annuli or rings. Those valves placed between the atria and ventricles are named atrioventricular valves (AV valves); those situated between the ventricles and outflow vessels are known as semilunar valves, because of the half-moon appearance of their cusps.

The AV valves open into the ventricular cavity in diastole and permit unobstructed blood flow from the atrium into the ventricle. In systole, rising pressure in the ventricular cavity forces the valve leaflets into a closed position. Each AV valve is attached to an ap-

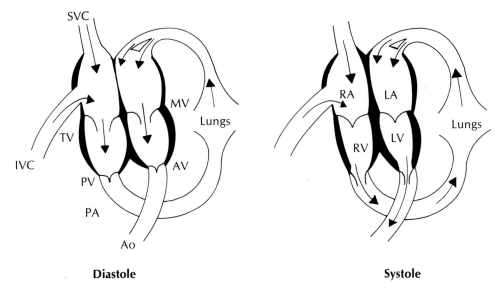

Diastole   **Systole**

Fig. 1-3. Normal circulation. Schematic representation of normal circulation shows inflow from venous orifices into atrial cavities and flow into ventricles through open AV valves in diastole. In systole, AV valves have closed, and blood is being ejected by ventricular contraction through open semilunar valves into aorta and lung. Note that diastolic inflow into atria continues throughout systole. SVC, superior vena cava; TV, tricuspid valve; MV, mitral valve; IVC, inferior vena cava; PV, pulmonary valve; AV, aortic valve; PA, pulmonary artery; Ao, aorta; RA, right atrium; LA, left atrium; RV, right ventricle; LV, left ventricle.

paratus that is intended to prevent inversion and therefore leakage during the high pressures achieved during systole (Fig. 1-4). Fingerlike projections of myocardium (the papillary muscles) extend from the ventricular walls toward the AV valves. Slender, cordlike bands, the chordae tendineae, connect the tips of the papillary muscles to the edges of the leaflets. The exact length of the chords and the systolic contraction of the papillary muscles ensure maintenance of tight closure of the AV valves. The semilunar valves are swept to an open position during systole, close in diastole, and maintain their diastolic closure as the result of their unique configuration. They are not associated with an apparatus that prevents inversion during closure.

The individual AV valves are named according to the number of leaflets they contain. The right-sided AV valve has three leaflets and is designated the tricuspid valve. The left-sided AV valve has two leaflets and is known as the bicuspid valve. Most often, however, it is called the mitral valve because of the resemblance to a bishop's mitre. The right-sided semilunar valve has been designated the pulmonic valve, since it lies at the junction of the right ventricle and the pulmonary artery. For similar reasons the left semilunar valve is known as the aortic valve.

Cardiac contraction occurs as the result of an electrical stimulus generated by a biologic pacemaker known as the sinoatrial (SA) node, located high in the right atrial wall. It spontaneously generates an impulse that spreads over the atrial walls and excites their contraction. Another node, the atrioventricular (AV) node, receives this impulse and passes it along a conduction system consisting of a single bundle of His and two branches, the right and left bundles, that spread out to form a network, Purkinje fibres, in the ventricles to conduct the impulse that excites ventricular contraction (Fig. 1-5).

The heart functions in a cyclic manner with

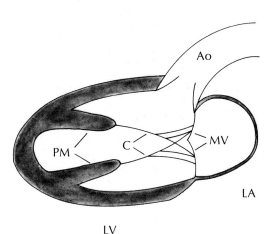

Fig. 1-4. Mitral apparatus. The papillary muscles (PM) and the chordae (C) anchor mitral valve leaflets during systole when pressure in ventricle is high, and outflow is occurring into aorta. The chordae are multiple and branch as they insert near edges of valve leaflets. They also cross over so that each papillary muscle is effective in stabilizing both mitral valve leaflets. Ao, aorta; MV, mitral valve; LA, left atrium; LV, left ventricle.

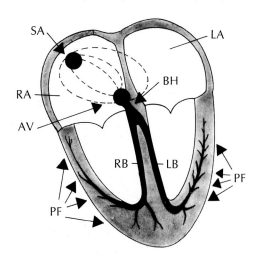

Fig. 1-5. Cardiac conduction system. The impulse that generates cardiac contraction originates in the sinoatrial node (SA) and spreads over the atria (dashed lines), causing them to contract. The impulse is received by atrioventricular node (AV) and is conducted through bundle of His (BH), which divides high in ventricular septum into right and left bundles (RB, LB). The bundles conduct impulse to ventricular myocardium through fine network of Purkinje fibers (PF), where the impulse stimulates ventricular myocardium to contract. RA, right atrium; LA, left atrium.

a phase of contraction (systole) and a phase of relaxation (diastole). Systole represents the time during which blood is ejected from the ventricle and occupies about one third of the cardiac cycle. Diastole denotes ventricular relaxation, during which the ventricle fills with blood from the atrium, and comprises the remaining two thirds of the cardiac cycle. It is convenient for echocardiographers to view a cardiac cycle as beginning just before the onset of ventricular diastole, when the atrial cavities are distended and the AV valves are still closed. The diastolic relaxation of the ventricles lowers the pressure in these cavities to a point below that in the atria, resulting in blood flow into the ventricle and a passive opening of the AV valve. Valve leaflet motion therefore reflects the pressure-flow pattern between the two chambers. Late in diastole, the atrial walls contract and expel additional blood into the ventricle. With the onset of systole the distended ventricles start to contract rapidly, raising cavity pressure above that in the atria and outflow vessels. As a result the AV valves close and the semilunar valves open, permitting efficient ejection of blood from the heart. During ejection, the atria are filling passively, receiving inflow from the venous orifices (openings). At the completion of ejection, ventricular pressure falls, the semilunar valves close, the AV valves open, and the cycle is repeated.

Detailed analysis of the contraction and relaxation process is useful in assessment of ventricular performance. The first phase of ventricular systole is called the isovolumetric contraction period, during which tension is being developed in the ventricular walls but there is no change in the volume of the ventricular cavity, since the semilunar valve is still closed. The isovolumetric relaxation period represents the interval between semilunar valve closure and the opening of the AV valve. During this period no blood is entering the ventricles, but the tension in the ventricular walls is decreasing.

Blood supply of heart

Two major arteries (left and right coronary arteries) arise from the base of the aorta just above the valve leaflets and branch out to supply the heart walls. The left coronary artery is distributed chiefly over left heart cavities and the interventricular septum, whereas the right supplies the right atrium and right ventricle. The two arterial networks are connected to each other by small peripheral interarterial channels (anastomoses), which can provide some cross-flow between the two systems (Fig. 1-6).

ABNORMAL CARDIAC ANATOMY AND FUNCTION
Structural abnormalities

Disease processes alter the orderly function of the heart in a variety of ways to decrease the pumping effectiveness or to place

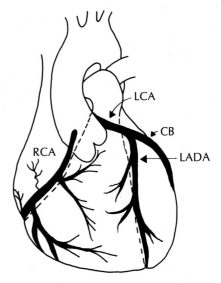

Fig. 1-6. Coronary circulation. Major coronary arteries are shown originating from base of aorta. Right coronary artery (RCA) runs in a groove on surface of heart between right atrium and right ventricle (dashed line). Left coronary artery (LCA) divides into a circumflex branch (CB) supplying the posterior wall of the left ventricle, and a left anterior descending artery (LADA) which supplies the apex and gives off branches to the interventricular septum. Groove between the right and left ventricles, in which the left anterior descending artery passes, is shown as a dashed line. The origin of left coronary artery is not visible on the surface of the heart, since it lies behind the right ventricular outflow tract, which is also shown by dashed lines.

an additional load on specific chambers through obstructions, intracardiac leaks, or combinations of these factors.

Obstructions are produced by a variety of mechanisms (Fig. 1-7). Most commonly, structural changes in valves limit normal opening and produce a stenosis. Congenital anomalies may give rise to fibrous ridges, membranes, or other deformities below (infravalvular) or above (supravalvular) otherwise normal valves. Masses may be located on valves or adjacent to valves to produce obstruction; overgrowth (hypertrophy) of a portion of a heart wall may contribute to obstruction. In some of these cases, abnormal valve motion projects normal leaflets into the outflow pathway during ejection. Functional or structural narrowing of the systemic or pulmonary small arteries leads to increased resistance against which the heart must work and raises pressure in these arteries (hypertension). The heart compensates for these obstructive changes by doing increased work, which results in symmetrical thickening of its walls (concentric hypertrophy) in the chambers lying behind the obstruction in the path of blood flow. The chambers involved show an increase in pressure (pressure overload), but the cavity size remains normal. The compensatory mechanism of hypertrophy may maintain an adequate level of function to permit virtually unrestricted activities, depending on the severity of the process. Long-standing pressure overload or the presence of other associated cardiac diseases may eventually result in myocardial damage and chamber enlargement. In atrioventricular valve obstruction, or stenosis, the forward (antegrade) flow of blood is decreased, and this may result in reduction of the size of the chamber beyond the obstruction. Stasis occurs and may give rise to clot formation in chambers proximal to obstruction. Clots may be hazardous, since portions may break off and be propelled out of the heart to lodge in the lung or systemic arteries, causing serious organ embarrassment or even death.

Valves may leak for a variety of reasons (Fig. 1-8). They may be deformed congenitally so that they do not close properly, or they may contain insufficient tissue to provide closure. Most commonly, valves leak because of acquired deformity secondary to some disease process. Thickening, calcification, or destruction of valve tissue may prohibit tight closure. The apparatus associated with the AV valve may be deformed congenitally (as in parachute mitral valve) or as a result of rheumatic fever, which thickens, distorts, and shortens the chordae tendineae and restricts the valve from moving into its proper position for closure. Dysfunction of the valve apparatus allows the valve to move too far during systole (mitral valve prolapse, coronary artery disease), so that closure is ineffective. In other instances the mitral valve may open during systole, possibly from abnormal traction by the papillary muscles or from rapid flow in the presence of a hypertrophied septum.

Injuries to the chest may tear a valve leaflet or portions of the valve apparatus. The valve may become flail so that it floats ineffectively with changes in chamber pressures and results in leakage and backflow. Processes producing chamber or great vessel enlargement may also dilate the annular areas

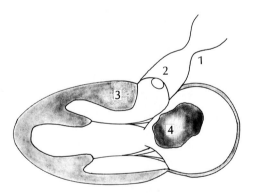

Fig. 1-7. Schematic demonstration of mechanisms that produce left heart obstructions. *1,* Supravalvular narrowing of aorta. *2,* Aortic valve stenosis, showing small circular valve orifice and upward doming of valve in systole. *3,* Asymmetric hypertrophy of the septum that encroaches on the left ventricular outflow space beneath the aortic valve. *4,* Tumor mass in left atrial cavity obstructing the mitral orifice.

to which the valves are attached. A normal valve contains enough extra tissue to compensate for a mild degree of ring dilatation, but a normal valve eventually becomes incompetent when dilatation progresses to a point beyond its ability to cover the orifice.

The apparatus requires the functional integrity of the atrium, annulus, leaflets, chordae tendineae, papillary muscles, and ventricular wall for its normal performance. Enlargement of the atrium may result in posterior displacement of its posterior wall so

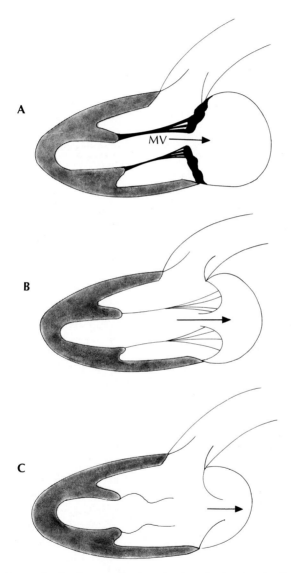

Fig. 1-8. Mechanisms of mitral regurgitation. In **A,** mitral valve leaflets are thickened and distorted by disease. Chordae tendineae are also thickened and shortened, resulting in incomplete closure of mitral valve in systole. In **B,** excessively long chordae permit mitral valve to balloon into left atrial cavity with inadequate closure of valve leaflets. In **C,** chordae have ruptured so that mitral valve becomes unstable and inverts into left atrial cavity. Note that left atrial cavity is largest in **A,** since the disease process is chronic.

that it exerts tension on the corresponding leaflet, preventing its proper coaptation and resulting in mitral incompetence.

Recent evidence suggests that mitral and tricuspid rings act as sphincters that contract and decrease their diameters by as much as 40% during atrial and ventricular systole. The rings also move downward and anteriorly during ventricular systole, probably due to the apex to base shortening of the ventricles. Ventricular dilatation results in lateral displacement of papillary muscles and prevents them from exerting their normal tension on the leaflets, thus producing improper leaflet coaptation and incompetence. Furthermore, impairment of ventricular contractility resulting from dilatation tends to minimize annular narrowing during ventricular systole and aggravates incompetence. In these instances the ring would also be expected to show decreased motion downward and anteriorly, and this may result in apparent flattening or sagging of the AV valve systolic segments on the echocardiogram. Abnormal left ventricular systolic contraction due to segmental myocardial disease may also aggravate mitral regurgitation in the same manner.

Valve regurgitation or incompetence produces backflow and disturbs the normal efficient forward pumping action of the heart. Additional volume is added to the chamber behind the incompetent valve with each cardiac cycle so that a volume overload results. The chamber receiving the regurgitant fraction dilates to accommodate the added blood volume. It also hypertrophies, since it must contract more vigorously to eject the increased volume. The thickness of the chamber walls is increased in the same proportion as the increase in the cavity diameter (Fig. 1-9). However this mechanism cannot compensate cardiac overloads indefinitely and eventually fails, depending on the severity and duration of the process.

Shunts between the cardiac chambers or great vessels are usually congenital in origin, though they may be acquired secondarily from infection, vascular injury to the ventricular septum, or from tunneling of leakage in a great vessel whose wall is diseased. A communication is produced from a high- to a low-pressure chamber with resultant shunting of blood. Shunts are usually named by the direction of blood flow (right to left) and by the level at which they occur (atrial or ventricular). Some are designated by the chambers or great vessels involved, beginning with the high pressure component (LV-RA shunt). Others are known by the persistence of a portion of fetal circulation that normally closes after birth (patent ductus arteriosus, patent foramen ovale).

Shunts may be bidirectional when pressures are nearly balanced, or they can be reversed when pressure in a chamber changes as part of the evolution of the disease process. Shunts produce mixing of nonoxygenated blood that is bluish in color with oxygenated bright red blood. This decreases the oxygen saturation of the systemic circulation and renders the skin and mucus membranes a dusky blue color (cyanosis, blue baby).

Chamber enlargement occurs in the portion of the circuit carrying the volume of the shunt that recirculates with each cardiac cycle. For instance, in atrial septal defect, the shunt flow occurs from the left atrium into the right atrium and is recirculated through the pulmonary circuit. As a result, right heart chambers and the pulmonary artery become enlarged. The left atrium may enlarge slightly, but the left ventricle and aorta may be normal or small (Fig. 1-10).

With time, increased volume in the pulmonary circuit may damage the small vessels, leading to narrowing and increased resistance to flow and elevated pressures in the pulmonary artery and right heart. This pressure change reverses the normal left to right direction of the atrial shunt when the pulmonary artery pressure reaches or exceeds systemic levels, and cyanosis results.

Cardiac malformations are often associated with other anomalies of development such as mongolism, cleft palate, extra or webbed fingers and toes, and so on. The position of internal organs may be reversed (situs inversus) so that the heart may be located in the right side of the chest (dextrocardia). A struc-

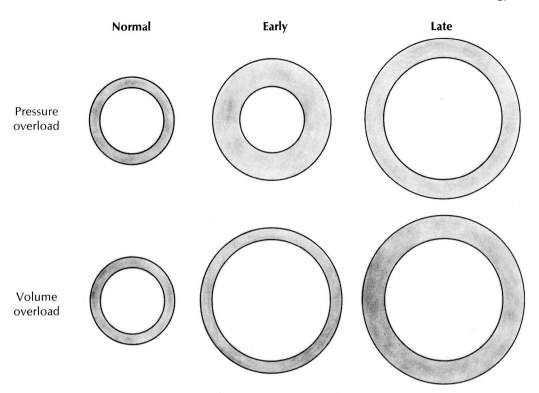

Fig. 1-9. Ventricular effects of pressure and volume overload. Pressure overload results in hypertrophy that first thickens wall of ventricle without alteration in chamber size. Late in the disease, chamber dilates without additional hypertrophy. In volume overload, chamber dilates early without hypertrophy of chamber wall. Later, hypertrophy ensues and wall becomes thickened.

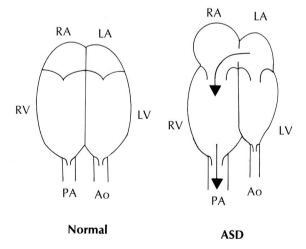

Fig. 1-10. Chamber enlargement as a result of intracardiac shunting. In an atrial septal defect (ASD), shunting occurs from left to right so that shunt volume *(arrows)* is added to volume of right heart chambers. As a result, right atrium (RA), right ventricle (RV), and pulmonary artery (PA) become enlarged. Left ventricle (LV) and aorta (Ao) are diminished in size. Left atrium (LA) usually remains normal.

ture such as a heart valve or great vessel may be absent (atretic), and the chamber or vessel distal to the atretic valve is usually absent or small. A septal defect must be present in the proximal chamber to permit its emptying, and a second communication must exist to bypass the obstruction and to establish some continuity of the pulmonary and systemic circuits to permit survival. A common pathway is the patent ductus arteriosus, which may remain open (patent) to serve as this important compensatory pathway (Fig. 1-11).

Complex malformations of importance to echocardiographers are discussed in the sections on clinical echocardiography. In general, they represent combinations of alterations in the origin of great vessels from cardiac chambers, underdevelopment or absence of valve or chambers, septal defects or total absence of septae, outflow stenoses, persistence of a single primitive undifferen-

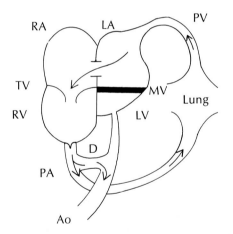

Fig. 1-11. Shunting as a compensatory mechanism for underdevelopment of cardiac structures. This is a schematic representation of mitral atresia with hypoplasia of left ventricle and proximal aorta. An atrial septal defect must be present to permit left atrium (LA) to empty. Blood flow to aorta is established by a patent ductus arteriosus (D), which permits blood flow from the pulmonary artery (PA) to normal distal aorta (Ao). RA, right atrium; TV, tricuspid valve; RV, right ventricle; PA, pulmonary artery; MV, atretic mitral valve; LV, left ventricle; PV, pulmonary veins.

tiated embryonic great vessel, and anomalies of pulmonary venous return. These conditions are the more severe forms of congenital heart disease in young children and frequently present with cyanosis, which is associated with an increase in the red blood cell content (hematocrit) of the blood as a compensatory mechanism to increase oxygen-carrying capacity. The thickened blood moves more sluggishly through smaller arteries and may result in clot formation (thrombosis). The arteries of the brain are often involved and may be complicated by infection with abscess formation. Pressure and volume changes within the heart vary, depending on the degree of filling of chambers and great vessels. Intracardiac flow patterns become complex, and there is marked distortion of normal anatomy. The growth and development of the child are adversely affected. Echocardiographic examination of these children requires great skill and flexibility on the part of the examiner to locate and identify structures and altered relationships.

Cardiac lining abnormalities

Infection may involve the inner lining of the heart (endocarditis) and is designated by the nature of the organism (bacterial, fungal) and the stage of the disease (acute, subacute, or healed). Organisms that enter the bloodstream tend to settle on abnormal areas such as diseased heart valves, the margins of septal defects, or where abnormal jets impinge on heart walls. The process produces thick, soft, friable masslike lesions (vegetations) that may shed portions with downstream seeding (emboli). When valves are involved, destruction of leaflets or of the valve apparatus is common, with resultant valvular regurgitation. Healed lesions may become calcified.

The endocardial lining of the heart may be congenitally thickened and produce changes in the function and configuration of the heart (endocardial fibroelastosis) much as those described later in cardiomyopathies.

The outer lining of the heart is frequently involved in inflammatory processes or by tumor invasion (pericardial effusion). When fluid accumulates rapidly (acute effusion), it may compress the heart (tamponade) acutely, reducing cardiac output. Slow accumulations (chronic effusion) may act as an impediment to cardiac filling (restrictive process) or produce no cardiac dysfunction. Healing of the inflamed pericardial surfaces may make them adherent to the heart and result in progressive cardiac constriction as the scar tissue contracts (constrictive pericarditis). The functional result is that of a restrictive process with embarrassment of chamber filling.

Myocardial dysfunction

Decreased muscle function may be generalized or segmental and results in impairment of cardiac performance and systemic perfusion (cardiac output).

Atherosclerosis produces thickening of the inner lining (intima) of the coronary vessels, and reduces the width of the channels. If mild, blood supply to the myocardium is reduced (ischemia) only during physical stress, resulting in chest pain during exertion (angina). More severe narrowing and occlusions deprive a segment of the myocardium of its blood supply and result in prolonged chest pain and muscle death (myocardial infarction).

The infarcted area loses its ability to contract normally and is gradually replaced by fibrosis and scarring, with eventual thinning of the wall. High ventricular pressure may balloon this area and produce a ventricular aneurysm (Fig. 1-12). Other complications depend on the location of the infarct. A weakened septum may perforate and create a ventricular septal defect, or the infarct may rupture into the pericardial cavity, producing sudden death. When papillary muscles are involved, they may become dysfunctional or may rupture. Both produce mitral regurgitation, which is more severe and often fatal in the presence of rupture.

Clots may form over infarcted areas or in ventricular aneurysms and may become detached and be carried into the systemic circulation to produce infarcts of other organs.

Functional loss occurs, depending on the location and extent of infarction. Initially, the involved segment may simply move less than normal heart muscle does (hypokinesis). In more advanced forms the heart wall may not move during systole (akinesis), or the motion pattern of the involved ventricular wall may be reversed so that paradoxical motion occurs and the segment bulges with each contraction (aneurysm).

The ischemic area around an infarcted segment may be an irritable area in the myocardium, producing serious and fatal arrhythmias. If sufficient muscle is damaged, the pumping action of the ventricle may be lost, with ensuing death. Intermediate degrees of muscle loss result in low cardiac output and poor systemic perfusion, depending on the site and extent of the abnormality.

When the infarct extends to the epicardial surface, a local pericarditis may be present and produce a pericardial effusion.

Surgery is used in the preinfarction phase of the disease or when angina is uncontrolled by medical therapy. The most common operation is bypass surgery in which a vein graft is inserted between the aorta and the involved coronary artery beyond the point of occlusion to increase blood flow in the involved segment. In some instances, surgical removal of the obstruction (endarterectomy) may be performed in conjunction with the bypass procedure.

Diseases producing diffuse involvement

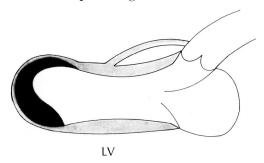

LV

Fig. 1-12. Left ventricular aneurysm. Apex of left ventricle has been involved in myocardial infarction that has thinned left ventricular wall (LV) with resultant bulging (aneurysm). A clot (thrombus) has formed in the area (black) and is adherent to inner aspect of thinned ventricular wall.

of cardiac muscle (cardiomyopathies) can be toxic in origin (alcohol, the result of systemic infection, myocarditis, post-infectious cardiomyopathy) or due to abnormal metabolism (infiltrative cardiomyopathies), endocrine disorders (myxedema), and unknown causes. Diffuse myocardial impairment from ischemic or hypertensive heart disease or chronic, advanced valvular lesions is not included under the term cardiomyopathy.

Cardiomyopathies may produce large dilated hearts, usually involving all chambers, with poor contraction of the walls and low cardiac output (Fig. 1-13). Valve motion is decreased, though the valves are structurally normal (congestive cardiomyopathy). When an infiltrative process stiffens the chamber walls, expansion during filling is limited. In the ventricles, diastolic filling is compromised and the slow atrial emptying alters the motion pattern of the AV valves. Cardiac enlargement is not a prominent feature in these cases (restrictive cardiomyopathy).

Other cardiomyopathies are typified by hypertrophy of the cardiac walls (hypertrophic cardiomyopathy), which may be symmetric or asymmetric. The latter is the most common variety seen in echocardiography. The septum is thickened disproportionately as compared to the posterior left ventricular wall and bulges into the outflow tract. Some of these patients manifest outflow obstruction secondary to the septal hypertrophy and to an abnormal protrusion of the mitral leaflets into the outflow during systole. The cause of this systolic anterior motion (SAM) is unknown but is probably related to a suction effect produced by rapid blood flow through an area of narrowing (Bernoulli or Venturi

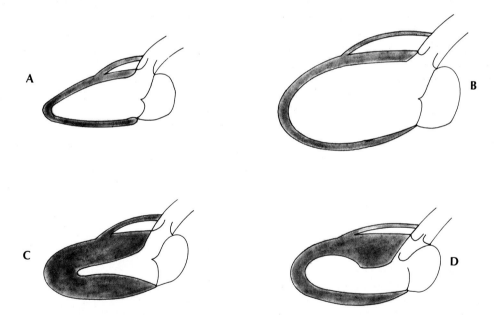

Fig. 1-13. Manifestations of cardiomyopathy. A normal ventricular contour is shown in **A.** Congestive cardiomyopathies **(B)** result in generalized dilatation of heart without significant thickening of heart walls. Hypertrophic cardiomyopathies **(C)** thicken ventricular walls symmetrically, reducing size of cavity. Asymmetric hypertrophic cardiomyopathy **(D)** produces massive thickening of ventricular septum while remaining ventricular walls are less hypertrophied or normal in thickness. In this condition there is left ventricular outflow tract obstruction related to the septal thickening as well as to an abnormal systolic anterior motion (SAM) of the mitral valve, which contributes to outflow obstruction. The ventricular cavity is generally small.

effect) or dysfunction of the papillary muscles, which pull the mitral valve up from the closed position. Mitral regurgitation is usually present. The left ventricular cavity is small and may obliterate in systole from vigorous contraction. This condition is commonly known as idiopathic hypertrophic subaortic stenosis (IHSS) or hypertrophic obstructive cardiomyopathy (HOCM).

Cardiac failure

When the heart is unable to maintain sufficient flow (cardiac output) to meet the metabolic needs of the body, cardiac failure occurs, since mechanisms such as hypertrophy and dilatation no longer compensate for the load placed on the heart. Predominant right heart failure results in incomplete transport of venous blood into the pulmonary artery. Peripheral venous engorgement occurs, leading to distention of neck veins, liver enlargement, edema (swelling) of dependent parts, and leakage of clear fluid into the abdominal cavity (ascites), thus producing distention. Isolated or predominant left heart failure results in incomplete clearing of pulmonary venous blood with pulmonary vascular congestion and edema of the lungs. The whole heart may usually fail, resulting in a combination of these findings (right and left heart failure). Pleural and pericardial fluid collections are frequently seen and can be detected by echocardiography (Fig. 1-14).

Disorders of rhythm

Disorders of rhythm change the rate or sequence of cardiac contraction. The SA node may fire more rapidly than normal under physiologic stress and produce a rapid heart rate (sinus tachycardia, 100/min or more), or it may beat more slowly (sinus bradycardia, less than 60/min). Abnormal foci of electrical activity may arise in the atrial or ventricular walls and produce premature contractions. Multiple foci in the atrium result in rapid, ineffective fluttering of the atrial walls (atrial flutter and fibrillation). The impulses are received by the AV node and produce rapid irregular ventricular contractions. Atrial systole is absent and, coupled with shortened diastolic filling of the ventricle, results in a decrease in the cardiac output. When similar foci are present in the ventricular walls, ventricular fibrillation follows and may lead to sudden death unless treated promptly, since effective ventricular contraction ceases. This is often preceded by repeated runs of ventricular premature beats (ventricular tachycardia).

The AV node may be blocked completely so that impulses arising from the SA node are not transmitted to the ventricles. These nodes then function independently at their own rates so that atrioventricular dissociation occurs with different intrinsic rates (complete heart block). Partial degrees of block result in delay between atrial and ventricular contractions or there is nonconduc-

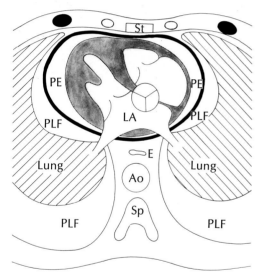

Fig. 1-14. Pleural and pericardial effusion. Pericardium is shown as heavy line surrounding heart and containing a pericardial effusion (PE). The pericardial space is generally widest laterally but can be seen anteriorly as well as posteriorly. It is obliterated where the pulmonary veins enter the heart, but there is a shallow space present behind left atrium (LA). Pleural fluid (PLF) does not extend anteriorly over the heart and cannot be seen behind the left atrium, since the mediastinal pleural reflections prevent pleural fluid from entering the mediastinal space. E, esophagus; Ao, aorta; Sp, spine; St, sternum.

tion of certain SA node impulses (incomplete heart block). Blocks in the bundle branches do not produce arrhythmias but delay the onset and duration of the contraction of the ventricle supplied by that branch (left or right bundle branch block).

CLINICAL INVESTIGATIONS
Electrocardiography

The generation and conduction of electrical impulses have been described. Electrocardiography is the recording and interpretation of the wave forms obtained. Routine recording requires the application of electrodes to the skin in a standardized manner to obtain comparable results. Electrocardiographic leads are combinations of electrodes from which the signal is obtained either as a difference from pairs of electrodes or directly from a single electrode. Different leads are used to emphasize the electrical signals obtained from different portions of the myocardium. Clinical evaluation of patients requires a 12-lead electrocardiogram that includes chest (precordial) and limb leads, but in echocardiography only one of the standard leads (I, II, or III) is routinely recorded (Fig. 1-15) with echocardiograms to provide landmarks to correlate the ultrasound recordings with the exact point in the cardiac cycle.

The size of deflection recorded with different leads varies, but all of them normally show three different complexes in every normal cardiac cycle. The first deflection (P wave) represents the spread of the excitation impulse over the atria. The second (QRS complex) consists of a large positive deflection (R wave) preceded and often followed by smaller deflections (the Q and S waves). This complex represents the passage of the electrical impulse through the network of conducting fibers of the ventricle after passage through the AV node and bundle of His; its normal duration usually ranges between 0.06 and 0.10 sec. The interval between the onset of the P wave and the onset of the QRS comples (P-R interval) measures the time of atrial propagation of the impulse and its normal delay at the AV node, generally between 0.12 and 0.20 sec.

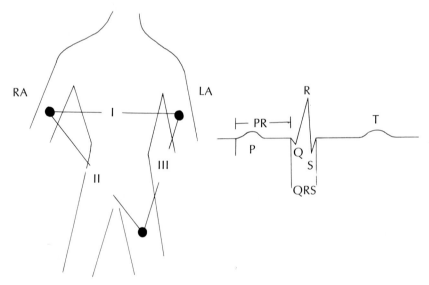

Fig. 1-15. Electrocardiographic leads used in echocardiography. Electrodes are shown attached to right arm (RA), left arm (LA), and to left leg. Leads represent potential differences between electrodes and are identified by Roman numerals commonly used. A typical ECG trace is shown with identification of waveforms. Intervals of interest in echocardiography are identified (PR, QRS). The shape of the QRS complex varies depending on leads recorded.

The third deflection that is always present is the T wave, a generally positive deflection whose termination closely approximates the end of ventricular systole. The T wave represents repolarization of the ventricular myocardium, a recharging phenomenon of the myocardial cells that prepares them to receive the next impulse (Fig. 1-15).

Clinical electrocardiography requires calibration of signal voltage and control of recording speed. Electrocardiographic diagnosis is obtained through precise measurement of time intervals, height of wave deflections, baseline displacement, and observation of alteration of waveforms. Diagnosis requires synthesis of information from multiple leads. In a given patient the heart rate can be measured by determining the time interval between two successive QRS complexes.

Electrocardiography is useful in a variety of clinical conditions. Abnormalities of rhythm and rate can be precisely characterized. Ventricular hypertrophy produces an increase in the size of the QRS complex, whereas atrial enlargement and hypertrophy results in amplitude and shape changes of the P wave. Myocardial infarction is recognized by shifts in ST segments and changes in the QRS complex and T waves from ischemia, muscle injury, or muscle death.

Premature beats from ectopic atrial or ventricular foci differ (Fig. 1-16). With supraventricular premature beats the involved cycle is shortened, but the QRS complex usually resembles that seen in normal sinus beats. The P waves may be present (with an atrial focus) or absent (when the focus is in the AV node). When the premature beat arises in the ventricular focus, the QRS complex becomes wide and bizarre in appearance, and the P waves are not visible. Premature beats are followed by a long interval (compensatory pause) before normal sinus rhythm is reestablished. Three or more successive premature beats constitute tachycardia, of which the ventricular variety is potentially life threatening.

In atrial fibrillation the P waves are replaced by irregular undulations of the base-

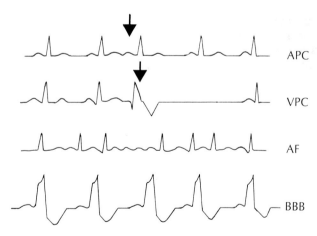

Fig. 1-16. Electrocardiographic traces obtained in rhythm and conduction disturbances. In atrial premature contraction (APC) the P wave *(arrow)* occurs early and is followed by a normal QRS complex and by a short pause before the next normal complex. In a ventricular premature contraction (VPC) an abnormal QRS complex *(arrow)* which is not preceded by a P wave, is generated, followed by a long compensatory pause. Atrial fibrillation (AF) results in rapid, irregularly spaced QRS complexes and small undulations of the baseline. Normal P waves are absent. When there is blockage of one of the branch bundles (BBB) the rhythm is undisturbed, but the individual QRS complexes are slurred and widened.

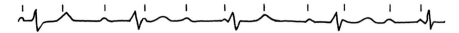

Fig. 1-17. Complete heart block. A complete block at level of AV node results in dissociation of atrial and ventricular complexes. The atrial rate is usually more rapid than the ventricular rate, and the P waves (marked by short lines) occur at regular intervals but without any relation to the QRS complexes.

line, and a rapid, irregular ventricular rate is present (Fig. 1-16).

Abnormal delay of the transmission of the impulse by the AV node prolongs the P-R interval and represents an incomplete heart block. With complete heart block, impulses are not transmitted by the AV node so that a focus distal to the block takes over generation of electrical impulses independently and at a slower rate. A typical tracing shows P waves with no fixed relation to the QRS complexes (Fig. 1-17).

The P-R interval may be abnormally short (less than 0.12 sec) when the impulse of the SA node bypasses the AV node and is conducted to the ventricle by anomalous pathways (Wolf-Parkinson-White, WPW, or pre-excitation syndrome).

When there is delay in conduction below the level of the His bundle, the duration of the QRS complex is increased and it exhibits slurring and notching (conduction defect, bundle branch block). When the block is complete, the QRS duration measures 0.12 sec or more (Fig. 1-16), whereas incomplete blocks are categorized by lesser delays. Inspection of precordial leads is necessary to distinguish left from right bundle branch block. In left bundle branch block (LBBB) the QRS complex in the right anterior precordial leads consists of a negative complex (QS wave) as opposed to right bundle branch block (RBBB), which has a prominent terminal R wave pattern.

Artificially implanted ventricular pacemakers produce an electrical impulse that stimulates the myocardium and is recorded as a vertical spike followed by a widened QRS complex.

Heart sounds, murmurs, and graphic recordings

Normally, two heart sounds are produced (Fig. 1-18). The first (S_1) occurs at the beginning of systole and is closely related to the closure of the mitral and tricuspid valves. The second heart sound (S_2) signifies the beginning of diastole and is generated by closure of the semilunar valves. Both heart sounds contain high- and low-frequency vibrations. S_2 can be separated into two major components originating from the aortic (A_2) and pulmonic (P_2) valves. A_2 is louder than P_2, and the interval between the two components lengthens during the inspiratory phase of respiration in normal subjects (physiologic splitting). The negative intrathoracic pressure during inspiration results in augmented systemic venous return into the right heart, producing an increase in the stroke volume and ejection time of the right ventricle. As a result, pulmonary valve closure is delayed. Since the pulmonary veins are intrathoracic structures, no significant alteration occurs in the left heart volume during the inspiratory phase (especially after a brief period of halted respiration), and aortic valve closure is not delayed. Recent studies suggest that the impedance characteristics of the pulmonary vascular bed are also involved in the mechanism of physiologic splitting of S_2.

Murmurs are produced by disease processes when abnormal blood flow forms jets and turbulence due to areas of narrowing or by increased flow through normal valves (Fig. 1-19). They are classified according to their time in the cardiac cycle (systole or diastole), their duration, loudness, and pitch. Stenotic and incompetent valves and septal

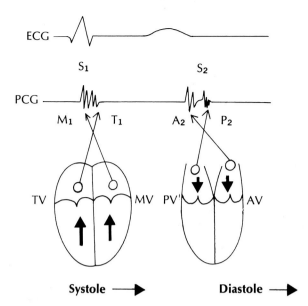

Fig. 1-18. Origin of heart sounds. The first heart sound (S₁) occurs mainly as the result of closure of the AV valves. M₁ is the component of the first heart sound related to mitral closure and T₁ relates to tricuspid valve closure. These components may not be separable on auscultation. The second heart sound (S₂) is produced by closure of the semilunar valves and can be more readily divided into two separate components, A₂ and P₂. A₂ is related to aortic valve closure and P₂ to pulmonic valve closure. ECG, electrocardiogram; PCG, phonocardiogram; TV, tricuspid valve; MV, mitral valve; PV, pulmonic valve; AV, aortic valve.

defects are responsible for most murmurs. Other abnormal heart sounds include midsystolic clicks related to mitral valve prolapse and early systolic sounds or clicks in patients with stenotic semilunar valves or outflow vessel dilatation. The stenotic mitral valve may produce a sound when it snaps open (opening snap). Rapid diastolic filling in the presence of a stiff or noncompliant ventricle may be associated with a middiastolic (S₃) or a late diastolic (S₄) sound (Fig. 1-19). Low-frequency rubbing sounds are produced by the roughened surfaces of the pericardium in pericarditis (pericardial rub).

The relations of individual murmurs to heart valves is obtained clinically by noting their location and pattern of radiation. Typically, mitral valve murmurs are heard medial to the apex, whereas aortic murmurs occur higher in the heart and may radiate into the neck (Table 1).

The technique used for recording heart sounds and murmurs is called phonocardiography (Fig. 1-19). Recordings are obtained on photosensitive paper using a microphone that is placed on the chest wall over the base of the heart, the left sternal border, and the apex area. Frequency filters are used to cut out background noise as well as to emphasize high- or low-pitched murmurs and other heart sounds. Analysis includes the time of onset in the cardiac cycle, duration, time-varying changes, location, the effects of respiration, body position, as well as minor interventions such as the Valsalva maneuver (breath holding and straining) and drugs like amyl nitrite. The interventions alter cardiac function and volume in a predictable manner and aid in the identification of the origin of certain murmurs. Phonocardiography documents clinically audible murmurs for teaching, research, and future comparison. When

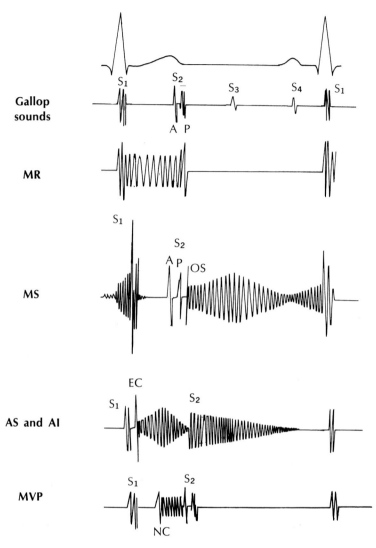

Fig. 1-19. Phonocardiographic representation of typical extra heart sounds and murmurs. Gallop sounds (S_3 and S_4) are shown in their usual diastolic position in the cardiac cycle. A murmur that extends throughout systole (pansystolic) is produced by mitral regurgitation (MR), whereas a diastolic murmur from mitral stenosis (MS) follows an opening snap (OS) and may be accentuated by atrial systole. The trace obtained in aortic stenosis and aortic insufficiency (AS and AI) reveals a diamond-shaped ejection murmur from the aortic stenosis and an early diastolic murmur resulting from aortic insufficiency. Ejection clicks (EC) occur early in systole and are seen in mild semilunar valve stenosis as well as in systemic or pulmonic hypertension. Mid to late nonejection systolic clicks (NC) occur in mitral valve prolapse (MVP) and may be followed by a systolic murmur of mitral regurgitation. S_1, first heart sound; S_2, second heart sound; A, aortic component; P, pulmonic component.

Table 1. Auscultatory and phonocardiographic findings in some clinical disease entities

Disease entity	Typical features
Mitral stenosis	Loud S_1; middiastolic rumbling murmur with presystolic accentuation at apex; opening snap occurs just before rumble; loud P_2 with pulmonary hypertension.
Mitral insufficiency	Loud pansystolic or holosystolic murmur (extends from S_1 to S_2) at apex; radiation to left axilla; S_3 and short middiastolic rumbling murmur due to increased flow through mitral orifice.
Mitral valve prolapse	Late systolic murmur associated with one or more midsystolic (non-ejection) clicks at apex; murmur may be pansystolic.
Aortic valve stenosis	Harsh diamond-shaped ejection systolic murmur (begins after S_1 and ends before A_2) at base and apex; peak intensity in midsystole or later; radiates to neck; early systolic (ejection) click may be present. When stenosis severe, click disappears and A_2 becomes soft and may occur after P_2, resulting in paradoxical splitting.
Idiopathic hypertrophic subaortic stenosis	Ejection systolic murmur at base (like aortic valve stenosis); variable intensity; increases with Valsalva maneuver and amyl nitrite inhalation; mitral insufficiency murmur at apex; prominent S_4 (due to hypertrophied and stiff left ventricle).
Aortic incompetence	High frequency, decrescendo blowing early diastolic murmur (starts with A_2) at base, left sternal border, or apex. Increased flow across valve may produce an ejection systolic murmur. When incompetence severe, middiastolic rumbling murmur (like mitral stenosis) may be present at apex (related to increased velocity of blood flow through a narrow mitral orifice resulting from the regurgitant jet partially closing the mitral valve [Austin-Flint murmur]).
Tricuspid stenosis	Middiastolic rumbling murmur at lower sternal border; increases in intensity with inspiration; may have presystolic accentuation.
Tricuspid insufficiency	Pansystolic murmur at left sternal border; increases in intensity with respiration; S_3 and middiastolic rumble may result from large flow across tricuspid valve.
Pulmonary stenosis	Harsh ejection systolic murmur (ends before P_2) over pulmonary area; wide (but not fixed) splitting of S_2 (P_2 closure delayed due to prolonged right ventricular ejection); P_2 soft when stenosis is severe; ejection click may be present when stenosis is not severe.
Pulmonary insufficiency	Blowing early diastolic murmur (starts with P_2) over pulmonary area.
Atrial septal defect	Ejection systolic murmur over pulmonary area (due to increased pulmonary blood flow); wide splitting of S_2 with no respiratory variations (fixed) due to fixed volume overload of the shunt; increased flow across tricuspid orifice may produce a middiastolic rumble; holosystolic murmur at apex in ostium primum defect.
Ventricular septal defect	Loud pansystolic murmur at left sternal border; physiologic or wide splitting of S_2; large shunting and large mitral flow may produce S_3 and middiastolic rumble; with pulmonary hypertension, P_2 loud.
Patent ductus arteriosus	Continuous murmur in systole and diastole over pulmonary area or under left clavicle; P_2 normal.

heart rates are rapid or when precise timing or duration of a sound is difficult to determine clinically, phonocardiography may play an important diagnostic role. Phonocardiography may be combined with echocardiography to provide correlation of the cardiac sounds with structure motion. It has provided better understanding of the origin of heart sounds and murmurs and has also been clinically useful in the investigation of the function of prosthetic valves.

Pulse waveform recording, apex cardiography, and the determination of systolic time intervals are other clinically useful noninvasive techniques for investigation of cardiac function. Pulse waveforms may be obtained by placing a small microphonelike probe over a pulsating vessel. The pulsations of a distended neck vein (jugular) or of the carotid artery (in the neck) contain information about cardiac function. The jugular venous pulse reflects function of right-sided structures, whereas the carotid pulse reflects some of the left ventricular and systemic ejection characteristics. It shows the onset, duration, and character of left ventricular ejection and may show some manifestations of aortic valve function.

Normally the carotid tracing shows a brisk initial upstroke reflecting the rapid rate of ejection of blood into the aorta and its large branches like the carotid artery at the beginning of systole. When the rate of ejection slows later in systole, a rounding at the top of the waveform occurs, and this is followed by a notch on the downslope that reflects cessation of ejection and reversal of blood flow in the aorta. The notch roughly coincides with the aortic component of the second heart sound (Fig. 1-20). The upstroke of the carotid pulse is delayed in the presence of

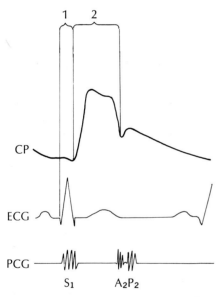

Fig. 1-20. Normal carotid pulse tracing. Carotid pulse (CP) is shown with simultaneously recorded ECG and phonocardiogram (PCG). Ventricular ejection results in rapid, brisk upstroke of carotid trace, which forms a peak followed by a decline in late systole. Rapid decline in late systole terminates in a notch that is related to aortic valve closure and is often used to identify the aortic component (A_2) of the second heart sound. The small notch following the peak is a normal finding. The interval (1) between the Q wave of the ECG and the beginning of the upstroke represents the pre-ejection period. Ventricular ejection occurs during interval 2.

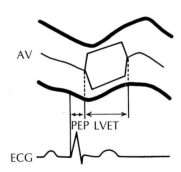

Fig. 1-21. Normal aortic valve echocardiogram. In schematic drawing, thick parallel lines represent walls of aortic root. The boxlike configuration in middle is formed by two cusps of the aortic valve (AV) in their open position during systole; closed position is represented by a central linear echo. The interval between beginning of QRS complex of the electrocardiogram (ECG) and the onset of aortic valve opening denotes the pre-ejection period (PEP); duration of valve opening is the left ventricular ejection time (LVET).

aortic valve stenosis, and the waveform may be bifid in IHSS.

Apex cardiography records the cardiac impulse at the apex of the heart and provides information concerning left ventricular filling and emptying.

The interval between the electrical excitation of the heart (beginning of QRS complex of the ECG) and the onset of ventricular ejection can be measured from simultaneously recorded aortic valve echocardiograms or carotid pulse traces (Fig. 1-21). The ratio between this interval (preejection) and the left ventricular ejection time is often called the systolic time interval and is useful in the clinical evaluation of left ventricular function.

Systolic time intervals are influenced by many factors. These include ventricular diastolic pressure, arterial diastolic pressure, the rate and sequence of intraventricular conduction, as well as the contractile state of the myocardium. Therefore the information obtained is of limited value.

Chest roentgenology and fluoroscopy

Chest roentgenograms provide images that show the size, position, and configuration of the heart, great vessels, and lungs. Heart size can be measured and followed serially. Individual chamber and great vessel size can also be evaluated. The degree of pulmonary vascular filling can be assessed from the size and density of the vascular markings and evidence of cardiac failure obtained. Pleural fluid and pulmonary diseases that influence cardiac function can be recognized.

Fluoroscopy uses x rays to image the heart in motion on a screen. It allows use of multiple oblique projections for better observation of the entire contour of the heart for determination of chamber size and pulsation. A barium swallow is routinely administered to visualize the relationship of the portions of the heart and great vessels that lie in the mediastinum (left atrium, segments of the aorta). Calcification of the pericardium, great vessels, and heart valves can be identified by their patterns of motion and location.

Radiologic techniques, such as chest roentgenology and fluoroscopy, may be inac-curate in the evaluation of chamber enlargement, since they rely on changes in cardiac contour and do not reveal the internal anatomy of the heart. For these reasons, an enlarged cardiac silhouette may be caused by enlargement of the heart or by pericardial effusion and cannot be readily differentiated by x-ray techniques. Ultrasound, on the other hand, is capable of delineating internal cardiac anatomy and recognizing cardiac silhouette enlargement from pericardial effusion.

Cardiac catheterization and angiocardiography

Cardiac catheterization involves the introduction of a slender catheter into the cardiac chambers through a peripheral vein or artery under fluoroscopic guidance. Right heart catheterization involves passing the catheter through an arm or leg vein and successively through the right atrium, right ventricle, the pulmonary artery, and finally lodging it snugly into a small peripheral pulmonary artery branch. The pressure in this wedged position closely approximates the pressures obtained in the left atrium and pulmonary veins. Left heart catheterization may be performed from the right heart by puncturing the atrial septum and passing the catheter into the left heart via the left atrium. Most often, a retrograde arterial approach is used from an arm or leg artery to pass the catheter into the aorta and left ventricle.

Cardiac catheterization determines the pressures in cardiac chambers and great vessels (Table 2). Abnormal elevations of pressures in specific chambers and altered pressure gradients between chambers are recorded. The shape of the pressure tracings may be of functional importance.

Cardiac output, which is the volume of blood ejected by the left ventricle per minute, can be measured by different techniques. The Fick principle utilizes the amount of oxygen consumption and the difference in oxygen content of venous and arterial blood. A green dye (cardio green, indocyanine green) can be injected into a heart chamber and sampled distally (indicator dilu-

Table 2. Normal pressures*

Area		Pressures (mm Hg)	
		Average	Range
Right atrium	Mean	2.8	1-5
Right ventricle	Peak systolic	25	17-32
	End-diastolic	4	1-7
Pulmonary artery	Mean	15	9-20
	Peak systolic	25	17-32
	End-diastolic	9	4-13
Pulmonary artery Wedge/left atrium	Mean	8	2-13
Left ventricle	Peak systolic	130	90-140
	End-diastolic	9	5-12
Systemic artery	Mean	85	70-105
	Peak systolic	130	90-140
	End-diastolic	70	60-90

*Modified from Fowler, N. O.: Cardiac diagnosis and treatment, New York, 1976, Harper & Row, Publishers.

tion technique). A time-concentration curve is obtained and used in the computation of cardiac output. The same principle is applied in thermodilution techniques in which a cold saline injection is used to produce a time-temperature curve. Normal cardiac output is 4 to 6 liters per minute; the volume ejected per heart beat (stroke volume) can be calculated by dividing the cardiac output by heart rate and ranges between 50 and 90 ml (average 70 ml) in normal persons.

Using the cardiac output, the area of the valve orifice can be calculated from the pressure gradient or differential pressure across the valve and from the flow through it. In an adult the normal mitral valve area is 4 to 6 cm², and functionally significant stenosis occurs when the area decreases to 2.5 cm² or less. The normal adult aortic valve area is 2.6 to 3.5 cm², and significant aortic stenosis usually shows a reduction to less than 50% of this value. Though useful clinically the calculated areas are unreliable in the presence of valvular incompetence.

In congenital heart disease the abnormal position and course of the catheter through heart chambers, great vessels, or into pulmonary vessels may reveal malposition of structures, the presence of anomalous veins, and deficiencies in atrial and ventricular sep-

ta. Monitoring of pressure and blood gas oxygen content is required for definitive identification of the type of chamber in which the catheter tip rests.

Analysis of blood gas content in various portions of the heart reveals the presence of mixing of blood from the right and left heart as well as the specific level at which the shunt occurs. The direction of the shunt (for example, R-L) and its size can also be evaluated. For instance, a left-to-right shunt at the atrial level adds volume to the right heart so that a ratio of flow through the pulmonic circuit, as compared to the systemic circuit, expresses the added volume in the right heart or shunt size.

Cardiac catheterization is a relatively safe procedure, and complications are uncommon. Cardiac arrhythmias, bleeding or thrombosis at the site of catheter introduction, and rarely, perforation of a heart wall or damage to a heart valve may occur. Along with angiocardiography, catheterization is the most valuable technique by which the nature and severity of cardiac disease is determined. The data obtained at cardiac catheterization have been the foundation upon which cardiac ultrasound interpretation is established.

Angiocardiography is often performed

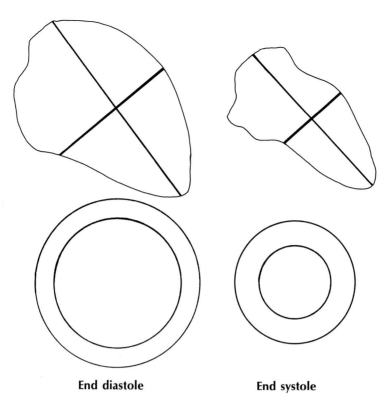

End diastole   **End systole**

Fig. 1-22. Left ventricular performance. Tracings made from left ventricular angiograms show cavity contours at end-diastole and end-systole. The long and short axes are shown. Beneath each contour is a representation of the cross section of each cavity made at level of short axis. Circumferences can be calculated from the cavity silhouettes and rate of circumferential change during contraction used to determine ventricular performance. Ventricular volume, stroke volume, and ejection fraction may also be measured.

during cardiac catheterization. X-ray visualization of cardiac anatomy, structure motion, and blood flow patterns are obtained by the injection of contrast agents through cardiac catheters to opacify heart chambers. Rapid serial filming techniques employing cine cameras or film changers record the passage of the contrast agent and the motion of heart walls and valves. Accurate depiction of great vessel and chamber size, position, shape, and wall motion is obtained. Valves are assessed for motion and thickness. Intracardiac masses and clots are demonstrated.

Left ventricular volume as it changes through the cardiac cycle can be accurately measured, and various indices of left ventricular performance can be derived. Left ven-

tricular volume is obtained by tracing a contour of the contrast-filled left ventricular cavity at end-diastole and end-systole (Fig. 1-22). The long and short axes are measured or derived mathematically. From these dimensions and the assumption that the ventricle is ellipsoidal in shape, a volume can be calculated.

Stroke volume is obtained by subtracting the systolic volume from the diastolic volume. Cardiac output is calculated by multiplying stroke volume by heart rate.

Ejection fraction expresses the efficiency of ventricular contraction as a percentage of the diastolic volume that is ejected with every cardiac cycle. It is calculated by dividing the stroke volume by the end-diastolic volume and is expressed as a percentage.

The rate at which the circumference of the left ventricle changes during systole at the level of the minor axis is another parameter of left ventricular function and is derived from muscle fiber shortening. The circumferential change between diastole and systole is divided by the ejection time and is expressed in centimeters per second. To correct for hearts of different sizes, the end-diastole circumference is incorporated into the formula so that the mean velocity of circumferential fiber shortening (MVCF) can be expressed in circumferences per second.

The mass of left ventricular muscle increases with hypertrophy and can be measured from cineangiocardiograms. The volume of the cavity is first calculated and subtracted from the volume of the entire ventricle, which includes the measured thickness of the left ventricular wall. Thus, the volume of the LV wall is determined and converted to mass by multiplying it by the specific gravity of cardiac muscle, which is 1.05.

Blood flow patterns observed during angiocardiography provide useful clinical information. A stenotic valve or a septal defect shapes the flowing contrast medium into a jet, which identifies the abnormality and may give an estimate of its size. Jets are also observed when valves are incompetent. The contrast injection site is selected to opacify only the chamber or great vessel downstream from the valve under examination. For instance, for mitral incompetence detection, the catheter is placed in the left ventricular cavity for contrast injection. An incompetent mitral valve allows backflow of the opacified blood from the left ventricle into the nonopacified left atrium. The degree of opacification and the rate of contrast clearance are aids in the semiquantitative assessment of the severity of mitral incompetence. The aortic valve is commonly evaluated in a similar fashion.

The technique for evaluation of valvular regurgitation is a useful application of angiocardiography, since at the present stage of development, echocardiographic techniques do not visualize regurgitation directly, but rely on secondary changes as indirect signs of valvular incompetence.

The tricuspid and pulmonic valves are less amenable to angiocardiographic evaluation of incompetence, since a retrograde approach to these valves is not feasible.

Coronary arteriography is an important angiocardiographic technique. Specially designed catheters are placed in the orifices of the left and right coronary arteries (just above the aortic valve) by retrograde insertion through an arm or leg artery. Contrast injections outline the coronary tree and reveal areas of narrowing—occlusion as well as cross-flow (collateral circulation)—between the two systems. This is important because the collateral circulation helps maintain perfusion in regions beyond areas of obstruction. Congenital variations in arterial distribution as well as size dominance of one system over the other determine the proportion of myocardium supplied by each vessel and, therefore, the relative significance of an obstruction involving one system.

A left ventriculogram is routinely performed to assess left ventricular function and to relate abnormalities of wall motion (hypokinesis, akinesis, paradoxical motion) with an obstructing lesion. The decision to perform bypass surgery is influenced not only by demonstration of an area of severe coronary artery narrowing but also by the effects on wall motion in the distribution of that artery.

Angiocardiography can also be accomplished using gas (CO_2) as the injected contrast agent, since gas is less opaque than blood or heart walls. The injected gas is limited to the right atrial cavity by proper patient positioning, since its free flow in large amounts through the right heart could produce adverse side effects. The thickness of the right atrial wall is measured and, when abnormally thick, indicates the presence of pericardial fluid applied to the right atrial wall. The CO_2 is rapidly removed from the blood and the method is very safe, although the use of echocardiography has generally replaced CO_2 angiocardiography in the diagnosis and evaluation of pericardial effusion. Routine opaque angiocardiograms can detect pericardial effusion as an abnormal thickening of the heart walls, but their routine use in the diagnosis of this condition is not justifiable in view of the success and accuracy of echocardiography.

Pathologic examinations

Pathologic examination of tissues obtained at surgery or biopsy provides useful information concerning cardiac structure and the diseases that alter structure. It does not, however, provide functional information equivalent to that obtained by the classic clinical techniques of cardiac catheterization and angiocardiography.

The cardiac surgeon may provide important observations regarding the pathologic status of the heart of a patient who has been examined by echocardiography. Though inspection of structures may be limited by surgical approach, the surgeon usually can provide important correlative data for the echocardiographer. For instance, the size of stenotic valves and of areas of narrowing in outflow tracts may be obtained. The degree and distribution of valvular calcification, the location, size, and related tissue destruction from infective vegetation, as well as the status of the supporting apparatus of AV valves, can be assessed at the time of surgery.

Congenital anomalies are occasionally delineated more completely during open heart surgery. In other instances the nature of the abnormality is verified or a previously unsuspected aspect of the condition is recognized; for example, an atrial septal defect may be revealed for the first time in a patient undergoing surgery for a valvular condition.

The causative process that produces pericarditis and effusion may be identified from fluid withdrawn by needles and examined bacteriologically (cultured) or by cytology (microscopic examination of cells in a fluid) when tumors involve the pericardium. In other instances, a pericardial specimen may be obtained during surgical drainage of pericardial effusion and examined pathologically.

At autopsy the entire heart may be examined grossly and evaluated for chamber and great vessel size and configuration, wall thickness, changes in valves and supporting apparatus, and the presence of congenital anomalies and other disease processes. Microscopic examination of tissue assesses the status of cardiac muscle fibers, degenerative or inflammatory processes in heart valves, and the nature of abnormal masses.

In myocardial infarction, study of underlying pathology reveals the size, stage of healing, and distribution of infarcts as well as the distribution and severity of coronary arterial lesions. Cardiomyopathies may be classified as to their etiologies.

BIBLIOGRAPHY

Fowler, N. O.: Cardiac diagnosis and treatment, New York, 1976, Harper & Row, Publishers.
Hurst, J. W., Logue, R. B., Schlant, R. D., and Wenger, N. K.: The heart, New York, 1978, McGraw-Hill Book Company.

2 Basic principles of ultrasound

PHYSICAL PRINCIPLES

Echocardiography involves concepts and techniques that are generally new in medicine, and the echocardiographer must understand the physical principles of ultrasound to carry out the examination successfully. The pulse echo technique, electronic instrumentation, beam formation, the interaction of sound and tissue, and the artifacts that result are important, since they influence the echocardiographic record and, therefore, its diagnostic content.

Ultrasound is the same form of energy that generates audible sound such as noise, music, or speech. It differs from ordinary sound in that its frequency is higher than the highest pitch (20,000 cycles per second) the human ear can perceive and is therefore inaudible. In echocardiography, frequencies of 1 to 7 million cycles per second (1 to 7 Megahertz [MHz]) are commonly employed.

Ultrasound is generated by certain crystals and ceramic materials that possess the property of piezoelectricity (pressure electricity) (Fig. 2-1). These materials, when stimulated by a voltage, change their shape, and conversely, when they are stressed by mechanical pressure, produce a voltage that can be detected. This mechanical energy can be made to propagate in tissues, where it behaves much like light in the ordinary environment. It can be transmitted through certain materials and it can be deviated in its

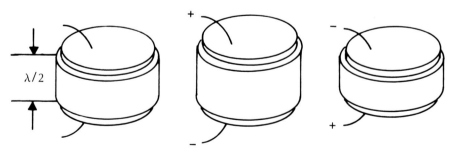

Fig. 2-1. Piezoelectric effect. *Left*, piezoelectric element with thickness of one half fundamental emission wavelength ($\lambda/2$) is shown relaxed. Application of voltage causes element to expand *(center)* or contract *(right)*, depending on its polarity relative to element. Mechanical deformations of piezoelectric element cause corresponding voltages. (From Gramiak, R., and Waag, R. C.: Cardiac ultrasound, St. Louis, 1975, The C. V. Mosby Co.)

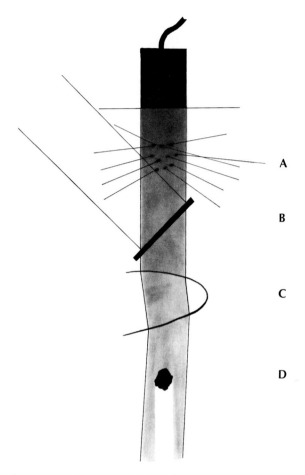

Fig. 2-2. Effects of tissues in ultrasonic beam. Ultrasonic energy interacts with tissues in a variety of ways. Scattering **(A)** occurs when the beam encounters small structures that deflect a portion of the energy in various directions. Scattering does not usually contribute to image formation in the heart but may result in the production of reverberation artifacts. Surfaces **(B)** that act as specular reflectors divert some of the sonic energy as a mirror reflects light. The shape of the reflected beam depends on the curvature of the surface, and its direction is a function of its angle in the beam. Reflections back to the transducer are the basis of imaging in echocardiography. Irregularly shaped tissue structures **(C)**, in which sound velocity differs from adjacent fluid or tissues, refract or bend the sound beam as a prism bends light. Deflections are usually minor in extent and usually do not produce recognizable errors in the position of structures. Substances such as calcium **(D)** may remove a large portion of the incident energy through high reflectivity and direct absorption. Acoustic shadows may result with total obliteration of image features in the shadowed area. In addition, throughout its passage, sonic energy is absorbed by direct interaction with tissue molecules. The sum total of the various processes that remove energy from the beam is called attenuation.

pathway (refracted). Certain materials absorb the energy and block its passage (shadowing), whereas others produce profuse scattering much as fog or smoke scatter light. Reflection also occurs and, along with transmission, forms the basis of echocardiographic imaging (Fig. 2-2).

The tissues of the cardiac window and the normal heart transmit sound well. Bone and calcified costal cartilages act as absorbers and therefore do not transmit the sonic energy. Lung is a poor transmitter since almost 100% of the energy is reflected.

Reflection of sonic energy occurs at points in tissue (interfaces) where the physical properties change. Differences in acoustic impedance (the product of tissue density times the speed of sound in that tissue) are responsible for reflection. Thus, two tissues of simi-

lar density (blood and myocardium) can be differentiated because an echo is produced when sound energy passes from blood into muscle or vice versa. This is the unique feature of ultrasound that permits soft tissue imaging; roentgenology, which recognizes differences in density alone, fails to provide information concerning the internal structure of the heart. In ultrasound systems, only a fraction of the energy is reflected, whereas the rest is transmitted and can be reflected repeatedly as the energy passes into deeper tissues.

If acoustic energy were to be transmitted continuously into the body and received energy were recorded, it would not be anatomically interpretable, since there would be no differentiation of reflectors by their depth. To resolve this problem, ultrasound systems

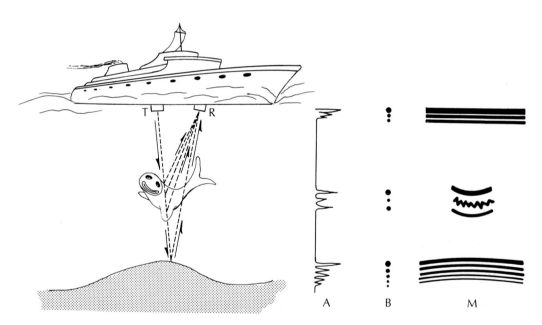

Fig. 2-3. Imaging modes in ultrasound. A sonar system illustrates propagation of a single pulse of ultrasound from a transmitter (T) and reflections from a moving fish and the ocean bottom to a receiver (R). A-mode display (A) features oscilloscopic baseline deflections whose amplitude varies with the intensity of the signal. In B-mode (B), spikes are converted into dots, whose brightness represents echo strength. When these dots are swept across a recording medium, motion derived from transit of ship or from targets within beam is presented as a variation in the position of reflectors as they change with time and is designated M-mode (M). The information contained in these modes is one-dimensional in nature. (From Gramiak, R., and Borg, S. A.: Advances in surgery, vol. 2, Chicago, 1977, Year Book Medical Publishers, Inc.)

are operated in a pulse-echo mode (Fig. 2-3). A very brief pulse of electrical energy, usually one or two millionths of a second in duration (one to two microseconds) is used to excite vibration in the crystal. The crystal then is quiescent and operates in a receive mode while echoes are returning. As a result, it is possible to measure precisely the time of arrival of individual echoes. The tissues in and around the heart transmit sound at about the same rate (1540 meters per second) so that the exact depth of an individual reflector can be determined and displayed. Pulses are repeated, usually at a rate of 1000 per second (pulse repetition frequency, or PRF), to provide continuity of observation of cardiac structure motion, even when it is very rapid, and to produce sufficient density of signals for satisfactory image formation.

An oscilloscope is used for display of cardiac ultrasound data. This device features a cathode ray tube, which has a surface much like the face of a television tube, on which the ultrasound information is shown in either of two forms. A-mode reveals the strength of the returning echoes by the size of a spike that occurs from a baseline. The depth of a reflector is indicated by the distance from left to right along the baseline measured from a large signal (the main bang), which represents the surface of the crystal. The designation A-mode is derived from the fact that the amplitude of the signal is presented. The other display mode is known as B-mode, in which the baseline signal is removed and the individual spikes that show the depth of reflectors are replaced by dots. The brightness of individual dots is meant to represent the intensity of the echo signal. In certain ultrasonic equipment the exact relationship between signal intensity and the size of the spike or brightness of the dot

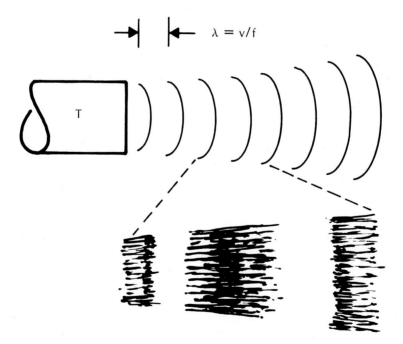

$$\lambda = v/f$$

Fig. 2-4. Wave principles. Transducer *(t)* is shown emitting beam. Wave-length (λ) of radiation is shown as spacing between regions of compression (shaded regions) and rarefaction (open region) produced by pistonlike motion of transducer element. Velocity, *(v),* of sound in medium and frequency *(f)* of vibration determines spacing between pressure peaks in beam. (From Gramiak, R., and Waag, R. C.: Cardiac ultrasound, St. Louis, 1975, The C. V. Mosby Co.)

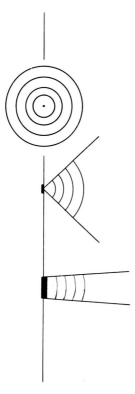

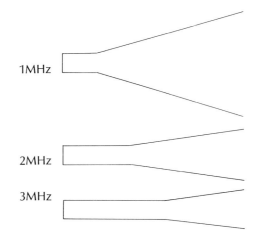

Fig. 2-6. Frequency and beam shape. The transition zone between the near and far field is demonstrated for three crystals of equal diameter but differing frequency characteristics. Note that transition zone shifts deeper with increasing frequency and that collimation in far field is also better at higher frequencies. In general, higher frequencies result in retention of beam collimation over greater distances for the same size transducer elements.

Fig. 2-5. Crystal size and beam pattern. A very small crystal, which functions as a point source *(top)*, radiates ultrasonic energy in all directions, much as a pebble generates waves when thrown into a pond. If crystal size is increased to diameter of 2 wave lengths *(middle)*, some directionality of energy is obtained but divergence is too great for clinical use. With larger crystals *(bottom)*, when the ratio of diameter to wave length approaches 20:1, a well-collimated beam is formed.

has been altered to produce better recordings with available systems.

Echocardiography has the special problem of recording the motion of reflectors in the ultrasonic beam. This is accomplished by using a B-mode display and sweeping a recording surface, such as light-sensitive paper or film, past the display at fixed speeds. In this mode the motion of reflectors is tracked (M-mode, or motion mode). Ultrasound instruments commonly contain a monitor oscilloscope on which the B-mode is swept repeatedly to provide an M-mode display ei-

ther by electronic storage of individual sweeps (storage oscilloscope) or through the use of special screens that retain a sizeable portion of the sweep (persistence oscilloscope).

An ultrasonic beam in tissue is composed of areas of high pressure in the molecules of tissue, resulting from the expansion of the crystal. When the crystal returns to its non-expanded size, a zone of low pressure occurs. The spacings between the high and low pressure zones depend on the frequency at which the crystal vibrates and is known as the wavelength (Fig. 2-4).

To obtain useful information in echocardiography, the sonic energy must be formed into a beam that examines only a limited portion of the heart. This is generally accomplished through the use of crystals that are wide in relation to the wavelength of the ultrasonic energy. To obtain a beam whose sides are nearly parallel and that does not spread out laterally in the area being examined, it is necessary to maintain a ratio of

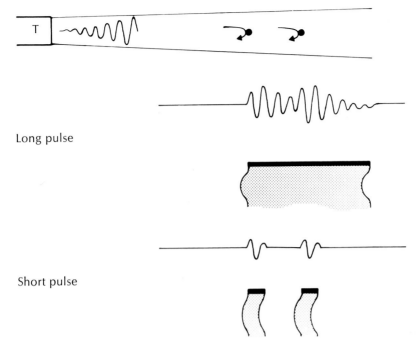

Long pulse

Short pulse

Fig. 2-7. Axial resolution. Long emitted pulse is shown traveling from transducer (T) and reflecting from two targets separated by less than pulse length. As a result, a single complex return is produced, and separation of structures in M-mode *(stippled)* is not possible. When short pulses of ultrasound are employed, targets can be resolved. (From Gramiak, R., and Waag, R. C.: Cardiac ultrasound, St. Louis, 1975, The C. V. Mosby Co.)

about 20:1 between the size of the crystal and the wavelength employed. Thus, crystals of 2 MHz frequency must be about 15 mm (½ inch) in diameter to produce well collimated beams. Smaller crystals are associated with beam divergence at increasing depths (Fig. 2-5).

The beam retains its good collimation in the near field and then diverges in the far field (Fig. 2-6). The transition point between the two fields is determined by the diameter of the crystal and the wavelength. A typical ½-inch crystal of 2.5 MHz has its transition point 6 cm from the crystal. At 5 MHz and ½ inch diameter, this transition point occurs at 10 cm. Higher frequencies therefore produce better beam collimation. However, attenuation of the beam increases with frequency so that it may not be practical to take advantage of the improved collimation and

resolution obtained with higher frequencies in large patients.

Resolution is defined as the ability to separate two reflectors that lie close to each other. High resolution provides details in closely spaced reflectors, whereas low resolution displays them as a single undifferentiated echo source. Two forms of resolution must be considered when describing an ultrasonic system, axial and lateral resolution. Axial resolution defines reflectors according to their depth from the crystal. The duration or length of the ultrasonic pulse controls axial resolution (Fig. 2-7).

A single ultrasonic reflector returns echoes as long as the pulse is passing through the reflector. The first returns from the traveling pulse accurately position the reflector in depth, but returns continue to be imaged until the tail of the pulse passes the posterior

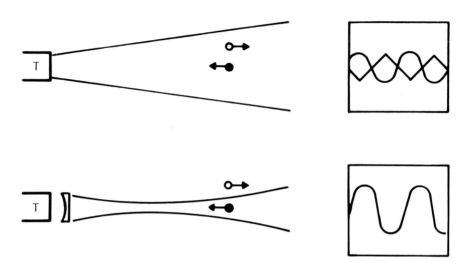

Fig. 2-8. Lateral resolution. Wide beam is shown encompassing two targets at same depth but with lateral separation and different motion patterns. Display superimposes these patterns as if they occurred on axis of beam. When beam is narrowed by focusing, as shown in lower panel, two closely spaced reflectors can be imaged independently and their motion patterns can be recorded individually. T, transducer. (From Gramiak, R., and Waag, R. C.: Cardiac ultrasound, St. Louis, 1975, The C. V. Mosby Co.)

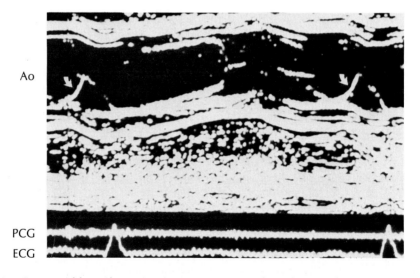

Fig. 2-9. Beam width artifacts. Aortic root (Ao) recording shows valve cusps in systole and in early diastole. Superimposed on this record is the A wave *(arrows)* of the mitral valve, produced by width of the ultrasonic beam. PCG, phonocardiogram; ECG, electrocardiogram.

margin of the reflector. Thus, the reflector is imaged as its true width plus the length of the pulse used. If a second reflector is present behind the first, the "tail" produced by the first reflector may fill in the space between them and combine the image of the second into that of the first.

Pulse length is controlled by the frequency used. The shortest pulses that can be formed must be one wavelength in duration. Higher frequencies therefore can produce shorter pulses. Crystals, like bells or gongs, tend to vibrate for long periods of time (ring down) unless they are mechanically or electrically stopped. Each crystal is therefore backed by a material that dampens this post-excitation ringing to produce the shortest possible pulses. The efficiency of this damping thus influences pulse length and resolution.

The degree of electronic amplification also influences effective pulse length. Since the terminal portions of the ring down of the crystal are of lower amplitude, high sensitivity detects the lower intensity echoes they produce and effectively results in wider pulses than are evident with lower gain. This reinforces the concept that the lowest possible gain that produces satisfactory images should be employed.

Ultrasonic beams are generally 10 to 15 mm in width. Ultrasonic systems image all returns as if the echo sources contained in the wide beam were positioned in the central axis of the beam (Figs. 2-8 and 2-9). The ability to differentiate structures that lie side by side (lateral resolution) is therefore a function of beam width. The narrowest possible beams are the most desirable. Acoustic lenses may be placed in front of the crystal to narrow the beam at a specific depth, much as a lens focuses light to a point. However, the beam tends to spread beyond the zone of best focus, and lateral resolution is degraded at greater depths. Systems employing electronic focusing of the beam using multielement transducers are under development and may solve this perplexing problem in the future.

The resolution of motion is dependent on the angle of the beam as it relates to the direction of structure motion (Fig. 2-10).

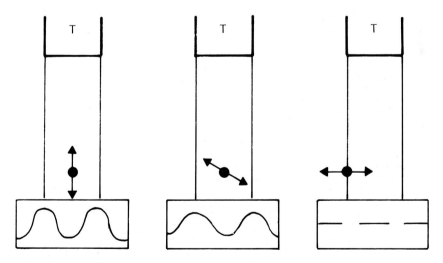

Fig. 2-10. Beam width and structure motion. *Left,* amplitude of structure motion that is along beam axis is displayed correctly. *Center,* when motion within beam is oblique, only that component occurring along beam axis is demonstrated. In extreme cases of motion across beam, record shows an apparently motionless echo, which may disappear if source is contained in beam during only a part of its movement *(right).* (From Gramiak, R., and Waag, R. C.: Cardiac ultrasound, St. Louis, 1975, The C. V. Mosby Co.)

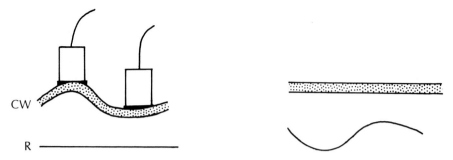

Fig. 2-11. Transducer motion during M-mode recording. M-mode echocardiograms are displayed without information concerning the position of the transducer during recording. A pulsating chest wall *(CW)* in front of a motionless reflector *(R)* alters distance between transducer and reflector, which the equipment will interpret and display as motion of the reflector.

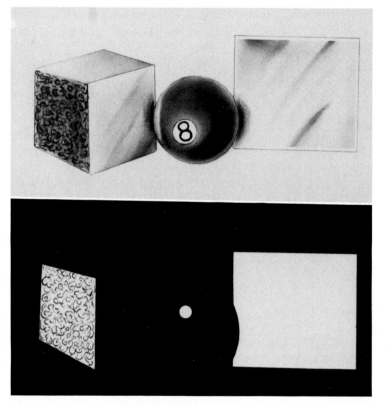

Fig. 2-12. Reflector characteristics. *Top,* diffuse optical illumination of polished planar surface, billiard ball and cube with one rough surface. *Bottom,* simulated sonic view of same objects when illumination beam is on axis of sight. Effects of specularity, shadowing, and diffuse reflection are illustrated. (From Gramiak, R., and Waag, R. C.: Cardiac ultrasound, St. Louis, 1975, The C. V. Mosby Co.)

Ideal motion representation is present when its direction is perpendicular to the beam axis. As the angle of the motion changes from the perpendicular, the recorded motion amplitude decreases. When motion occurs across an ultrasonic beam, there is no change in depth of the structure so that the equipment recognizes only the presence of a reflector in the beam. When this structure moves out of the beam, its echo disappears. The system is incapable of recognizing the direction of transverse motions.

The greatest amplitude of motion, as recorded in an echocardiogram, therefore most closely approximates the motion of a structure and should be sought in every echocardiographic examination of heart valves and walls.

Other motion artifacts occur when the transducer is placed on a moving surface such as a chest wall lying over a strongly pulsating heart. The instrumentation does not register movement of the transducer, so the chest wall is recorded as a stationary echo complex. The elevation of the transducer with each beat increases the distance to deeper reflectors with each pulsation so that a relatively stationary surface appears to change its depth, or to move, in a cyclical manner with each heart beat. Beam scanning over a thin, bumpy chest wall can also introduce similar artifacts (Fig. 2-11).

Reflecting tissues in the beam have certain structure-related characteristics (Fig. 2-12). Those containing fibrous tissue produce strong reflections (heart valves and pericardium). When they are smooth and oriented in sheetlike configurations, they act as specular or mirrorlike reflectors. They tend to return the ultrasonic energy in a narrow, compact beam much like that which was received (Fig. 2-13). Typically, they produce

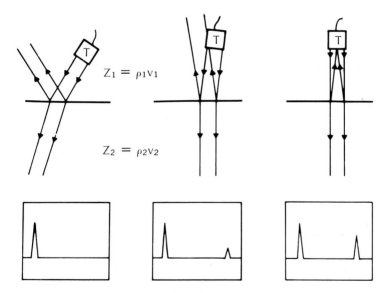

Fig. 2-13. Principles of reflection and refraction. Sound is shown reflected and refracted at boundary between two media of different acoustical impedances, Z, which is product of medium density (ρ) and velocity, V. Angle of incidence is equal to angle of reflection so that received signal intensity depends on angular relationship between transducer and boundary. Maximum signal strength *(right)* is obtained when beam is perpendicular to reflecting interface. In other instances, reflected beam may be only partially received *(center)* by transducer or not received at all *(left)*. Refraction is not important in medical imaging of heart. (From Gramiak, R., and Waag, R. C.: Cardiac ultrasound, St. Louis, 1975, The C. V. Mosby Co.)

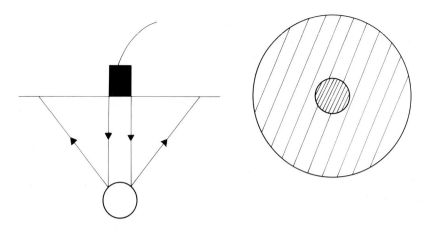

Fig. 2-14. Reflector shape and returning beam pattern. A curved reflecting surface in an ultrasonic beam will return a broad pattern of reflections to the surface. Diagram shows a spherical reflector and circular area of returns around the centrally located transducer. Spherical reflectors are easy to detect with ultrasound, since the wide returning beam virtually eliminates dropouts. A rough or diffuse reflector acts in a similar manner, but the pattern of return is more difficult to predict.

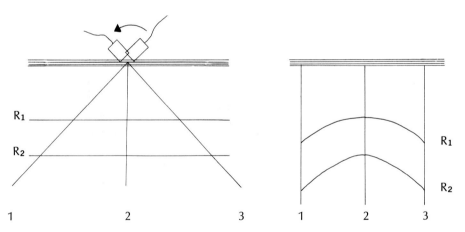

Fig. 2-15. Beam angulation and structure size and position. Beam angulation used to image two straight and parallel reflectors, R_1 and R_2, uses different path lengths and encounters different dimensions at the extremes of angulation (*1* and *3*). A perpendicular beam angle *(2)* demonstrates true size and position. A time-motion display, which is always perpendicular, shows artifactual curvature of reflectors and apparent increase in separation between R_1 and R_2 at extremes of angulation. This effect is limited with highly specular reflectors.

very strong echoes whose amplitude is dependent on the angle between the crystal and the reflector. When this relationship is perpendicular, amplitudes are highest but tend to diminish as the reflector tilts in the beam. Tilting is often great enough that the returning echoes miss the crystal receiver. This results in apparent disappearance of the structure and a discontinuity in its recording (dropouts). Dropouts are avoided

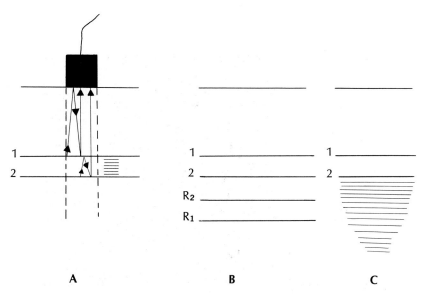

Fig. 2-16. Mechanism of reverberation artifacts. Incident beam is shown in dotted lines **(A),** while reflections between interface *1* and the transducer surface and between interface *2* and *1* are demonstrated as solid lines with arrowheads to delineate reverberation pathways. Elongated sound path produced by re-reflection between interface *1* and the transducer is twice length of true distance and positions a reverberation (R_1) at twice the correct depth **(B).** Similarly, the added path length produced by reflection between interface *2* and *1* results in a reverberation (R_2), which is imaged behind interface 2. When multiple small interfaces are present within a structure **(A),** reverberation pattern becomes extremely complex, and a shower of deep reverberations is produced **(C).**

by selection of the particular transducer angle and position that captures the reflector in an entire cardiac cycle.

Curved surfaces return echoes in a broad beam so that signal strength is reduced, but dropouts are less frequent than are those from flat surfaces (Fig. 2-14).

Diffuse reflectors are those that are composed of small multiple internal interfaces (muscle) or roughened surfaces such as diseased or calcified heart valves. Diffuse reflectors are less direction-sensitive for detection since they return the ultrasonic energy in a broad, diffuse manner.

Detection is easier than with specular reflectors, but amplitude of echoes is less, since the received energy is spread over a wider area. When calcification is present, however, the returning signals are of high amplitude as a result of the higher degree of reflectivity produced by the high acoustic impedance

difference (acoustic mismatch) at the calcification-blood interface.

Measurement of the size of cardiac chambers or great vessels is influenced to some degree by beam angle (Fig. 2-15). Oblique beams may depict a cavity diameter or a heart wall thickness to be greater than it really is. Specular reflectors tend to control this problem somewhat, since perpendicularity is required for dropout-free imaging. However, variations in apparent structure size are commonly observed as a result of this phenomenon.

Acoustic artifacts are present in almost all ultrasonic studies and can be controlled in part by careful selection of recording sensitivity parameters. The most common are reverberations or re-echoes, which occur as the pulses return to the crystal and are reflected back away from the crystal as they encounter acoustic impedance mismatches

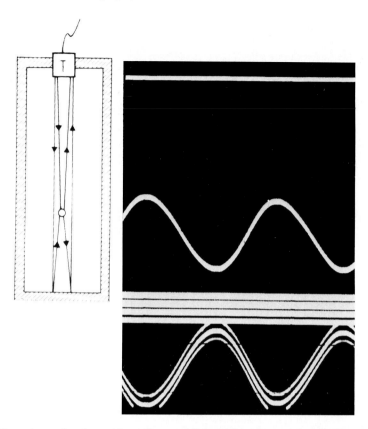

Fig. 2-17. Complex reflections. M-mode recording *(right)* of moving ball in water column shows (from top) transducer position, sinusoidal motion pattern of ball, bottom of tank and reverberations from within it, and motion pattern positioned beyond water column. Latter motion pattern, which is out of phase with actual ball motion, arises from path that is lengthened by distance from ball to end of water column. (From Gramiak, R., and Waag, R. C.: Cardiac ultrasound, St. Louis, 1975, The C. V. Mosby Co.)

(Figs. 2-16 and 2-17). Re-echoing produces elongated or complex sound pathways so that the returning signal is delayed in respect to the initial point of origin and is therefore imaged deep to it. Reverberation occurs between tissues and the skin or face of the crystal and from multiple points within the tissue. For instance, a pulse may be reflected from a point within the chest wall, reflected back to the skin surface, reflected again back into the chest wall, and be reflected to the receiver. The delayed return is interpreted by the equipment as a deeper position so that a signal that has no cardiac structure relationship is positioned over the heart cavity. This results in a shower of signals and de-

posits multiple dots or short linear echo sources over the heart cavities. These near-tissue reverberations have dictated the need for electronic suppression in the near field. They also occur in more deeply situated tissues, but their longer returning paths may image them behind areas of interest, or multiple reflections and absorption by tissue may reduce them to levels that are not recognized. However, when pericardial effusion is suspected, they could be of importance, since high-gain recording images them and obscures the echo-free nature of the clear fluid present in effusions. In other instances, such as the interventricular septum, sound may reverberate within the structure (ring

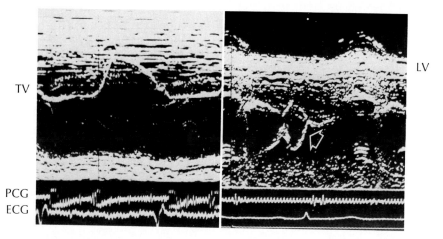

Fig. 2-18. Reverberations in echocardiographic examinations. *Right,* inverted image *(arrow)* of mitral valve behind left ventricular wall, *LV.* This pattern is produced by reflections from posterior wall through a mechanism similar to that illustrated in Fig. 2-17. *Left,* tricuspid valve, *TV,* is partially obscured by reverberations that probably originate in chest wall. Reverberations, which are similar to those from bottom of water column in Fig. 2-17, are positioned in range of right ventricle. PCG, phonocardiogram; ECG, electrocardiogram. (From Gramiak, R., and Waag, R. C.: Cardiac ultrasound, St. Louis, 1975, The C. V. Mosby Co.)

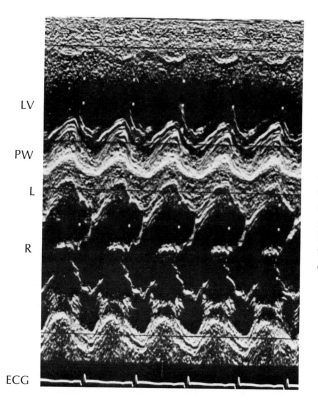

Fig. 2-19. Reverberations during echocardiographic examinations. Ultrasonic beam as it exits through left ventricular posterior wall (PW) is reflected off surface of lung (L) without significant penetration of lung tissue. Multiple linear moving echoes are observed in the space posteriorly and represent reverberatory artifacts (R) from cardiac structures. LV, left ventricle; EGG, electrocardiogram.

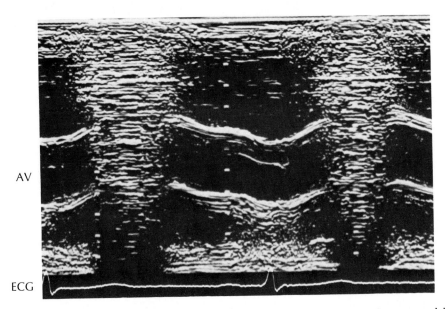

AV

ECG

Fig. 2-20. Lung-induced image loss. Routine aortic valve recording is interrupted by lung that slips between the chest wall and heart with each cardiac contraction. The shower of echoes represents reverberations that occur in the first few millimeters of lung and does not represent significant penetration. Acoustic shadowing also occurs, and no structural information is recorded when lung enters the beam. AV, aortic valve; ECG, electrocardiogram.

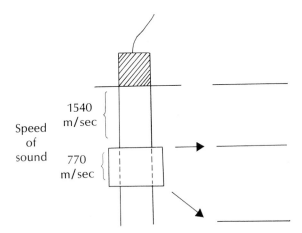

Speed
of
sound

1540
m/sec

770
m/sec

Fig. 2-21. Speed of sound and imaging. Ultrasonic instruments are calibrated to position reflectors correctly in a medium that has a uniform speed of sound. In tissue imaging, an average figure of about 1540 m/sec is used and produces satisfactory results, despite small variations in the speed of sound in different tissues. If a substance having half the speed of sound of tissue is introduced into the beam, the longer time required for passage of the ultrasonic energy is interpreted by the equipment as a structure twice its original size.

around), thereby lengthening the sound path only by a relatively small amount. These reverberations are imaged as a diffuse haze of small echoes lying just behind the septum.

Long-range reverberations may occur in a direct path between a strong reflector such as the mitral valve and the crystal. This effectively doubles the return time so that a phantom image of the moving valve is recorded at twice its normal depth. The recorded motion amplitude of the phantom is twice that of the normal valve and its image may be inverted, depending on the sound path used during reverberation. Reverberations are among the most common artifacts present in ultrasonic records (Figs. 2-18 and 2-19).

Shadowing may occur when the reflector in the sound path attenuates the beam. This occurs whenever lung slips into the sound path between the chest wall and the heart (Fig. 2-20). It may occur with every cardiac pulsation or with respiration. In either case, useful information from the heart cannot be obtained while the lung is in the sound beam. A heavily calcified valve or annulus may also produce shadowing.

Artificial heart valves made of silastic may produce artifacts because of the slower speed of sound in the prosthesis (Fig. 2-21). Since the speed of sound in the silastic is slower than in tissue, the equipment images portions of the prosthesis to be apparently much larger than they really are. Demagnification of any measurements by a factor of 0.64 corrects for this distortion. The apparent deep position of the poppet (ball portion of the valve) behind the prosthesis is an artifact of the same process and should not arouse suspicion of abnormal alteration of the prosthetic valve.

INSTRUMENTATION

An echocardiographic instrument typically is sufficiently compact and is mounted on wheels for portability. It consists of electronics that generate and receive the signal, a transducer, monitor oscilloscopes, and a recorder, usually a paper strip chart or a camera.

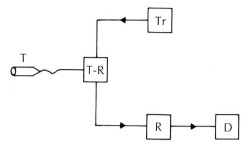

Fig. 2-22. Basic pulse-echo ultrasound system. Transducer is excited by transmitter, *Tr*, through transmit-receive switch, *T-R*, which protects sensitive receiver from high-voltage excitation signal. Receiver, *R*, amplifies and processes echoes for display, *D*. (From Gramiak, R., and Waag, R. C.: Cardiac ultrasound, St. Louis, 1975, The C. V. Mosby Co.)

The electronics can be viewed according to the major components present (Fig. 2-22). A transmitter generates the short, high-voltage pulses that excite the crystal. A transmit-receive switch is placed in the system to protect the highly sensitive receiver from the relatively high voltages used in excitation. The receiver amplifies the low-amplitude electrical signals from the crystal, which may be as small as a hundred-thousandth of the original pulse, and processes them into a form suitable for display on an oscilloscope.

The crystal is housed in a protective casing containing the electrical leads that conduct the pulse and returning signals, a damping material that mechanically controls postexcitation ringing of the crystal, and a tuning element that increases sensitivity for a given frequency (Fig. 2-23). However, this tuning and the manner in which the crystal is excited differ among manufacturers so that transducers from different units may not be interchangeable. Also, the make of the equipment must be specified when a new transducer is ordered.

The frequency emitted by a crystal is governed by its thickness, and thinner crystals generate higher frequencies. A transducer is selected for an examination, depending on patient size and chest wall configuration. In an adult, a ½-inch, 2- to 2.5-MHz transducer

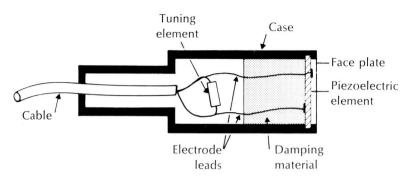

Fig. 2-23. Transducer construction. Piezoelectric element is mounted in case that provides electrical isolation. Case also contains damping material, electrical connections, tuning element, and face plate. (From Gramiak, R., and Waag, R. C.: Cardiac ultrasound, St. Louis, 1975, The C. V. Mosby Co.)

offers the best compromise between resolution and penetration for adequate recording of cardiac structures at all depths. In exceptional cases where the chest wall is particularly thick or the heart may be very large, use of a 1.0 MHz transducer may be the only way to obtain useful information.

Larger crystals are more sensitive, since they present a larger surface to receive the echo return and may be used when even more sensitivity is required. Three-quarter-inch, 2.25 MHz transducers are commonly used in abdominal B-scanning. Smaller crystals may be required in thin or emaciated patients to ensure adequate coupling in narrow or concave intercostal spaces. A large deposit of contact gel is usually necessary. Focusing depth is selected to position the best portion of the beam near the mitral valve or the posterior wall. A 7.5-cm focus point serves well in most adult patients.

A large child or an adult with a thin chest wall may be successfully examined with a 3.5-MHz transducer; a 5-MHz, ¼-inch transducer may produce better records in toddlers and infants. A 5-cm focus is preferred in small patients.

If a variety of transducers is not available, a ½-inch, 2.25-MHz unfocused transducer can be used in all patients. Though some loss in image quality occurs, the records are usually adequate for interpretation. A special transducer has been manufactured for cardiac examination from the suprasternal notch. The crystal is relatively small and is positioned at right angles to the handle of the transducer, which allows easy insertion and angling when placed in the suprasternal notch.

INSTRUMENT CONTROLS

Instrument controls are provided for the operator to adjust image quality. They allow manipulation of the sensitivity characteristics of the receiver as well as the power output of the transducer to manage those patient factors and physical aspects of ultrasound that are important in clinical examinations.

Control settings of ultrasonic instruments are calibrated in decibels (dB), a unit commonly used to describe the loudness of sounds. The decibel is a ratio of one intensity to another and is used to describe relative loudness or a range of loudnesses rather than absolute values. It is convenient to use, since the ratios are expressed logarithmically so that large intensity differences, such as those occurring in ultrasound (1:1,000,000), are reduced to numbers that are easy to handle. Decibels are employed in ultrasound to characterize the intensity range over which amplifiers operate and to indicate the power range of transducer outputs. They are also useful to compare one gain setting or power output to another. In clinical operation they are valuable instrument control landmarks that allow some standardization of the examination procedure.

Decibels are calculated on the following formula:

$$dB = 10 \times \log_{10} \frac{I_2}{I_1}$$

where dB = decibels, 10 is a correction factor for a larger unit (the Bel used in the original formula), and I_2 and I_1 are two different intensities being compared.

Commonly encountered intensity ratios and their decibel designations are shown in Table 3.

A control is generally present to adjust the overall sensitivity of the receiver. Increasing sensitivity is required for the detection of weak echo returns from poor reflectors or those situated at great depth. This control is identified in various ways by different manufacturers and may be called sensitivity or coarse gain (Fig. 2-24). Its function is apparent, since adjustment reveals increasing or decreasing signal amplitude (A-mode) or brightness (B-mode) over the entire area being examined.

Another control is provided to compensate for the attenuation of the sonic energy in relation to the depth of the signal. As the returning echoes diminish in intensity relative to their depth, they can be selectively amplified according to their time of arrival at the transducer. For this reason, this control is usually identified by inclusion of the word *time*, for example, *time-v*aried gain, or TVG, or in other instruments, *time* gain *c*ompensa-

tion, or TGC. Increasing the gain of this control selectively amplifies weak, deeply originating signals more than it amplifies the stronger signals that come from superficial targets. It is usually operated in conjunction with a control that selectively attenuates the signals originating in the near field, where reverberation artifacts are prominent and require suppression. This control is usually used to keep the signal level in the anterior region lower than is usually possible with an unmodified time-varied gain. Commonly, this control is identified as near gain, suppression, or TGC initial. In addition to the level of amplification the depth over which the effect is produced can be controlled. This feature is usually designated delay. The rate at which the amplification level recovers from the suppression may also be adjusted to provide a smooth blending of signals in the image. Depth compensation rate or slope is generally used to identify this aspect of gain adjustment. Modern instrumentation provides display of the gain characteristics in the form of a curve whose amplitude is proportional to sensitivity. The effect of manipulation of the various gain controls can be readily appreciated by observing changes in the displayed gain curve (Fig. 2-25).

A reject control is present to selectively remove echoes of low amplitude from the recording and to emphasize stronger echoes. This allows discrimination against the low-amplitude signals that arise from electronic noise and from reverberations that have been attenuated by multiple passes through tissue. High reject levels decrease the overall sensitivity of the system.

A damping control electrically affects postexcitation ringing of the crystal by increasing energy loss of the voltage that causes the crystal to vibrate. This results in a decrease in the power emitted by the crystal and shortens pulse length. Generally, this control operates in a stepwise fashion, and the power decreases are noted in decibels. Increased damping has the same system effect as decreased sensitivity.

The instrument may also have other controls that operate to alter the display after it

Table 3. Commonly encountered intensity ratios and their decibel designations

Intensity ratio	Log$_{10}$ of ratio	dB
1	0	0
10	1	10
100	2	20
1000	3	30
10,000	4	40
100,000	5	50
1,000,000	6	60

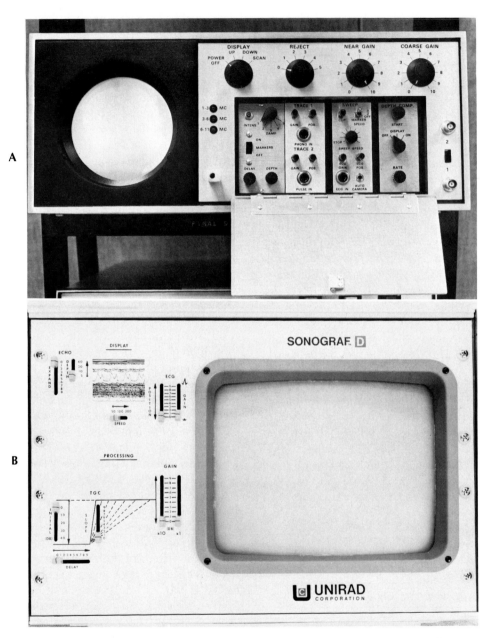

Fig. 2-24. Instrument controls. The instrument control panel and display oscilloscopes of two commercially available ultrasonoscopes are shown. **A,** Instrument utilizes controls that are rotated to change amplifier characteristics, and the gain settings are arbitrarily numbered. **B,** Slide controls are featured, and gain settings are indicated in decibels (dB). Both make provisions for ECG recording; **A** also contains an accessory panel for including PCG.

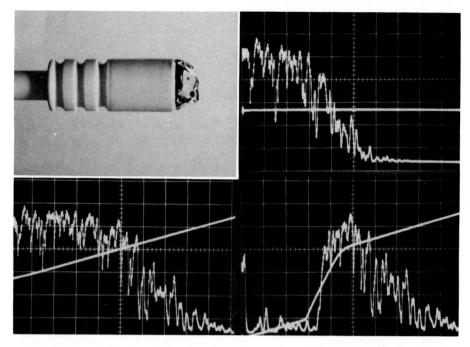

Fig. 2-25. Effect of instrument controls on echo imaging. Echoes obtained from reverberations within gel are presented with different control settings. Each A-mode display contains a line that characterizes gain employed as function of range. *Upper right,* uniform gain is shown. *Lower left,* addition of amplification of echoes arriving later. *Lower right,* suppression of echoes in near field is illustrated. (From Gramiak, R., and Waag, R. C.: Cardiac ultrasound, St. Louis, 1975, The C. V. Mosby Co.)

has been properly amplified. One controls the size of the display, which permits imaging of various depths of tissue. The echo depth display may be controlled by click stops or by a continuously variable knob. In addition, the speed of the M-mode sweep may be adjusted and scale marks may be added to the display. Conventional oscilloscopic adjustments such as focus, brightness, and astigmatism (a form of focus) may also be included to optimize the quality of the oscilloscopic image. They do not, however, influence the image that is recorded. Separate controls are also included for the position and gain of the phonocardiogram and ECG.

Certain manufacturers have produced instruments that depart from some of these traditional equipment features. In one the overall sensitivity, suppression, and time-varied gain controls have been replaced by a series of individual gain controls for each 2 cm of tissue depth. Gain curves can be easily tailored in a manner not possible with traditional systems. Templates can be generated for reproducibility of examinations (Fig. 2-26). Another supplier has recently developed an instrument with automated gain control that requires little operator selection of examination control features. This device also promises reproducibility and should decrease the amount of skill needed for clinical echocardiography. It has not yet had adequate clinical use for evaluation of its potential.

Each echocardiographer should read and understand the manual supplied by the manufacturer and should consult the company representative when questions arise. Thorough knowledge of instrument function and operation is of vital importance to physicians and technicians involved in echocardiography.

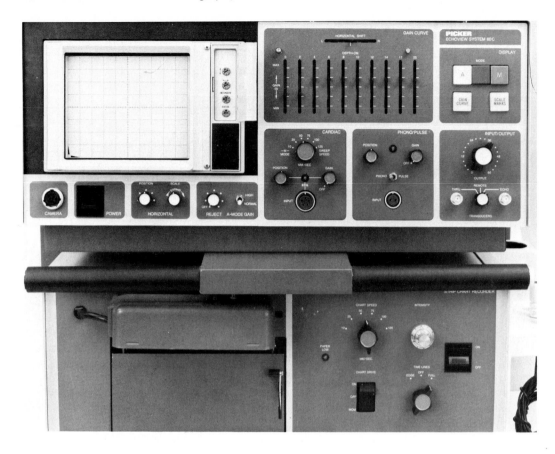

Fig. 2-26. Segmental gain control. This instrument has a series of individual controls, each of which specifies gain over a 2 cm segment of the displayed field. This allows manipulation of sensitivity at any selected depth without affecting gain in the rest of the field. A strip chart recorder is present under the control panel.

SIGNAL PROCESSING

Signal processing in echocardiography extends beyond the regulation of displayed echo intensity by adjustment of instrument controls. The electronics of the instrument process the ultrasound signals to keep them within the capabilities of the oscilloscopes that present the image for recording. If signal amplitudes were to be displayed in a linear fashion (an echo that is twice the strength of another is shown as twice as bright as the weaker), the brightness range of the oscilloscope would not be able to encompass the differences in intensity of echoes, which may be greater than 10,000:1 (dynamic range). The signal amplitudes can be compressed logarithmically to permit imaging of the weakest and brightest sources. Since the $\log_{10}$ of signal amplitude is used to control brightness, a dynamic range of 10,000:1 would be reduced to a display brightness of 4:1 ($\log_{10}$ of 10,000 = 4). This produces images of low contrast, so most commercial instruments employ dynamic range compression that is intermediate between linear display and logarithmic compression.

Signal processing is also used to make the image more acceptable for diagnosis and mainly consists of techniques that image structure margins more sharply and removes small echoes that represent insignificant structure information, electronic noise, and low-level reverberation artifacts.

The signal generated by the transducer

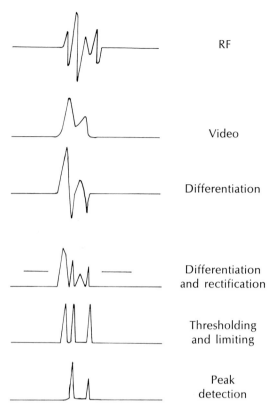

RF

Video

Differentiation

Differentiation
and rectification

Thresholding
and limiting

Peak
detection

Fig. 2-27. A-mode displays of signal processing in ultrasound. In this illustration, an RF waveform is sequentially processed by commonly employed techniques to show envelope detection (video), differentiation, differentiation and rectification, and thresholding and limiting. The threshold used to create the limited display is shown in horizontal lines on the rectified waveform. Peak detection is shown as derived from the video signals. It may also be added to the differentiated and rectified processing to generate added image detail and quality.

consists of multiple high-frequency oscillations (RF, or radio frequency) and contains both positive and negative deflections (Fig. 2-27). RF is not commonly employed as a display source because it is more convenient to derive a more simple waveform from the RF signal by first discarding the negative portion and then tracing the contour of individual bursts of RF that indicate reflector position. This outlining technique is known as envelope or video detection and is the display used in A-mode presentations. Images derived from unprocessed video signals tend to be fuzzy because the peaks have sloping contours that produce broad echo patterns with indefinite margins. To overcome this difficulty, differentiation (sometimes

called fast-time constant) was introduced to sharpen the configuration of echo complexes. Differentiation uses the rate or velocity at which signal amplitude is increasing or decreasing to produce deflections from the baseline. The tip of a peak is a point at which the signal is neither increasing nor decreasing in amplitude, so velocity at that instant is zero, returning the trace to baseline. Downward slopes produce negative deflections in differentiated records. As a result, two peaks are produced by a single spike in a video display. Since an oscilloscope is incapable of displaying negative deflections (zero amplitude is represented as zero brightness), the techniques of rectification or DC restoration have been applied to invert the negative deflections and to present them as positive waveforms, thereby producing more numerous and sharper echoes.

Most echocardiographic instruments have been developed to show structure margins with the greatest possible clarity. To achieve this goal the technique of thresholding and limiting has been added to rectified differentiation. A threshold defines the level below which all echoes are rejected, whereas those echoes that surpass the threshold are amplified to the limit of the system's ability to produce brightness (limiting). This processing "cleans up" the record and assures the imaging of solid portions of the heart with a uniform brightness, although signal amplitude may vary from changes in angular orientation of the reflector. The records produced are detailed and sharply contrasted but lack gray scale information.

Another signal-processing mode that sharpens waveforms and may provide better structure characterization is peak detection. Simply, the peaks of waveforms are detected and presented as sharply defined individual deflections (an opposite concept from differentiation, which reduces peaks to zero). Peak detection is usually combined with thresholding and limiting and may be superimposed on the previously described forms of signal presentation.

Signal processing produces records that appear to contain more detail that probably arises in the content and character of the tissues being examined with ultrasound. Clinical use has not identified the superiority of one signal-processing mode, although highly differentiated, thresholded, and limited processing, which essentially detects structure edges, appears superior to other processing modes.

BIOLOGIC EFFECTS

Biologic effects can be produced in tissues by ultrasound, depending on the power level used and the duration of exposure. The effects arise from the conversion of ultrasonic energy to heat by tissue absorption, cavitation that produces bubbles in tissue and local tissue fragmentation from extensive localized negative pressures present in the beam, and from less completely understood nonthermal effects. Ionization in tissue associated with x-ray exposure does not occur to produce damage to the elements of cells that control cell growth and reproduction.

The measurement of the quantity of ultrasonic energy that interacts with tissue is a difficult laboratory procedure and is not carried out in patient studies. For investigational purposes the elevation of temperature arising from sound absorption in tissue may be measured, and delicate pressure-sensitive devices, similar to analytic balances, may be employed to measure the pressure produced by the ultrasonic beam.

The power used in clinical systems is described as the electrical loading of a unit area of the crystal and is expressed in watts (W) per square centimeter (cm). Peak values are determined during the electrical excitation of the crystal and are generally under 10 W/cm^2. The duration of the pulse and the pulse-repetition frequency result in a reduction of peak power to an average power of about 1/1000 of the peak, generally under 10 mW/cm^2.

Doppler devices that operate in a continuous wave (CW) mode (nonpulsed) have peak and average intensities that are the same and are generally around 15 mW/cm^2 for obstetrical use and can be as high as 400 mW/cm^2 in vascular diagnosis.

In therapeutic devices that depend on a tissue heating effect for physiotherapy, CW ultrasound is used at power levels of about 1 W/cm^2.

In diagnostic and physiotherapy applications, there have been no reported instances of early or late tissue damage from patient examination or treatment.

High-power levels can produce biologic effects. For instance, an ultrasonic cleaner operating at 50 W/cm^2 produces pain if the hand is inserted into the cleaner, but tissue damage does not occur before the induction of pain.

High-power levels can destroy tissues and have found application in medicine as a surgical tool. The power levels are around 1000

W/cm². The mechanism of tissue destruction involves thermal effects, cavitation, and nonthermal effects.

Scientists concerned with the biologic effects of ultrasound recognize that immediate or delayed tissue damage has not occurred after more than 20 years of clinical usage. However, it is generally conceded that more research is required to establish the power levels and exposure durations that can be positively stated to be safe. For this reason, an attitude of caution is generally recommended during patient examination to minimize exposure, especially to developing fetuses whose tissues are recognized as more sensitive to extraneous energies.

RECORDING TECHNIQUES

Permanent records are required in echocardiography to preserve the motion pattern of rapidly moving structures, to permit measurement of structure size, and to provide comparison with previous examinations. Methods initially employed included still camera photography and analog gate devices. Still cameras may photograph an image of an M-mode sweep retained on a storage oscilloscope, or they may use an open shutter technique to record a B-mode as it sweeps across an oscilloscope without storage. These methods have fallen into disuse since the film cost may be high and because the records contain only a short period of cardiac activity.

The analog gate was introduced to allow continuous recording of the motion of one reflector such as the anterior leaflet of the mitral valve along with physiologic data. The system required specification of a range or depth beyond which the position of the first reflector was detected and recorded (gate). Artifacts produced by dropouts as well as those arising from other structures entering the gate produced major alterations in the trace obtained, so that these devices are seldom used except for special research applications.

Strip chart records have been in large part responsible for the elevation of echocardiography from a highly specialized laboratory curiosity to its present position of a reliable clinical tool. They have freed the examiner from the burden of camera operation, which detracted from concentration on precise transducer positioning, allowed the capture of fleeting echo patterns, and permitted the recording of sequences of cardiac motion, including motion of the transducer during recording to document the relationship of structures in a semianatomic format.

Strip chart recorders originally were cameras that photographed a stationary B-mode display onto 35-mm film that was moved continuously during exposure to produce M-mode records. A few centers continue to use this technique, which has certain advantages and disadvantages. In our estimation, based on approximately 10,000 patient examinations recorded on 35-mm film, the advantages justify continued use of film recording. The film image is reduced to size to about 1 inch vertically. This compression of about 6:1 in image size also reduces the length of the record by the same factor. Thus, a 40-foot length of film, a typical patient record, represents about 250 feet of paper from a strip chart recorder. This compression also reduces cost by a factor of about 10, permits high-speed recording (equivalent to 125 mm/sec or more on strip charts), provides easy storage of patient files, and makes individual examinations readily accessible, since conventional motion picture rewinding devices are available to handle the film. Projection is required for viewing and has proved to be an excellent teaching medium for groups of trainees. The film record has excellent resolution and gray scale capability and can record any signal offered to it in echocardiography. The images are permanent, and the film is not easily damaged. Prints and slides are made quickly and inexpensively. The cameras are inexpensive (about $2000) compared to strip chart recorders and have proved reliable over many years of use.

The equipment requires a slave oscilloscope (cost about $2000) for the camera to view, and some electronic expertise is necessary to conduct the output of the ultrasonoscope to the slave. Commercial packages are not available. A facility to process 35-mm film is required, and the record is not available for immediate inspection during the examination. Prints are necessary for comparative studies, and this involves additional personnel time.

Paper strip chart recorders may be part of the physiologic recorders present in cardiac catheterization and noninvasive diagnostic laboratories. An electronic interface must be purchased to present the ultrasonic signal to the recorder in proper electronic form. The physiologic recorders are not mobile in a form that allows bedside examination of patients, and there may be competition for

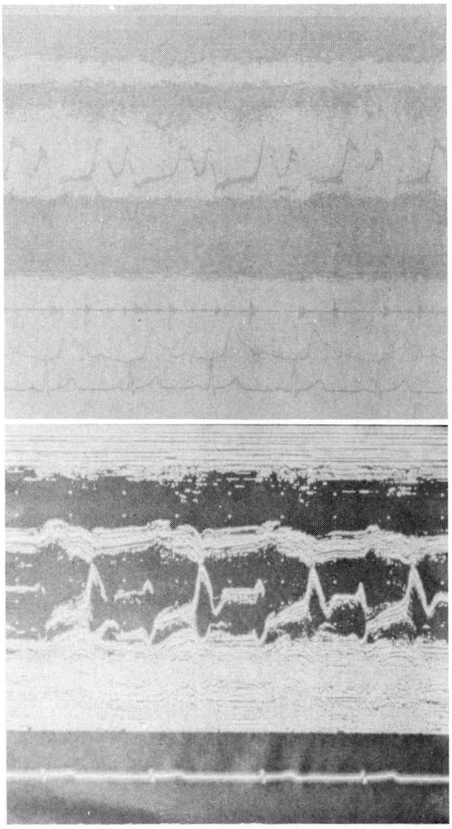

Fig. 2-28. Examples of recordings made with direct print paper. **A,** Unprocessed record. **B,** Chemically processed record. (From Gramiak, R., and Waag, R. C.: Cardiac ultrasound, St. Louis, 1975, The C. V. Mosby Co.)

their use since they usually have a nonechocardiographic work load.

Independent strip chart recorders (cost about $10,000) are compact and are packaged with the ultrasonoscope for ready mobility to the bedside. Their advantages have made them the most popular form of recording in echocardiography. The record is large and requires no projection. It is easily labeled, and measurements can be made directly. The recorder is activated by a foot switch so that the examiner's hands are free to operate equipment controls. The record may not require processing, depending on the paper employed, so that the images can be seen quickly enough to allow adjustment of techniques as the examination is in progress.

The disadvantages are mostly related to the light-sensitive paper employed. The most popular variety of paper develops to a bluish image when exposed to ultraviolet light. The contrast is low, and the image tends to fade when exposed to more light. Chemical processing in a photographic developer such as Dektol increases the contrast considerably and improves the permanence of the recording (Fig. 2-28). The paper is thin, tears easily, and may be loaded into the recorder incorrectly so that it is exposed through the back and produces examinations that appear backward.

Other papers are intended for chemical processing in certain recorders. These are of fairly good contrast, with gray echoes on a greenish background. They can also be raised to high contrast by photographic development.

A third type of paper develops its image following heat exposure. The exposed paper passes over a hot drum to produce contrasty images in black and white. The heat required to develop these papers is high, and there have been problems in processing, especially when continuous recordings are attempted (Table 4).

All papers suffer from the common disadvantage of their size. Strip chart recordings must be folded to fit into file folders so that an important portion of the record could be destroyed.

Table 4. Strip chart recorder paper types

	Light developed	Chemically developed	Heat developed
Resolution	High	High	High
Contrast	Low	Moderate	High
Delay to viewing at 25 mm/sec	5 to 30 sec	10 to 30 sec	12 sec
Paper cost per foot	18 cents	6 to 8 cents	8 cents
Color	Pink	Gray on green	Black and white
Further processing	Yes	Yes	No
Paper width	6 to 8 in	5 to 7 in	8½ in
Writing speed	Fast	Fast	Slow

Magnetic tape recording is clinically feasible only with videotape recorders. A complete echocardiographic examination may be recorded on videotape but requires playback and subsequent rerecording on a strip chart or a camera system to obtain hard copy. Their use has not been widespread.

BIBLIOGRAPHY

Taylor, K. J. W.: Current status of toxicity investigations, J. Clin. Ultrasound **2:**149, 1974.

Carlsen, E. N.: Ultrasound physics for the physician: a brief review, J. Clin. Ultrasound **3:**69, 1975.

Wells, P. N. T.: Absorption and dispersion of ultrasound in biological tissue, Ultrasound Med. Biol. **1:**369, 1975.

Wells, P. N. T.: Ultrasonics in clinical diagnosis, New York, 1977, Churchill-Livingstone.

3 Echocardiographic examination technique

GENERAL CONSIDERATIONS

Echocardiograms can be obtained in a laboratory designated for these studies or at the bedside. Better examinations are possible in the laboratory, since space can be arranged for easy and repeatable operation. Light levels can be controlled, and a standard examination table used.

The procedure should be explained briefly to the patient to allay anxiety concerning the examination. Small children, especially, require reassurance and usually lose their apprehension if they are allowed to hold the transducer briefly before the examination is begun. The presence of a parent in the room during the echocardiogram often allays the apprehension of young children.

A pacifier may be useful in small infants, who should ideally be fed before the examination. If struggling cannot be controlled, it may be necessary to postpone the examination until the patient is sedated.

The condition of the patient's chest wall may produce difficulty during the examination. Skeletal deformities, such as severe scoliosis or pectus excavatum, may be associated with rotation and displacement of the heart and may make the examination difficult or occasionally impossible. Surgical removal of the breast, especially when followed by x-ray therapy, may produce a chest wall that is so taut that the soft tissues are inadequate to obtain good transducer seating, making angulation difficult.

The position of the echocardiographer during patient examination is largely a matter of personal preference and equipment configuration. The examiner usually faces the head of the patient and may prefer to sit or to stand, but in either case comfort and a stable position are important. The transducer may be held in the left hand or the right, while the free hand is used to adjust instrument controls. Once the pattern of examination is established, it should be maintained as closely as possible in all future studies. The development of echocardiographic skills is more rapid if the examination conditions are not varied.

The equipment should be positioned so that the monitor oscilloscope is clearly visible without too much need for the examiner to turn his head, is shielded from strong light sources, and at a distance that allows manipulation of the controls (Fig. 3-1). The availability of a helper who is familiar with the instrument controls may be important when these conditions cannot be met (bedside studies) or when the examiner must use two hands to hold the transducer (Fig. 3-2).

Many echocardiographic examinations can be performed with the patient lying flat on his back. If difficulty is experienced in target location, it is useful to place him in a decubi-

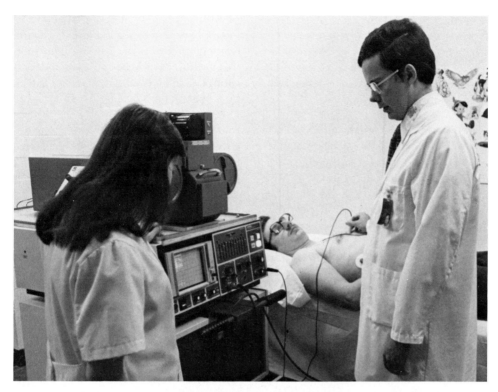

Fig. 3-1. Echocardiographic examination. The position of the examiner and his assistant in relation to the equipment and patient are shown during an echocardiographic examination in our laboratory. Continuous recordings are made on 35 mm film by means of a camera and slave oscilloscope mounted over the equipment.

tus position, partly or completely on his left side. Gravity then tends to displace the heart further to the left, thereby enlarging the ultrasonic window. Some rotation of the heart may also take place, and the examination may be easier to perform. A pillow or bolster should be used to support the patient in this position.

When examining the base of the heart (aortic and pulmonic valves), turning the patient's head to the left pulls the base of the heart in this direction and improves the accessibility of these structures.

Breathless patients may not tolerate lying flat for an echocardiogram and should be propped into a semisitting position by adjusting the examining table or providing extra pillows for their comfort. It is possible to obtain some information with the patient sitting in a chair, but the records are not as meaningful as those taken when the patient is in a relatively flat position. Standing studies are experimental and should be used only to supplement a conventional echocardiogram.

An electrocardiogram should be recorded with each echocardiogram without exception. Adhesive electrodes that snap onto the ECG cables provide excellent contact, are convenient to use, and minimize interference from patient motion (especially in pediatrics). The lead that is displayed and the size of the deflection in the ECG (controlled by a separate ECG sensitivity control) should be selected to produce easily visible waveforms. A separate control is present in the ECG amplifier to position the trace so that it does not interfere with the echocardiogram. This may be above or below the ultrasound display. With some instruments it is necessary to position the trace in the echo-free portion of the echocardiogram so that it is not lost in echoes from the heart. In other instances the ECG may be associated with electronics that blank out all other signals in a narrow band adjacent to the trace so that cardiac echo sources do not mask the trace.

The phonocardiogram may be recorded along with the echocardiogram and the ECG. This requires the placement of a contact microphone, which is held on the chest wall by an elastic band encircling the chest. The microphone should be positioned so that it or the belt does not interfere with the transducer. A position just below the apex of the heart or higher on the chest over the pulmonic valve area is usually satisfactory. Care should be exercised during the examination, since the contact gel used in echocardiog-

raphy (see below) may seep between the microphone and skin and degrade the phonocardiographic record. The amplifier used in phonocardiography has volume and position control similar to the ECG, and the same trace positioning technique should be followed. A filtration control is also present to remove unwanted frequencies from the recording, and specific filtration levels may be required for ideal recordings of specific sounds and murmurs. Carotid and jugular venous pulsations may also be recorded by applying a special pickup over the vessels.

Patient examination requires the application of a substance to the chest wall to provide good contact (coupling) with the transducer for efficient transmission of the ultrasonic energy into the body. Water and oils

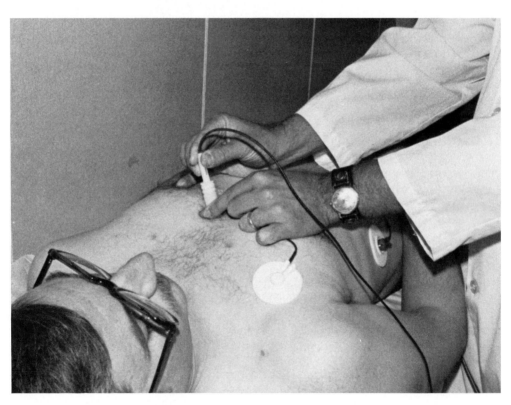

Fig. 3-2. Two-handed transducer-holding technique. The hand that ordinarily operates the instrument controls is placed on the chest wall, and the thumb and index finger are used to hold the lower end of the transducer firmly. The examining hand is placed higher on the transducer for beam angulation maneuvers. This technique is useful for examining a breathless or restless patient.

may be used but are less effective than commercially available gels. These gels contain methyl cellulose and water with other ingredients that serve as preservatives and prevent drying. They do not stain clothing, and residues dry to a harmless powder. Repeated application may be required as the gel thins or dries. A loss of sound transmission (seen as an apparent loss of sensitivity in the equipment) indicates the need for reapplication. In some cases a thick layer of gel is required to correct for chest wall irregularities or to permit transducer tilting when chest wall tissues are sparse.

The transducer selected for the examination is placed on the gel applied to the chest wall. The exact point of placement cannot be predicted, since there is considerable variation in the size and shape of patients' chests. A good starting place is along the left sternal border in the third to fifth intercostal space. The transducer should be held firmly and pressed gently against the chest wall. Excessive pressure can cause discomfort or pain.

Transducer manipulation is the greatest skill that the echocardiographer must master. It involves steady holding over an area of interest and minute angulations to obtain maximal excursions of motion or to sweep the beam through the length of a structure such as the mitral valve. Bolder angulations or sliding motions over the chest wall are used to relate structures to each other (mitral-aortic, mitral-tricuspid sweep). The extent of these motions cannot be described clearly and must be learned by practice. When attempting bold angulation or slides, it is useful to first identify the angle and position of the target structures at both ends of the sweep and to start and stop with the transducer in this position. A few practice sweeps made with monitor observation develops the coordination and timing that result in satisfactory records. Above all, attention should be fixed on the monitor oscilloscope; looking at the transducer has little if any value.

A two-handed holding technique may be required if the chest wall is heaving during

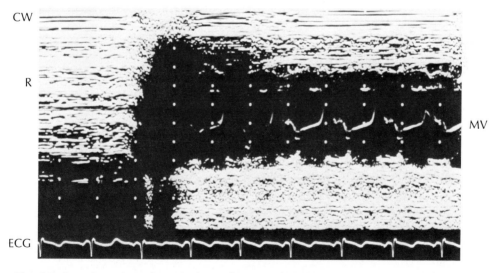

Fig. 3-3. Location of cardiac window. The recording begins over lung that produced typical reverberations (R). As the beam is moved beyond the lung margin, echo-free spaces, which represent cardiac cavities, rhythmically moving linear complexes from heart walls, and rapidly moving thin line echoes from valves are encountered. Their motion is repetitive and related to the cardiac cycle. CW, chest wall; MV, mitral valve; ECG, electrocardiogram.

respiration or if a restless patient is being examined (Fig. 3-2). The hand that ordinarily operates the instrument controls is placed on the chest wall, gripping the transducer between the thumb and index finger at the point where it touches the chest. This assures stability of the contact with the transducer. The examining hand is placed higher on the stem of the transducer and used to angulate the beam.

If target identification is not relatively easy in the initial try, do not hesitate to move the transducer to other areas. In tall, slender patients the heart may be lower in the chest, and cardiac enlargement may displace structures considerably to the left. In obese patients or pregnant women the heart may be more horizontal, and a transducer position higher on the chest wall may be required. Only the presence of lung or bone should

limit exploration, and even these can be partially avoided by angling under them.

Early in development, every echocardiographer should explore the size of the cardiac window to develop an appreciation of the variations encountered. It may be surprisingly large when hearts are enlarged, or it may be exceedingly small when the lungs are overinflated by emphysema. The normal range includes considerable variation, and babies and young children have cardiac windows that are relatively large. This variation occurs because the sternum, which is not calcified, is only a minimal barrier, and because of the relative widening of the mediastinum produced by the normal thymus which is larger in children than in adults. The cardiac window may be mapped by sliding the transducer over the chest wall and observing the echo patterns. When the beam is

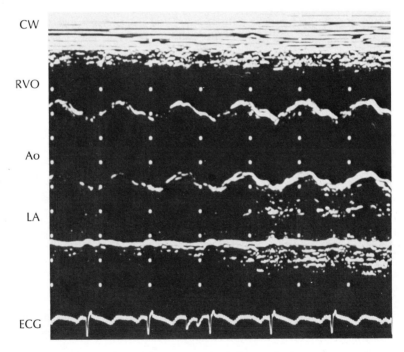

Fig. 3-4. Gain settings. A low-gain setting, on left, results in an incomplete recording of both aortic walls, and the posterior wall shows more dropouts, since it is located farther from the transducer than is the anterior wall. An increase in the overall and time-varied gain *(right)* results in a more complete recording of both walls, which demonstrates nearly equal signal intensity. CW, chest wall; RVO, right ventricular outflow; Ao, Aortic root; LA, left atrium; ECG, electrocardiogram.

passing into the lung, a dense, nonmoving echo pattern is displayed over a few centimeters of depth, beyond which no reflections are detected. These signals arise from the first few millimeters of lung, and the deeper display is produced by reverberation artifacts. No significant penetration occurs in air-containing lung. More medial sliding of the transducer directs the beam into the heart, which is recognized by the rhythmic motion in the cardiac cycle of its walls or contained structures. Further sliding toward the midline directs the beam into the sternum, which absorbs most of the sonic energy and can be recognized by the fact that moving heart structures disappear. The cardiac window, therefore, is that area where heart echoes can be obtained (Fig. 3-3).

An understanding of the operation of instrument controls is vital at this point, since searching for the cardiac window may be fruitless if control settings are grossly inadequate. The first experience with an ultrasonic device should begin by setting the re-ceiver gain at a high position, with no TVG, reject, or damping. This assures that signals will be present. A-mode is useful during high-gain searching to recognize a rapidly moving target such as a valve leaflet in the presence of high-amplitude background echoes. In lower-gain situations, A-mode is mainly used to assess signal amplitude for adjustment of TVG for proper recording of signals. Observation of A-mode displays should be used in conjunction with the more familiar M-mode, which shows the motion of structures. The following steps can then be followed to produce an ideal record (Figs. 3-4 to 3-9).

1. Move the transducer until a moving portion of the heart is detected.
2. Decrease the gain until the moving structure becomes evident with an echo-free cardiac cavity next to it. At this time it should be evident that there are moving echoes near the top (anterior) as well as near the bottom (posterior) of the display. The anterior

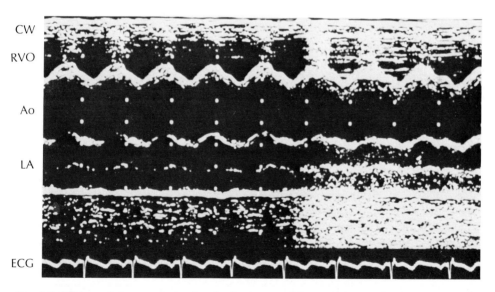

Fig. 3-5. Effects of time-varied gain. An improper time-varied gain used in aortic root (Ao) recording images the anterior wall well but fails to demonstrate deeper structures *(left)*. When corrected *(right)* the aortic wall echoes are of equal intensity, and deeper structures are better imaged. The linear echo in the left atrium (LA) is an unknown finding that may be related to the entrance of pulmonary veins into the left atrium. CW, chest wall; RVO, right ventricular outflow tract; ECG, electrocardiogram.

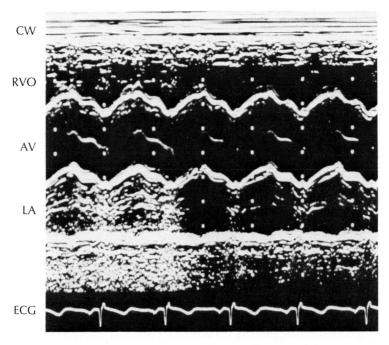

CW

RVO

AV

LA

ECG

Fig. 3-6. Artifact of time-varied gain. A high time-varied gain produces reverberatory clutter that obscures the left atrial cavity (LA) recorded behind the aortic valve (AV). The posterior aortic wall is also more prominently recorded than is the anterior. Decrease in the time-varied gain *(right)* results in clearing of the left atrial cavity and tends to equalize the intensity of both anterior and posterior aortic wall images. CW, chest wall; RVO, right ventricular outflow; ECG, electrocardiogram.

echoes will probably be brighter or more prominent than those that lie deeper.

3. Increase the TVG until the deep and superficial structures begin to appear as equal in brightness. (It may not be necessary to use this control.) At this point the cavities of the heart that were previously echo-free will fill with echoes again.

4. Decrease overall gain until the posterior cavity is clear. The walls of the heart should be imaged as strong echo sources.

5. The cavities in the anterior portion of the record will probably not be clear at this time. Introduce some delay in the suppression control and begin suppressing near-field gain until the anterior wall of the heart can be seen as it moves. Advance the delay until the anterior heart cavity clears. This is usually the right ventricle, and the delay should terminate at its posterior margin, the interventricular septum.

6. The reject control may now be activated if further cleanup of the cardiac cavity is required.

7. Adjust beam position and angle until a standard target such as the mitral valve or aortic root is encountered.

8. Touch up any controls that can improve the image. This requires considerable expertise, which comes with experience. However, the control positions at this time are excellent starting points for the next patient and subsequent examinations. Additional technique descriptions are included in the sections dealing with clinical echocardiography.

Bedside examination is one of the unique capabilities of cardiac ultrasound, and every

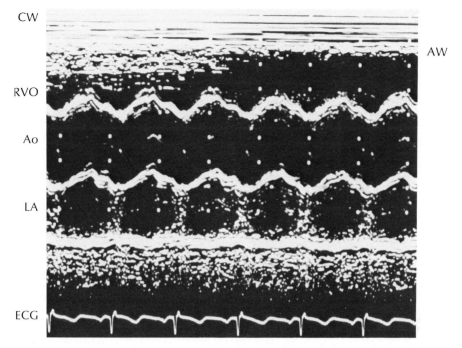

Fig. 3-7. Use of near-gain suppression. The reverberatory clutter present in front of the aortic root (Ao) is removed, and the anterior right ventricular wall (AW) is seen as a linear moving echo just beneath the chest wall (CW) on the right. LA, left atrium; RVO, right ventricular outflow; ECG, electrocardiogram.

echocardiographer must be prepared to examine patients out of the familiar surroundings of the laboratory. Bedside examinations may be complicated by cramped space, the necessity to move furniture and the bed, to make room for the equipment, and high light levels that may interfere with the viewing of monitor oscilloscopes. Mechanical ventilators used to assist the patient's respiration may produce interference during lung inflation so that it may be necessary to record the heart's activity between cycles of lung inflation.

Examination of patients in isolation may require cleaning the transducer before contact with the patient. Sterilization after its use in a patient with a communicable disease must be accomplished with gas sterilization, since heat will damage the transducer.

In the coronary care unit, we have found it desirable to have a special connecting cable fabricated to obtain the ECG directly from the monitor oscilloscope to obviate the need to attach additional electrodes.

Ultrasonic studies are occasionally performed in the cardiac catheterization laboratory as part of a research effort, to evaluate clinical problems arising from cardiac catheterization (such as a question of pericardial effusion from inadvertent perforation of the heart and escape of blood into the pericardial space), or to study the flow of intracardiac ultrasonic contrast agents in congenital heart disease to obtain flow pattern information in the presence of intracardiac shunts. Since the examiner's position relative to the patient may be different from that in laboratory examination, target detection is more difficult. It is helpful to study these patients before cardiac catheterization to become familiar with their individual anatomy.

Ultrasonic contrast agents may be injected into the heart during cardiac catheterization for structure identification and to record

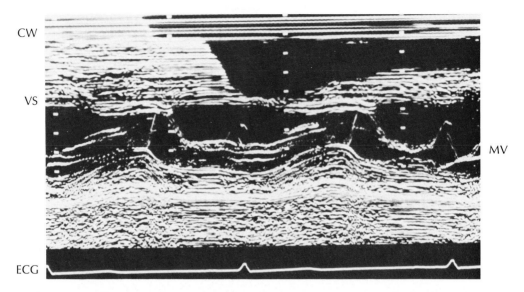

Fig. 3-8. Suppression control errors. Initially, no suppression results in clutter imaging, which obscures the ventricular septum (VS). Excessive delay is then used and destroys almost all of the septal image. Corrective attempt *(right)* fails to clear the right side of the septum, which may be poorly seen moving within the clutter. A change to the decubitus position of the patient may help to image the septum more clearly and to minimize the need for manipulation of the controls. CW, chest wall; MV, mitral valve; ECG, electrocardiogram.

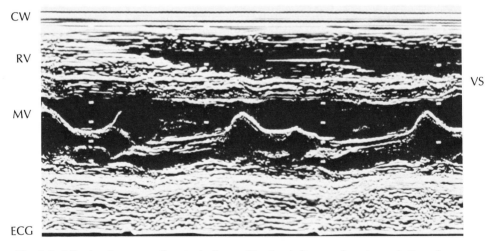

Fig. 3-9. Mitral valve recording technique. On the left, reverberatory clutter obscures the right ventricular cavity (RV). However, the right side of the ventricular septum (VS) is visible and can be delineated by maneuvering the near gain to suppress reverberations in front of it. Ideal suppression allows the demonstration of a few background echoes in the right ventricle to assure that structurally important echo sources are not masked. CW, chest wall; MV, mitral valve; ECG, electrocardiogram.

blood flow patterns (Fig. 3-10). These agents contain small amounts of gas distributed in minute bubbles, or they may produce small bubbles as a result of the very rapid injection (cavitation). The amount of gas required is very small, usually about .02 ml, and no harm is produced by this procedure. Indocyanine green (a dye used for cardiac output studies) is commonly used, though saline or other fluids, which derive their contrast from rapid injection rates or from small bubbles present in the fluid, catheters, or in stopcocks, may be employed.

A typical contrast study may be used to demonstrate presence or absence of a shunt, the level at which it occurs, or to show leakage of an incompetent valve (Fig. 3-11). The transducer position is selected to image the chamber into which the abnormal flow takes place. When possible, the chamber receiving the injection should be included. The record should begin before injection and continue until the contrast has cleared. (The contrast effect may be a dense cloud of echoes, or it may take the form of numerous small individual reflectors that appear to float upward toward the transducer.) If no contrast effect is noted, it may be necessary to check the position of the catheter by fluoroscopy or to try another injection. The contrast effect may not be consistent from injection to injection. It is important to indicate the moment of injection on the ultrasound record by deflecting an unused channel (such as the phonocardiographic channel) when the injection is made.

We have found it useful to do contrast injections in patients who have had septal defects closed surgically. The surgeon usually leaves a catheter whose tip is in the appropriate chamber for pressure monitoring. It can be used for contrast injection in the intensive care unit in the immediate postoperative period. Contrast injection reveals the completeness of surgical closure of the defect or any residual leak that may be present.

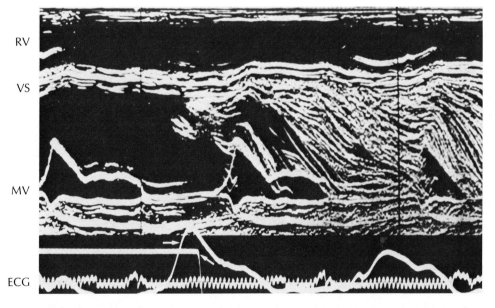

Fig. 3-10. Left ventricular contrast injection. Indocyanine green was injected into the left ventricle during ventricular systole. The ventricular septum (VS) contains the contrast material, and absence of right ventricular filling indicates an intact septum with no left-to-right shunting. The signals below the echocardiogram are a damped aortic pressure curve *(horizontal arrow),* an indicator of the time of injection *(oblique arrow),* and an electrocardiogram (ECG). RV, right ventricle; MV mitral valve.

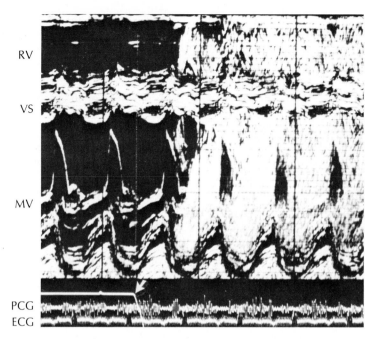

Fig. 3-11. Contrast study in ventricular septal defect. Injection of indocyanine green in the aortic root during cardiac catheterization shows filling of the left ventricular cavity, as well as appearance of contrast material into the right ventricle, which reveals the presence of aortic incompetence and ventricular septal defect. The endocardial surface of the left ventricular posterior wall can also be identified by noting the posterior limitation of contrast effect. RV, right ventricle; VS, ventricular septum; MV, mitral valve; PCG, phonocardiogram; ECG, electrocardiogram. Arrow denotes timing of injection.

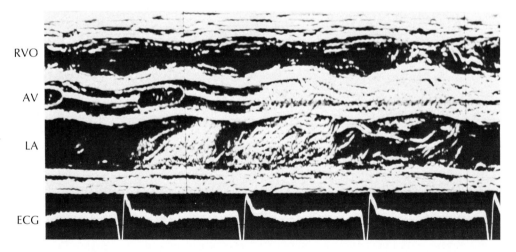

Fig. 3-12. Contrast studies following surgical closure of a ventricular septal defect. Injection of saline into left atrium (via a surgically placed catheter) reveals contrast echoes in the aortic root with appearance in the right ventricular outflow (RVO), indicating incomplete closure of the defect. AV, aortic valve; LA, left atrium; ECG, electrocardiogram.

(Fig. 3-12). Despite adequate surgical repair, small leaks along suture lines may be detected immediately after operation, but unlike a residual leak they are sealed by tissue reaction and disappear over the next few days.

The presence of a catheter in the heart provides a pathway by which electrical energy may reach the heart directly. Extremely small amounts of electricity pose a hazard to the heart, since they may induce life-threatening arrhythmias. Recently manufactured ultrasonic equipment complies with regulation U.L. 544, which specifies regulations for electrical safety in hospitals, and is therefore safe to use during cardiac catheterization. Older devices may have unacceptably large ground current leakage, which will trigger safety devices in the cardiac catheterization laboratory when plugged into electrical outlets. Consult a physicist, engineer, or technician who is responsible for electrical safety in the hospital if there is any question concerning the electrical safety of equipment before its use in areas such as the cardiac catheterization laboratory.

Echocardiographic equipment is not approved for use in an explosive atmosphere. Therefore, if general anesthesia is to be used during catheterization, it is necessary to check with the anesthesiologist before attempting echocardiography.

Echocardiographic equipment should be checked periodically to ensure a high level of performance. Sensitivity may be evaluated by placing a plastic block about 1 inch thick under the transducer (be sure to use coupling gel and to achieve good contact) with maximum receiver gain and no TVG suppression or reject. Count and record the number of reverberations that can be observed (A-mode is more useful here than M-mode). If sensitivity decreases with time, the number of reverberations detected will also diminish. This tests both the transducer and instrument electronics so that the test should be repeated with each transducer used.

The accuracy of depth determination can be checked by placing the same plastic block in a water bath at a fixed measured distance from the transducer. Comparison of actual and recorded depth reveals calibration errors if present. Consult the manufacturer's representative or service representative for additional suggestions regarding performance testing or if you detect changes that suggest instrument or transducer malfunction.

CARDIAC TARGET CHARACTERISTICS

The way in which portions of the heart are imaged is an important factor in their identification and in establishing orientation of the structures the beam is passing through. Ventricular walls, including the septum, are usually fairly thick (the scale marks projected on the image at 1-cm spacings are useful for this purpose), and the walls move in a rhythmic manner with excursions of about 1 or 2 cm or less. Heart valves, when normal, are thin reflectors only a millimeter or two in thickness and show rapid and slow motions that may be as much as 30 mm in amplitude and trace a pattern that contains peaks and angles during a cardiac cycle. Heart chambers are echo-free spaces, bounded by heart walls and containing the rapidly moving patterns of valves. Calcifications present as echoes that are more intense than cardiac walls or valves. They may be quite thick when involving a valve, or they may be composed of multiple, thin, linear echoes. The motion of calcified valves is usually markedly reduced as compared to normal valves, and they are identified by their position in the heart relative to the other normal structures. Masses such as tumors and infective endocarditis result in clumps of dots or short lines that appear in a chamber that should be echo-free or that are attached to a moving heart valve. Masses move to a variable degree with the blood flow in the chamber in which they are located. Those attached to valves may move rapidly with the valve or may show exaggerated motion, particularly if destruction of valve tissue is present. In other instances, valves may show relatively normal motion but exhibit a fuzzy multilinear pattern produced by smaller vegetations present on valve leaflets. Clear spaces outside the heart walls occur in pericardial effusion. The clear fluid present in this condition produces no echoes, and an additional space is found in front of or behind the ventricular walls.

ECHOCARDIOGRAPHIC ANATOMY

Echocardiographic anatomy is the foundation of echocardiography and is one of the most difficult concepts to grasp. The difficulties arise from the fact that the heart is a complex structure that is viewed echocardiographically along a single line of sight at a particular time. Echocardiograms have been described as "icepick" views, which are obtained by passing a single line through the heart and showing the position, thickness, and motion of solid structures as they lie in the path of the line. There is no information about structures that lie next to the line. To obtain this information the beam must be moved, in which case the original information disappears and must be remembered to establish anatomic relationships. Patterns of structure position and motion often change rapidly with minimal beam motion, thereby rendering anatomic orientation more difficult. However, knowledge of cardiac anatomy and experience in performing echocardiography, with time, allow the examiner to recognize the structures being examined and to develop in his mind the anatomic relationships that are important in echocardiographic diagnosis. His responsibility is to provide meaningful recordings that show cardiac anatomy clearly and with a maximum of diagnostic content.

Chest wall (precordial) transducer placement is most commonly used and therefore is the best starting point for description of echocardiographic anatomy (Fig. 3-13). The mitral valve is the most commonly used structure to begin description of echocardiographic anatomy, since it is relatively easily found because its motion and position readily identify it. After the mitral valve is located, it becomes a landmark to which the examiner can return when maneuvers to locate other structures fail.

The mitral valve is located by placing the transducer perpendicularly on the chest wall in the left third to fifth intercostal spaces at the left sternal border and angling it slightly

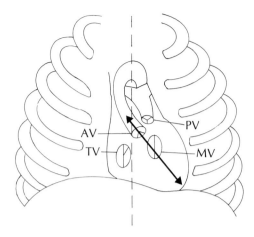

Fig. 3-13. Position of echocardiographic targets. This frontal display shows the superior-inferior and lateral relationships of the valve rings. The long axis of the left ventricle is demonstrated by the double-pointed arrow. In depth the pulmonic valve (PV) and tricuspid valve (TV) are most superficial, the aortic valve (AV) lies somewhat deeper, while the mitral valve (MV) is most posterior in the heart. Note that the long axis of the left ventricle passes through aortic and mitral valves. Dotted line represents midline of chest; tricuspid valve lies to the right in substernal position (sternum is not shown). Aortic valve is often partially under the sternum.

medially. In adults, it lies about 5 to 8 cm (using the range markers displayed on the oscilloscope) in depth and has the previously described characteristics of a valve. If the valve echo is not obtained, angle the transducer slowly toward the apex beat and look for rapidly moving echoes. Do not hesitate to reposition the transducer higher or lower than the starting point or further medially or laterally. A very large heart may require considerable lateral displacement.

Failure to find the mitral valve after these initial efforts requires an examination of the echo pattern to determine the portion of the heart through which the beam may be passing so that a more deliberate effort can be made to locate the mitral valve. When the beam is too low, it passes through the left ventricular cavity beyond the tip of the mitral

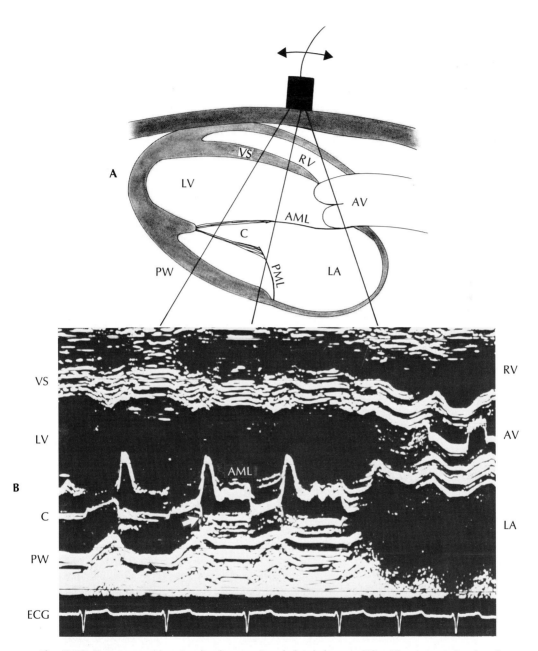

Fig. 3-14. Beam scanning in the long axis of the left ventricle. The anatomic sketch (**A**) shows three commonly used beam positions and the anatomic structures they routinely detect. The echocardiogram (**B**) demonstrates typical ultrasonic appearance as obtained by scanning beam through this portion of heart. *Arrow* indicates posterior leaflet of mitral valve. RV, right ventricle; VS, ventricular septum; LV, left ventricular cavity; AV, aortic valve; AML, anterior leaflet of mitral valve; PML, posterior leaflet of the mitral valve; C, chordae; LA, left atrium; PW, left ventricular posterior wall; ECG, electrocardiogram.

valve. The cavity can be recognized by the characteristic thickness and motion of its walls. Angling the beam toward the patient's feet and left hip reveals that the cavity space narrows as the cardiac apex is approached. Multiple, linear echoes from the papillary muscles or chordae are often found within the cavity with this maneuver. Scanning backward toward the patient's head and right shoulder directs the beam into the mitral valve. Further scanning upward encounters the aortic root, whose walls present as strong, parallel linear echo sources, somewhat thicker than valve leaflets. The posterior margin of the aortic root is continuous with the mitral valve. The linear scan described defines the long axis of the left ventricle and includes the mitral valve (Fig. 3-14). A beam position and angle that is much too medial may detect the tricuspid valve, whereas lesser degrees of medial overangulation show an anterior chamber wall with exaggerated motion. Decreasing the extent of medial beam angulation or moving the beam laterally should reveal the mitral valve or papillary muscles echoes from which the long axis search pattern can be initiated.

When the mitral valve is successfully detected, the structures in the beam can be described in a sequence that begins at the chest wall. The first cardiac structure is the anterior wall of the right ventricle, which is relatively thin (5 mm or less in width) and is just under the chest wall (Fig. 3-15). Immediately deeper to it lies the right ventricular cavity, which is bounded posteriorly by the interventricular septum. It is usually necessary to adjust the suppression control so that the delay ends at the posterior margin of the right ventricular cavity and also shows it as an echo-free space. The interventricular septum, next in line in the beam, shows the characteristics of a heart wall and usually measures approximately a centimeter in thickness. The beam next enters the outflow portion of the left ventricular cavity in which the mitral valve is shown to be moving. Behind the mitral valve is the left atrial cavity, followed by the left atrial wall. Solid-appearing echoes behind the left atrial wall and arising in mediastinal structures mask the thickness of the atrial wall, but the motion pattern here is relatively flat and differs from the wall of the left ventricle. Sometimes,

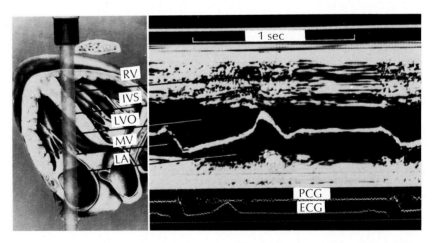

Fig. 3-15. Normal mitral valve (echocardiographic anatomy). Right ventricular cavity is not well represented, probably because beam passes through it and interventricular septum tangentially. Left atrium is shown behind mitral valve. Left ventricle may also be found behind mitral valve when ultrasonic beam is directed more laterally and inferiorly. PCG, phonocardiogram; ECG, electrocardiogram. (From Gramiak, R., and Shah, P. M.: Radiol. Clin. North Am. **9:**472, 1971.)

especially when the left ventricle is enlarged, the beam exits from the heart through the posterior left ventricular wall. Its thickness (around 1 cm) and active, rhythmic motion pattern differentiate it from the left atrial wall. The pericardium and lung, lying behind the left ventricular wall, form a strong reflecting interface beyond which useful signals are not detected.

The length of the mitral valve and left ventricular outflow tract should be scanned as part of every echocardiographic examination. The long axis pathway is used for this purpose (Fig. 3-13). It is useful to perform all scanning maneuvers using slower recording speeds (for instance, 25 mm/sec) for adequate appreciation of various structural relationships.

The left ventricular cavity imaged near the region of the cardiac apex often shows rather thick linear echoes, which represent papillary muscle components. As the ultrasonic beam is slowly moved medially and cephalad and just before the mitral valve leaflets are encountered, papillary muscle echoes are replaced by those obtained from the chordae of the mitral valve apparatus. These are slender echoes that lie usually about 1 cm in front of the posterior left ventricular wall and have a motion pattern that follows that of the endocardium but is slightly slower in systole. At the junction of the chords and the mitral leaflets, rapid opening motion of one or both leaflets is present with the onset of diastole, but complete diastolic traces are not obtained. Progressing more cephalad, the tip of the anterior mitral leaflet is recorded and shows a typical double-peaked diastolic configuration that is generally diminished in amplitude but may show prominence of the terminal peak (produced by atrial systole). The posterior leaflet of the mitral valve is also usually recorded completely at about this point in the scan and shows a motion pattern opposite that of the anterior leaflet in diastole and has less amplitude that that of the anterior leaflet, since the posterior leaflet is the smaller of the two. When both the anterior and posterior leaflets are recorded, the beam generally exits

through the posterior left ventricular wall. Further scanning along the long axis of the left ventricle next detects the body of the anterior leaflet (midportion). This portion shows the maximum diastolic motion of the anterior leaflet. The beam then exits from the heart through the left atrial wall. Progression of scanning shows the attachment of the anterior leaflet to the posterior margin of the aortic root. This portion is the base of the mitral leaflet and the site of attachment in the anterior portion of the mitral ring. The amplitude of motion of the anterior leaflet in diastole continues to diminish until it is replaced by the motion of the aortic root, which moves posteriorly in diastole and anteriorly in systole.

This scanning maneuver also images the interventricular septum, whose point of attachment to the anterior margin of the aortic root can be shown. At the beginning of the scan the interventricular septum shows a thickness of around 10 mm but tapers abruptly to a few millimeters just before it attaches to the aortic root. This thin portion of the septum is composed mainly of fibrous tissue and represents the membranous portion. The motion pattern of the mitral valve and septum are discussed in subsequent sections.

The scan from the mitral valve to the aortic root is the most convenient method to locate the aortic valve. Occasionally the medial and cephalic angulation of the beam must be very steep when the transducer is placed over the body of the anterior mitral leaflet. In these cases, moving the transducer one interspace toward the patient's head and angling the beam medially will detect the aortic root and valve. The aortic valve is recognized as slender echoes that move rapidly toward the periphery of the aortic root in systole and occupy a position midway in the aortic root in diastole. The ideal aortic valve detection position shows the aortic root margins with equal amplitudes of motion. A beam that is angled too far medially demonstrates exaggerated motion amplitude of the anterior aortic margin as compared to the posterior and is an exception to the rule that maximal structure motion amplitude must be sought

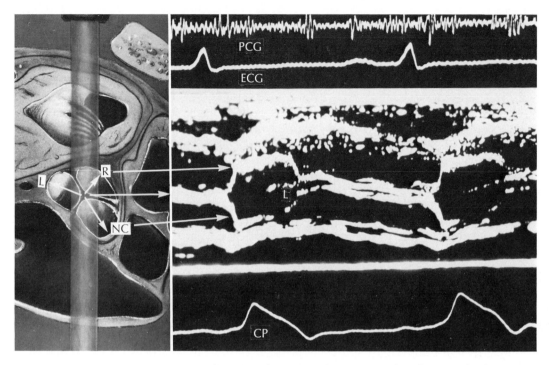

Fig. 3-16. Ultrasonic anatomy of aortic valve cusps. In cross-sectional anatomic view, ultrasonic beam passes through aortic valve. The cross section has been rotated to depict beam as vertical for better orientation with echocardiogram. Note that cusps in diastole produce a central linear echo configuration. In systole the right coronary cusp *(R)* moves anteriorly, while the noncoronary cusp *(NC)* moves posteriorly. Left coronary cusp *(L)* moves laterally in relation to ultrasonic beam and therefore shows little or no motion on ultrasonic record. PCG, phonocardiogram; ECG, electrocardiogram; CP, carotid pulse. (From Gramiak, R., and others: Radiology **96:**1-8, 1970.)

during examination. The exact mechanism of this exaggerated motion is not understood but could be related to the complex motion of the aortic root, which occurs in a plane but is studied along a single line.

In correct beam position the structures examined in sequence from the chest wall are the anterior wall of the outflow portion of the right ventricle, the right ventricular outflow tract, the aortic root and valve cusps, the left atrial cavity, and finally, the posterior left atrial wall with mediastinal contents behind (Figs. 3-16 and 3-17).

A variable segment of the aorta can usually be examined above the aortic valve. This can be accomplished by cephalic angulation from the aortic valve recording position or by displacing the transducer one interspace above the aortic valve and angling the beam medially. Recordings obtained in this position show the margins of the aortic root in a more anterior position than at the level of the valve as a consequence of the normal anterior arching of the aorta as it leaves the heart. Since this recording is obtained above the level of the right ventricle, the right ventricular outflow tract is not imaged, and the anterior aortic wall is the first structure encountered under the chest wall. Valve leaflets, of course, are not present, and the left atrium lies behind the aorta. Sweeps from the aortic valve into the ascending aorta are useful to show any areas of supravalvular stenosis, aneurysms, poststenotic dilatations resulting from abnormal blood flow through a stenotic aortic valve, and the normal anterior

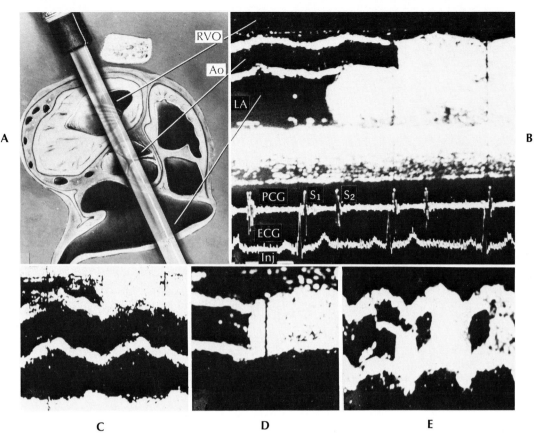

Fig. 3-17. Ultrasonic anatomy during aortic valve recording. **A,** Anatomic sketch illustrates path of ultrasonic beam and structures encountered during aortic valve recording. **B,** Injection (Inj) was made into left atrial cavity (LA) with filling of space behind aortic root (Ao) and demonstration of aorta during subsequent ventricular systole. **C,** Right ventricular outflow tract (RVO) is identified anterior to aortic root after right ventricular contrast injection. **D,** Aortic root is filled after left ventricular contrast injection. **E,** Injection was made in supravalvular position and identifies valve cusps. Rectangular defects in contrast pattern result from ejection of noncontrast blood from left ventricle, which lies at the plane below ultrasonic study. S_1, first heart sound; S_2, second heart sound; PCG, phonocardiogram; ECG, echocardiogram. (From Gramiak, R., Shah, P. M., and Kramer, D. H.: Radiology **92:**939, 1969.)

arching of the aorta, which may be useful in the differential diagnosis of patients with congenital heart disease. The ability to make these scans may be severely limited in patients with small cardiac windows.

Detection of the tricuspid valve may begin from an aortic valve beam position. To image the tricuspid valve, the beam is directed caudally and more medially under the sternum (Figs. 3-18 and 3-19). Landmarks such as those present in the left ventricle are of less use in tricuspid valve detection and it is usual to scan the beam around, slowly using the angulation described until a reflector is found at about the same depth as the anterior aortic margin. Its motion pattern may be slow and rhythmic, but minor adjustments of beam angle (usually more medial and more caudal) pass the beam through the tricuspid valve, which is recognized by

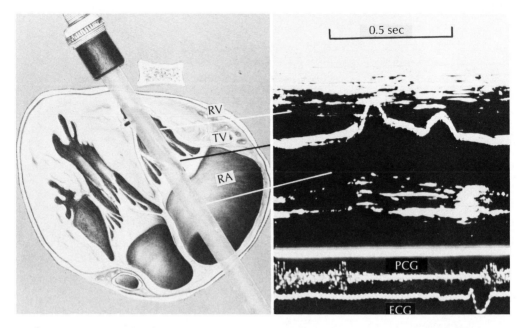

Fig. 3-18. Tricuspid valve echocardiographic anatomy. Waveform of tricuspid valve (TV) is similar to that of mitral valve. Best tricuspid echoes are obtained in patients with a large right ventricle (RV); right atrium (RA) lies behind tricuspid valve. PCG, phonocardiogram; ECG, electrocardiogram. (From Gramiak, R., and Shah, P. M.: Radiol. Clin. North Am. **9:**483, 1971.)

its rapid anterior fling at the onset of diastole. This results in a trace that shows a relatively flat systolic position followed by rapid anterior movement in diastole (gull wing appearance) and may represent the only recording possible in a normal patient. In young children, normal adults studied in a decubitus position, and in patients with enlarged right hearts, a complete tracing of the tricuspid valve may be obtained, and it resembles a mitral valve image. However, the depth of the trace is more superficial, and the chamber anatomy around these valves differs.

In tricuspid valve recordings the beam first encounters the right ventricular wall and passes through the right ventricular cavity. The tricuspid leaflet marks the boundary between the right ventricle and the right atrium, which lies behind the systolic position of the tricuspid valve. The beam then passes through the right atrial cavity until it reaches the right atrial wall, which has lung lying behind it. In other instances, a thin line or echo

is found just behind the tricuspid valve, especially when somewhat less medial angulation is used as compared to that previously described. This echo moves rhythmically in a pattern similar to that of the aortic root and represents the interatrial septum. The left atrial cavity lies deep to the interatrial septum, and the beam exits from the heart through the left atrial wall and into the mediastinum (Fig. 3-20).

The tricuspid valve may be located beginning with the beam passing through the mitral valve. Steep medial and caudal angulation is used, and the landmarks, search patterns, and anatomy are similar to those already described. This sweep between the mitral and tricuspid valve should be practiced, since it provides important anatomic information in patients with congenital heart disease (Fig. 3-21).

The tricuspid valve is more difficult to examine than either the mitral or aortic valves. Ordinarily, it is difficult to obtain complete

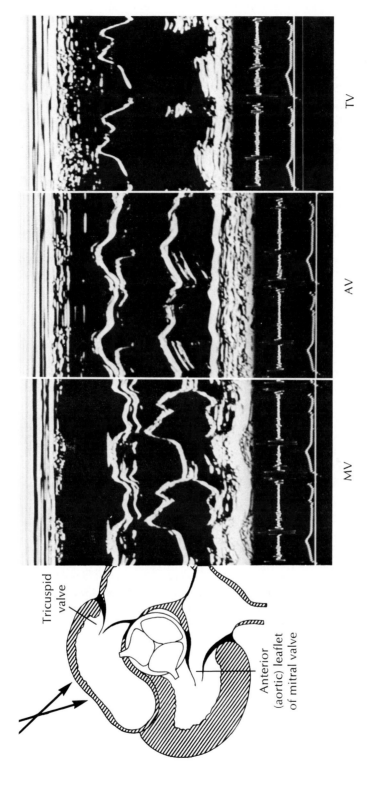

Fig. 3-19. Echocardiographic relationships of tricuspid valve. Mitral valve (MV) occupies deepest position, and its systolic segment is at the level of posterior margin of aortic root. The ventricular septum is recorded in front of the mitral valve and lies at the same depth as the anterior aortic margin. The tricuspid valve (TV) is more anteriorly situated, and its depth is approximately that of the anterior aortic margin or ventricular septum. The anatomic sketch indicates the beam direction for mitral and tricuspid valve recording. Aortic valve (AV) records are obtained by an intermediate position. These discontinuous echocardiographic tracings from the three valves were obtained from a patient with an atrial septal defect and a dilated right ventricle.

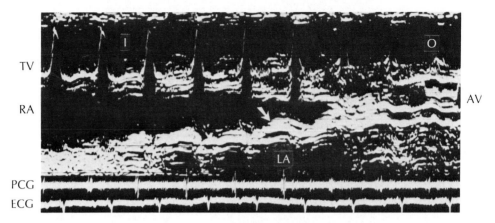

Fig. 3-20. Beam scanning from tricuspid to aortic valve in a patient with right heart enlargement. The echo-free space in front of tricuspid valve *(TV)* systolic segment represents right ventricular inflow *(I)*; area in front of aortic root is right ventricular outflow tract *(O)*. Right atrial cavity *(RA)* is recorded behind the tricuspid valve, and the beam exits through posterior right atrial wall at extreme left. As scan progresses, the right atrial wall, which is flat, merges with a moving echo *(arrow)*, which represents interatrial septum and separates right atrial cavity from left atrium *(LA)*. The interatrial septum ends at level of posterior aortic margin. AV, aortic valve; PCG, phonocardiogram; ECG, electrocardiogram.

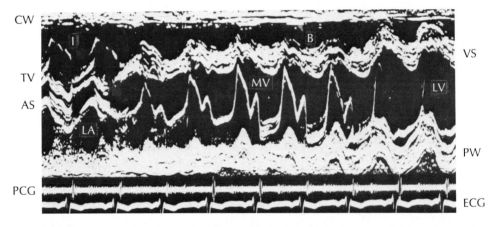

Fig. 3-21. Beam scanning from tricuspid valve to left ventricle. Tricuspid valve *(TV)* is seen at approximately same level as ventricular septum *(VS)*. Atrial septum *(AS)* is recorded behind tricuspid valve and is in continuity with the anterior mitral leaflet. As beam is scanned laterally and inferiorly, posterior leaflet of mitral valve *(MV)* is also recorded, and beam exits through left ventricular posterior wall *(PW)*. Further transducer angulation results in ultrasonic beam passing through short axis of left ventricle *(LV)* immediately past tip of mitral valve. Echoes from chordae tendineae and fragments of mitral leaflets are present in this region. CW, chest wall; I, right ventricular inflow; B, right ventricular body; LA, left atrium; PCG, phonocardiogram; ECG, electrocardiogram.

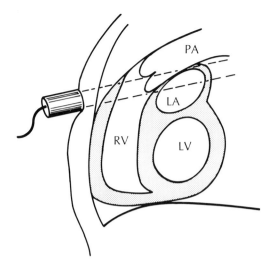

Fig. 3-22. Schematic representation of pathway of ultrasonic beam as it obliquely traverses right ventricular outflow–pulmonary artery area during pulmonic valve detection. The upward oblique beam direction explains why usually only a single posterior valve cusp is detected and illustrates how elevation of valve cusp toward opening produces posterior deflection on echogram. PA, pulmonary artery; RV, right ventricle; LA, left atrium; LV, left ventricle (From Nanda, N. C. and others; Circulation **50:**575, 1974.)

sweeps of tricuspid valve anatomy, and the examination may consist of records obtained in only one beam position. The tricuspid valve apparatus is seldom detected, and sweeps to the pulmonic valve are not obtained in the normal adult, since the outflow tract of the right ventricle is long and cannot be followed at this stage in echocardiographic development. However, as mentioned earlier, in patients with right-sided enlargement, the tricuspid valve is displaced leftward and can be easily and more completely recorded. Also, the right side of the heart, including the outflow tract, can be surveyed more fully and scans to other valves readily obtained.

The pulmonic valve is the most difficult cardiac valve to detect, probably because of the proximity of lung and because of rather steep transducer angulation required to find it (Fig. 3-22). The most rewarding approach begins with the transducer placed at the level used to record the aortic valve. The beam is then angled very slowly toward the patient's left shoulder (cephalad and laterally) while the examiner observes the monitor display. The aortic root pattern disappears and is replaced by an anterior space whose pos-

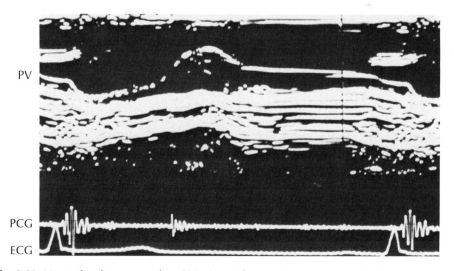

Fig. 3-23. Normal pulmonary valve (PV). A rapid posterior movement is observed in early diastole followed by a further circumscribed posterior movement (A dip) following atrial systole. The valve opening movements are relatively slow. PCG, phonocardiogram; ECG, electrocardiogram.

terior margin is three to four times wider than an aortic wall. The cusps of the pulmonic valve are found in this space. Very small changes in beam angle are required to image valve leaflet motion, and most beginners do not direct the beam high enough. The valve may appear intermittently as the patient breathes. Do not make beam adjustments under these conditions, but wait for the valve image to reappear on the next respiratory cycle. It is possible to develop a rhythmic pattern of beam angulation in time with patient respiration to track the pulmonic valve as it moves up and down in the patient's chest. This is a difficult technique and should be reserved for later phases of echocardiographic skill development.

If the cardiac window is small at this level and the chest wall sufficiently thick, we have found it useful to begin beam angulation from a transducer position over the edge of the sternum. The beam passes through soft tissue and skims over bone, thereby allowing examination of the pulmonic valve through smaller windows.

The pulmonic valve may also be found beginning from the mitral valve recording position. Angulation of the beam or transducer displacement toward the patient's head along a line that parallels the midline often detects the pulmonic valve. It will be recognized by the characteristic patterns already described and requires the same meticulous beam adjustments.

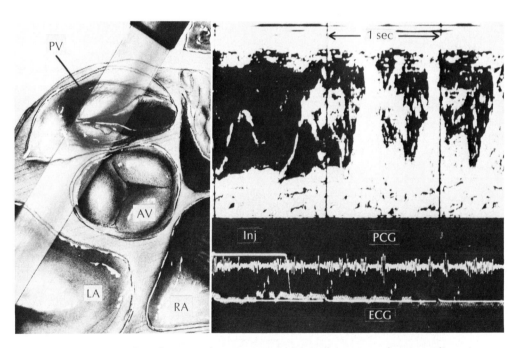

Fig. 3-24. Contrast identification of structures during pulmonary valve recording. Anatomic sketch demonstrates lateral beam angulation used for pulmonary valve (PV) detection but does not convey that upward angulation is also required. Pulmonary artery contrast injection (Inj) fills space behind valve cusp with dense echoes and shows some irregular filling of right ventricular outflow tract, which lies in front of pulmonary valve. This is probably due to catheter-induced pulmonary regurgitation. Barlike echoes that extend anteriorly from valve cusps in diastole probably represent other contrast-filled cusps that descend into beam only briefly. Other contrast injections have identified left atrium (LA) as the chamber lying deep to pulmonary valve. AV, aortic valve. RA, right atrium; PCG, phonocardiogram; ECG, electrocardiogram. (From Gramiak, R., Nanda, N. C., and Shah, P. M.: Radiology **102:**153, 1972.)

The normal pulmonic valve recorded from either of these positions is a thin echo that describes an oblique path in diastole and makes a rapid posterior movement when it opens in systole. (Figs. 3-23 and 3-24). Its position during systole is not recorded as consistently as during diastole.

In infants and young children the examination technique may differ, since the cardiac window in these cases is usually wider at the level of the pulmonic valve. The transducer may be placed higher than in adults (often the second intercostal space directly over the pulmonic valve, 1 or 2 cm from the sternal edge). The beam is directed straight posteriorly, and the valve cusps are identified by their motion pattern, which generally resembles an aortic valve when this high position is used. Both walls of the pulmonary artery are also identified and move like the aortic root (Fig. 3-25).

Pulmonic valve recording is usually from one position only, and beam sweeping is generally not used to obtain additional information concerning this valve. It is useful, however, to become adept at sweeping the beam from the aortic to the pulmonic valve to develop an appreciation of the normal lateral and anterior position of the pulmonic valve in respect to the aortic. This relationship is reversed in certain cases of congenital heart disease (transposition of the great vessels). Scanning maneuvers are useful in relating the pulmonary valve to other valves as well as in the regional examination of right heart chambers, especially when they are enlarged (Figs. 3-26 and 3-27). The echocardiographic anatomy of the pulmonic valve recording is summarized beginning at the anterior portion of the record. The beam first passes through the right ventricular outflow tract, which represents the cavity present in

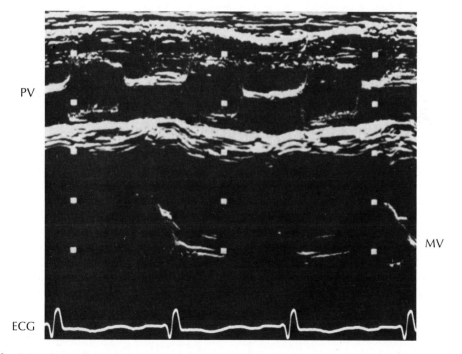

Fig. 3-25. Recording of pulmonary artery in infant. Both walls of pulmonary artery as well as anterior and posterior cusps are recorded. The high transducer position and caudal beam angulation occasionally detect mitral valve *(MV)* in same recording. PV, pulmonary valve; MV, mitral valve; ECG, electrocardiogram.

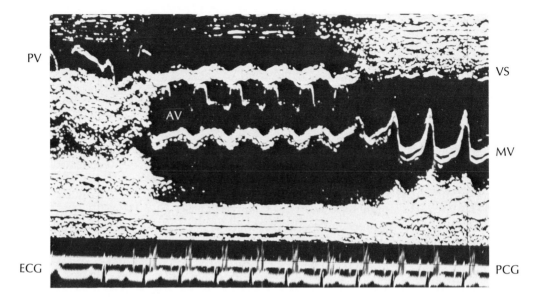

Fig. 3-26. Relationship of aortic *(AV)* and mitral *(MV)* valves to the pulmonic valve *(PV)*. Beam sweeping shows that the pulmonary valve is situated more anteriorly as compared to the aortic and mitral valves. VS, ventricular septum; PCG, phonocardiogram; ECG, electrocardiogram.

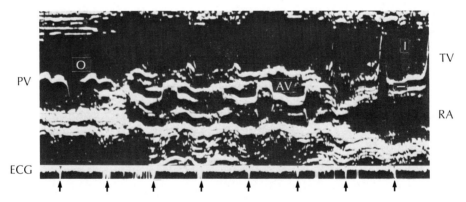

Fig. 3-27. Right ventricular scan in patient with enlarged right heart. Ultrasonic beam is moved from pulmonary to aortic valve *(AV)* and thence to tricuspid valve *(TV)*. Space in front of tricuspid valve represents inflow area of right ventricle *(I)*, whereas echo-free zone in front of aortic valve is right ventricular outflow area. Space in front of pulmonary valve *(PV)* denotes upper portion of right ventricular outflow *(O)* immediately beneath pulmonary valve. RA, right atrium; ECG, electrocardiogram. The QRS complexes are indicated by arrows.

front of the pulmonic valve cusp image. The pulmonic artery is shown only as a space behind the cusp. The wide echo pattern that originates behind the posterior wall of the pulmonary artery is a complex space that separates the vessel from the left atrium. Anatomically, this space is also just to the left of the aortic root (this can be shown by aortic-pulmonic sweeping) and contains the left main coronary artery as well as fat and

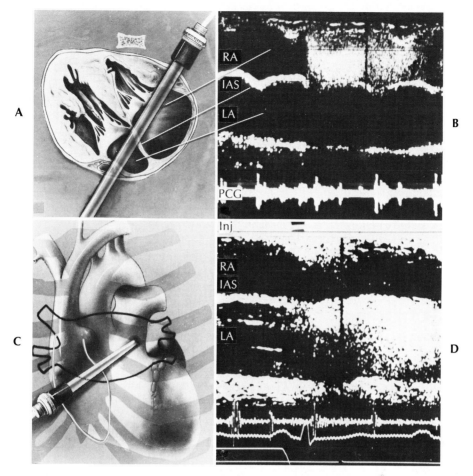

Fig. 3-28. Ultrasonic anatomy during atrial septal recording. **A** and **C,** Anatomic structures encountered by ultrasonic beam, which is placed in right parasternal position in angulation required to detect atrial septum. **B,** Right atrial contrast injection, showing filling of space in front of atrial septum. **D,** Left atrial contrast injection fills space behind septum. RA, right atrium; IAS, interatrial septum; LA, left atrium; PCG, phonocardiogram; Inj, injection signal.

connective tissue that are ordinarily found around the heart. The left coronary artery is only rarely recognized in recordings obtained from this space (the atriopulmonic sulcus). After passing through the atriopulmonic sulcus, the beam enters the left atrium and exits through the left atrial posterior wall into the mediastinum. In infants and occasionally in adults with right heart enlargement, the ultrasonic beam may pass through both walls of the pulmonary root directly without first traversing the right ventricular outflow.

The transducer may be placed to the right of the sternum when the heart is sufficiently enlarged or displaced to create a window on the right (Fig. 3-28). This beam position is seldom used routinely, but in a special case may provide information about the atrial cavities and tricuspid valve. To show the atrial cavities the beam is placed one interspace below the level of the mitral valve and directed upward and medially. Careful beam angulation demonstrates the atrial septum as a relatively thin echo pattern that shows rhythmic motions similar to those of the aortic root at a depth of 4 to 6 cm in adults. The anterior right atrial wall is the first structure demonstrated with the right atrial cavity beneath it. The atrial septum forms the posterior margin of the right atrium and divides it from the left atrium lying behind the septum. The beam leaves the heart through the left atrial posterior wall and enters the mediastinum. Fat is often located between the right atrial and chest walls and may produce a sonolucent space, which is a normal finding in this location.

A subxiphoid technique has been developed and is useful when emphysema pushes the diaphragm inferiorly, carrying the heart with it (Fig. 3-29). The usual cardiac window is obliterated or so compromised that routine precordial examination is not rewarding. The

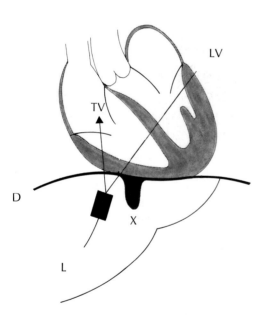

Fig. 3-29. Subxiphoid echocardiogram. Anatomic sketch shows cross section of heart in relation to xiphoid process (X), diaphragm (D), and liver (L). Structures most amenable to study from a subxiphoid position are tricuspid valve (TV) and left ventricular cavity (LV). This technique is most useful when usual precordial window approach provides inadequate information. In some cases, a transducer position to the left of the xiphoid process produces similar information.

transducer is placed just to the right of midline next to the xiphoid process, and the beam is directed upward toward the base of the neck or angled toward the left shoulder. Beam direction toward the neck records the tricuspid valve and may provide some useful information concerning the right ventricular cavity and aorta. Theoretically, the pulmonary valve can be detected. Direction of the beam to the left identifies the interventricular septum and left ventricular cavity. Experienced workers have had difficulty obtaining mitral valve echoes and demonstrating the left atrium. Elevation of the patient's head by 20 to 30 degrees relaxes the abdominal muscles and facilitates transducer placement. The records produced are similar in content to those obtained from a left precordial position, though structures are more deeply placed and echoes originating from the abdomen (usually liver) are imaged as a wide band of echoes before the heart walls. Be willing to try various low transducer locations and to modify precordial techniques in an attempt to define intracardiac structures.

Information that differs from that obtained by precordial transducer placement may be recorded from a suprasternal or supraclavicular position (Fig. 3-30). The beam is directed downward toward the heart using ordinary transducers or those with a right angle handle designed especially for this purpose. The greatest difficulty, especially with standard transducers, is in angling the beam sufficiently under the chest wall and not toward the patient's back. A pillow under the back to produce extension of the head and neck is useful, as is turning the patient's head.

The sound path from which most useful information is derived passes successively through the arch of the aorta, the right pulmonary artery, and the left atrial cavity. These structures are identified by their expected wall thicknesses, motion, and position. The aortic arch is typically about 25 mm wide, whereas the right pulmonary artery is somewhat smaller (about 20 mm) and the left atrial cavity is considerably deeper (around 50 to 55 mm). On some occasions the innominate vein is imaged as a narrow band lying in front of the aorta. A typical record therefore shows these spaces lying adjacent to each other with shallow pulsatile movement of the arterial structures. These studies are most useful to obtain the size of the aortic arch and of the right pulmonary artery. They also are another means by which left atrial size can be measured or an abnormal mass in the left atrial cavity demonstrated. A variant of the suprasternal view has been shown to have some utility in examining the aortic prosthesis. Landmarks for beam direction are lacking, and the examiner looks for the typical angular trace of the moving portion of the valve (ball or poppet), which lies at the expected depth of the aortic valve or at about 12 to 14 cm from the transducer. This beam position is ideally suited to this purpose, since the sound path is directed down the lumen of the ascending aorta and is nearly perpendicular to poppet motion, thereby demonstrating its range of motion. Though conceptually attractive, use has been limited because of difficulty in obtaining recordings.

RECORDING PHILOSOPHY

The philosophy of individual echocardiographers influences the successful operation of a cardiac ultrasound laboratory as much as skill in transducer and instrument manipulation. Leading echocardiographers have been characterized by their determination, flexibility, and intensity in pursuit of excellence. Compromises, shortcuts, undue haste and indifference are milestones to mediocrity. The candidate who feels that excellence can be compromised should not enter this challenging field but should seek a less demanding activity.

The first and most important concept in excellence is a complete echocardiographic examination. This should routinely include recording of all four heart valves, the diameter of the left ventricle, and evaluation of potential echo-free spaces adjacent to the anterior and posterior heart walls. These should be recorded so that solid structures are well differentiated from cardiac cavities with complete cycle recording of the mitral valve, including the maximal diastolic excursion as determined by altering beam position during recording. A sweep of as much of the left ventricular cavity as possible and extending into the aortic root should be obtained in every patient. When congenital heart disease is present, mitral to tricuspid and aortic to pulmonic scans are also necessary. Valve motion should be recorded at a speed that clearly demonstrates the motion complexes (50 to 150 mm/sec), whereas scans that relate structures or evaluate cavity configurations are better represented at slower paper speeds (10 to 25 mm/sec).

The ECG and PCG (if desired) should be of sufficient amplitude for easy observation and placed so that they do not conflict with the echo pattern. Sufficient length of recording should be used to assure accurate depiction of all portions of a structure as well as enough cardiac cycles (10 to 20 as a minimum) for evaluation of beat-to-beat changes in function. More than one transducer

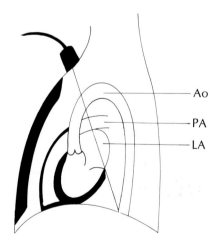

Fig. 3-30. Suprasternal technique. Structures encountered in this transducer position are shown. Since main pulmonary artery lies to left of midline, beam usually detects right branch of pulmonary artery (PA). This technique provides the opportunity to demonstrate different portions of heart and great vessels than does usual precordial position. Ao, aorta; LA, left atrium.

position should be used, where possible, to provide assurance that maximal valve motion is recorded.

The sequence in which structures are recorded usually follows the intracardiac routes that begin with the mitral valve and are extended in a maplike fashion to other structures. When convenient, this is a good routine but can be altered if difficulties are encountered. Certainly, the unexpected location of the transducer over a target out of sequence should prompt the examiner to record the target, since it may be difficult to find it again.

The record must contain sufficient information to answer the clinical question as well as to demonstrate any associated changes in chamber size. Recording from nonstandard positions (for example, suprasternal, subxiphoid, right of sternum) should be added when information from these sites will clarify the clinical conditions more fully. The echocardiographer must use knowledge of cardiac anatomy and the nature of disease processes to fulfill the role as an *examiner* of the heart rather than an individual carrying out a routinized test.

Some patients are notoriously easy to examine and produce recordings that are exemplary with minimal effort (Fig. 3-31). These are usually slender, young individuals whose heart is vertically placed beneath the chest wall and offers easily attained perpendicular relationships of structures to the examining beam. Cardiac enlargement also tends to make examination easy, but the obese, elderly patient may be difficult to examine. This difficulty most likely arises from a combination of factors. The thick chest wall probably produces more reverberation artifacts than does that of thin subjects, and obesity elevates the diaphragm so that the axis of the heart is changed from an easy vertical to a difficult, near-horizontal position. The perpendicular relationship that makes structure detection easy is lost, and it may not

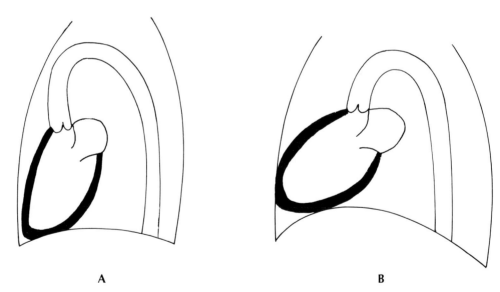

A   B

Fig. 3-31. Heart orientation and ultrasound recording. Position and angle of left heart are shown in lateral projection in relationship to anterior chest wall and diaphragm. Vertical heart **(A)** is usually found in slender young individuals and allows easy and more complete recording of cardiac structures. Horizontal heart **(B)** is usually found in obese and older patients and makes echocardiography difficult. Access to heart may be limited to apex, and optimal perpendicular beam-structure relationships are difficult to obtain, especially in region of base of heart.

be possible to obtain meaningful information from all cardiac structures.

Patient factors that influence the echocardiogram may require acceptance of less than ideal studies and consequently lowered diagnostic confidence. It may not be possible to circumvent the previously described effects that degrade record quality; however some diagnostic information can usually be extracted from records that are less than ideal and may not represent "textbook" examples of disease processes. Records of this type are common in all laboratories, though they may not be on public display.

INTERVENTIONS

Interventions are used during echocardiography to alter heart rate and ventricular volume mainly in patients with cardiomyopathies with obstruction (IHSS, HOCM) and occasionally in mitral valve prolapse. The commonly used interventions are hand grip, the Valsalva maneuver, and inhalation of amyl nitrite.

The ultrasonic recording may be difficult with the Valsalva maneuver, since the position of the heart usually shifts, and the target (the mitral valve) may slip out of the beam. Recording should be continuous beginning before the Valsalva maneuver and include 20 or 30 seconds after the pressure is released and normal breathing takes place.

Before use of amyl nitrite it is important to describe the effects the patient will experience from the drug. These may be summarized as follows:

1. The odor is mildly unpleasant, somewhat like ether or paint thinner. Some patients describe it as "old gym shoes," "sneakers," or "a pungent locker room odor."
2. There is always a strong blush of the skin and a sensation of warmth.
3. The heart pounds rapidly.
4. There may be light-headedness and dizziness.
5. There is a tendency for very deep breathing and coughing from the medication. The patient should be alerted to this effect so that every effort can be made to control this reaction, which makes recording of the echocardiogram difficult and occasionally impossible.
6. The reaction to the medication is transient and lasts only 30 to 60 seconds with no permanent effects.
7. Repeat administration of the drug may be necessary if the desired response of tachycardia is not obtained. Lack of response may occasionally be due to outdated medication. You may have to try a new batch.

Recording should begin with a normal baseline trace and be continuous through the periods of inhalation, tachycardia, and recovery, since the changes induced are transient and difficult to capture ultrasonically.

More vigorous interventions like the Valsalva maneuver and amyl nitrite inhalation may be hazardous in certain patients, since a decrease in cardiac output may result. Its use is avoided in patients with advanced arterial disease, particularly if the blood supply to the brain is affected. It should not be used in advanced diseases that are already associated with lower cardiac output nor in the presence of severe myocardial ischemia, since a myocardial infarct might be precipitated.

Respirations produce minor changes in cardiac function. The negative pressures within the chest required to draw air into the lungs also draw in increased quantities of blood into the right heart during inspiration. During expiration the inflow is reduced, and this may be dramatic during forced expiration. Since inspiration requires a downward motion of the diaphragm, the heart moves downward with inspiration and returns upward on expiration. In some patients this movement may be sufficiently large to remove a target structure from the beam. If transducer position is not changed, the target will return. It may be necessary in these cases to make recordings during suspended respiration (usually expiration produces the best record) or to learn to track the target by rhythmically angling the beam downward on inspiration and upward on expiration.

Recordings made with a stationary beam

during respiration may show apparent changes in the size of the heart cavities or in the pattern of valve motion. The respiratory displacement of the heart changes the region being examined by the beam so that a different cavity diameter may enter the beam or a different portion of a heart valve recorded. The effects of respiration on cardiac function are therefore best determined with the respiratory scanning procedure described above.

COMMENTS

1. Ask for help from a more experienced echocardiographer if you cannot find all targets or if you find nothing after ten minutes of trying.
2. Do not let examinations extend beyond 30 minutes as a general rule.
3. Use beam sweeps when recording the mitral valve to observe the entire length of the leaflet and its relationship to the aorta. Also obtain mitral-to-tricuspid sweeps in congenital heart disease.
4. Learn to track targets that move with respiration by angling the beam as the patient breathes.
5. Use all of the cardiac window and feel free to move the transducer around if you cannot find the target.
6. Remember to use nonstandard beam positions (suprasternal, right of sternum, subxiphoid) to provide additional information to characterize a disease process.
7. Do not divert your gaze from the monitor oscilloscope during searching to look at the transducer, especially when a target is difficult to find. The information you are seeking may appear on the monitor when you look away.
8. Be willing to repeat any portions of an examination that were missed or unsatisfactory. You will be surprised how much easier a second examination can be.
9. Do not forget to put the transducer on the right side of the chest if an adequate examination cannot be performed from the left side. This may be necessary in dextrocardia or in conditions where the heart is displaced to the right.

BIBLIOGRAPHY

Gramiak, R., and Waag, R. C., editors: Cardiac ultrasound, St. Louis, 1975, The C. V. Mosby Co.

Chang, S.: M-mode echocardiographic techniques and pattern recognition, Philadelphia, 1976, Lea & Febiger.

Feigenbaum, H.: Echocardiography, Philadelphia, 1976, Lea & Febiger.

PART TWO
Clinical echocardiography

This section has been organized to correspond to the usual detection techniques employed in echocardiography. Valves are the major examination landmarks that are individually examined and require a comprehensive grasp of all disease conditions that affect them and alter structure and motion. These landmarks provide the bulk of echocardiographic diagnostic information. Chambers are studied by their relationship to valves in most instances. Changes in their size, wall motion, and thickness are related usually to the severity of valvular disease. In coronary artery disease the left ventricle is altered without primary valve abnormality. This entity, as well as pericardial effusion, is therefore described separately.

Congenital heart lesions that are identified by abnormalities in the motion of a single heart valve are included in the sections dealing primarily with valvular disease. Complex malformations use information derived from valve studies but require recognition of changes in chamber and great vessel size and position as well as alterations in continuity between chambers and great vessels. The absence of structures also plays an important diagnostic role. For this reason, complex anomalies are also discussed in a separate section.

4 Mitral valve

STRUCTURES IN BEAM

The following are structures in the beam, beginning at the chest wall.

1. Anterior wall of right ventricle.
2. Right ventricular cavity
3. Interventricular septum
4. Left ventricular outflow tract
5. Anterior leaflet
6. Left atrial cavity
7. Left atrial posterior wall
8. When the posterior leaflet is detected, it lies behind the anterior cusp, and the beam generally exits through the posterior left ventricular wall.

NORMAL TRACING

A normal mitral valve executes a series of repeated motions that are produced by blood flow through the open valve in diastole. A normal mitral valve trace is shown in Fig. 4-1, in which the anterior leaflet waveform is labeled by a convention that identifies the major hemodynamic events that result in valve motion. Typically, two peaks are produced in diastole and, in keeping with electrocardiographic and functional considerations, the description begins with atrial systole. Contraction of the atrial walls raises the pressure in the left atrium and accelerates blood flow into the left ventricle (atrial kick) at the end of diastole. The mitral valve moves in response to this flow, and the anterior leaflet moves anteriorly and forms a peak (A) when this motion reaches its maximum and then begins to decline as the flow de-

creases. Ventricular contraction starts raising the pressure in the left ventricle at point B (coincident with the R wave), driving the mitral valve even further posteriorly, often at a greater speed so that the trace may show a slight angulation at B. Posterior motion continues to point C when the leaflets of the mitral valve come together in closure. Point C is normally the deepest position of the anterior leaflet in the heart. The period between B and C represents isovolumic contraction. The first heart sound follows point C very closely. Ventricular ejection takes place between C and D while the mitral valve moves anteriorly in a steady fashion. This movement is the result of anterior and downward displacement of the mitral ring or annulus produced by ventricular contraction. The end of ejection and the beginning of diastole occur at point D, which comes at about the end of the T wave of the ECG and when the second heart sound is produced. The mitral valve begins its opening motion (D-E) when left ventricular pressure drops below that in the left atrium and left atrial blood begins its motion into the left ventricle and reaches its fully opened position at E. D-E represents the phase of rapid diastolic filling of the left ventricle. Lowering of pressure in the left atrium results in the mitral valve returning to a position of semiclosure, F. Alternatively, vortex (eddy) formation in the left ventricle produced by blood entering it in diastole may be responsible for this motion. The slope of the line between points

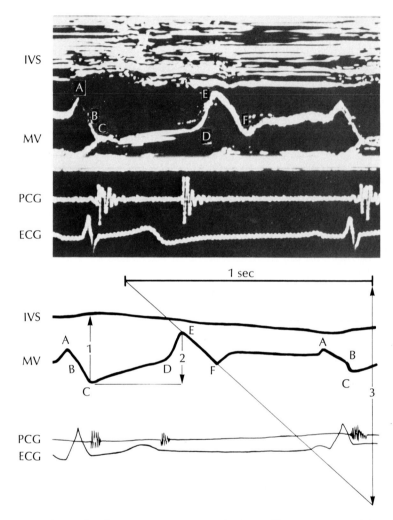

Fig. 4-1. Normal mitral valve. Measurement technique. The upper panel is a normal mitral valve study in which, by convention, anterior structures are represented at the top of the record and posterior structures at the bottom. Echoes are shown as white areas, absence of echoes as black. Physiologic events are labeled by letters. Note that the posterior leaflet moves in a direction opposite to the anterior leaflet at the time of atrial systole and during the movement toward closure (C). The line drawing in the lower panel illustrates the measurement technique used to obtain important diameters and rates of movement. A, Peak produced by atrial systole. B, Beginning of ventricular systole. C, Point of mitral valve closure. D, Beginning opening movement of mitral valve. E, Fully opened position of valve. F, End of rapid ventricular filling phase. 1, Width of left ventricular outflow tract. 2, Amplitude of mitral valve motion. 3, Distance mitral valve would have moved in 1 sec, or rate of EF slope in millimeters per second. IVS, interventricular septum; MV, mitral valve; PCG, phonocardiogram; ECG, electrocardiogram.

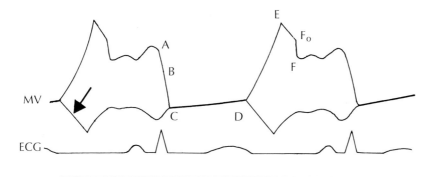

Fig. 4-2. Normal mitral valve. The schematic representation of the normal mitral valve (MV) echocardiogram shows an intermediate point F$_0$ between E and F as well as a small anterior deflection before atrial systole (between F and A). Their origin is not known, but they represent normal findings. The posterior leaflet *(arrow)* moves in a direction opposite to the anterior cusp and has a smaller amplitude of motion. ECG, electrocardiogram.

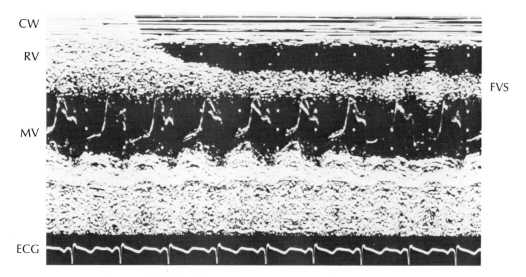

Fig. 4-3. Mitral valve recording technique. The mitral valve (MV) recording on the left demonstrates the presence of intense reverberatory clutter over the right ventricle. The ventricular septal margins are not delineated. The use of anterior suppression can result in the creation of a false ventricular septum (FVS) separating the right ventricle (RV) from the mitral valve. CW, chest wall; ECG, electrocardiogram.

E and F expresses the rate at which left atrial emptying takes place. This is an important echocardiographic landmark since it is slowed or flattened by conditions that result in slow left atrial emptying. Occasionally an intermediate point (F_0) may be identified between E and F (Fig. 4-2). A quiescent pe-

riod follows F, during which the mitral valve does not exhibit any significant motion and the atrial and ventricular musculature are not active (diastasis). However, flow from the left atrium into the ventricle continues since the pulmonary veins are emptying into the left atrium without interruption. There may be a

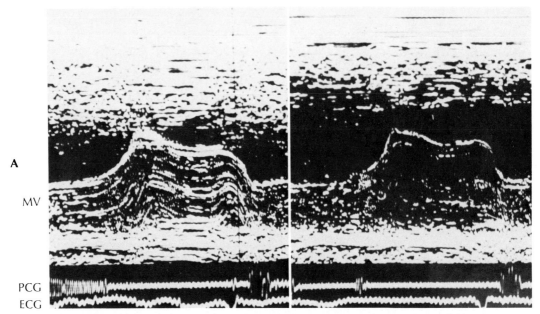

Fig. 4-4. A, Left atrial myxoma. Linear and punctate echoes arising in the myxoma are present behind the mitral valve (MV) in systole and diastole. **B** was recorded at insufficient instrument insensitivity, so that echoes from the tumor mass itself are poorly seen. At operation, a myxoma was found attached to the atrial wall near the left atrial appendage by a short thick stalk. PCG, phonocardiogram; ECG, electrocardiogram. (From Gramiak, R., Nanda, N. C., Gross, C. M.: Semin. Roentgenol. **10:**291-297, 1975.)

Table 5. Useful mitral valve echocardiographic measurements

EF slope	Normal	80-150 mm/sec
	Possible mild rheumatic involvement	35-55 mm/sec
	Mitral stenosis range	Under 35 mm/sec
AC slope	Normal	125-250 mm/sec
	Mitral stenosis	350-600 mm/sec
CE amplitude	Normal valve mobility	20-30 mm
	Restricted valve mobility	16-19 mm
	Poor valve mobility	15 mm or less
Left atrial dimension (end-systole)	Normal	10-20 (mm/M² body surface area)
	Mild enlargement	20-30 (mm/M² body surface area)
	Moderate enlargement	30-40 (mm/M² body surface area)
	Severe enlargement	Over 40 (mm/M² body surface area)
LVO dimension	Normal	20-35 mm (caged ball prosthesis acceptable for valve replacement)
	Narrow	Under 20 mm (low profile prosthesis recommended for valve replacement)

short shallow bulge in the anterior leaflet recording at this time, which has no current diagnostic significance and whose etiology is probably related to flow. Atrial systole follows and reinitiates the cyclic pattern described. The normal posterior leaflet produces a smaller but inverted pattern in diastole. In systole, it blends into the echo of the anterior leaflet and cannot be distinguished from it in normal patients.

The normal leaflet is a thin structure and produces one or possibly two echoes. More than two echoes usually indicates some thickening of the valve. The wide beams used in echocardiography may image portions of the mitral apparatus or the aortic root over the mitral valve image, producing extra lines that may be confusing but should not be interpreted as evidence of an abnormality.

TECHNICAL CONSIDERATIONS

The general scheme described earlier for the setting of sensitivity controls usually yields satisfactory recording of the mitral valve. We usually employ little or no TVG and suppress anterior echoes to the point that a fine speckle is present in the right ventricular cavity. This assures detection of any structurally important echoes present in the right ventricle and decreases the size of the step that is produced when suppression ends. Large suppression steps may mask the right side of the ventricular septum or produce an artifactual recording of clutter echoes as a straight line that can be mistaken for the right side of the septum (Fig. 4-3). Delays longer than ideal, especially with a high degree of suppression, may destroy all or part of the ventricular septal image.

It is desirable to record or at least observe the mitral valve at gains higher than those used for optimal imaging. This may reveal the presence of structures of low reflectance (vegetations, tumors), which could pass unnoticed at gains too low for their detection (Fig. 4-4).

Measurement of various amplitudes and rates of motion of the mitral valve trace can be made; their utility is discussed in subsequent sections dealing with individual disease processes. Ideally, ultrasonic records should be measured from the leading edge of one echo source to the leading edge of another so that pulse length, which broadens ultrasonic images, does not enter into the measurements. When this is not possible and a measurement must be made from the trailing edge of one echo to the leading edge of another, an error of 1 to 2 mm may be introduced, depending on pulse length.

Amplitude or dimensions are measured using a caliper to determine the spacing between the two echoes. This is translated into a numerical value by placing the caliper on the scale markers, which are produced on the record at 1-cm intervals. Millimeters must be estimated because these are not indicated directly, and small inaccuracies of measurement may occur as a result.

The rate at which a structure moves can be determined by drawing a line that extends the excursion of that part of the record so that the amplitude over a projected excursion of 1 second can be obtained. The amplitude of this extended motion is the rate of motion and is usually expressed in millimeters per second.

The EF slope of the mitral valve is commonly measured and can present some difficulty if the trace does not extend from point E to F in a straight line. The meaning of slower slopes, which are occasionally seen during this interval (EF_0 slope), is not entirely clear. We have preferred to connect points E and F and consider only the rate of the straight line.

Useful mitral valve echocardiographic measurements are presented in Table 5.

ECHOCARDIOGRAPHIC FINDINGS IN DISEASE
Mitral stenosis

Anatomic and functional changes. Mitral stenosis is a common manifestation of rheumatic heart disease. Rheumatic heart disease is a delayed sequel of rheumatic fever and commonly results in mitral and aortic valve disease. It begins in childhood with rheumatic fever (fever, joint pains, myocarditis), which occurs weeks or months following streptococcal infection in the upper respiratory tract. After an interval of years, damage to heart valves becomes evident. The valve tissues develop an inflammatory reaction, which involves the leaflets and chordae and results in scarring and, later, calcification. The scarring thickens the valve leaflets and joins them together at their commissures so that stenosis results. The thickening, scarring, and calcification may deform

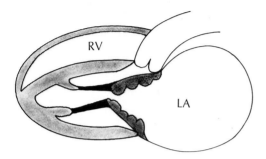

Fig. 4-5. Mitral stenosis. Both leaflets of the mitral valve as well as the chordae are thickened and fused, resulting in a narrow funnel-shaped mitral orifice. The obstructed orifice has produced enlargement of the left atrium (LA) and later of the right ventricle (RV) and pulmonary artery.

the leaflets (Figs. 4-5 and 4-6) and the chordae, or the leaflets, may remain relatively thin and pliable. The size of the orifice determines the degree of obstruction to left atrial emptying.

Left atrial pressure increases, a pressure gradient develops between the left atrium and the left ventricle in diastole, and the left atrium enlarges. The elevated pressure is transmitted backward through the pulmonary vascular bed and raises pressure in the small vessels (wedge pressure), the main pulmonary artery, and in the right ventricle. Forward flow through the stenotic valve is usually decreased so that the left ventricle and aorta remain normal or become small.

Surgical relief of the obstruction usually reverses the changes produced by mitral stenosis, unless severe damage has occurred to the small vessels of the lung as the result of chronic, severe pulmonary hypertension.

Clinical summary

• Typical middiastolic rumbling murmur increases in intensity during atrial contraction (presystolic accentuation) when the patient is in sinus rhythm. The presystolic accentuation of the diastolic murmur usually disappears when atrial fibrillation develops.

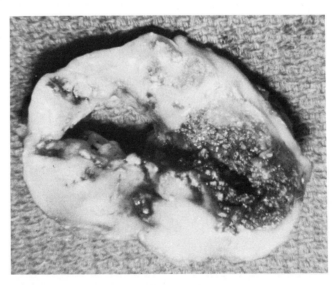

Fig. 4-6. Surgically resected mitral valve. Heavy calcification (dense white areas) and ulceration are present in both leaflets, which are fused at the commissures.

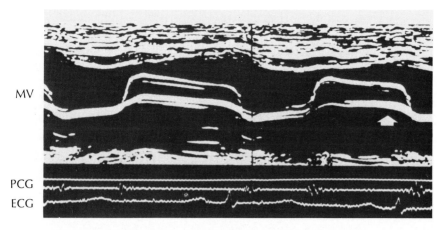

Fig. 4-7. Typical mitral stenosis. The diastolic slope is reduced, and leaflets are minimally thickened. A wave is absent, and posterior leaflet *(arrow)* moves parallel to anterior leaflet in diastole. MV, mitral valve; PCG, phonocardiogram; ECG, electrocardiogram. (From Gross, C. M., Gramiak, R., and Nanda, N. C.: Chest **68:**570, 1975. By permission of the American Heart Assn., Inc.)

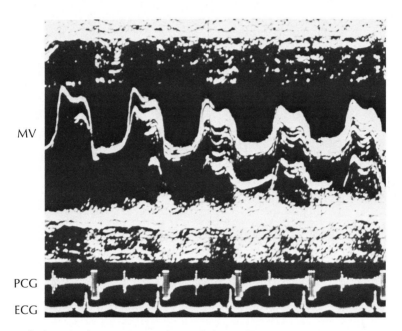

Fig. 4-8. Calcific mitral stenosis simulating left atrial myxoma. At the beginning of the trace, EF slopes are rapid, shallow A waves are present, and the posterior cusp is in an anterior position in diastole. As the beam is angled deeper into the left ventricular cavity, the leaflet image thickens from calcification. The echoes behind the mitral valve (MV) simulate a myxoma on a short stalk. However, the left atrial cavity was free of mass echoes and cardiac catheterization and angiocardiography documented the presence of mild mitral stenosis. There was no indication of a left atrial myxoma. The origin of the masslike echoes is difficult to ascertain but could be related to calcification in the posterior papillary muscle or chordae. PCG, phonocardiogram; ECG, electrocardiogram.

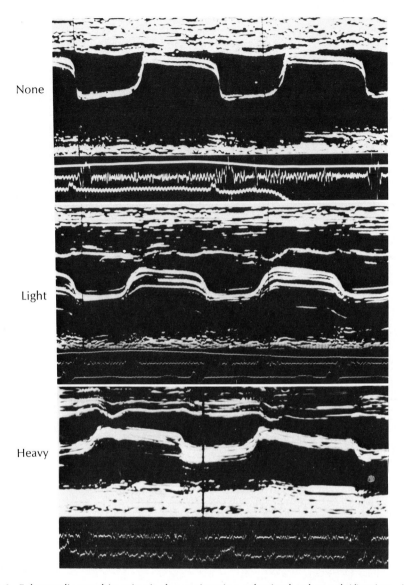

None

Light

Heavy

Fig. 4-9. Echocardiographic criteria for estimation of mitral valve calcification. In the absence of leaflet calcification *(upper panel),* valve echoes are thin and are regularly comprised of one or two linear signals. In the presence of light calcification *(middle panel)* multiple and discrete echo sources can be elicited in the valve. Heavy calcification *(lower panel)* results in thick conglomerate patterns without separation of individual linear components. (From Nanda, N. C., and others: Circulation **51:**263, 1975. By permission of the American Heart Assn., Inc.)

- A history of rheumatic fever may or may not be elicited. The pulmonic component of the second heart sound is loud when pulmonary hypertension is present.
- Distended pulmonary vasculature and enlarged left atrium on chest roentgenograms. (Barium swallow provides more definitive evidence of left atrial enlargement.)
- Fluoroscopy may reveal calcification of valve cusps or of the left atrial wall.

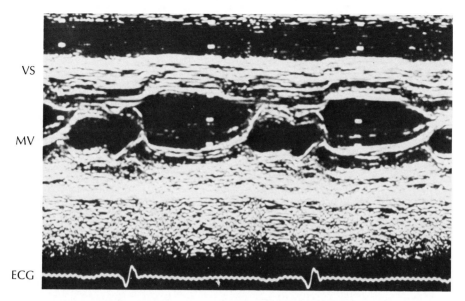

Fig. 4-10. Mitral valve in pulmonary hypertension. The mitral valve (MV) shows prolonged diastolic apposition with the ventricular septum (VS) indicative of a narrow, compressed left ventricular outflow tract. The mitral valve also shows pansystolic sagging. The ventricular septum is thickened. The patient had severe primary pulmonary hypertension. ECG, electrocardiogram.

• Cardiac catheterization shows pressure gradient across the mitral valve in diastole. The calculated valve area is decreased.

• Angiocardiography shows a large left atrium, evidence of obstruction at the mitral valve, and a jet through the stenotic orifice. Clots in the left atrium may be imaged as filling defects. (These are very rarely found on echocardiography.)

Echo features in mitral stenosis (Fig. 4-7)

• Diminished EF slope. Significant mitral stenosis has slopes under 35 mm/sec related to slow left atrial emptying produced by stenosis. Very mild stenosis may present with slopes between 35 and 55 mm/sec.

• Absence of A waves. This could be secondary to atrial fibrillation or to high pressure behind the valve, which masks the effects of atrial contraction when normal sinus rhythm is present. A waves may be clearly visible in mild cases (Fig. 4-8).

• Abnormal motion of the posterior cusp. The commissural fusion pulls the posterior cusp forward in diastole with the anterior cusp. A second echo source is imaged parallel and behind the anterior cusp. This occurs in approximately 90% of patients.

• The valve image may be thin (one or two lines) when uncalcified and composed of multiple, relatively thin parallel lines (light scattered calcification) or very thick from large deposits of heavy calcium (Fig. 4-9).

• The amplitude of motion is decreased when the subvalvular apparatus is involved in the rheumatic process or when the cusp is heavily calcified.

• The left atrium is enlarged (best shown in aortic valve recording position).

• An increase in the rate of mitral valve closure (AC slope) is also commonly observed. A slow AC slope in the absence of mitral valve calcification is strong evidence against mitral stenosis.

Comments

• Record with varied sensitivity to be sure an obstructing mass is not present that produces a valve motion that mimics mitral stenosis.

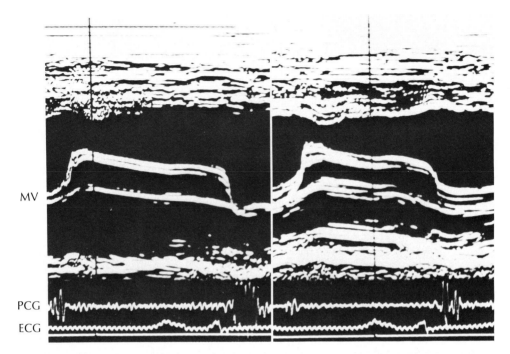

Fig. 4-11. Effect of instrument sensitivity in the evaluation of mitral valve calcification. Low instrument sensitivity *(left)* can mask the presence of calcification. Failure to record the left side of the ventricular septum indicates insufficient sensitivity during the examination. Optimal recording *(right)* shows light calcification in the valve leaflets. The left side of the ventricular septum is clearly shown. MV, mitral valve; PCG, phonocardiogram; ECG, electrocardiogram. (From Nanda, N. C., and others: Circulation **51:**263, 1975. By permission of the American Heart Assn., Inc.)

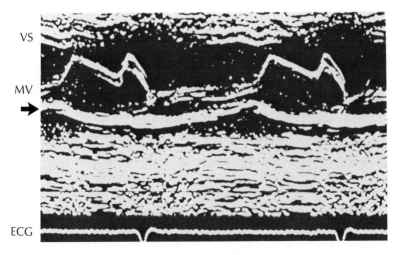

Fig. 4-12. Mitral annular calcification. This isolated image of the mitral valve (MV) shows a complete trace of the anterior leaflet and fragmentary late diastolic echoes from the posterior leaflet. The thick echo pattern *(arrow)* behind the mitral complex corresponds to calcification of the mitral annulus identified fluoroscopically. VS, ventricular septum; ECG, electrocardiogram.

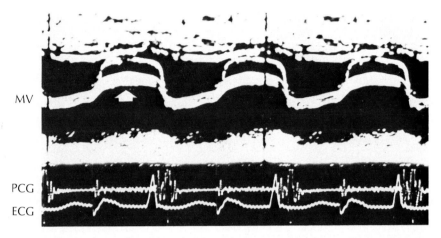

Fig. 4-13. Mitral stenosis. Heavily calcified posterior cusp *(arrow)* with a relatively mobile, noncalcified anterior leaflet, confirmed at surgery. *MV*, mitral valve; *PCG*, phonocardiogram; *ECG*, electrocardiogram. (From Nanda, N. C., and others: Circulation **51**:263, 1975. By permission of the American Heart Assn., Inc.)

- Slow EF slopes alone do not indicate mitral stenosis. They may be the result of a hypertrophied left ventricle that is so stiff it does not permit rapid left atrial emptying. They may also result from pulmonary hypertension (Fig. 4-10). However, distinction from mitral stenosis is not difficult because the valve images are not thickened and the posterior leaflet moves normally. Patients with systemic lupus erythematosis may have nonbacterial outgrowths on the mitral valve, and the echocardiographic picture may resemble mitral stenosis.
- A waves disappear with atrial fibrillation without mitral stenosis.
- Angle the beam so that a recording of the posterior cusp is obtained.
- Evaluate cusp calcification with a sensitivity setting that images the left side of the ventricular septum but does not record small background echoes in the outflow tract of the left ventricle (Fig. 4-11).
- The mitral annulus calcifies in older patients as the result of aging. It is usually not an indicator of heart disease, though mitral regurgitation may occur when the calcification is sufficiently severe and interferes with the mitral ring contraction during systole. The leaflets are not usually involved. Fluoroscopy and chest roentgenography reveal a typical reversed C- or U-shaped distribution of calcium in the position of the mitral annulus. The echocardiogram shows a normal anterior leaflet with a dense band of echoes behind it (Fig. 4-12). The posterior leaflet may be obscured, and shadowing behind the calcium may block recording of the posterior heart wall.
- Heavy posterior leaflet calcification may be deeply placed behind the anterior leaflet echo, mimicking annular calcification or a calcified left atrial clot (Fig. 4-13).
- The extent and severity of fibrosis and calcification in rheumatic mitral valve disease go hand in hand. A heavily calcified valve also has extensive fibrosis, and a noncalcified leaflet is usually associated with mild fibrosis. In vitro experiments in our laboratory, using resected mitral valves, suggest that the thick and multilayered echoes present in rheumatic valves originate from calcification rather than from fibrosis, which is a much weaker reflector of ultrasound (Fig. 4-14).
- Vary the beam position to be sure that maximal EF slopes and amplitudes of motion are recorded. This also allows selection of the narrowest portion of the LVO for measurement (obtained during beam sweeping from the mitral to the aortic valve (Fig. 4-15).

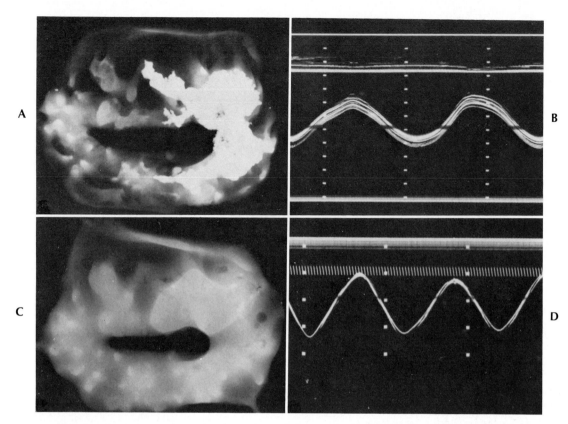

Fig. 4-14. In vitro studies of mitral valve calcification. A surgically excised mitral valve was placed in a waterbath and moved during recording. When the ultrasonic beam was passed through the calcified portion (**A,** radiograph of specimen), the echo pattern showed multiple, thick lines (**B**). After the valve was decalcified in an acid solution, the specimen radiograph (**C**) shows complete clearance of calcification. The ultrasonic recording was repeated with identical gain settings (**D**) and revealed a dramatic reduction in the thickness of the echo complex despite a ×2 magnification of the lower image as compared to the upper (**B**). This study indicates that calcification is the major factor responsible for the production of thick echo complexes in valves involved in rheumatic heart disease. Fibrotic valves, on the other hand, show only small differences when compared to normal valves. (Unpublished data courtesy of Ronald Schwartz, fourth-year student, University of Rochester School of Medicine, 1977.)

• A narrow left ventricular outflow tract observed in some patients with mitral stenosis is related to the small size of the left ventricular cavity. This results from reduced filling of the left ventricle produced by orifice obstruction and "compression" resulting from enlargement of the right ventricle, which is secondary to pulmonary hypertension (Fig. 4-16).

• Be sure that a good left atrial recording, including its posterior wall, is obtained.

• The entire cycle of tricuspid valve motion may be present from right ventricular enlargement.

• Study the pulmonic valve closely for evidence of pulmonary hypertension.

• The aortic valve may be abnormal because it is commonly involved in the rheumatic process.

• Mitral valve flutter seen in aortic regurgitation (see subsequent discussion on p. 144) is usually masked in the presence of mitral stenosis. However, subtle fluttering of the left side of the septum may be observed.

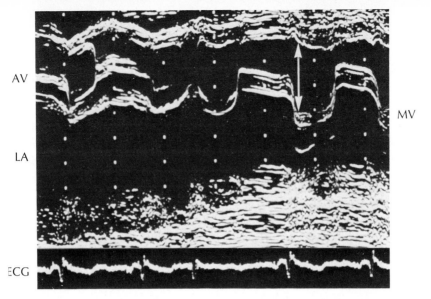

Fig. 4-15. Beam scanning from the mitral to the aortic valve for determination of the left ventricular outflow dimension in mitral stenosis. The space between the left side of the ventricular septum and the mitral valve immediately below the aortic valve represents the outflow area, and its dimension is measured at the beginning of systole *(arrow)*. AV, aortic valve; MV, mitral valve; LA, left atrium; ECG, electrocardiogram.

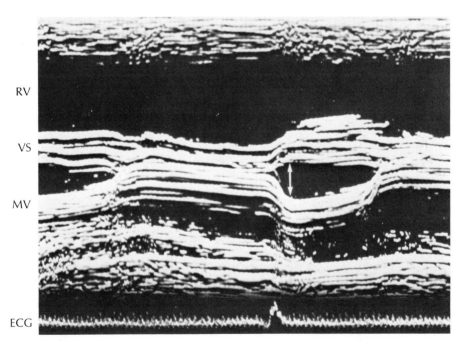

Fig. 4-16. Narrow left ventricular outflow tract in mitral stenosis. A heavily calcified mitral valve (MV) is shown in the presence of a very narrow left ventricular outflow tract *(arrow)*, which measured 15 mm. In diastole the calcified mitral valve is in contact with the ventricular septum (VS), which is displaced posteriorly by an enlarged right ventricle (RV) secondary to pulmonary hypertension. A confusing picture such as this can be resolved by beam scanning, which reveals the expected relationships of the mitral valve and septum to the aortic root and to the left ventricular cavity toward the apex. ECG, electrocardiogram.

• Though clots may occur in the left atrium with mitral stenosis, they are rarely recognized on the echocardiogram.

Rheumatic mitral regurgitation

Anatomic and functional changes. Thickening and calcification at the edges of the leaflets distort and roughen the surface so that a water-tight closure cannot be achieved. In extreme cases the leaflets may be so immobile that the orifice is fixed in a semiopen position. Varying degrees of mitral stenosis are almost always present with rheumatic mitral regurgitation. Occasionally, the leaflets are relatively pliable and uncalcified, but the chordae may be heavily involved and shortened so that closure is incomplete. The left atrium enlarges, usually more than in pure mitral stenosis and especially when the mitral regurgitation is chronic and severe. A giant left atrium may be produced. The left ventricle enlarges and shows hyperdynamic motion of the walls secondary to an increase in the volume the ventricle must pump forward through the aorta and repeatedly backward into the left atrium through the leaking valve. The pulmonary and right heart changes described in mitral stenosis are present.

Clinical summary
• A typical pansystolic murmur is present.
• The apex beat may be forceful and sustained from left ventricular enlargement.
• At cardiac catheterization the pressure in the left atrium is elevated with a prominent systolic component (V wave), produced by the regurgitant jet. If stenosis is minimal, a gradient may not be present or the findings of mitral regurgitation are superimposed on those of mitral stenosis.
• Chest roentgenograms are similar to mitral stenosis, but the left atrium and left ventricle are usually larger. Fluoroscopy may reveal an expansile pulsation of the left atrium during systole from the regurgitation.
• Left ventricular angiograms show contrast backflow into the left atrium through the incompetent valve. The degree of opacification of the left atrium is used as a semiquantitative estimate of severity, usually expressed in grades of 1 to 4+.

Echocardiographic features
• The findings are generally indistinguishable from mitral stenosis, and the presence of mitral regurgitation generally is not recognized.
• Severe leaflet calcification is frequently present.
• With primary involvement of the chor-

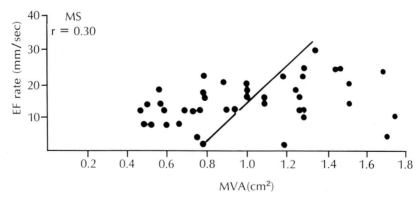

Fig. 4-17. Relationship of the mitral EF slope to the severity of mitral stenosis. This study demonstrates a poor correlation (r = 0.30) between the mitral EF slope and the mitral valve area determined by cardiac catheterization This is in contrast to earlier work that suggested that the EF slope could be used to assess the severity of mitral stenosis. MS, mitral stenosis; MVA, mitral valve area determined by Gorlin's formula. (Nanda, N. C., and others: unpublished data, 1971.)

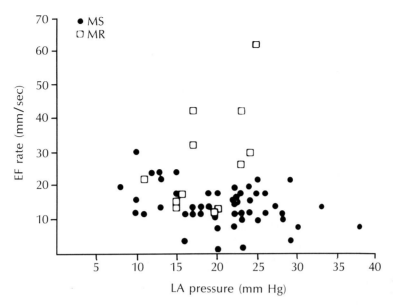

Fig. 4-18. Mitral EF slopes in rheumatic mitral regurgitation. The mitral EF slope is not useful in distinguishing mitral stenosis from mitral regurgitation in patients with rheumatic mitral valve involvement. A majority of patients with predominant mitral regurgitation have slow EF slopes (35 mm/sec or less), which are usually considered indicative of significant mitral stenosis. MS, pure or predominant mitral stenosis; MR, predominant mitral regurgitation (rheumatic); LA pressure, mean left atrial pressure. (Nanda, N. C., and others: unpublished data, 1971.)

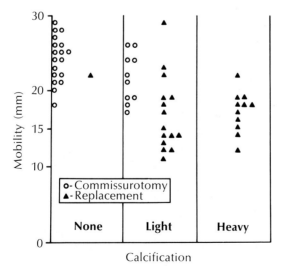

Fig. 4-19. Ultrasound evaluation of the status of the mitral valve and the type of surgery. (From Nanda, N. C., and others: Circulation **51**:263, 1975. By permission of the American Heart Assn., Inc.)

dae the leaflet echo may be only slightly abnormal. These cases may represent early descriptions of mitral regurgitation, which featured a rapid early diastolic slope with flattening later in diastole. This is a relatively uncommon finding and is generally not observed in most patients with rheumatic mitral regurgitation.

• Increase in gain may reveal the presence of systolic intracavitary echoes in the left atrial cavity recorded behind the aortic root and probably represent turbulence created by the regurgitant jet. In the normal patient, these echoes are seen in presystole and are most likely related to turbulence following atrial contraction.

• The left atrium may be very large and may exhibit systolic expansion of its posterior wall.

• The ventricular septum may show increased amplitude of motion caused by left ventricular volume overload. The left ventricular cavity is enlarged.

Comments

• The separation of pure rheumatic mitral stenosis from predominant mitral regurgitation is practically impossible by echocardiography.

• Be sure to record all the secondary features described under mitral stenosis.

• An enlarged, hyperdynamic left ventricle and an unusually large left atrium may be clues to the presence of mitral regurgitation.

Role of echocardiography

• M-mode echocardiography does not determine the severity of mitral stenosis, nor does it recognize the presence of associated mitral regurgitation (Figs. 4-17 and 4-18).

• Echocardiography is a sensitive detector of calcification and can semiquantitate its severity. This may be more accurate than radiologic techniques. The surgeon may be aided in the selection of the surgical procedure preoperatively, since uncalcified valves are amenable to commissurotomy and heavily calcified valves require valve replacement. Lightly calcified valves require inspection at the time of surgery to determine the distribution of calcific deposits. When the commissures are uninvolved, commissurotomy may be performed without the complication of mitral regurgitation.

• Echocardiography is also useful in evaluating the mobility of the mitral valve, and this is of considerable importance in preoperative planning. Mobility in the normal range (20 mm or more) is generally correlated with the feasibility of commissurotomy, whereas poor mobility (15 mm or less) is a reliable predictor for valve replacement, even in the absence of heavy cusp calcification (Fig. 4-19). The conventional method for measuring the mobility of the mitral valve (CE amplitude) generally overestimates it because it also includes ring motion. Although DE amplitude should more closely approximate true cusp movement, evaluation of mitral valve mobility for surgical planning has not been improved by separate consideration of DE rather than total CE amplitude.

• The width of the left ventricular outflow tract (measured from the left side of the septum to the C point of the mitral valve) is useful in the selection of the type of valve prosthesis to be inserted. Narrow left ventricular outflow tracts (under 20 mm) require the insertion of a low profile (disc type) prosthesis. A large prosthesis (ball valve type) may produce serious obstruction to left ventricular outflow and should be used only in patients with left ventricular outflow dimensions over 20 mm (Fig. 4-20).

• Commissurotomy returns the mitral valve trace toward normal with an increase in the EF slopes and reappearance of A waves. Patients can be followed postoperatively for changes in the echo, which indicate restenosis.

• A normal mitral valve trace virtually excludes rheumatic involvement of the mitral valve.

• Pulmonary hypertension may be recognized from pulmonary valve recording and followed during the postoperative period for evaluation of the relief of pressure on the pulmonary vascular bed.

• Lesions that clinically may resemble mitral stenosis, such as atrial myxomas and aor-

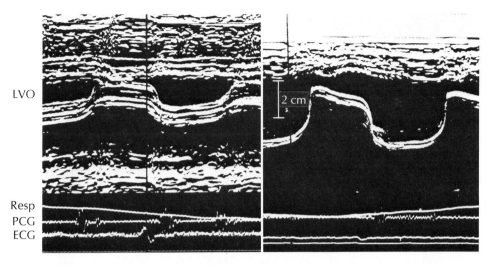

LVO

2 cm

Resp
PCG
ECG

Fig. 4-20. Mitral valve echocardiograms from two patients with mitral stenosis. The echogram on the left demonstrates a narrow left ventricular outflow tract (LVO); the one on the right illustrates a normal-sized outflow tract. Resp, respirations; PCG, phonocardiogram; ECG, electrocardiogram. (From Nanda, N. C., and others: Circulation **48:**1208, 1973. By permission of the American Heart Assn., Inc.)

tic regurgitation, can be detected. Myxomas result in echoes that fill in the space behind the anterior leaflet, and aortic regurgitation produces rapid diastolic fluttering of the mitral valve leaflets (see subsequent discussions for more complete description).

• Nonrheumatic lesions, such as mitral valve prolapse, IHSS, and chordae rupture, which present with clinical evidence of mitral regurgitation, can be detected and their nonrheumatic nature recognized (see subsequent discussions).

• Coexistent involvement of the aortic valve by the rheumatic process may produce calcification of the valve leaflets and alterations of the motion pattern of the aortic leaflets.

Mitral valve prolapse

Anatomic changes and clinical summary. This is an exceedingly common condition found frequently in young persons. There are usually no clinical symptoms, though some patients may experience atypical chest pains and skipped heart beats. The arrhythmias may be severe and rarely result in sudden death. The involved mitral leaflet becomes elongated, redundant, and thickened by myxomatous degeneration (Fig. 4-21). The chordae become elongated and allow one or both leaflets to buckle into the left atrium in mid or late systole. The buckling produces a sharp heart sound (click), usually in mid to late systole, and it may be followed by a murmur of mitral regurgitation (also known as midsystolic click-murmur syndrome, Barlow's syndrome, billowing mitral valve, floppy mitral valve). Occasionally more than one click may be audible. The click and murmur may change with patient position and may be loudest when the patient is lying on his left side, sitting, or standing. It may be useful to examine these patients echocardiographically in a position that produces the loudest clicks and murmurs, but usually the typical echocardiographic findings can be recognized by examining the patients flat or on their left sides.

The degenerated valve tissue is susceptible to infection so that antibiotic prophylaxis is often recommended in these patients during dental work or surgical procedures to prevent bacterial endocarditis.

Interventions, such as the Valsalva ma-

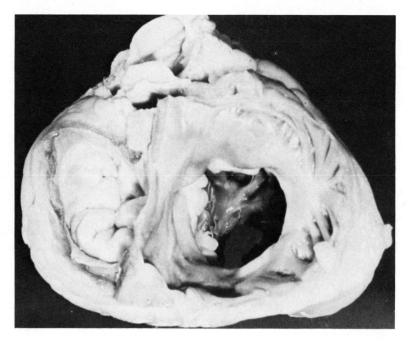

Fig. 4-21. Myxomatous degeneration of the mitral valve. Cross section of the heart at the level of the mitral valve demonstrating multiple, redundant folds from myxomatous degeneration *(left)*. The tricuspid valve is partially seen on the right and exhibits similar changes. This autopsy specimen was obtained from a 62-year-old woman with Turner's syndrome, who showed myxomatous changes of all four cardiac valves. (Courtesy Dr. DeLa Torre, Jacksonville, Fla.)

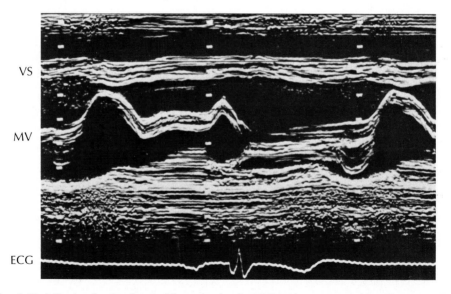

Fig. 4-22. Mitral valve prolapse. The mitral valve (MV) shows a steplike posterior displacement in mid to late systole typical of valve prolapse. VS, ventricular septum; ECG, electrocardiogram.

neuver and amyl nitrite inhalation, reduce left ventricular volume and move the onset of valve prolapse (including the click and murmur) earlier into systole. However, this is of limited value in diagnosis because the condition can generally be recognized without these interventions.

The ECG may show evidence of arrhythmias and changes in the configurations of the T waves. Chest roentgenograms may reveal a narrowing of the distance between the sternum and the spine but generally are normal. Cardiac catheterization and left ventricular angiography are performed only in symptomatic patients and show buckling of the mitral valve in systole as well as evidence of mitral regurgitation. Most often, one or more scallops of the posterior mitral valve leaflet may be observed to prolapse, though the anterior leaflet may be involved alone or in combination with the posterior leaflet.

Echocardiographic features

• A mid to late systolic steplike posterior displacement of 2 mm or more below the mitral closure point is considered diagnostic of prolapse (Figs. 4-22 and 4-23). Equally reliable is a gradual downhill movement of the mitral valve throughout systole (Fig. 4-24). Pansystolic sagging or hammocking of the mitral valve of at least 3 mm below the closure position is also highly suggestive of prolapse in the absence of left ventricular dilatation. Lesser degrees of posterior displacement, flattening, or sagging are suggestive but not diagnostic of prolapse and require assessment of clinical and phonocardiographic findings for a more definitive diagnosis. Another suggestive but not diagnostic finding is the presence of localized systolic bulges of the mitral valve (Fig. 4-25) similar to those seen in IHSS (see below). In a given patient the above findings may occur singly or in combination.

• The EF slope and valve motion amplitude may be increased (over 35 mm) because of increased blood flow when significant mitral regurgitation is present, or it may reflect the increased excursion of a large, redundant leaflet. This is a nonspecific finding and not diagnostically useful.

• The valve trace usually shows a multilayered character in systole and diastole. The individual echo sources probably originate in the thickened and degenerated leaflet or

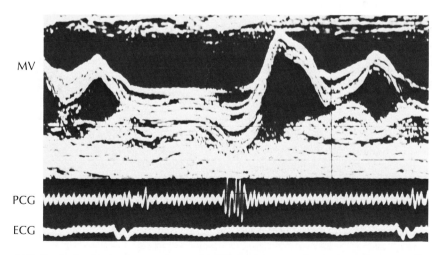

Fig. 4-23. Typical mitral valve prolapse. Multilayering as well as a large late systolic posterior displacement are observed. The patient was a 19-year-old woman who presented with ventricular premature contractions. She was lost to clinical follow-up and died suddenly two years after this echocardiogram was taken. MV, mitral valve; PCG, phonocardiogram; ECG, electrocardiogram.

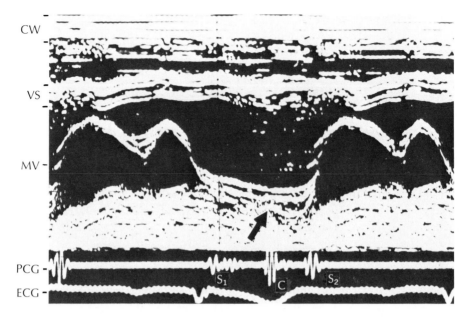

Fig. 4-24. Mitral valve prolapse. Mitral valve echocardiogram demonstrates generalized sagging of the systolic segment as well as the typical mid-to-late posterior systolic displacement *(arrow)*, coinciding with the nonejection click (C), S_1, first heart sound; CW, chest wall; VS, ventricular septum; MV, mitral valve; PCG, phonocardiogram; ECG, electrocardiogram; S_2, second heart sound. (From Winters, S. J., Schreiner, B., Griggs, R., and Nanda, N. C.: Ann. Intern. Med. **85:**19-22, 1976.)

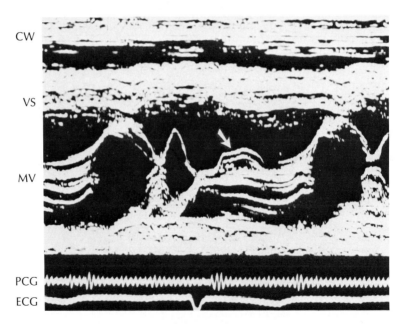

Fig. 4-25. Systolic anterior motion (SAM) in mitral valve prolapse. A midsystolic hump *(arrow)* is observed in addition to a late systolic prolapse pattern. The SAM probably originates in a portion of leaflets away from the prolapsing segment, and beam width is responsible for imaging both patterns simultaneously. CW, chest wall; VS, ventricular septum; MV, mitral valve; PCG, phonocardiogram; ECG, electrocardiogram.

from folds and wrinkles related to the elongation and redundancy. This is also a nonspecific finding.

Comments

• Always scan the entire length of the leaflet to find the abnormal process. Some portions of the valve may move normally, and the findings change depending on the portion of the leaflet studied. Thus, during patient examination, a careful and systematic search of all portions of the mitral valve for evidence of prolapse and a beat-by-beat perusal of the record obtained are mandatory before prolapse can be excluded with a reasonable degree of certainty. In general, recordings obtained at the body or tip of the mitral leaflets tend to show the prolapse findings at their best. Also, it is more rewarding to examine the mitral valve when the beam is exiting through the left atrial wall rather than through the left ventricular posterior wall.

• Always try to record posterior leaflet motion because this leaflet is most often involved. However, anterior leaflet motion is usually abnormal, even though an angiocardiogram may indicate isolated posterior cusp prolapse.

. • Be sure to place the transducer low on the chest wall. High transducer placement with angulation toward the feet to find the mitral valve has been shown to be a source of false-positives in normal subjects.

• Be careful in making the diagnosis of thickening secondary to vegetations because the myxomatous degeneration usually present in prolapse can cause confusion.

• Do differentiate the multilinear pattern of myxomatous degeneration from calcification by the fact that the multiple lines found in mitral valve prolapse are usually very thin, tend to show fine undulations in their motion pattern with a tendency toward a lacy appearance, and are not associated with changes in the motion pattern of the leaflet characteristic of rheumatic involvement.

• Be careful in patients with chordae rupture (see p. 112) because mitral valve prolapse and chordae rupture may have echocardiographic features in common, both produced by systolic instability of the mitral valve. The systolic posterior motion in chordae rupture is usually more severe, the leaflets may invert completely so that they are echoed in the left atrial cavity, and there may be coarse diastolic fluttering secondary to loss of stability in diastole.

• Do not attempt to separate the anterior leaflet from the posterior during systole. The multiple lines commonly present make this difficult.

• Do not try to diagnose the presence of mitral regurgitation by an apparent separation of leaflet echoes during prolapse. Valves that close tightly may appear to separate when a portion of the leaflet other than the apposed edges is recorded.

• Mitral valve prolapse may not be diagnosed if the cardiac window is small.

• A large prolapse is unlikely to be missed by echocardiography.

• In the normal patient a premature ventricular contraction may produce a pattern of mitral valve prolapse, especially pansystolic sagging (Fig. 4-26).

• Occasionally we have seen mitral valve prolapse in a setting of narrow left ventricular outflow tract and a small left ventricular cavity in the absence of a thickened septum.

• Systolic anterior motion usually occurs near the base of the leaflet. Some investigators believe that anterior billowing is an artifact produced by recording the posterior wall of aortic root with the mitral valve since the valve leaflets tend to bulge behind the aorta. However, we have seen anterior motion patterns that differ markedly from superimposed aortic root traces, and we believe that this process is secondary to the prolapse pattern occurring at the tip of the leaflet. Systolic humps on the mitral valve may be observed in apparently normal patients in the standing position and do not necessarily hint at the possibility of prolapse. The etiology is not known.

• Reduplication of C points may be observed in some patients and may cause confusion when assessing the presence or the degree of posterior displacement of the mitral valve. In the presence of multiple sys-

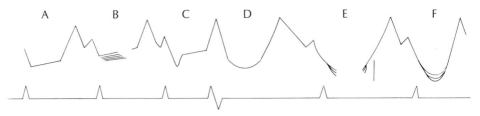

Fig. 4-26. Schematic representation of variety of findings encountered in evaluation of mitral valve prolapse. A normal systolic segment is shown in A. B is a nonspecific finding resulting from late systolic dropouts and, alone, is not diagnostic of prolapse. The early systolic plunge in C is of unknown etiology but is not part of the diagnostic pattern of prolapse. In D there is holosystolic sagging following a premature ventricular contraction. This is a normal finding. E is a prolapse pattern similar to F but is complicated by mid systolic dropouts. The vertical bar shown in early diastole is a nonspecific finding, though it appears more frequently in prolapse than in normal patients.

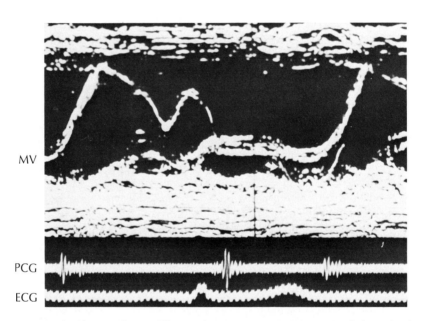

Fig. 4-27. Mitral valve prolapse. The prolapsing segment *(arrow)* of the mitral valve (MV) may be subtle and poorly seen, especially when it merges with the image of the posterior left atrial wall. Some increase in the amount of time-varied gain has been useful to detect these subtle changes. PCG, phonocardiogram; ECG, electrocardiogram.

tolic echoes, strategically occurring dropouts may give the false appearance of prolapse on cursory examination (Fig. 4-26).

• Vertical linear echoes behind the anterior cusp of the mitral valve in early diastole occur in patients with valve prolapse as well as in some normal patients. Their significance is not known (Fig. 4-26).

• In patients with mitral valve prolapse, systolic dropouts may mask the abnormality because the prolapsing segments may move out of the beam. A clue to the diagnosis may be found in the form of multiple short brushlike lines moving posteriorly at the beginning of systole. Varying the beam position usually displays the full extent of the prolapsing systolic segment. The prolapsing segment may be incompletely recorded and appear faint (Fig. 4-27). Posterior displacement of the mitral valve limited to early systole does not have any diagnostic significance (Fig. 4-26).

• Mitral regurgitation may also be produced by a congenitally cleft leaflet occurring as an isolated abnormality. The echocardiographic features resemble valve prolapse (multilayered echoes, systolic sagging).

• The left atrial posterior wall may be mistaken for the posterior mitral leaflet because of their proximity in some records. Its normal posterior movement in systole may be misdiagnosed as valve prolapse (Fig. 4-28).

• Tricuspid valve prolapse may be associated and should be looked for in all cases.

• Mitral valve prolapse is commonly seen in association with musculoskeletal deformities such as scoliosis and pectus excavatum, neuromuscular disorders (myotonia and oth-

er dystrophies), Marfan's syndrome, and in apparently healthy young women. Since mitral valve prolapse may be familial, other members of the family of a patient presenting with prolapse may need to be studied echocardiographically.

• A prolapsing mitral valve that is involved in old or recent infective endocarditis may show a rapid systolic fluttering of the leaflets during prolapse (Fig. 4-29). The flutter is probably produced during mitral regurgitation by turbulent blood flow across structurally abnormal but flexible leaflets. Detection of flutter may serve as a valuable clue to the presence of infective endocarditis, since other diagnostic features of vegetation may be absent and multilayered echoes due to myxoid degeneration may be difficult to distinguish from bacterial vegetations. Serial echocardiograms in patients with mitral valve prolapse have shown the develop-

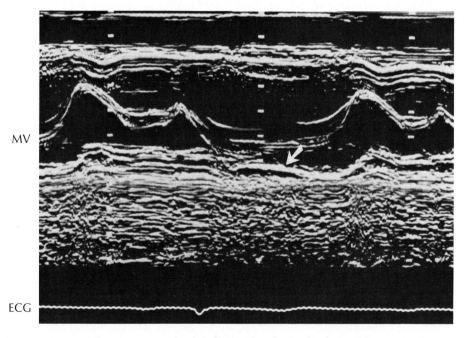

MV

ECG

Fig. 4-28. Potential error source in the diagnosis of mitral valve prolapse. An inexperienced echocardiographer may mistake the posterior wall of the left atrium *(arrow)* for the systolic segment of the mitral valve (MV) when the AC segment is poorly recorded and lies near the posterior wall. Dropouts in the systolic portion of the trace may heighten the illusion that continuity between the AC segment and the left atrial wall is present. Though this patient was referred for the question of mitral valve prolapse, other portions of the record were entirely normal. ECG, electrocardiogram.

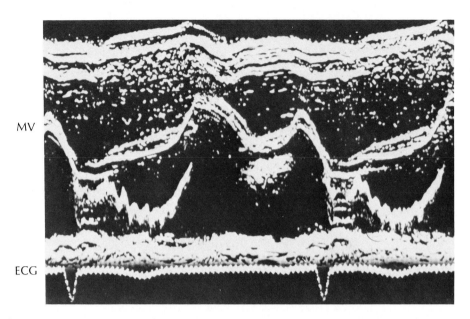

Fig. 4-29. Systolic flutter of the mitral valve in a patient with mitral valve prolapse and healed bacterial endocarditis. The flutter is seen predominantly on the prolapsing mitral segment. MV, mitral valve; ECG, electrocardiogram.

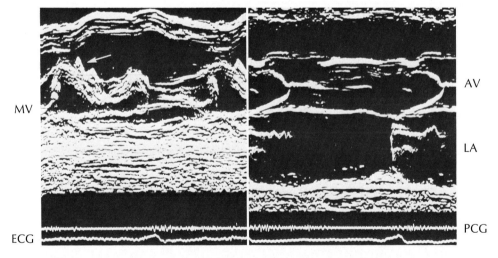

Fig. 4-30. Chordae rupture secondary to endocarditis. The mitral valve (MV) is thickened by fuzzy, multilinear echoes arising from bacterial vegetations. In diastole the anterior leaflet exhibits erratic fluttering motions *(arrow)*. In systole the mitral valve trace sags posteriorly, and mitral leaflets can also be seen fluttering in the left atrial cavity (LA) behind the aortic valve (AV). The diastolic instability and systolic inversion of leaflets into the left atrium are the results of chordae rupture secondary to the bacterial endocarditis. PCG, phonocardiogram; ECG, electrocardiogram. (From Nanda, N. C.: Mod. Concepts Cardiovasc. Dis. **45:**135, 1976. By permission of the American Heart Assn., Inc.)

ment of systolic flutter following bacterial endocarditis. Be sure to expand this valve image and use a high recording speed to show high frequency fluttering during prolapse when infective endocarditis is suspected in a patient with mitral valve prolapse, Systolic fluttering is uncommon in chordae rupture without previous bacterial infection.

• Hammocklike sagging of the mitral systolic segment may be unreliable evidence of prolapse in the presence of a large left ventricle. Impairment of left ventricular performance associated with ventricular dilatation diminishes the apex-to-base shortening of the ventricle in systole and results in reduction

or abolition of the downward and anterior motion of the mitral annulus so that the mitral tracing appears flat or sags during systole.

Role of echocardiography

• Echocardiography is useful in confirming or excluding the presence of mitral valve prolapse in clinically suspected cases.

• Diagnostic accuracy is not well documented since left ventricular angiograms are performed infrequently. However, experienced echocardiographers believe that around 85% of clinically typical cases are detected. Careful transducer placement reduces the incidence of overdiagnosis where-

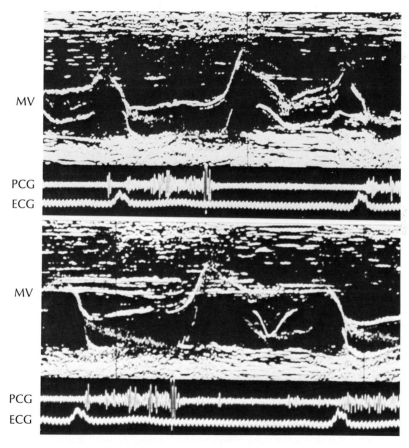

Fig. 4-31. Chordae rupture. The systolic segment shows three different types of patterns: relatively normal systolic motion, a deep vertical systolic plunge, and a gradual downhill fluttering motion *(lower panel)*. During diastole the posterior valve cusp executes an erratic movement pattern that is at times parallel to the anterior leaflet. MV, mitral valve; PCG, phonocardiogram; ECG, electrocardiogram.

as false-negatives are avoided by diligent and extensive scanning of the mitral leaflets in individuals suspected of having this entity.

• When mitral valve prolapse is identified, antibiotic prophylaxis may be used during dental and surgical procedures to prevent bacterial endocarditis.

• Systolic fluttering of the prolapsing segment of the mitral valve suggests the presence of healed or active endocarditis.

Rupture of the mitral apparatus

Anatomic and functional changes

• The two papillary muscles divide into two to five individual heads from which the chordae tendineae arise. The cords are numerous and branch near the mitral leaflets, where they insert mainly into the edges of the cusps, though some insert further toward the body of the leaflet. The cords from each papillary muscle are distributed into

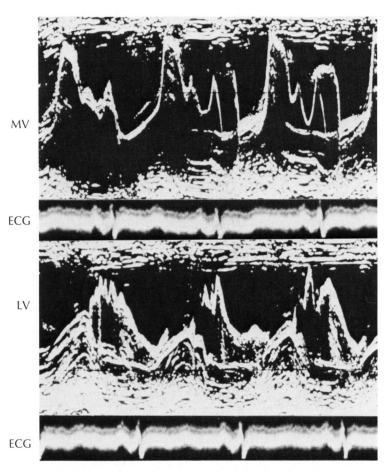

Fig. 4-32. Mitral valve and left ventricular cavity recordings in a patient with healed subacute bacterial endocarditis and chordae rupture. With the beam directed at the mitral valve (MV) an abnormal linear echo source appears in the left ventricular outflow tract in late diastole and moves rapidly posteriorly in early systole until it blends with the image of the closed mitral valve. In the left ventricular cavity (LV) a widely flapping echo source is seen mostly in diastole. These abnormal echoes probably are derived from flail ruptured chordae that move into the body of the left ventricle in diastole and reach the limit of their excursion in the left ventricular outflow tract in systole. Series of isolated mitral valve recordings appeared entirely normal and an extended search was required to elicit the true findings. ECG, electrocardiogram.

both mitral leaflets so that some overlap occurs and rupture of one papillary muscle may affect the support of both leaflets.

• Rupture of a papillary muscle occurs as the result of myocardial infarction and death of the papillary muscle or from chest injury. This results in massive, life-threatening mitral regurgitation, which may require surgical intervention on an emergency basis so that echocardiography may not be performed. Chordae rupture, on the other hand, is a less emergent condition whose severity varies, depending on the number of cords ruptured and their distribution. In the more severe cases the cords to both leaflets rupture, allowing both leaflets to invert into the left atrial cavity. Mitral regurgitation is severe in these cases. The cause may be endocarditis or trauma, but many patients with chordae rupture present with no previous history of heart disease.

• Chordae rupture is a relatively uncommon condition but occurs with sufficient frequency to be encountered occasionally in every echocardiographic laboratory.

Clinical summary. The patient history may reveal chest trauma or infective endocarditis. A murmur of mitral regurgitation is always present. The patient is generally seen in the acute phase when the left atrium has not had time to dilate, and it may appear to be normal fluoroscopically. Cardiac catheterization and left ventricular angiography demonstrate mitral regurgitation and an erratic movement of the mitral leaflet may be seen.

Echocardiographic features

• The findings can be normal (if unsupported segments are not imaged in the plane of the beam) or those of mitral valve prolapse.

• In diastole the unsupported leaflet may show a coarse, erratic movement that produces an irregular series of peaks along with fine fluttering (Fig. 4-30).

• In systole, dropouts are common, or the unsupported leaflet may be seen to plunge far posteriorly with the onset of systole, remain in a deep position, and then move anteriorly with the onset of diastole. An unsupported posterior leaflet appears to float be-

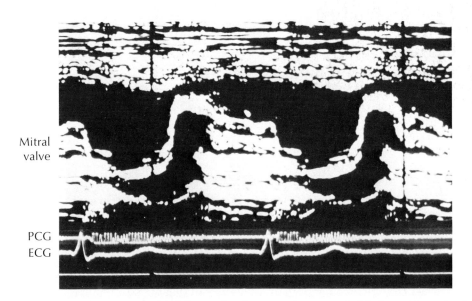

Mitral valve

PCG
ECG

Fig. 4-33. Chordae rupture. Multilayered echo complex seen behind anterior mitral leaflet in diastole is probably another indicator of poorly supported posterior leaflet, which is folded and probably upright within ultrasonic beam to produce multilayered echo pattern. Left atrial cavity contained no unusual echoes, and at surgery, chordae to posterior leaflet were ruptured. PCG, phonocardiogram; ECG, electrocardiogram.

hind the anterior leaflet and may parallel its motion in diastole (Fig. 4-31).

• Mitral valve leaflets may be observed as rapidly fluttering linear echoes in the left atrial cavity when systolic inversion occurs (Fig. 4-30).

• Systolic fluttering observed in the normal recording position or in cases with inversion of leaflets into the left atrium has occurred generally when bacterial endocarditis has involved the valve. Systolic flutter in the absence of endocarditis is observed in less than 15% of patients with chordae or papillary muscle rupture.

• When a sizable length of a cord is detached from the papillary muscle, it will be seen as an erratically moving echo source in the left ventricle, which is imaged along with the trace of the mitral leaflet (Fig. 4-32). Its motion pattern may change from beat to beat, and it may disappear abruptly as it leaves the examining beam. It may present as a vertical, linear echo in contact with the mitral valve in mid systole and should not be regarded as an artifact.

• Rarely, an unsupported posterior leaflet produces multiple echoes behind the anterior leaflet in a pattern that mimics an atrial myxoma (Fig. 4-33). This pattern is probably the result of echoing the posterior leaflet as it stands vertically in the beam with multiple folds or wrinkles representing the echo sources. The left atrium is free of echoes, thereby ruling out a left atrial tumor.

Comments

• Be sure to examine the left ventricular cavity, the entire mitral leaflet, and the left atrial cavity. Multiple scans in these areas may be helpful.

• Use a variety of beam positions to be cer-

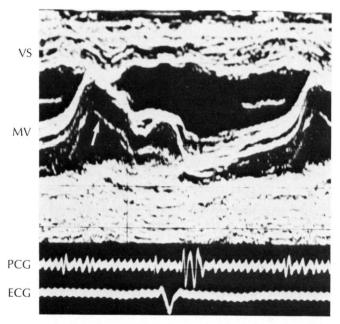

Fig. 4-34. Mitral "ghost" echoes. A relatively thin linear echo *(arrow)* parallels the motion of the anterior leaflet in a pattern that mimics a flail posterior leaflet. The posterior leaflet here and in other portions of the record shows normal motion, and the patient presented with no evidence of mitral regurgitation. This thin echo as well as the short horizontal line present in the left ventricular outflow tract may represent intracardiac reverberations. However, follow-up echocardiograms are planned for further evaluation. VS, ventricular septum; MV, mitral valve; PCG, phonocardiogram; ECG, electrocardiogram.

tain that adequate records of the systolic and diastolic motion of the mitral valve are obtained.

• Use a high recording speed and image expansion to ensure demonstration of fine flutter.

• Record all unusual patterns, even if they do not appear typical of chordae rupture or are poorly understood at the time of examination.

• High sensitivity may be useful since the unsupported leaflets are prone to unusual tilting that will decrease signal amplitude.

• "Ghost" echoes, which probably represent intracardiac reverberations, should not be mistaken for mitral valve prolapse or chordae rupture (Fig. 4-34).

• Surgical treatment usually consists of valve replacement. In mild cases, it may be possible to repair the valve (valvuloplasty), in which case, postoperative echocardiograms show diminution of the EF slopes, usually in the range of 50 mm/sec.

Role of echocardiography. The diagnosis is usually made clinically, and echocardiography supports the clinical diagnosis. Endocarditis may be demonstrated as the underlying cause, and it may be possible to show which leaflets are involved in the process.

Mitral valve vegetations

Anatomic and functional changes
• Vegetations are small masslike lesions that tend to involve heart valves that are structurally abnormal.

• These lesions are soft in the acute phase and may break, producing emboli.

• Destruction of valve tissue and chordae commonly occurs.

• Fungal vegetations are usually larger than are bacterial ones.

• Healing is associated with fibrosis, scarring, and calcification.

• Functionally, the lesions may commonly produce valve incompetence, rarely obstruction.

Clinical summary. Fever, changing heart murmur, signs of embolization, and positive blood cultures are diagnostic. Cardiac

catheterization and angiocardiography may be dangerous, since the catheter may dislodge a portion of the mass. Chest roentgenograms may provide findings related to the nature of the complications produced, for example, mitral regurgitation.

Echocardiographic features
• The mitral valve may appear normal.

• Shaggy, fuzzy echoes are present on the mitral valve, which retains a normal motion pattern. (Fig. 4-35).

• Mitral valve motion is altered when obstruction by a large vegetation (mitral stenosis pattern) or chordae rupture occurs.

Comments
• A normal mitral valve recording does not rule out vegetations, since only about 50% of those present at surgery or autopsy are detected by ultrasound. Those smaller than 2 mm are usually missed.

• Be sure to record both leaflets, including a complete scan of the mitral valve to prevent missing a lesion. For instance, only the basal portion of the mitral valve may appear abnormal.

• Active and healed vegetations may not be differentiated by echocardiography.

• Healed lesions containing calcium look much larger on the echocardiogram than their actual size.

• A large mitral vegetation may mimic a left atrial myxoma.

• Serial studies are useful to show progression of structural and functional changes.

• A vegetation may disappear on serial studies when a large portion of the mass breaks away and embolizes.

Role of echocardiography. Echocardiography may confirm the clinical diagnosis and localize the process to a specific valve. It also shows associated structural changes, especially progression over a period of time. Extension of the infection into contiguous structures such as a heart wall may be demonstrated. Rarely, the infectious nature of disease may be hidden, and the echocardiogram may be the first source of the true diagnosis, thereby avoiding a potentially hazardous catheterization. Echocardiographic detection of vegetations usually signifies fairly ad-

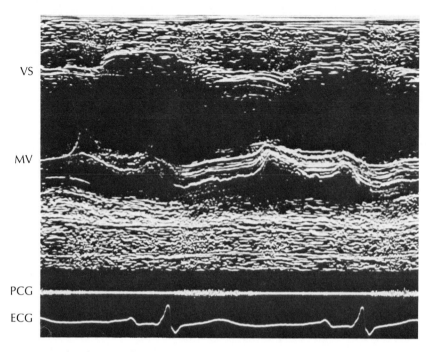

Fig. 4-35. Mitral valve involvement with bacterial endocarditis. The anterior leaflet image is thickened by a multilayered echo complex present in systole and diastole *(right)*. The mitral valve (MV) image on the left is unimpressive and emphasizes the importance of careful beam scanning along the entire length of the mitral valve in the diagnosis of this condition. VS, ventricular septum; PCG, phonocardiogram; ECG, electrocardiogram.

vanced disease so that surgical intervention may be required.

Idiopathic hypertrophic subaortic stenosis (IHSS)

Anatomic and functional changes. This condition is characterized by marked hypertrophy of the ventricular septum that is often localized, producing a bulge that encroaches on the outflow tract of the left ventricle, thus narrowing it. The entire septum may not be affected, and the posterior wall of the left ventricle is usually normal in thickness. Microscopic examination of the septum shows a bizarre arrangement of the muscle fibers characteristic of this condition. The ventricle is small, irregularly shaped, and hyperactive. Arrhythmias and sudden death may occur. Mitral valve function is altered, leading to systolic obstruction to left ventricular outflow and mitral regurgitation.

The mitral valve closes normally at the beginning of systole, and the anterior leaflet begins an anterior motion soon after closure that often reaches the ventricular septum. The leaflet remains in this anterior open position during about 50% of the ejection time, then returns to a closed position before diastolic reopening. This systolic anterior motion (SAM), along with outflow narrowing from septal hypertrophy, is responsible for the functional outflow tract obstruction characteristic of this disease. Mitral regurgitation occurs commonly. The aortic valve may move toward closure during the obstructive phase, or it may flutter coarsely from the turbulent flow produced. The carotid pulse usually shows a brisk upstroke and a notch in the waveform related to decreased flow during obstruction.

The cause of the abnormal mitral valve motion is poorly understood. It may be related

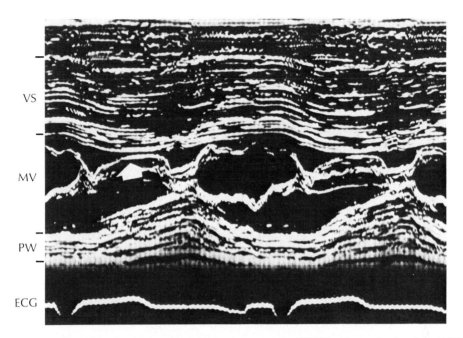

Fig. 4-36. Idiopathic hypertrophic subaortic stenosis (IHSS). The mitral valve (MV) shows an abnormal systolic anterior movement (SAM; *arrow*), which almost touches the left side of the ventricular septum (VS). The left ventricular outflow tract is narrowed, and the ventricular septum is markedly thickened as compared to the left ventricular posterior wall (PW). ECG, electrocardiogram. (From Nanda, N. C.: Mod. Concepts Cardiovasc. Dis. **45**:135, 1976. By permission of the American Heart Assn., Inc.)

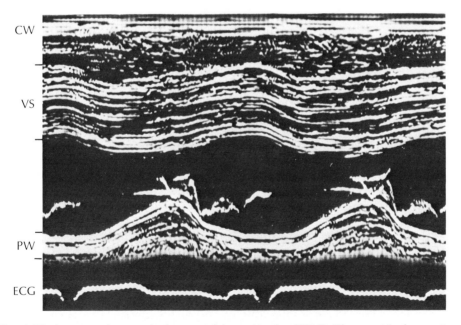

Fig. 4-37. Asymmetric ventricular septal hypertrophy (ASH). The ventricular septum (VS) in this patient with IHSS is thickened to more than twice the width of the left ventricular posterior wall (PW). ECG, electrocardiogram; CW, chest wall.

to the rapid flow, which sucks the mitral valve into the open position (Bernoulli effect) or to abnormal function of the papillary muscles.

Clinical summary. The clinical presentation may be typical or atypical. When typical, there are murmurs suggestive of outflow obstruction and mitral regurgitation. A fourth heart sound is present. The ECG may show evidence of conduction defects, left ventricular hypertrophy, or signs of myocardial ischemia or damage. The clinical findings may be atypical, and the patient may present with a nonejection click and a soft murmur suggestive of mitral valve prolapse, or the presence of anginal pains may simulate coronary artery disease.

Interventions such as the Valsalva maneuver or amyl nitrite inhalation increase the degree of obstruction and hence the intensity

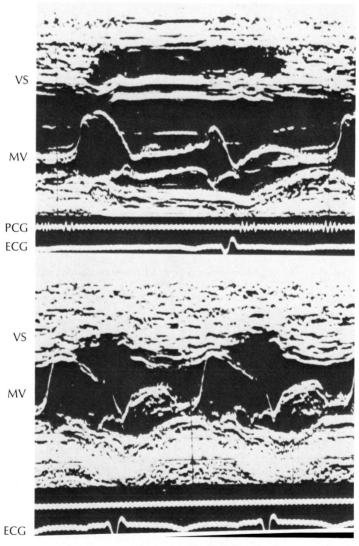

Fig. 4-38. Systolic abnormalities of the mitral valve (MV). A small, resting systolic anterior movement of the mitral valve (MV, *upper panel*) becomes large and very prominent following the administration of amyl nitrite *(lower panel)*. PCG, phonocardiogram; ECG, electrocardiogram; VS, interventricular septum. (From Scovil, J. A., and others: Circulation **53:**953, 1976. By permission of the American Heart Assn., Inc.)

of the murmur, making the clinical diagnosis more definite. Cardiac catheterization shows evidence of a gradient in the left ventricular outflow tract or, more conveniently, between the body of the left ventricle and a systemic artery. Chest roentgenograms are of little diagnostic value, but angiocardiography generally shows mitral regurgitation and a small irregular left ventricular cavity with a prominent indentation produced by the bulging septum. The ventricle may be hyperdynamic and may empty almost completely with systolic obliteration of the cavity. The mitral valve moves into the outflow tract during systole with the most active motion occurring at the tip of the leaflet.

Echocardiographic features (Figs. 4-36 to 4-37)

• The septum is thick (15 to 35 mm) and may or may not show poor excursion (less than 3 mm), whereas the posterior left ven-

tricular wall is usually normal in width (10 to 12 mm) or only slightly hypertrophied, asymmetric septal hypertrophy (ASH).

• The left ventricular outflow tract is narrow (under 20 mm).

• The anterior mitral leaflet shows an abnormal systolic anterior motion (SAM). This movement may be accentuated by Valsalva maneuver or amyl nitrite inhalation (Fig. 4-38).

• The EF slope is usually very flat.

• The posterior leaflet moves away from the anterior in diastole as in the normal and may bulge forward to some extent in systole.

• The aortic valve may close in midsystole and reopen in late systole (Fig. 4-39). Most often it exhibits a coarse undulation (about 4 to 10 cycles/sec).

• Systolic thickening of the ventricular septum (normal, 30%) may be reduced.

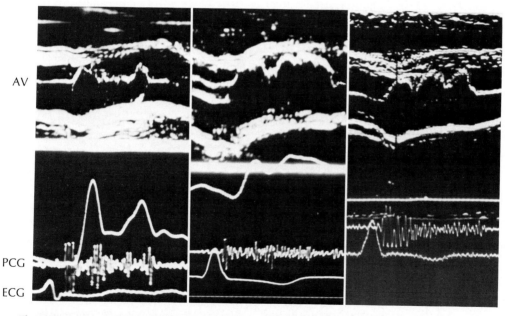

Fig. 4-39. Aortic valve movements in the presence of idiopathic hypertrophic subaortic stenosis (IHSS). The records represent three different patients, all of whom showed hemodynamic and echocardiographic evidence of IHSS. The panel on the left shows extensive midsystolic closure of the valve. In the central panel the valve appears to close briefly in midsystole and then executes some coarse flutters upon reopening. In the panel on the right, three coarse rolling motions of the valve cusp can be seen in systole. The carotid pulse, seen on the left above the PCG, is also typical for IHSS. AV, aortic valve; PCG, phonocardiogram; ECG, electrocardiogram.

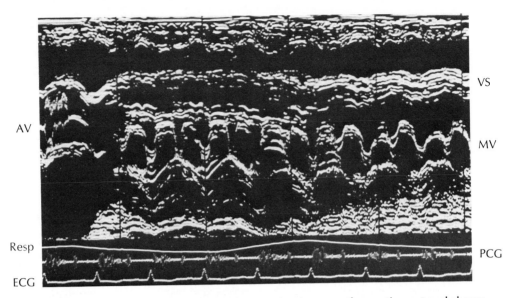

Fig. 4-40. Left ventricular scan in IHSS. The scan begins over the aortic root and shows erratic movements of the aortic valve (AV). As the beam is progressively passed through the ventricular septum (VS), marked thickening is encountered, which encroaches on the left ventricular outflow tract. The localized nature of this thickening can be seen when the beam passes deeper into the left ventricular cavity and reveals a septum of relatively normal thickness. Systolic anterior movements of the mitral valve (MV) are also evident. Dropouts occurring in the central portion of the thickened area of the septum illustrate how its width can be midjudged. Resp, respiration; PCG, phonocardiogram; ECG, electrocardiogram.

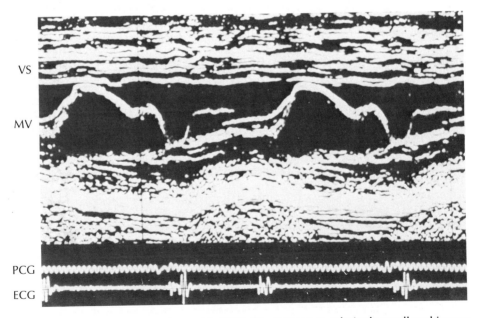

Fig. 4-41. Partial SAMs in a patient with IHSS. The SAMs are relatively small and incomplete and do not touch the ventricular septum (VS), which is hypertrophied. MV, mitral valve; ECG, electrocardiogram; PCG, phonocardiogram.

Comments

• This condition is also known as hypertrophic obstructive cardiomyopathy (HOCM) and muscular subaortic stenosis (MSS).

• An iron-clad echocardiographic diagnosis requires all elements described, not just isolated findings such as a thick septum, SAM, or a narrow left ventricular outflow tract.

• Diagnosis may be difficult for beginners, since the narrow left ventricular outflow tract and both systolic and diastolic anterior motion of the mitral leaflets can be confusing.

• The bulge in the septum may be localized (Fig. 4-40), and beam scanning helps to identify the narrowest portion of the left ventricular outflow tract, which may not be present immediately underneath the aortic valve. Be sure to make recordings at this point. Recordings made away from the bulge may be confusing since the septum does not appear thick and the LVO may appear of normal width, although SAMs could be present.

• The SAM of the anterior leaflet varies in size according to the severity of the obstruction. SAMs may be partial (Fig. 4-41), small, fragmentary, or present only on occasional beats when there is no resting obstruction (latent or labile IHSS). When obstruction is present at rest, SAMs reach the ventricular septum and are observed in every cardiac cycle. Amyl nitrite inhalation (Valsalva maneuver may also be useful) should be used whenever a SAM is poorly seen or is absent in a patient with suspected IHSS. Intervention increases the obstruction and results in large typical SAMs, which may reach the septum. The best recordings of SAM are obtained from the tip of the mitral leaflet. Recordings from the base of the leaflet may show no SAM or an erroneously small SAM.

• Artifacts that superficially resemble SAMs (Fig. 4-42) are commonly observed. Frequently, one of the walls of the aortic root may seem to be superimposed on a normal mitral echo, but the anterior movement of the aortic root during systole is gradual and is never seen to descend to the mitral base-

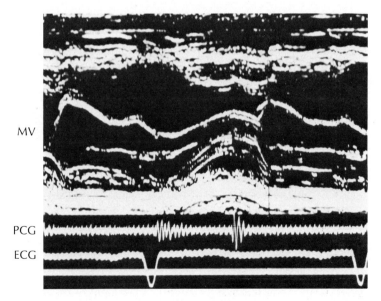

Fig. 4-42. Chordae motion mimicking SAM. A mitral valve (MV) recording made near the tips of the leaflets shows a prominent anterior bulging during systole, which may originate in chordae recorded with portions of the mitral valve. Other mitral valve recordings in this patient revealed normal systolic segments and no evidence of IHSS. PCG, phonocardiogram; ECG, electrocardiogram.

line before the opening of the mitral valve. A more confusing artifact is produced by simultaneously echoing both the mitral valve and the chordae or the papillary muscle. However, in this case the pseudo-SAM thus produced is seen to move parallel with the left ventricular endocardium and may cross the mitral valve as it opens in diastole, a feature atypical of the true SAM. Although artifacts may be mistaken for the true SAM, the converse is also possible. Occasionally in IHSS, the SAM may not appear to return to the mitral baseline before the onset of diastole. In these instances a careful exploration of the tips of the mitral leaflets usually demonstrates typical SAMs.

• Although SAMs are characteristic of IHSS, they are not specific for it and have been observed in other conditions. Most often they are found in mitral valve prolapse

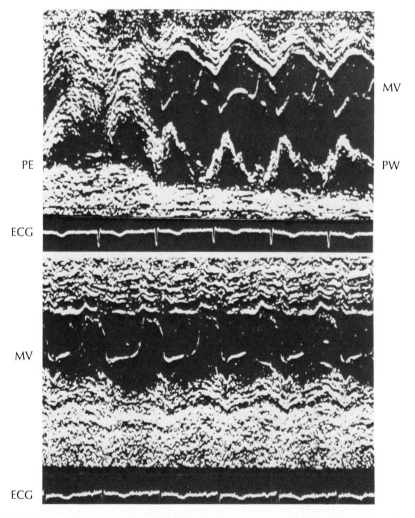

Fig. 4-43. *Upper panel,* Abnormal systolic anterior movement of the mitral valve (MV) observed with large pericardial effusion (PE). The posterior left atrial wall (PW) recorded behind the mitral valve shows hyperdynamic motion and early systolic peak formation. *Lower panel,* Normal mitral valve systolic tracing obtained following resolution of effusion. ECG, electrocardiogram. (From Nanda, N. C., and others: Circulation **54:**500, 1976. By permission of the American Heart Assn., Inc.)

and large pericardial effusions. The mechanism for their production in mitral valve prolapse is incompletely understood but appears to be caused by anterior bulging of the proximal portion of the leaflet during the phase of prolapse involving the distal half of the leaflet. In pericardial effusion, SAM is an artifact produced by swinging of the heart in the large pericardial effusion space (Fig. 4-43) and disappears following resolution of the effusion.

SAMs are also uncommonly seen in instances in which their origin and clinical significance are not clear. These include myocardial infarction, acute aortic incompetence (from rapid ventricular ejection in systole, Bernoulli or Venturi effect; Fig. 4-44), left ventricular aneurysms, severe primary or secondary pulmonary hypertension, secundum atrial septal defect, parachute mitral valve, dextrotransposition of the great vessels with or without left ventricular outflow obstruction, discrete subaortic membranous

stenosis, systemic hypertension associated with concentric left ventricular hypertrophy, shock syndrome (hypovolemia and rapid ejection), and normal volunteers, especially when examined in the standing position. It should be emphasized that generally the SAMs seen in these conditions are not large and do not become prominent with provocative tests. Also, asymmetric ventricular septal hypertrophy and narrow outflow tract dimensions are not present in the majority of these patients, and these features assist in excluding the presence of IHSS.

• We have seen previously documented SAMs disappear in proven cases of IHSS when the disease becomes advanced and is associated with cardiac failure.

• Asymmetric septal hypertrophy (ASH) may be present without other obstructive features. No SAM of the mitral valve is present. The ratio of the thickness of the septum to the posterior wall exceeds 1.3 or 1.5 measured at end-diastole. Interventions

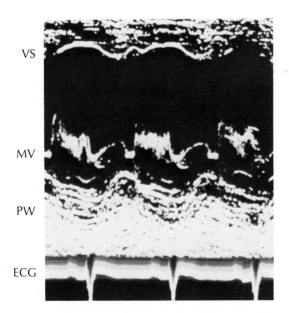

Fig. 4-44. SAMs in aortic incompetence. The systolic segments of the mitral valve (MV) bulge anteriorly in a pattern like that seen in IHSS. However, the left ventricle is dilated, and the ventricular septum (VS, partially seen) is of normal thickness. Ventricular outflow obstruction does not occur. This finding probably results from rapid flow and an associated Bernoulli effect, which pulls the mitral leaflet anteriorly. PW, posterior left ventricular wall; ECG, electrocardiogram.

should be used to differentiate this condition from latent IHSS.

False-positive ASH may been seen when the right ventricular side of the septum becomes thickened in conditions such as pulmonary hypertension or in congenital heart disease when pressure or volume overload hypertrophies the right ventricle. It is also observed in normal neonates and is probably related to the presence of high pulmonary vascular resistance.

Though patients with IHSS usually also show ASH, concentric hypertrophy of the ventricle may occur in a later phase of IHSS, so that this element may not be present in the diagnostic picture.

• Successful surgical treatment of IHSS by excision of a portion of the thickened septum (myectomy) results in the disappearance of SAM and the obstructive features of the disease but generally does not appreciably alter septal thickness nor the width of the LVO.

• The flat EF slope of the mitral valve reflects decreased left ventricular compliance or mechanical limitation of mitral valve motion in the narrow outflow tract. Do not attempt to diagnose coexisting mitral stenosis; it almost never occurs with IHSS. Countermotion of the posterior leaflet in diastole helps to identify this "false" mitral stenosis.

• IHSS may be present in association with conditions that produce obstruction to left ventricular emptying, such as aortic valve disease (Fig. 4-45), coarctation of the aorta, and subaortic membrane. In these cases the presence of SAM indicates a second point of obstruction and may require direct surgical removal of the hypertrophied septal muscle when the primary or fixed obstruction is corrected. In the presence of a fixed distal obstruction the SAMs may be relatively small and the use of interventions to increase their size may be disappointing. These patients also have narrow outflow tracts and asymmetric ventricular septal hypertrophy. Isolated, severe aortic valve stenosis by itself is not generally associated with narrow outflow measurement.

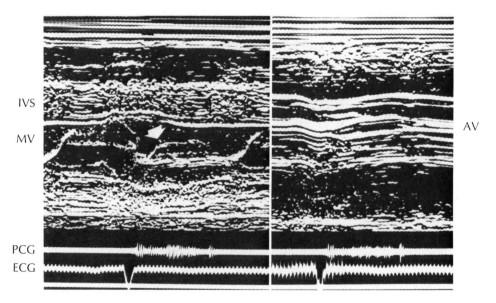

Fig. 4-45. Co-existing aortic valve stenosis and IHSS. The mitral valve study (MV) shows a relatively shallow systolic anterior movement *(arrow)* of the mitral leaflet *(left panel).* The aortic valve (AV) is calcified, and its systolic motion is markedly restricted *(right panel).* IVS, ventricular septum; PCG, phonocardiogram; ECG, electrocardiogram. (From Nanda, N. C., and others: Circulation **50:**752, 1974. By permission of the American Heart Assn., Inc.)

The presence of aortic valve disease tends to mask the clinical and cardiac catheterization findings of coexisting IHSS. Echocardiographic suggestion of the coexistence of these two entities should prompt careful evaluation at the time of cardiac catheterization, surgery, or both.

IHSS has been observed in as many as 10% of patients with coarctation of the aorta. Generally, the SAMs are large, show an expected increase in size with amyl nitrite and are associated with asymmetric septal hypertrophy. However, the left ventricular outflow may not be narrowed, probably from the effects of long-standing obstruction produced by the coarctation. The ventricular septum also generally shows normal or hyperdynamic excursion in contrast to isolated IHSS.

• A narrow left ventricular outflow tract may be quickly recognized without measurement by observing diastolic mitral-septal apposition or by scanning the beam from the mitral to the aortic valve. The thickened septum can be seen bulging into the left ventricular outflow tract and narrowing it. There may be a normal-appearing septum in the area just below the aortic valve.

• Infants of diabetic mothers may show asymmetric septal hypertrophy, SAMs, and clinical evidence of left ventricular outflow obstruction. The SAMs possibly result from hypovolemia and metabolic imbalance commonly seen in these infants, and they often disappear as the child gets older.

• The anterior right ventricular wall may also be thickened (more than 1 cm) in some patients with IHSS. The left atrium may be enlarged, and the pulmonary valve may show evidence of pulmonary hypertension.

• The left ventricular cavity may be so small in advanced cases that the mitral valve may not be easily recognized and may be difficult to find.

• An occasional patient may present with mid-left ventricular cavity obstruction—the left ventricle has an "hourglass" appearance (Fig. 4-46). The chamber distal to the hypertrophied septal muscle is prevented from discharging its function as a muscular pump, which results in low cardiac output. SAMs are not generally present or may be small and atypical. However, a transient but dramatic decrease in the size of the left ventricle beyond the tip of the mitral valve produced by massive septal hypertrophy may be observed during beam scanning of the left ventricular cavity (Fig. 4-47).

• In children with IHSS the septal motion may not be compromised, and the left ventricular outflow tract dimensions may be in the normal range (see Fig. 4-38).

• SAMs have been reported to disappear

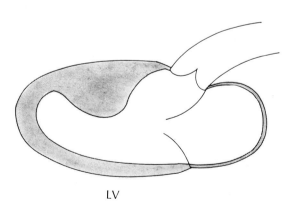

LV

Fig. 4-46. Mid-left ventricular cavity obstruction. The ventricular septum is hypertrophied in its midportion, producing a constriction at that level and giving an hourglass appearance to the left ventricular cavity (LV). In IHSS the septum is generally hypertrophied in the subaortic region.

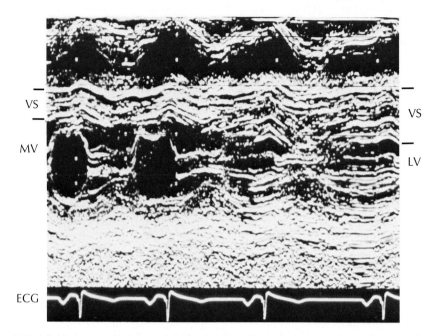

Fig. 4-47. Mid-left ventricular cavity obstruction. Beam scanning from the mitral valve (MV) to the left ventricular cavity (LV) demonstrates marked thickening of the ventricular septum (VS, horizontal bars on either side of the illustration) with almost complete systolic obliteration of the distal portion of the left ventricular cavity. Angiography revealed a constriction at the midventricular level, producing a typical hourglass configuration. At surgery the septum was found to be massively hypertrophied in the midventricular area and myectomy was performed. Postoperatively the patient showed clinical improvement and the echocardiogram showed widening of the left ventricular cavity. ECG, electrocardiogram.

or become smaller in an occasional IHSS patient when the patient is placed on propranolol therapy. Interventions may not produce the desired increase in heart rate, and obstruction may be difficult to document in these patients.

• We have noted the development of characteristic features of IHSS in a patient with Fabry's disease. Rheumatoid arthritis, amyloid disease, and a congenital bicuspid aortic valve have also been associated with IHSS.

• IHSS may be familial, and examination of other family members of an affected individual may be indicated.

• SAMs occurring in late systole are often associated with milder degrees of obstruction.

• The left ventricular posterior wall thickness may vary with minimal changes in beam angulation. A more reliable estimate of its thickness may be obtained if the transducer is moved in a transverse plane perpendicular to that used for scanning from the mitral to the aortic valve and taking the thickness at the point where the left ventricular end-diastolic dimension is at its maximum. This method (T-scan technique), although theoretically attractive, requires further evaluation.

Role of echocardiography

• The diagnosis of IHSS requires demonstration of the entire anatomic-functional complex, which includes SAMs, ASH, and a narrow left ventricular outflow tract. No single finding is specific for IHSS. Provocative tests like inhalation of amyl nitrite are useful in the presence of atypical findings and add greater specificity to the diagnosis.

- Echocardiography is probably the best noninvasive method for documentation of this entity. In some institutions it has displaced or eliminated invasive procedures for diagnosis when the echocardiographic and clinical pictures are typical.
- Echocardiography is capable of recognizing IHSS when it coexists with distal fixed left ventricular outflow obstruction such as aortic valve stenosis, coarctation of the aorta, discrete subaortic membranous stenosis, which may effectively mask its clinical and hymodynamic manifestations. In adults and children with these conditions it is especially important to search diligently for evidence of coexisting IHSS, since their treatment and management may differ when both conditions are present.
- Clinically suspected but echocardiographically atypical cases of IHSS should be followed at extended intervals to see if the full-blown picture develops.

Myxomas

Anatomic and functional changes. Myxomas are benign, noncancerous tumors that develop in cardiac cavities. The most common site is the left atrium. Myxomas are mostly composed of semiclear gelatinous material, fibrous tissue, and blood vessels and often contain areas of hemorrhage and occasionally calcification. The soft nature of these masses predisposes them to break off pieces that may embolize to distant arterial sites. Most often myxomas are attached to the atrial septum by a stalk, which permits the mass to move with the blood flow pattern. In diastole, therefore, these masses usually move into the mitral orifice and produce obstruction that clinically mimics mitral stenosis. In systole, they are pushed back into the left atrial cavity as the mitral valve closes.

Myxomas may also be attached to the free wall of the atrium, in which case they usually have shorter stalks and move less with blood flow. Myxomas attached to valve leaflets have also been described. They vary considerably in size, but they may be so large that they virtually fill the left atrial cavity

completely. Though benign, they may recur after surgery and are known to be present in more than one cardiac chamber. Though relatively uncommon, they represent a lesion that is accurately detected and characterized by ultrasound.

Clinical summary. The first suspicion of the presence of a myxoma may be in the form of emboli in a patient with signs of mitral stenosis plus constitutional symptoms such as low-grade fever, malaise, and weakness. Catheterization of left heart chambers may be dangerous and is usually avoided, since it may result in dislodging a portion of the tumor or producing hemorrhage into it. Angiocardiograms made following pulmonary artery injection are therefore performed and reveal a mass in the left atrial cavity.

Echocardiographic features (Fig. 4-48)
- An abnormal grouping of linear and punctate echoes is present behind the anterior leaflet of the mitral valve in diastole.
- The space behind the systolic segments is clear if a long stalk is present (atrial septal attachment).
- The systolic and diastolic spaces behind the mitral valve contain tumor echoes when the site of attachment is nearer the outflow of the left atrium, on the atrial wall (short stalk), or when the myxoma attached to the atrial septum is very large.
- The left atrium (recorded behind the aortic root) always contains abnormal echoes that resemble those found behind the mitral valve.
- The EF slope of the mitral valve is usually reduced, and the A waves are diminished or absent as a result of the obstruction produced by the mass.

Comments
- Vary instrument sensitivity so that the mass will not be missed and an erroneous diagnosis of mitral stenosis made (Fig. 4-49).
- Be sure to examine the left atrial cavity, since moving tumor echoes are always present unless the mass fills the left atrial cavity so that motion of the tumor is markedly reduced or absent.
- Do not diagnose a left atrial myxoma un-

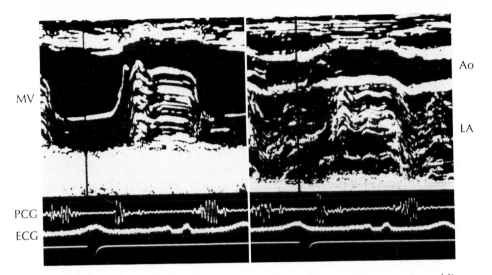

MV

Ao

LA

PCG
ECG

Fig. 4-48. Atrial myxoma. Recording on left shows a characteristic grouping of linear echoes behind mitral valve. Note clear space in early diastole and lack of similar echoes during systole. Examination of left atrium is shown on right. Abnormal echoes are present in left atrial cavity, and their diastolic motion pattern mimics mitral pattern. Diagnosis may be more difficult when an area of heavy calcification situated anteriorly produces sufficient shadowing to obscure a major portion of the mass. This can be avoided by use of multiple beam positions and angles. Ao, aortic root. (From King, D. L., editor: Diagnostic ultrasound, St. Louis, 1974, The C. V. Mosby Co.)

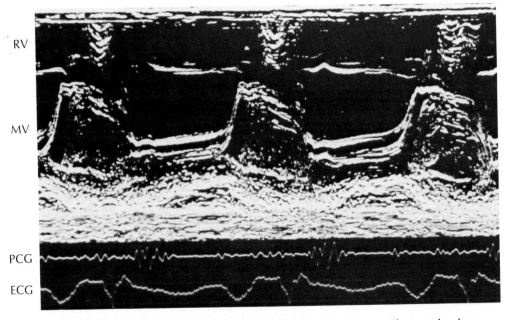

RV

MV

PCG

ECG

Fig. 4-49. Mitral valve recording in a patient with biatrial myxoma. Abnormal echoes are present in the right ventricle anterior to the ventricular septum and represent the portion of the right atrial myxoma prolapsing into the right ventricle. Low gain recordings of the mitral valve *(left)* appear innocent and require an increase in sensitivity or change in beam position for delineation of the abnormal grouping of echoes behind the mitral valve arising in the left atrial myxoma *(right)*. RV, right ventricle; MV, mitral valve; PCG, phonocardiogram; ECG, electrocardiogram.

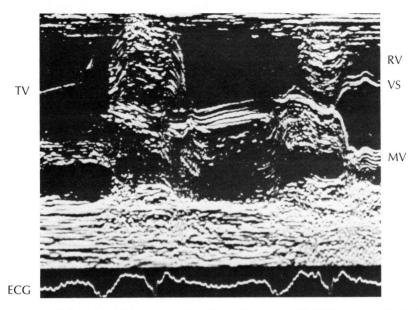

Fig. 4-50. Biatrial myxoma. Beam scanning from the tricuspid (TV) to the mitral (MV) valve reveals abnormal grouping of echoes behind both valves typical of atrial myxomas. The abnormal echoes observed in front of the ventricular septum (VS) represent the right atrial mass prolapsing further into the body of the right ventricle (RV) during atrial systole. ECG, electrocardiogram.

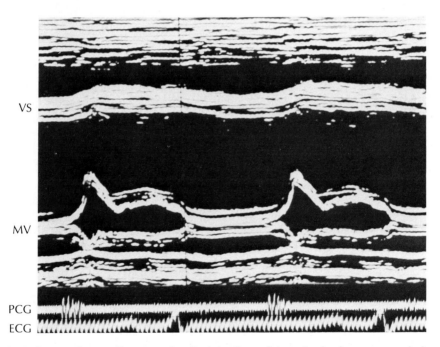

Fig. 4-51. Congestive cardiomyopathy. Both leaflets of the mitral valve are recorded and show diminished excursions. The systolic segment shows flattening and minimal sagging. The left ventricular cavity is dilated. The ventricular septum does not show significant systolic thickening. VS, ventricular septum; MV, mitral valve; PCG, phonocardiogram; ECG, electrocardiogram.

less there are tumor echoes in the left atrium, since a calcified mitral valve may resemble a myxoma (see Fig. 4-8).

• Examine the left ventricle and right heart cavities since myxomas may be multiple (Fig. 4-50).

• Large vegetations may mimic myxomas, and myxomas may become infected so that differentiation between these two entities may be impossible.

• A calcified mobile blood clot in the left atrium (ball valve thrombus) may also be indistinguishable from a myxoma.

Role of echocardiography. Echocardiography is the best diagnostic technique for the detection of atrial myxomas. In some centers, patients are sent to surgery without additional diagnostic examinations. Patients who present with vague cardiac symptoms and findings should be carefully examined in search of an obscure myxoma.

Congestive cardiomyopathies

Anatomic and functional changes. Though this category represents primary muscle disease, it is included in the mitral valve discussion, since the diagnostic characteristics are usually first encountered during examination of the mitral valve. A variety of generalized cardiac disorders can seriously hamper cardiac muscle function and produce the same echocardiographic features, so it is convenient to discuss them as if they were a single entity.

The most obvious anatomic change is cardiac dilatation, which is best seen in the left ventricle but may involve other chambers. Heart walls are not particularly thickened and may show poor motion indicating low cardiac output. Heart valves remain structurally normal, but their motion may be altered in keeping with low cardiac output. Clots may occur in dilated ventricles.

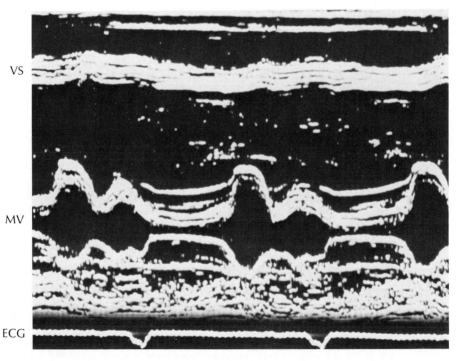

VS

MV

ECG

Fig. 4-52. Systolic separation of mitral leaflets. This patient with congestive cardiomyopathy shows an apparent separation of mitral valve (MV) leaflets during systole, though there was no clinical evidence of mitral regurgitation. This effect was probably produced by passing the beam through a more proximal portion of the leaflets, away from the distal apposed edges. VS, ventricular septum; ECG, electrocardiogram.

Clinical summary. The patient's history may point to an etiologic condition such as chronic alcoholism. There may be murmurs of mitral and tricuspid regurgitation from dilatation of the AV rings. Third and fourth heart sounds may be present along with indicators of low cardiac output. The chest roentgenogram reveals generalized cardiac enlargement. Cardiac catheterization shows no gradients across the valves. Angiocardiography demonstrates generalized cardiac dilatation and reduced contractility of the left ventricular walls.

Echocardiographic features (Figs. 4-51 and 4-52)

• Mitral valve opening amplitude is diminished from low cardiac output, but leaflets are not thickened.

• EF slopes are fairly rapid—around 100 mm/sec.

• Anterior and posterior leaflets are recorded simultaneously, almost always, probably due to left ventricular enlargement.

• Systolic segments are often flattened, or they may sag from reduced annular motion secondary to impaired performance of a dilated left ventricle.

• Extra lines are commonly observed superimposed on the mitral trace. These are probably from the chordae or the aortic root and are imaged with the mitral valve because of beam width and a more vertical mitral ring position secondary to left ventricular enlargement (Fig. 4-53).

• The left ventricular outflow tract is very wide and may measure 50 to 60 mm. This

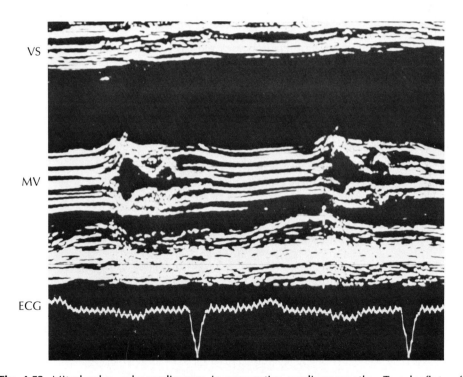

Fig. 4-53. Mitral valve echocardiogram in congestive cardiomyopathy. Two leaflets of the mitral valve (MV) are demonstrated and show a diminished separation of leaflets related to decreased flow through the mitral valve. The prominent, multilayered echoes surrounding the mitral valve in systole and diastole probably arise from different portions of the valve and from chordae. This finding may be related to a more vertical orientation of the valve in the beam produced by left ventricular enlargement and displacement of the atrioventricular junction superiorly.

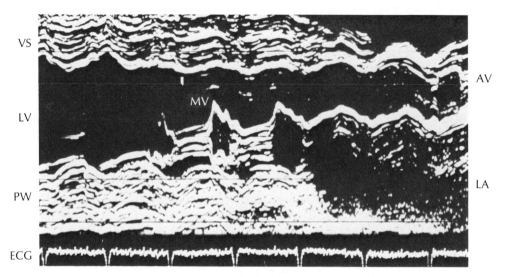

Fig. 4-54. Concentric left ventricular hypertrophy in cardiomyopathy. Beam scanning from the left ventricular cavity (LV) to the aortic valve (AV) demonstrates tapering of the ventricular septum (VS) as it attaches to the anterior wall of the aorta. Both the ventricular septum and the left ventricular posterior wall (PW) are symmetrically hypertrophied. The left ventricular cavity is normal in size while the left atrium (LA) is enlarged. MV, mitral valve; ECG, electrocardiogram.

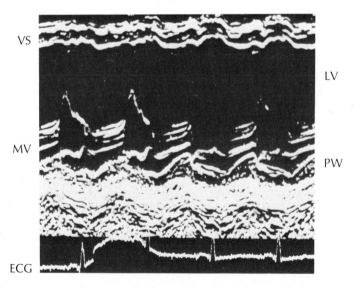

Fig. 4-55. Congestive cardiomyopathy in a child. The left ventricular cavity (LV) is dilated, and both the ventricular septum (VS) and the left ventricular posterior wall (PW) show diminished excursions. MV, mitral valve; ECG, electrocardiogram.

finding is often the first clue to the presence of a congestive cardiomyopathy.

• The septum is of normal thickness, its motion amplitude may be reduced (less than 3 mm), and the degree of systolic thickening is also less than normal (less than 30% increase over diastolic).

• Aortic root motion is also flattened, and the degree of opening of the aortic leaflets is reduced (less than 15 mm). Both represent indicators of decreased cardiac output.

• The tricuspid valve is easily recorded with complete traces of the diastolic waveform, and two cusps are commonly seen. These are indicators of right ventricular enlargement.

• The pulmonic valve is easily recorded.

• All chambers appear enlarged.

Comments

• End-stage diffuse coronary artery or valvular disease such as aortic incompetence and mitral incompetence may show identical changes in the heart cavities.

• Frequently, echocardiography is required to differentiate cardiomyopathies from pericardial effusion, since the clinical and roentgenographic findings of a large heart may be in both. Be certain to look for echo-free spaces that arise from pericardial fluid adjacent to the heart walls.

• Other types of cardiomyopathies may show normal or concentric posterior wall and septal hypertrophy with small, normal, or large chambers and do not fit into the groups of IHSS or congestive cardiomyopathy (Fig. 4-54).

• Patients with congestive cardiomyopathies are among the easiest to examine with ultrasound because the cardiac window is large (the enlarged heart displaces some of the overlying lung), and right heart enlargement positions the tricuspid and pulmonic valves for easy accessibility.

Role of echocardiography. Though the etiology of the myocardial disease cannot be shown, the functional impairment is evident on the echocardiogram. The exclusion of pericardial effusion is important clinical information.

Congenital heart disease

Mitral stenosis and incompetence, mitral valve prolapse, IHSS, congestive cardiomyopathy (Fig. 4-55), and myxomas occur in children and have the same echocardiographic appearance as when found in adults.

Parachute mitral valve is a condition in which the papillary muscles are fused into a single muscle group (Fig. 4-56). The chordae are thickened and sometimes fused. Obstruc-

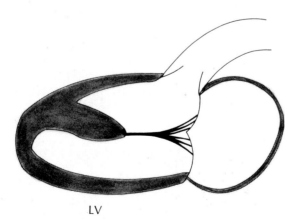

LV

Fig. 4-56. Parachute mitral valve. This entity is characterized by a large single papillary muscle and by thickened and shortened chordae, which draw the mitral leaflets and commissures together resulting in mitral orifice obstruction. Mitral incompetence may also be present. The left atrium is enlarged. LV, left ventricle.

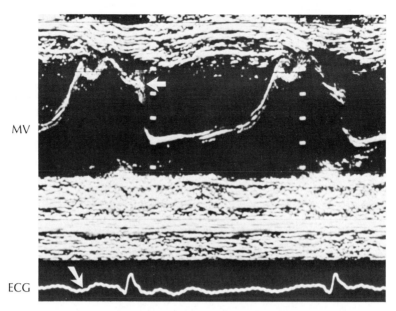

Fig. 4-57. Mitral valve recording in a patient with parachute mitral valve. This mitral valve (MV) recording is not specific for the diagnosis of parachute mitral valve and is presented to demonstrate a variety of findings in this rare entity. The major finding is a prominent A wave positioned near the E point. This proximity results from a delayed opening movement of the valve and prolongation of the AC interval, which produces a plateau *(arrow)* in the AC segment. Both phenomena are related to an increase in left ventricular diastolic pressure observed in this patient, who had predominant mitral regurgitation. The short EF slopes are rapid and not in the mitral stenosis range. There are no findings that mimic IHSS. The arrow on the electrocardiogram (ECG) denotes the P wave (PR interval was 200 msec).

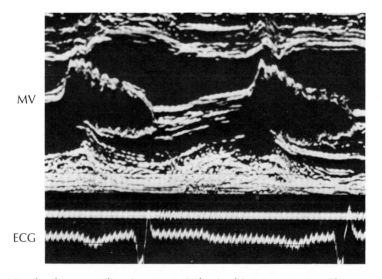

Fig. 4-58. Mitral valve recording in congenital mitral incompetence. The most prominent finding is diastolic undulations of the mitral valve (MV). The mitral leaflets in this patient were small and thickened, and the subvalvular apparatus deformed. There was no evidence of aortic regurgitation. MV, mitral valve; ECG, electrocardiogram.

tion to left atrial emptying is produced, and the lesion is often associated with congenital mitral stenosis. Mitral incompetence may also be present. In one reported case the echocardiographic pattern was indistinguishable from IHSS, though microscopic examination of the ventricular septal musculature failed to show the disordered, bizarre pattern of the muscle fibers seen in typical IHSS. In one patient studied by us recently, the mitral valve showed good amplitude of motion with only slight diminution of EF slopes, a prominent B point (Fig. 4-57), which correlated with increased left ventricular diastolic pressure, and a hypercontractile septum (more than 100% thickening in systole). The patient had predominant mitral regurgitation. A prominent diastolic flutter of the mitral valve may be seen in congenital mitral incompetence when the leaflets are small and thickened and the subvalvular apparatus deformed (Fig. 4-58).

Mitral valve abnormalities are associated with ostium primum atrial septal defects located low in the atrial septum. The anterior leaflet is often cleft, producing mitral re-

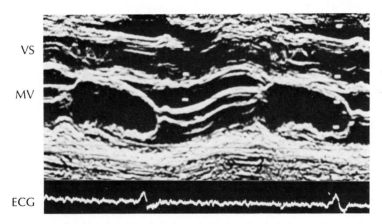

Fig. 4-59. The mitral valve (MV) in this patient with an ostium primum atrial septal defect exhibits prolonged diastolic apposition with the ventricular septum (VS) indicating the presence of a narrow left ventricular outflow tract. ECG, electrocardiogram.

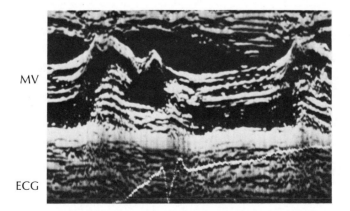

Fig. 4-60. Mitral valve recording in a patient with ostium primum atrial septal defect. Multilayered echoes in systole and diastole are consistent with the presence of a cleft anterior mitral leaflet present in this patient. MV, mitral valve; ECG, electrocardiogram.

gurgitation. The attachment of the anterior leaflet is abnormal, resulting in a narrow left ventricular outflow tract, which can be detected echocardiographically (Fig. 4-59). The left ventricular outflow narrowing is often recognized by a prolonged apposition of the anterior mitral leaflet with the ventricular septum in diastole. This finding may be especially useful in children, in whom direct measurement of the outflow width varies with the size of the patient and has not been systematically evaluated.

Cleft leaflets are usually not recognized, though some layering and duplication of images have been seen. (Fig. 4-60). Other atrial septal defects of the ostium secundum variety (these occur higher in the atrial septum) are not associated with clefts of the

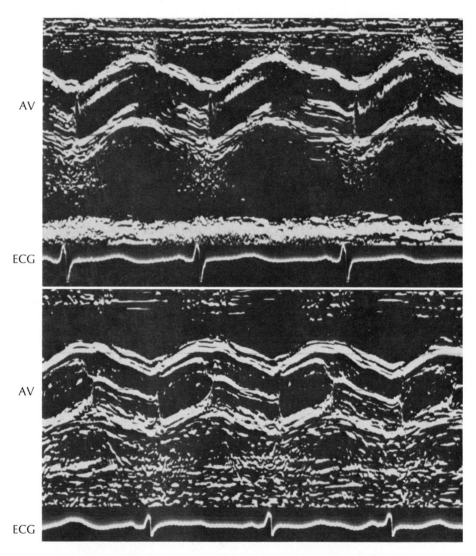

Fig. 4-61. Discrete membranous subaortic stenosis. *Upper panel,* The aortic valve (AV) shows a prominent motion toward closure of the right coronary cusp immediately after opening typical of this entity. Rapid systolic fluttering of the valve cusp is also present. The preclosure peak practically disappeared following surgical resection of the membrane *(lower panel).* ECG, electrocardiogram.

mitral valve, although an increased incidence of mitral valve prolapse has been reported. Atrial septal defects are discussed more fully in the section dealing with complex malformations.

Subaortic obstruction

Anatomic and functional changes. Congenital subaortic obstruction may be produced by fibromuscular ridges or thin membranes that are present immediately below

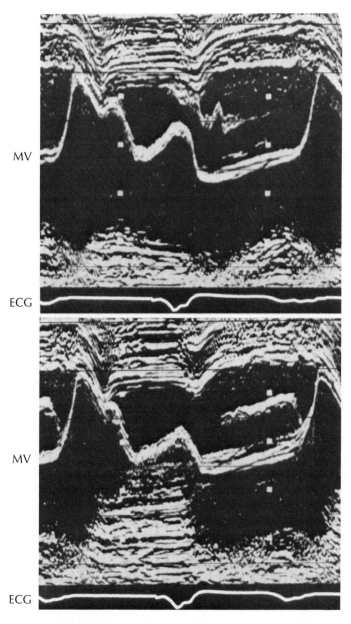

Fig. 4-62. Mitral valve recordings in discrete subaortic stenosis. Abnormal echoes are seen in the left ventricular outflow space and arise from the subaortic membrane. *Upper panel,* Undulating echo appears to be in contact with the ventricular septum. *Lower panel,* Images make a movement toward the mitral baseline in late systole mimicking a SAM. MV, mitral valve; ECG, electrocardiogram.

the aortic valve and are attached to the interventricular septum and to the anterior leaflet of the mitral valve. They may be localized and discrete (common) or diffuse (rare), in which case a tunnellike narrowing is produced by the fibromuscular thickening of the endocardial tissue. They impede left ventricular emptying, and a close proximity to the aortic valve often results in aortic incompetence by interfering with valve motion, or the valve may be damaged by the jet produced by the narrowing.

Clinical summary. Systolic and diastolic murmurs are present from the outflow obstruction and aortic incompetence. Cardiac catheterization reveals a gradient in the subaortic area. Angiocardiography demonstrates the anatomy and defines the type of subaortic obstruction.

Echocardiographic features (Fig. 4-61)

• The motion of aortic valve cusps is altered by the turbulent flow produced in the LVO. In all of our 20 cases of discrete membranous subaortic stenosis, a prominent finding has been an abrupt motion toward closure

of one or both aortic leaflets occurring immediately after opening and often followed by rapid fluttering throughout the remainder of systole. Reopening movements of the cusp are uncommon. Generally the size of these early systolic peaks correlates with the severity of obstruction. When the amplitude of the preclosure movement is 50% or more of the initial opening excursion, the gradient in the left ventricular outflow tract is usually 50 mm Hg or more. These preclosure peaks disappear or diminish markedly after surgical removal of the membrane (Fig. 4-61).

• Echocardiograms may occasionally show abnormal linear echoes in the outflow tract arising from the membrane, which may move in a pattern that parallels portions of the mitral trace (Fig. 4-62).

• In about half the patients the membranes may be represented by curved linear echoes (having a flaglike configuration), which appear in the outflow tract in systole (Fig. 4-63) and occasionally may seem to be attached to the anterior mitral leaflet in diastole. They may be seen to merge with the

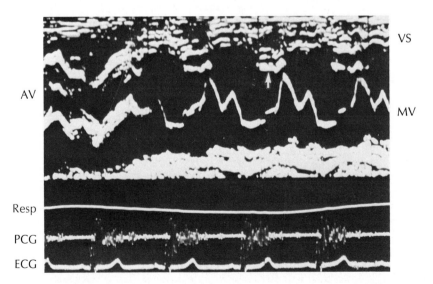

Fig. 4-63. Mitral valve recordings in subaortic membranous stenosis. Beam scanning from the aortic to the mitral valve (MV) demonstrates the presence of abnormal linear echoes *(arrow)* in the left ventricular outflow tract in the vicinity of the mitral valve in a patient with discrete subaortic stenosis. The echoes arise from the subaortic membrane, which is often attached to the anterior mitral leaflet. AV, aortic valve; VS, ventricular septum; Resp, respiration; PCG, phonocardiogram; ECG, electrocardiogram.

aortic valve cusps when the transducer is angled toward the aortic root because of their subaortic position. These echoes may persist following surgery, since the mitral attachment of the membrane may not be removed to prevent damage to the mitral valve.

• Beam scanning from the aortic to the mitral valve may reveal a narrow left ventricular outflow tract.

Comments

• Use a variety of transducer positions and make multiple scans from the left ventricle to the aortic valve to obtain the particular angle that images the maximum preclosure of the aortic valve, a thin membrane, or a tunnel. Aortic valve preclosure may appear insignificantly small in some beam angles (Fig. 4-64). It may not be visualized at all if the early systolic portion of the cusp is not well recorded. It is easy to miss this entity if you are not specifically looking for it.

• A false impression of a tunnel may be produced in scans where the beam is too lateral or too medial and misses the true width of the LVO.

• Vary gain to obtain echoes from a membrane that may be delicate and thin.

• Aortic valve preclosure occurs in other conditions, but it is found regularly in subaortic stenosis.

• Early systolic aortic preclosure is frequently observed with aortic root dilatation, such as that seen with aortic aneurysms, but the aortic root image will be markedly dilated and will differentiate it from subaortic membranous stenosis (Fig. 4-65). It may also be observed in atrial fibrillation when the preceding R-R interval is short (due to incomplete ventricular filling and hence low forward flow) and in other low cardiac output states. Aortic valve preclosure has also been observed in patients with Fallot's tetralogy following surgical repair and probably results from turbulence or bulging of the patch into the left ventricular outflow. Minimal preclosure of the aortic valve in early systole is observed in many conditions and is nonspecific.

• Subaortic membranous stenosis in the presence of aortic valve disease may show a

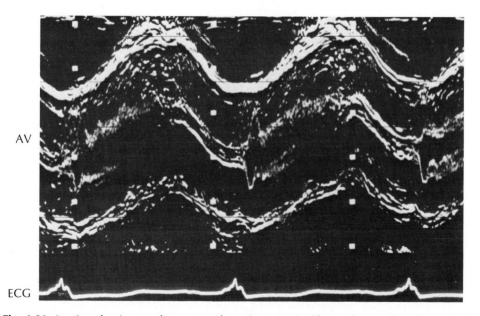

Fig. 4-64. Aortic valve in membranous subaortic stenosis. The early systolic rebound of the aortic leaflets toward closure may be difficult to record because of dropouts. This illustration is a portion of a record that included many cardiac cycles, most of which failed to demonstrate this important finding. AV, aortic valve; ECG, electrocardiogram.

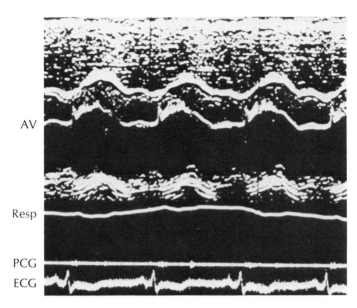

Fig. 4-65. Aortic valve preclosure in aortic aneurysm. The aortic root is dilated, and the right coronary cusp shows a prominent closing movement in early systole. There was no evidence of a subaortic membrane. AV, aortic valve; Resp, respirations; PCG, phonocardiogram; ECG, electrocardiogram.

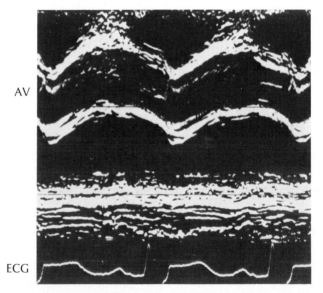

Fig. 4-66. Effect of aortic root motion on aortic cusp systolic preclosure. The right coronary cusp demonstrates systolic preclosure with abrupt, early systolic posterior motion of the cusp at a time when the aortic root is also moving posteriorly. The observed magnitude of right coronary cusp preclosure in this patient represents the vector sum of the intrinsic posterior motion toward closure of the cusp and the motion imparted to the cusp by the simultaneous posterior motion of the aortic root. This provides an explanation for the prominent preclosure pattern. The patient has an ostium secundum atrial septal defect with no evidence of subaortic obstruction. Abnormal motion of the aortic root may be related to the altered hemodynamics in the contiguously situated right ventricle. AV, aortic valve; ECG, electrocardiogram.

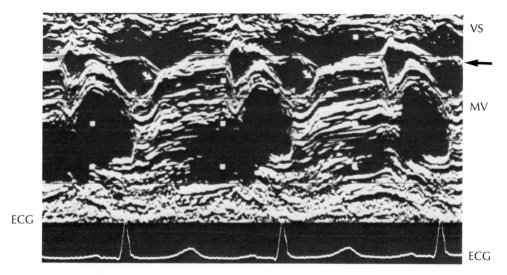

Fig. 4-67. Discrete subaortic membranous obstruction and IHSS in the same patient. The SAMs *(white arrow)* are in contact with the membrane *(horizontal arrow)*, which is seen as a linear echo in the left ventricular outflow. At surgery the membrane was resected, and septal myectomy was performed. VS, ventricular septum; MV, mitral valve; ECG, electrocardiogram.

small early systolic aortic valve preclosure since the cusps are relatively rigid.

• Aortic valve preclosure may be explained in terms of the Bernoulli effect. As the left ventricular outflow tract becomes narrow, the pressure head of the subaortic jet increases, but the lateral pressure across it diminishes distal to the obstruction and results in valve preclosure.

• Occasionally, transient abnormal posterior motion of the aortic walls in systole may result in a spurious preclosure of the right coronary cusp since the cusp follows the motion of the walls (Fig. 4-66).

• Mitral valve diastolic flutter from aortic regurgitation is common.

• True IHSS may coexist with subaortic obstruction. Be sure to obtain a record that shows all the features of IHSS. Associated IHSS may show preclosures characteristic of either or both types of obstruction. The SAM may be observed to be in contact with the membrane (Fig. 4-67).

• SAMs of the mitral valve also occur rarely in both the tunnel and membrane variety without associated IHSS and are usually incomplete and small (Fig. 4-68).

• A subaortic membrane imaged in the left ventricular outflow tract may masquerade as a mitral valve SAM.

• Left ventricular outflow narrowing as judged by prolonged mitral-septal diastolic apposition occurs in approximately 75% of patients with discrete subaortic membranous stenosis.

• Tunnel narrowings are best demonstrated by scans made from the mitral valve to the aortic root (Fig. 4-69). Varying degrees of tunnel formation can be recognized in the subaortic region by comparing LVO width at its narrowest point to the diameter of the aorta. Early systolic preclosure of the aortic valve is not generally observed with tunnel narrowings, but coarse systolic flutter is common.

Role of echocardiography

• Echocardiographic findings of subaortic stenosis are very useful, since the clinical presentation may be difficult to differentiate from aortic valve disease. This is especially true in the occasional adult patient in whom a possible congenital lesion may be overlooked. The finding of aortic valve preclosure should alert one to the possibility that ap-

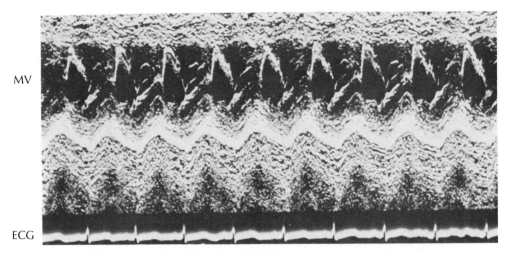

Fig. 4-68. Mitral valve recordings in a patient with discrete subaortic membranous stenosis. The record was obtained at the tip of the mitral valve (MV) and shows the presence of partial SAMs reminiscent of IHSS. The SAMs did not become prominent during provocation with amyl nitrite, and no evidence of IHSS was found during cardiac catheterization and subsequent surgery. ECG, electrocardiogram.

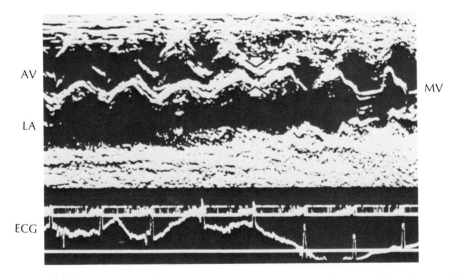

Fig. 4-69. Tunnel narrowing in subaortic obstruction. A beam sweep from the aortic valve (AV) to the mitral valve (MV) shows a tunnellike area of narrowing of the left ventricular outflow tract *(arrows)*. The aortic valve is only partially seen but exhibits an early systolic rebound toward closure. LA, left atrium; ECG, electrocardiogram.

parent acquired aortic valve disease may actually be the result of discrete subaortic obstruction.

• Echocardiography is more useful in the diagnosis of discrete subaortic stenosis than in the diffuse tunnel-type of obstruction, which may be difficult to distinguish from IHSS.

Aortic regurgitation

Anatomic and functional changes. Thickening, destruction, or eversion of the edges

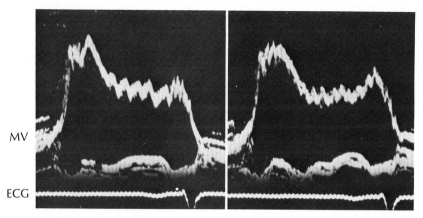

Fig. 4-70. Diastolic flutter of the mitral valve in aortic incompetence. Coarse and fine undulations of the anterior leaflet of the mitral valve (MV) begin at the E point, extend throughout diastole, involve the A wave, and continue during the A-C interval. This pandiastolic flutter has been seen in the more severe cases of aortic regurgitation. The two mitral wave forms were selected from the same patient to show variations in the form of the E point, character of the flutter, and extension of fluttering to the C point. ECG, electrocardiogram.

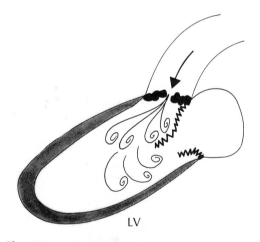

Fig. 4-71. Aortic incompetence. The aortic valve is thickened, and its edges fail to coapt with each other in diastole, resulting in aortic incompetence. The regurgitant jet strikes the open mitral leaflets, producing fine mitral diastolic oscillations that can be detected by echocardiography. LV, left ventricle.

of the aortic leaflets associated with a congenital or rheumatic process may produce leakage of blood into the left ventricle from the aorta if the valve cusps fail to coapt normally in diastole. Aortic regurgitation may also result from traumatic cusp rupture, bacterial infection, or aortic annulus dilatation produced by aortic root enlargement. Cusp perforation (congenital or following bacterial infection) also leads to aortic regurgitation, even though leaflet coaptation is relatively unaffected.

Clinical summary. In aortic regurgitation, leakage of the incompetent valve lowers the systemic blood pressure in diastole so that the pulse pressure is widened. Palpation of a peripheral artery reveals a "water-hammer" or collapsing pulse. A typical blowing early diastolic murmur along the left sternal border identifies the process. However, a separate mitral diastolic murmur that resembles mitral stenosis (Austin-Flint murmur) may be present even though the mitral valve is structurally normal. The murmur is related to increased velocity of blood flow through a narrow mitral orifice resulting from the regurgitant jet partially closing the mitral valve. It may be difficult, therefore, to ascertain clinically if both the aortic and mitral valves are abnormal or if the mitral murmur is secondary to aortic regurgitation.

The left ventricle dilates and shows an increased amplitude of wall motion, since the volume of blood that leaks back in diastole (regurgitant fraction) is an added burden to the left ventricle (volume overload).

Cardiac catheterization rules out mitral valve disease and determines left ventricular diastolic pressure, which is elevated when the regurgitant fraction is large and the left ventricular performance impaired. Retrograde injection of radiopaque contrast agents into the ascending aorta reveals the degree of aortic regurgitation semiquantitatively and provides information concerning the status of the aortic valve.

Echocardiographic features
• The mitral valve flutters rapidly in diastole from the regurgitant jet striking the open leaflets (Figs. 4-70 and 4-71). The frequency of flutter is usually in the 35 to 135 cycles per second range. Flutter amplitude may be small or as large as 10 mm. A low gain setting and examination of the tips of the mitral leaflets are useful in the determination of subtle diastolic mitral valve flutter. Diastolic flutter may be absent in an occasional patient with very mild incompetence.

• The mitral valve waveform may show a limited opening amplitude, a slow EF slope, and a large A wave from elevation of left ventricular diastolic pressure (Fig. 4-72).
• The mitral valve may preclose in diastole (be sure the P-R interval is not prolonged). (Fig. 4-73.) This finding occurs in very severe acute aortic regurgitation but is also seen occasionally in the chronic case.
• The left ventricular outflow tract and the body of the left ventricle may be enlarged. The outflow tract may measure as much as 5.0 cm in width, and left ventricular end-diastolic dimensions of 7.0 cm are common.
• The septum and left ventricular posterior wall are very active and show an increased amplitude of motion (an indication of increased left ventricular overload from the regurgitant fraction). (See Fig. 4-74.)
• The left atrium may enlarge in the advanced stage of the disease process when the left heart fails.
• The aortic valve may show evidence of calcification (thick echoes replacing normal

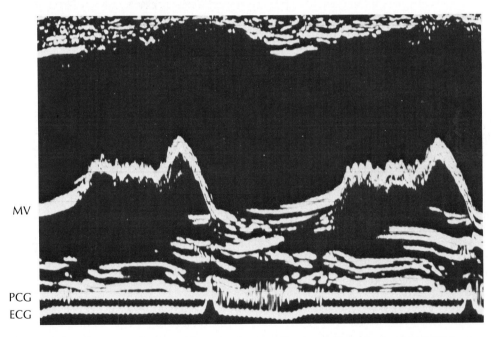

Fig. 4-72. Aortic incompetence. The opening amplitude of the mitral valve (MV) is reduced and the EF slope flattened from elevation of the left ventricular diastolic pressure. Atrial systole opens the valve more completely and produces a large A wave. The fine diastolic fluttering is produced by the regurgitant jet striking the anterior leaflet. The left ventricle is enlarged. PCG, phonocardiogram; ECG, electrocardiogram.

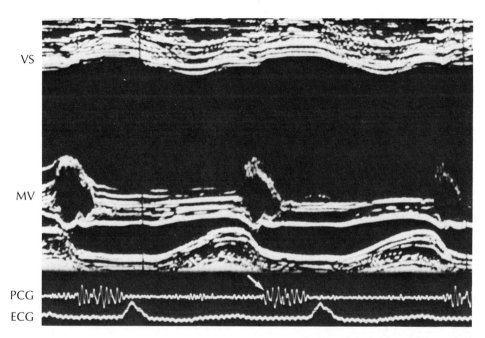

Fig. 4-73. Austin-Flint murmur in aortic incompetence. The phonocardiogram (PCG) shows a prominent, low-frequency murmur in late diastole *(arrow)*. Note that the mitral valve (MV) closes in diastole before the onset of the QRS complex of the electrocardiogram (ECG). Subtle diastolic fluttering of the mitral valve could be seen in other portions of the record. VS, ventricular septum.

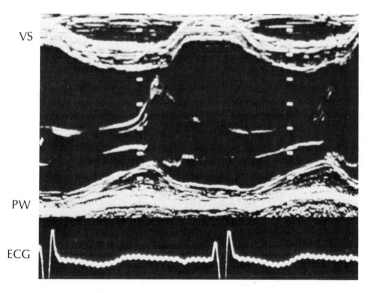

Fig. 4-74. Left ventricular cavity echo in a patient with left ventricular volume overload, demonstrating hyperdynamic motion of the ventricular septum (VS). PW, left ventricular posterior wall; ECG, electrocardiogram.

slender cusps), but there is usually fairly good motion.

• There may be evidence of a bicuspid aortic valve (see discussion on p. 169) or a subaortic membrane (described previously).

Comments

• The mitral valve may flutter in the absence of aortic regurgitation. In infants the mitral valve may flutter in a pattern indistinguishable from that of aortic regurgitation. Flutter is also a common finding in dextrotransposition of the great vessels following balloon septostomy in the absence of associated semilunar valve incompetence. The flutter has been noted to become prominent or to appear as a new finding following placement of an intra-atrial baffle to achieve physiologic correction. Bidirectional shunting across the newly created atrial septal defect and turbulence produced by altered pathways of blood resulting from the baffle have been implicated in its genesis. Chordae rupture shows diastolic fluttering, but there is usually a very coarse component not seen in aortic regurgitation. Rarely, the mitral valve flutters in the presence of mitral regurgitation. Very fine and shallow flutters are occasionally seen in cases in which the cause is not apparent.

• Both leaflets and chordae as well as the left side of the ventricular septum may flutter in aortic incompetence.

• When mitral stenosis is present, the mitral leaflet may be too thick or too tense to flutter. Look at the left side of the interventricular septum for subtle flutter to identify coexisting aortic incompetence.

• Severity of aortic incompetence is difficult to judge from echocardiograms. Large amplitude pandiastolic flutters, large left ventricles (6 to 7 cm), a dilated outflow tract (5 cm) and dilated aortic root, or mitral valve preclosure indicate severe incompetence.

• With very severe aortic regurgitation, the left ventricular diastolic pressure may transiently exceed that in the aortic root resulting in actual opening of the aortic valve in diastole.

• There may be SAMs of the mitral valve, probably from increased and rapid flow. Because the left ventricular outflow is large,

the SAMs do not touch the ventricular septum and are not associated with outflow obstruction. IHSS can coexist with aortic valve disease but should be diagnosed only when the entire echocardiographic picture of IHSS is present.

• The aortic leaflets may appear structurally normal when the disease process is mild, when they have been perforated from previous endocarditis, or when aortic root dilatation is responsible for the aortic incompetence.

• Diastolic flutter of the aortic valve may be observed in patients with unsupported, flail cusps resulting from bacterial endocarditis or trauma.

Role of echocardiography

• Almost all patients with aortic regurgitation show mitral diastolic flutter. Notable exceptions are the presence of calcific mitral valve disease and a large vegetation involving the aortic valve, which may reduce the impact of the regurgitant jet on the mitral leaflets by altering its direction.

• Echocardiography can rule out mitral stenosis coexisting with aortic incompetence and show that the mitral diastolic murmur is of the Austin-Flint variety and produced by abnormal flow (Fig. 4-73).

• The size of the left ventricular cavity and the status of the aortic valve can also be evaluated.

FUNCTIONAL OBSERVATIONS

Alterations in cardiac function can change the waveform of the mitral valve echocardiogram and should not be confused with intrinsic disease of the mitral valve or of the supporting apparatus.

• Very rapid heart rates shorten the length of diastole so that the A wave blends with the EF slope and therefore appears to be absent.

• In atrial fibrillation the A waves disappear, and there may be a rolling undulation of the anterior mitral leaflet in diastole (Fig. 4-75). This should not be confused with the rapid flutters seen in aortic regurgitation. High recording speeds are useful in the differentiation. The posterior left atrial wall may show coarse undulations in atrial fibrillation.

• When atrial fibrillation is relatively slow,

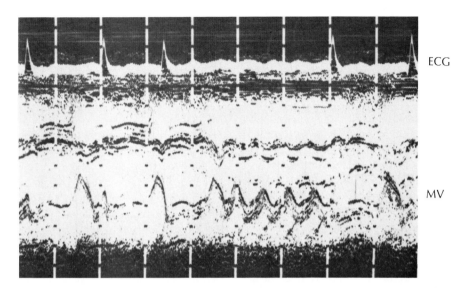

Fig. 4-75. Mitral valve recording in atrial flutter–fibrillation. Both leaflets of the mitral valve (MV) show coarse undulations in diastole resulting from rapid and irregular atrial activity. ECG, electrocardiogram. (Courtesy Cardiology Division, Genesee Hospital, Rochester, N.Y.)

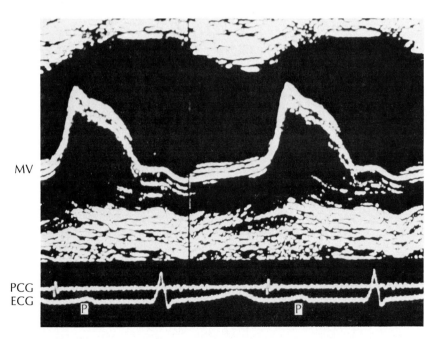

Fig. 4-76. Mitral valve recording in first-degree heart block. The PR interval is elongated, and atrial systole moves the mitral valve to a closed position. An additional posterior deflection of the trace is recorded during the isometric ventricular contraction, followed by normal gradual anterior motion during systole. This pattern could be easily confused with mitral valve prolapse if no reference is made to a simultaneously recorded electrocardiogram.

the mitral valve may exhibit several peaks in diastole that may have the appearance of A waves. They are, however, often multiple and can occur earlier in diastole than true A waves.

• Premature ventricular contraction closing the valve in diastole in a patient with mitral stenosis can create the impression that a rapid EF slope is present. EF slopes should never be evaluated under these circumstances. This may also be commonly seen with atrial fibrillation (short R-R intervals) when ventricular contraction occurs just after the opening movement of the mitral valve, bringing the valve to an early and abrupt closure.

• Heart block lengthens the interval between atrial and ventricular contraction (Fig. 4-76). If the P-R interval exceeds the upper normal value of 200 msec, the mitral valve may move to closure as the result of atrial systole alone. There is often a short plateau before additional posterior motion of the leaflet occurs from the onset of ventricular systole. The pattern may resemble mitral valve prolapse if careful attention is not paid to the simultaneously recorded ECG.

• In complete heart block, atrial systole may occur at any time during the cardiac cycle. In diastole, it may result in brief anterior motion of the mitral valve. During ventricular systole, no displacement or a shallow localized bulge may be present. The bulge probably results from augmentation of the normal anterior motion of the annulus produced by atrial systole.

• The amount of blood flowing through the mitral valve in diastole varies the amplitude of opening of a normal leaflet (Fig. 4-77). Recording of both valve leaflets is required to make a semiquantitative estimate of the volume transported. Large flows separate the

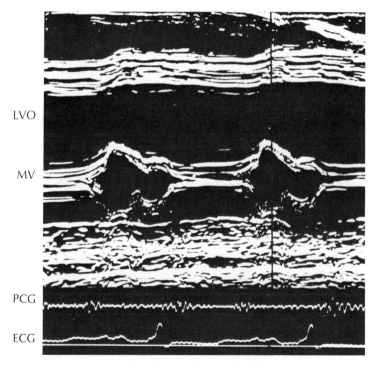

Fig. 4-77. The mitral valve (MV) shows decreased separation of the leaflets in diastole from reduced flow through the mitral orifice. The EF slopes are not significantly reduced, and A waves are present. The patient presented with congestive cardiomyopathy. LVO, left ventricular outflow; PCG, phonocardiogram; ECG, electrocardiogram.

leaflets widely, whereas low flows show decreased separation. This technique is largely experimental and has not gained clinical utility.

• Elevations of diastolic pressure in the left ventricle influence the mitral valve waveforms (Fig. 4-78). When pressure is elevated early in diastole, the mitral valve must open against an increased pressure load. The amplitude as well as the rate of mitral opening are markedly reduced, and the E-F slope flattened. Atrial systole accounts for most of the flow from the left atrium into the left ventricle, so that the A waves become very prominent and often exceed the E point in amplitude. This pattern is commonly seen in the presence of grossly dilated, failing ventricles such as those seen with severe aortic regurgitation. In ventricles that are stiff and noncompliant (usually from hypertrophy or fibrosis of the musculature) the pressure increases rapidly with atrial systole, since the stiff ventricle does not expand readily. As the result of increased pressure, the mitral valve begins to move posteriorly toward closure earlier than normally so that the peak of this motion (point A) occurs relatively earlier in the cardiac cycle. Consequently a short but prominent plateau or notch occurs in the mitral trace between A and C points and serves as a useful indicator of increased left ventricular end-diastolic pressure. A difference of less than 60 msec between the P-R interval of the ECG and the A-C interval has been shown to indicate elevations of left ventricular diastolic pressure of 20 mm Hg or more, provided the P-R intervals are 0.14 second or more in duration.

• A prominent plateau may also be seen in first-degree heart block in the absence of elevated left ventricular end-diastolic pressure. In these patients the P-R minus A-C interval is generally greater than 60 msec.

• In pulmonary hypertension the rate at

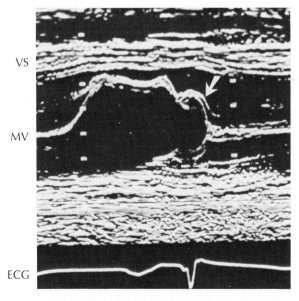

Fig. 4-78. Mitral valve recording in a patient with elevated left ventricular end-diastolic pressure. The usual smooth downstroke of the mitral valve (MV) between points A and C has been interrupted and shows a short plateau *(arrow)* in its midpoint. The A wave is shortened, and the AC interval prolonged (138 msec). The difference between the PR interval (175 msec) and the AC interval is 37 msec, well below the accepted normal value of 60 msec or more. Note that both leaflets show similar findings and that the EF slopes are flattened. VS, ventricular septum; ECG, electrocardiogram.

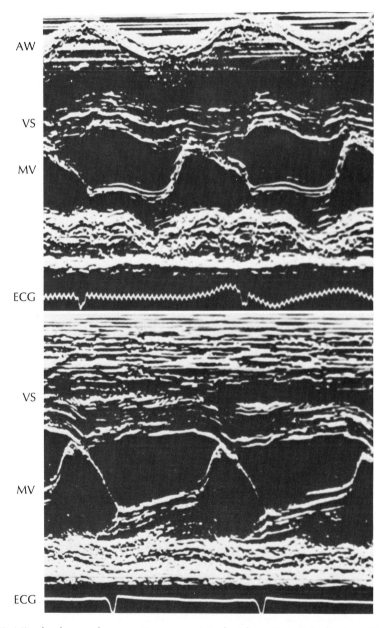

Fig. 4-79. Mitral valve prolapse pattern associated with pericardial effusion. The upper panel was recorded in the presence of a large effusion; the lower panel shows the same patient after resolution of fluid and return of normal valve motion pattern. AW, anterior right ventricular wall; VS, ventricular septum; MV, mitral valve; ECG, electrocardiogram.

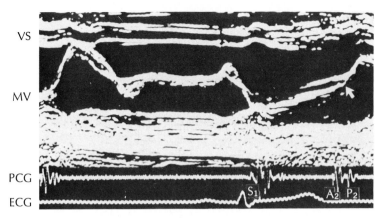

Fig. 4-80. Simultaneous recording of the mitral valve (MV) and phonocardiogram (PCG). The first heart sound (S_1) is closely related to mitral valve closure; the aortic component of the second heart sound (A_2) begins before mitral valve opening in diastole *(arrow)*. The interval between the onset of A_2 and mitral valve opening represents the isovolumic relaxation period of left ventricle. VS, ventricular septum; P_2, pulmonic component of the second heart sound; ECG, electrocardiogram.

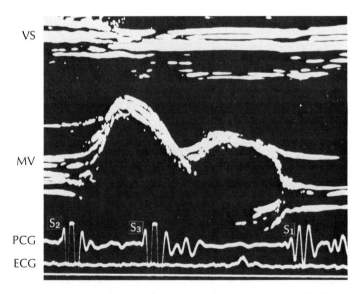

Fig. 4-81. Simultaneous recording of the mitral valve (MV) and phonocardiogram (PCG), demonstrating the presence of a prominent third heart sound (S_3) occurring during the mitral EF slope when the mitral valve is making a movement toward closure against antegrade flow from the left atrium. VS, ventricular septum; S_1, first heart sound; S_2, second heart sound; ECG, electrocardiogram.

which the mitral valve opens, the CE amplitude, and the EF slope are commonly reduced and do not indicate primary disease of the left ventricle. The etiology of this change is not clear, though we have specu-

lated that it may represent a variant of the noncompliant ventricle, since one wall of the left ventricle (the septum) may be functionally stiffened by the high pressures present in the right heart. Caution is advised, therefore, in diagnosing coexisting left heart disease when clinical or echocardiographic evidence of pulmonary hypertension is present.

• Pericardial effusions may be sufficiently large so that the heart swings in the fluid with each contraction. This motion of the entire heart is superimposed on the intrinsic motion of heart valves in systole, so that patterns simulating SAM or mitral valve prolapse are commonly seen. Do not attempt to make diagnoses related to systolic abnormalities of mitral valve motion in the presence of a large pericardial effusion, since the findings disappear when the effusion is removed or clears following medical treatment (Fig. 4-79).

• Mitral valve motion may be correlated with acoustic events by simultaneously recording a phonocardiogram with the mitral valve echocardiogram (Figs. 4-80 and 4-81).

BIBLIOGRAPHY
Mitral stenosis

Edler, I., and Gustafson, A.: Ultrasonic cardiogram in mitral stenosis, Acta Med. Scand. **159**:85, 1957.

Joyner, C. R., Reid, J. M., and Bond, J. P.: Reflected ultrasound in the assessment of mitral valve disease, Circulation **27**:506, 1963.

Segal, B. L., Likoff, W., and Kingsley, B.: Echocardiography; clinical application in mitral stenosis, J.A.M.A. **193**:161, 1966.

Effert, S.: Pre- and post-operative evaluation of mitral stenosis by ultrasound, Am. J. Cardiol. **19**:59, 1967.

Gustafson, A.: Correlation between ultrasound-cardiography, haemodynamics and surgical findings in mitral stenosis, Am. J. Cardiol. **19**:32, 1967.

Zaky, A., Nasser, W. K., and Feigenbaum, H.: Study of mitral valve action recorded by reflected ultrasound and its application in the diagnosis of mitral stenosis, Circulation **37**:789, 1968.

Silver, W., Rodriquez-Torres, R., and Newfelt, E.: The echocardiogram in a case of mitral stenosis before and after surgery, Am. Heart J. **78**:811, 1969.

Duchak, J. M., Jr., Chang, S., and Feigenbaum, H.: The posterior mitral valve echo and the echocardiographic diagnosis of mitral stenosis, Am. J. Cardiol. **29**:628, 1972.

Freeman, J. J., Hitt, J. S., and Rinaldo, J. A.: Mitral leaflet velocity in the determination of mitral stenosis, Med. Res. Eng. **11**:4-6, 1972.

Lundstrom, N. R.: Echocardiography in the diagnosis of congenital mitral stenosis and an evaluation of the results of mitral valvolotomy, Circulation **46**:44, 1972.

Nanda, N. C., Gramiak, R., Shah, P. M., and Lipchik,

E. O.: Ultrasound evaluation of mitral valve calcification, Circulation **46**(suppl 2):20, 1972 (abstract).

McLaurin, L. P., Gibson, T. C., Waider, W., Grossman, W., and Craige, E.: An appraisal of mitral valve echocardiograms mimicking mitral stenosis in conditions with right ventricular pressure overload, Circulation **48**:801, 1973.

Abbasi, A. S., Ellis, N., and Levisman, J. A.: Normal posterior mitral leaflet motion in mitral stenosis, J. Clin. Ultrasound **2**:221, 1974 (abstract).

Quinones, M. A., Gaasch, W. H., Waisser, E., and Alexander, J. K.: Reduction in the rate of diastolic descent of the mitral valve echogram in patients with altered left ventricular diastolic pressure—volume relations, Circulation **49**:246, 1974.

Bellin, H., and Towe, J.: Ultrasonic-cardiographic long-term observations in patients with operated stenosis of the mitral valve, Bibl. Cardiol. **33**:191-194, 1975.

Berman, N. D., Gilbert, B. W., McLaughlin, P. R., and Morch, J. E.: Mitral stenosis with posterior diastolic movement of posterior leaflet, Can. Med. Assoc. J. **112**:976-979, 1975.

Cope, G. D., Kisslo, J. A., Johnson, M. L., and Behar, V. S.: A reassessment of the echocardiogram in mitral stenosis, Circulation **52**:664, 1975.

Dashkoff, N., Karakushensky, M., and Fortuin, N. J.: Echocardiographic features of mitral annulus calcification, Circulation **52**(suppl 2):34, 1975 (abstract).

Flaherty, J. T., Livengood, S., and Fortuin, N. J.: Atypical posterior leaflet motion in echocardiogram in mitral stenosis, Am. J. Cardiol. **35**:675-678, 1975.

Gross, C. M., Gramiak, R., and Nanda, N. C.: Echocardiography in chronic rheumatic mitral valve disease, Chest **68**:569-572, 1975.

Henry, W. L., Griffith, J. M., Michaelis, L. L., McIntosh, C. L., Morrow, A. G., and Epstein, S. F.: Measurement of mitral orifice area in patients with mitral valve disease by real-time, two-dimensional echocardiography, Circulation **51**:827-831, 1975.

Hirschfeld, D. S., and Emilson, B. B.: Echocardiogram in calcified mitral annulus, Am. J. Cardiol. **36**:354-356, 1975.

Krueger, S., Starke, H., Miscia, V. F., and Forker, A. D.: Echocardiographic diagnosis of silent mitral stenosis, Nebr. Med. J. **60**:159-161, 1975.

Nanda, N. C., Gramiak, R., and Shah, P. M.: Echocardiographic misdiagnosis of the severity of mitral stenosis, Clin. Res. **23**:199A, 1975 (abstract).

Nanda, N. C., Gramiak, R., Shah, P. M., and DeWeese, J. A.: Mitral commissurotomy versus replacement; pre-operative evaluation by echocardiography, Circulation **51**:263, 1975.

Starek, P. J. K., Gibson, T. C., Wilcox, B. R., and Murray, G. F.: The echocardiogram in the assessment of mitral valve area, Am. J. Cardiol. **35**:170, 1975 (abstract).

Ticzon, A. R., Demato, A. N., Caracta, A. R., Lau, S. H., and Gross, L.: Echocardiographic manifestation of "false" mitral stenosis that was, Ann. Intern. Med. **83**:503, 1975.

Yousof, A. M., Endrys, J., and Zyka, I.: The effect of atrial pacing on the mitral echocardiogram of mitral stenosis recorded simultaneously with haemodynamic data, Cor. Vasa 17:262-268, 1975.

Cachfra, J. P., Brun, P., Laurent, F., Loisance, D., Bloch, G., and Galey, J. J.: Surgery for mitral stenosis; comparative evaluation of the different procedures; interest of pre- and post-operative echocardiography. In Kalmanson, D., editor: The mitral valve, Acton, Mass., 1976, Publishing Sciences Group, Inc., pp. 559-568.

Gabor, G. E., Mohr, B. D., Goel, P. C., and Cohen, B.: Echocardiographic and clinical spectrum of mitral annular calcification, Am. J. Cardiol. 38:836-842, 1976.

Lundstrom, N. R.: Proceedings; value of echocardiography in diagnosis of congenital mitral stenosis, Br. Heart J. 38:534-535, 1976.

Pathak, L., Pai, R. R., and Nair, K. G.: Pre and post operative evaluation of mitral stenosis by echocardiography, Indian Heart J. 28:158-164, 1976.

Raj, M. V. J., Bennett, D. H., Stovin, P. G. I., and Evans, D. W.: Echocardiographic assessment of mitral valve calcification, Br. Heart J. 38:81, 1976.

Nichol, P. M., Gilbert, B. W., and Kisslo, J. A.: Two-dimensional echocardiographic assessment of mitral stenosis, Circulation 55:120-128, 1977.

Ridges, J. D., Pryor, T. A., and Parker, D. L.: Intraventricular septal motion in mitral stenosis. In White, D. N., and Brown, R. E., editors: Ultrasound in medicine, Vol. 3, New York, 1977, Plenum Publishing Corporation, p. 227.

Toutouzas, P., Velimezis, A., Karayannis, E., and Avgoustakis, D.: End-diastolic amplitude of mitral valve echogram in mitral stenosis, Br. Heart J. 39: 73-79, 1977.

Mitral valve prolapse/mitral regurgitation

Joyner, C. R., Dyrda, I., Barrett, J. S., and Reid, J. M.: Preoperative determination of the functional anatomy of the mitral valve, Circulation 32(suppl 2):120, 1965 (abstract).

Joyner, C. R., and Reid, J. M.: Ultrasound cardiogram in the selection of patients for mitral valve surgery, Ann. N. Y. Acad. Sci. 118:512, 1965.

Segal, B. L., Likoff, W., and Kingsley, B.: Echocardiography: clinical application in mitral regurgitation, Am. J. Cardiol. 19:50, 1967.

Winters, W. L., Jr., Hafer, J., Jr., and Soloff, L. A.: Abnormal mitral valve motion as demonstrated by the ultrasound technique in apparent pure mitral insufficiency, Am. Heart J. 77:196, 1969.

Dillon, J. C., Haine, C. L., Chang, S., and Feigenbaum, H.: Use of echocardiography in patients with prolapsed mitral valve, Am. J. Cardiol. 26:630, 1970 (abstract).

Shah, P. M., and Gramiak, R.: Echocardiographic recognition of mitral valve prolapse, Circulation 42(suppl 3):45, 1970 (abstract).

Dillon, J. C., Haine, C. L., Chang, S., and Feigenbaum, H.: Use of echocardiography in patients with prolapsed mitral valve, Circulation 43:503, 1971.

Kerber, R. E., Isaeff, D. M., and Hancock, E. W.: Echocardiographic patterns in patients with the syndrome of systolic click and late systolic murmur, N. Engl. J. Med. 284:691, 1971.

Duchak, J. M., Jr., Chang, S., and Feigenbaum, H.: Echocardiographic features of torn chordae tendineae, Am. J. Cardiol. 29:260, 1972 (abstract).

Sweatman, T., Selzer, A., Kamagaki, M., and Cohn, K.: Echocardiographic diagnosis of mitral regurgitation due to ruptured chordae tendineae, Circulation 46:580, 1972.

Tallury, V. K., DePasquale, N. P., and Burch, G. E.: The echocardiogram in papillary muscle dysfunction, Am. Heart J. 83:12, 1972.

Burgess, J., Clark, R., Kamigaki, M., and Cohn, K.: Echocardiographic findings in different types of mitral regurgitation, Circulation 48:97, 1973.

Kim, H., Kinoshita, M., Shirahama, Y., Tomonaga, G., and Kusukawa, R.: An attempt to correlate the mitral valve echogram with the hemodynamics of patients with pure mitral insufficiency, Jpn. Circ. J. 37:403, 1973.

Millward, D. K., McLaurin, L. P., and Craige, E.: Echocardiographic studies of the mitral valve in patients with congestive cardiomyopathy and mitral regurgitation, Am. Heart J. 85:413, 1973.

Nanda, N. C., Shah, P. M., Robinson, T. I., and Gramiak, R.: Echocardiographic evaluation of valve dysfunction in mitral regurgitation, Clin. Res. 21:71A, 1973.

DeMaria, A. N., King, J. F., Bogren, H. G., Lies, J. E., and Mason, D. T.: The variable spectrum of echocardiographic manifestations of the mitral valve prolapse syndrome, Circulation 50:33, 1974.

Giles, T. D., Burch, G. E., and Martinez, E. C.: Value of exploratory "scanning" in the echocardiographic diagnosis of ruptured chordae tendineae, Circulation 49:678, 1974.

Popp, R. L., Brown, O. R., Silverman, J. F., and Harrison, D. C.: Echocardiographic abnormalities in the mitral valve prolapse syndrome, Circulation 49:428, 1974.

Brown, O. R., Kloster, F. E., and DeMots, H.: Incidence of mitral valve prolapse in the asymptomatic normal, Circulation 53(suppl. 2):77, 1975 (abstract).

Brown, O. R., and Kloster, F. E.: Echocardiographic criteria for mitral valve prolapse: effect of transducer position, Circulation 52(suppl. 2):165, 1975.

Hirschfeld, D. S., and Emilson, B. B.: Echocardiogram in calcified mitral annulus, Am. J. Cardiol. 36:354, 1975.

Jeresaty, R. M., Landry, A. B., Jr., and Liss, J. P.: "Silent" mitral valve prolapse, analysis of 32 cases, Am. J. Cardiol. 35:146, 1975 (abstract).

Markiewicz, W., Stoner, J., London, E., Hunt, S. A., and Popp, R. L.: Mitral valve prolapse in one hundred presumably healthy females, Circulation 52(suppl. 2): 77, 1975 (abstract).

Pasquale, M. P., Savran, S. V., Schreiter, S. L., and Bryson, A. L.: Clinical frequency and implications of mitral valve prolapse in the female population, Circulation **52**(suppl. 2):78, 1975 (abstract).

Roye, J. A., and Lotfy, L. B.: Echographic pattern of mitral valve prolapse produced with special maneuvers in healthy individuals, Circulation **52**(suppl. 2):235, 1975.

Sahn, D. J., and Friedman, W. F.: Cross-sectional echocardiographic evaluation of mitral valve prolapse in children, Am. J. Cardiol. **35**:179, 1975 (abstract).

Schwartz, D. C., Kaplan, S., and Meyer, R. A.: Mitral valve prolapse in children; clinical, echocardiographic, and cine-angiographic findings in 81 cases, Am. J. Cardiol. **35**:169, 1975 (abstract).

Weiss, A. N., Mimbs, J. W., Ludbrook, P. A., and Sobel, B. E.: Echocardiographic detection of mitral valve prolapse; exclusion of false positive diagnosis and determination of inheritance, Circulation **52**:1091, 1975.

Winkle, R. A., Goodman, D. J., and Popp, R. L.: Simultaneous echocardiographic–phonocardiographic recordings at rest and during amyl nitrite administration in patients with mitral valve prolapse, Circulation **51**:522, 1975.

Yoshikawa, J., Kato, H., Owaki, T., and Tanaka, K.: Study of posterior left atrial wall motion by echocardiography and its clinical application, Jpn. Heart J. **16**:683-693, 1975.

Desser, K. B., Benchimol, A., and Sheasby, C.: Apexcardiographic-echocardiographic correlation in mitral valve prolapse, Chest **70**:68-69, 1976.

Gilbert, B. W., Schatz, R. A., Vonramm, O. T., Behar, V. S., and Kisslo, J. A.: Mitral valve prolapse, two-dimensional echocardiographic and angiographic correlation, Circulation **54**:716-723, 1976.

Owens, J. S., Kotler, M. N., Segal, B. L., and Parry, W.: Pseudoprolapse of the mitral valve in a patient with pericardial effusion, Chest **69**:214-215, 1976.

Patton, R., Dragatakis, L., and Sniderman, A.: Augmented left atrial filling—a new echocardiographic sign of mitral insufficiency, Circulation **54**(suppl. 2):169, 1976.

Reeves, W., Griggs, R., Nanda, N. C., and Gramiak, R.: Echocardiographic demonstration of mitral valve prolapse in muscular dystrophy, Circulation **54**(suppl. 2):97, 1976.

Sahn, D. J., Allen, H. D., Goldberg, S. J., and Friedman, W. F.: Mitral valve prolapse in children, a problem defined by real-time cross-sectional echocardiography, Circulation **53**:651, 1976.

Winters, S. J., Schreiner, B., Griggs, R. C., Rowley, P., and Nanda, N. C.: Familial mitral valve prolapse and myotonic dystrophy, Ann. Intern. Med. **85**:19, 1976.

Chandraratna, P. A. N., Tolentino, A. O., and Mutucumarana, W.: Echocardiographic observations on the association between mitral valve prolapse and asymmetric septal hypertrophy. In White, D. N., and Brown, R. E., editors: Ultrasound in medicine, vol. 3, New York, 1977, Plenum Publishing Corporation, p. 231.

Levisman, J. A.: Echocardiographic diagnosis of mitral regurgitation in congestive cardiomyopathy, Am. Heart J. **93**:33-39, 1977.

Meyer, J. F., Frank, M. J., Goldberg, S., and Cheng, T. O.: Systolic mitral flutter, an echocardiographic clue to the diagnosis of ruptured chordae tendineae, Am. Heart J. **93**:3-8, 1977.

Reiffel, J. A., Green, W. M., King, D. L., and Manni, C.: Augmentation of auscultatory and echocardiographic mitral valve prolapse by atrial premature depolarizations, Am. Heart J. **93**:533, 1977.

Sahn, D. J., Wood, J., Allen, H. D., Peoples, W., and Goldberg, S. J.: Echocardiographic spectrum of mitral valve motion in children with and without mitral valve prolapse; the nature of false positive diagnosis, Am. J. Cardiol. **39**:422-431, 1977.

Ticzon, A. R., Damato, A. N., Kennedy, F. B., Francis, L. J., Leonard, B. J., and Moran, H. E.: The effects of arrhythmias on the echocardiographic findings of patients with and without mitral valve prolapse, Clin. Res. **25**:258A, 1977.

Mitral valve vegetations

Dillon, J. C., Feigenbaum, H., Konecke, L. L., Davis, R. H., and Chang, S.: Echocardiographic manifestations of valvular vegetations, Am. Heart J. **86**:698, 1973.

Spangler, R. D., Johnson, M. D., Holmes, J. H., and Blount, S. G., Jr.: Echocardiographic demonstration of bacterial vegetations in active infective endocarditis, J. Clin. Ultrasound, **1**:126, 1973.

Estevez, C. M., and Corya, B. C.: Serial echocardiographic abnormalities in nonbacterial thrombotic endocarditis of the mitral valve, Chest **69**:801-804, 1976.

Gomes, J. A., Calderon, J., Lajam, F., Sakurai, H., and Friedman, H. S.: Echocardiographic detection of fungal vegetations in Candida Parasilopsis endocarditis, Am. J. Med. **61**:273-276, 1976.

Nomeir, A. M., Watts, E., and Philp, J. R.: Bacterial endocarditis, echocardiographic and clinical evaluation during therapy, J. Clin. Ultrasound **4**:23-27, 1976.

Sutton, R., Petch, M., and Parker, J.: Echocardiography in infective endocarditis, Br. Heart J. **38**:312, 1976.

Wann, L. S., Dillon, J. C., Weyman, A. E., and Feigenbaum, H.: Echocardiography in bacterial endocarditis, N. Engl. J. Med. **295**:135-139, 1976.

Bouchner, C. A., Tallon, J. T., Myers, G. S., Hutter, A. M., and Buckley, M. J.: The value and limitations of echocardiography in recording mitral valve vegetations, Am. Heart J. **84**:37, 1977.

Gilbert, B. W., Haney, R. S., Crawford, F., McClellan, J., Gallis, H. A., Johnson, M. L., and Kisslo, J. A.: Two-dimensional echocardiographic assessment of vegetative endocarditis, Circulation **55**:346-353, 1977.

Sze, K. C., Nanda, N. C., and Gramiak, R.: Systolic

flutter of the mitral valve, Circulation **56**(suppl. 3): 50, 1977.

Thomson, K. R., Nanda, N. C., and Gramiak, R.: The reliability of echocardiography in the diagnosis of infective endocarditis. In White, D. N., and Brown, R. E., editors: Ultrasound in medicine, vol. 3, New York, 1977, Plenum Publishing Corporation, p. 53.

Idiopathic hypertrophic subaortic stenosis

Popp, R. L., and Harrison, D. C.: Ultrasound in the diagnosis and evaluation of therapy of idiopathic hypertrophic subaortic stenosis, Circulation **40**:905, 1969.

Shah, P. M., Gramiak, R., and Kramer, D. H.: Ultrasound localization of left ventricular outflow obstruction in hypertrophic obstructive cardiomyopathy, Circulation **40**:3, 1969.

Pridie, R. B., and Oakley, C. M.: Mechanism of mitral regurgitation in hypertrophic obstructive cardiomyopathy, Br. Heart J. **32**:203, 1970.

Shah, P. M., Gramiak, R., Adelman, A. G., and Wigle, E. D.: Role of echocardiography in diagnostic and hemodynamic assessment of hypertrophic subaortic stenosis, Circulation **44**:891, 1971.

Abbasi, A. S., MacAlpin, R. N., Eber, L. M., and Pearce, M. L.: Echocardiographic diagnosis of idiopathic hypertrophic cardiomyopathy without outflow obstruction, Circulation **46**:897, 1972.

Shah, P. M., Gramiak, R., Adelman, A. G., and Wigle, E. D.: Echocardiographic assessment of the effects of surgery and propranolol on the dynamics of outflow obstruction and hypertrophic subaortic stenosis, Circulation **45**:516, 1972.

Tajik, A. J., Gau, G. T., and Schattenberg, T. T.: Echocardiographic pseudo IHSS pattern in atrial septal defect, Chest **62**:324, 1972.

Clark, C. E., Henry, W. L., and Epstein, S. E.: Familial prevalence and genetic transmission of idiopathic hypertrophic subaortic stenosis, N. Engl. J. Med. **289**:709, 1973.

Hardarson, T., and Curiel, R.: Study of clinical pharmacology of hypertrophic obstructive cardiomyopathy by noninvasive diagnostic investigations, Br. Heart J. **35**:865, 1973.

Henry, W. L., Clark, C. E., and Epstein, S. E.: Asymmetric septal hypertrophy (ASH); echocardiographic identification of the pathognomonic anatomic abnormality of IHSS, Circulation **47**:225, 1973.

Henry, W. L., Clark, C. E., and Epstein, S. E.: Asymmetric septal hypertrophy; the unifying link in the IHSS disease spectrum; observations regarding its pathogenesis, pathophysiology, and course, Circulation **47**:827, 1973.

Henry, W. L., Clark, C. E., Glancy, D. L., and Epstein, S. E.: Echocardiographic measurement of the left ventricular outflow gradient in idiopathic hypertrophic subaortic stenosis, N. Engl. J. Med. **288**:989, 1973.

King, J. F., DeMaria, A. N., Reis, R. L., Bolton, M. R., Dunn, M. I., and Mason, D. T.: Echocardiographic assessment of idiopathic hypertrophic subaortic stenosis, Chest **64**:723, 1973.

Allen, H. D., Larter, W., and Goldberg, S. J.: Further differentiation of the asymmetrically thickened septum, Circulation **50**(suppl. 3):29, 1974 (abstract).

Bolton, M. R., Jr., King, J. F., Polumbo, R. A., Mason, D., Pugh, D. M., Reis, R. L., and Dunn, M. I.: The effects of operation on the echocardiographic features of idiopathic hypertrophic subaortic stenosis, Circulation **50**:897, 1974.

Chung, K. J., Manning, J. A., and Gramiak, R.: Echocardiography in coexisting hypertrophic subaortic stenosis and fixed left ventricular outflow obstruction, Circulation **49**:673, 1974.

Cooperman, L. B., Rosenblum, R., and Cohen, M. V.: Abnormal septal contraction in idiopathic hypertrophic subaortic stenosis, Circulation **50**(suppl. 3):29, 1974 (abstract).

Epstein, S. E., Henry, W. L., Clark, C. E., Roberts, W. C., Maron, B. J., Ferrans, V. J., Redwood, D. R., and Morrow, A. G.: Asymmetric septal hypertrophy, Ann. Intern. Med. **81**:650, 1974.

Henry, W. L., Clark, C. E., Roberts, W. C., Morrow, A. G., and Epstein, S. E.: Differences in distribution of myocardial abnormalities in patients with obstructive and non-obstructive asymmetric septal hypertrophy (ASH); echocardiographic and gross anatomic findings, Circulation **50**:447, 1974.

King, J. F., DeMaria, A. N., Miller, R. R., Hilliard, G. K., Zelis, R., and Mason, D. T.: Markedly abnormal mitral valve motion without simultaneous intraventricular pressure gradient due to uneven mitral-septal contact in idiopathic hypertrophic subaortic stenosis, Am. J. Cardiol. **34**:360, 1974.

Nanda, N. C., Gramiak, R., Shah, P. M., Stewart, S., and DeWeese, J. A.: Echocardiography in the diagnosis of idiopathic hypertrophic subaortic stenosis coexisting with aortic valve disease, Circulation **50**:752, 1974.

Rossen, R. M., Goodman, D. J., Ingham, R. E., and Popp, R. L.: Echocardiographic criteria in the diagnosis of idiopathic hypertrophic subaortic stenosis, Circulation **50**:747, 1974.

Rossen, R. M., Goodman, D. J., Ingham, R. E., and Popp, R. L.: Ventricular septal thickening and excursion in idiopathic hypertrophic subaortic stenosis, Circulation **50**(suppl. 3):29, 1974 (abstract).

TenCate, F. J., Roelandt, J., Vletter, W. B., and Hugenholtz, P. G.: Asymmetric septal hypertrophy; entirely a familial disease? Circulation **50**(suppl. 3): 17, 1974 (abstract).

Boughner, D. R., Schuld, R. L., and Persaud, J. A.: Hypertrophic obstructive cardiomyopathy; assessment by echocardiographic and doppler ultrasound techniques, Br. Heart J. **37**:917, 1975.

Cohen, M. V., Cooperman, L. B., and Rosenblum, R.: Regional myocardial function in idiopathic hypertrophic subaortic stenosis; an echocardiographic study, Circulation **52**:842, 1975.

Feizi, O., and Emanuel, R.: Echocardiographic spectrum of hypertrophic cardiomyopathy, Br. Heart J. 37:1286, 1975.

Greenwald, J., Yap, J. F., Franklin, M., and Licktman, A. M.: Echocardiographic mitral systolic motion in left ventricular aneurysm, Br. Heart J. 37:684, 1975.

Henry, W. L., Clark, C. E., Griffith, J. M., and Epstein, S. E.: Mechanism of left ventricular outflow obstruction in patients with obstructive asymmetric septal hypertrophy (idiopathic hypertrophic subaortic stenosis), Am. J. Cardiol. 35:337, 1975.

Johnson, A. D., Lonky, S. A., and Carleton, R. A.: Combined hypertrophic subaortic stenosis and calcific aortic vascular stenosis, Am. J. Cardiol. 35:706, 1975.

Shah, P. M.: IHSS—HOCM—MSS—ASH? Editorial on the naming of disease states. Circulation 51:577, 1975.

Smith, E. R., and Flemington, C. S.: Systolic muscle thickening and excursion in patients with asymmetric septal hypertrophy, Circulation 52(suppl. 2):141, 1975 (abstract).

Stewart, S., Nanda, N. C., and DeWeese, J. A.:Simultaneous operative correction of aortic valve stenosis and idiopathic hypertrophic subaortic stenosis, Circulation 52(suppl. 1):34, 1975.

Wise, D. E., Livengood, S., and Fortuin, N. J.: Clinical and echocardiographic aspects of asymmetric septal hypertrophy, Am. J. Cardiol. 35:178, 1975 (abstract).

Boughner, D. R., and Persaud, J. A.: Parachute mitral valve; echocardiographic findings resembling idiopathic hypertrophic subaortic stenosis, J. Clin. Ultrasound 4:213-217, 1976.

Cohen, M. V., Teichholz, L. F., and Gorlin, R.: B-scan ultrasonography in idiopathic hypertrophic subaortic stenosis; study of left ventricular outflow tract and mechanism of obstruction, Br. Heart J. 38:595-604, 1976.

Frazien, L. J., Talano, J. V., Stephanide, L., Loeb, H. S., and Gunnar, R. M.: Esophageal echocardiography for evaluation of left ventricular outflow obstruction, Clin. Res. 24:218A, 1976.

Gehrke, J. Proceedings; new observations on systolic anterior motion of mitral valve leaflets in hypertrophic cardiomyopathy, Br. Heart J. 38:314, 1976.

Gehrke, J., and Leeman, S.: Proceedings; Grey scale, a valuable tool in the differential diagnosis of hypertrophic cardiomyopathy, Br. J. Radiol. 49:730, 1976.

Larter, W. E., Allen, H. D., Sahn, D. J., and Goldberg, S. J.: The asymmetrically hypertrophied septum; further differentiation of its causes, Circulation 53:19, 1976.

Sze, K. C., and Shah, P. M.: Pseudoejection sound in hypertrophic subaortic stenosis; an echocardiographic correlative study, Circulation 54:504-509, 1976.

Toshima, H., Koga, Y., Uemura, S., Zinnouchi, J., and Kimura, N.: Echocardiographic study on hypertrophic cardiomyopathy, Jpn. Heart J. 17:275-289, 1976.

Weyman, A. E., Feigenbaum, H., Hurwitz, R. A., Girod, D. A., Dillon, J. C., and Chang, S.: Localization of left ventricular outflow obstruction by cross-sectional echocardiography, Am. J. Med. 60:33-38, 1976.

Williams, D. E., Sahn, D. J., and Friedman, W. F.: Cross-sectional echocardiographic localization of sites of left ventricular outflow tract obstruction, Am. J. Cardiol. 37:250, 1976.

Lombardi, A., Nanda, N., and Gramiak, R.: Significance of abnormal mitral systolic anterior movements; echocardiographic observations. In White, D. M., and Brown, R. E., editors: Ultrasound in medicine, vol. 3, New York, 1977, Plenum Publishing Corporation, p. 81.

Nanda, N. C., Reeves, W. C., and Gramiak, R.: Abnormal systolic anterior motion of atrioventricular valves in complete heart block; echocardiographic studies. In White, D. N., and Brown, R. E., editors: Ultrasound in medicine, vol. 3, New York, 1977, Plenum Publishing Corporation, p. 113.

Reeves, W. C., Shah, P. M., Lever, H. M., Nanda, N. C., and Gramiak, R.: Clinical and echocardiographic progression of hypertrophic subaortic stenosis, Clin. Res. 25:248A, 1977.

Spilkin, S., Mitha, A. S., Matisonn, R. E., and Chesler, E.: Complete heart block in a case of idiopathic hypertrophic subaortic stenosis; noninvasive correlates with the timing of atrial systole, Circulation 55:418-422, 1977.

Other cardiomyopathies

Abbasi, A. S., Ellis, N., and Child, J.: Echocardiographic features of infiltrative cardiomyopathy, J. Clin. Ultrasound 2:221, 1974 (abstract).

Borer, J. S., Henry, W. L., and Epstein, S. E.: Echocardiographic characteristics of infiltrative cardiomyopathy, Circulation 50(suppl. 3):217, 1974 (abstract).

Nimura, Y., Nagata, S., Matsumoto, M., Beppu, S., and Tamai, M.: An unusual pattern of the mitral echocardiogram observed in cases of congestive cardiomyopathy and other myocardial diseases, Jpn. Heart J. 16:500-511, 1975.

Borer, J. S., Henry, W. L., and Epstein, S. E.: Echocardiographic observations in patients with systemic infiltrative disease involving the heart, Am. J. Cardiol. 39:184-188, 1977.

Gottdiener, J. S., Sherber, H. S., Hawley, R. J., and Engle, W. K.: Cardiac involvement in polymyositis; a non-invasive study, Clin. Res. 25:224A, 1977.

Left atrium

Hirata, T., Wolfe, S. B., Popp, R. L., Helmen, C. H., and Feigenbaum, H.: Estimation of left atrial size using ultrasound, Am. Heart J. 78:43, 1969.

Allen, H. D., and Goldberg, S. J.: Usefulness of biaxial

left atrial dimension measurements by echocardiography, J. Clin. Ultrasound 2:222, 1974 (abstract).

Brown, O. R., Harrison, D. C., and Popp, R. L.: An improved method for echographic detection of left atrial enlargement, Circulation 50:58, 1974.

Francis, G. S., and Hagan, A. D.: Echocardiographic criteria of normal left atrial size in adults, Circulation 50(suppl. 3):76, 1974 (abstract).

Lundstrom, N. R., and Mortensson, W.: Clinical applications of echocardiography in infants and children. II. Estimation of aortic root diameter and left atrial size; a comparison between echocardiography and angiocardiography, Acta Paediatr. Scand. 63:33, 1974.

Sasse, L.: Echocardiography of left atrial wall, J.A.M.A. 228:1667, 1974.

TenCate, F. J., Kloster, F. E., VanDorp, W. G., Meester, G. T., and Roelandt, J.: Dimensions and volumes of left atrium and ventricle determined by single beam echocardiography, Br. Heart J. 36:737, 1974.

Chirife, R., Feitosa, G. S., Frankl, W. S.: Electrocardiographic detection of left atrial enlargement, correlation of P wave with left atrial dimension by echocardiography, Br. Heart J. 37:1281-1285, 1975.

Termini, B. A., and Lee, Y. C.: Echocardiographic and electrocardiographic criteria for diagnosing left atrial enlargement, South Med. J. 68:161-165, 1975.

Chandraratna, P. A., Nanda, N. C., Shah, P. M., Hodges, M., and Gramiak, R.: Echocardiographic study of the effects of acute left atrial hypertension on left atrial size, J. Clin. Ultrasound 4:15-18, 1976.

Garber, E. B., Morgan, M. G., and Glasser, S. P.: Left atrial size in patients with atrial fibrillation; an echocardiographic study, Am. J. Med. Sci. 272:57-64, 1976.

Henry, W. L., Morganroth, J., Pearlman, A. S., Clark, C. E., Redwood, D. R., Itscoitz, S. B., and Epstein, S. E.: Relation between echocardiographically determined left atrial size and atrial fibrillation, Circulation 53:273-279, 1976.

Lemire, F., Tajik, A. J., and Hagler, D. J.: Asymmetric left atrial enlargement; an echocardiographic observation, Chest 69:779-781, 1976.

Waggoner, A. D., Adyanthaya, A. V., Quinones, M. A., Alexander, J. K.: Left atrial enlargement; echocardiographic assessment of electrocardiographic criteria, Circulation 54:553-557, 1976.

Josephson, M. E., Kastor, J. A., Morganroth, J.: Electrocardiographic left atrial enlargement; electrophysiologic, echocardiographic and hemodynamic correlates, Am. J. Cardiol. 39:967, 1977.

Left atrial tumor

Effert, S., and Domanig, E.: The diagnosis of intra-atrial tumor and thrombi by the ultrasonic echo method, Ger. Med. 4:1, 1959.

Schattenberg, T. T.: Echocardiographic diagnosis of left atrial myxoma, Mayo Clin. Proc. 43:620, 1968.

Popp, R. L., and Harrison, D. C.: Ultrasound in the diagnosis of atrial tumor, Ann. Intern. Med. 71:785, 1969.

Wolfe, S. B., Popp, R. L., and Feigenbaum, H.: Diagnosis of atrial tumors by ultrasound, Circulation 39:615, 1969.

Finegan, R. E., and Harrison, D. C.: Diagnosis of left atrial myxoma by echocardiography, N. Engl. J. Med. 282:1022, 1970.

Kostis, J. B., and Moghadam, A. N.: Echocardiographic diagnosis of left atrial myxoma, Chest 58:550, 1970.

Matsumoto, M., Matsuo, H., Nagata, S., Oyama, S., Nimura, Y., Asoh, M., Miyazaki, H., Hamaji, M., Nakata, T., Kobayashi, Y., and Shimada, H.: Left atrial myxoma detected by ultrasound cardiogram, Med. Ultrason. 10:9, 1972.

Nasser, W. K., Davis, R. H., Dillon, J. C., and others: Atrial myxoma. I: Clinical and pathologic features in nine cases, Am. Heart J. 83:694, 1972.

Nasser, W. K., Davis, R. H., Dillon, J. C., and others: Atrial myxoma. II: Phonocardiographic, echocardiographic, hemodynamic and angiographic features in nine cases, Am. Heart J. 83:810, 1972.

Bass, N. M., and Sharratt, G. P.: Left atrial myxoma diagnosed by echocardiography, with observations on tumour movement, Br. Heart J. 35:1332, 1973.

Gustafson, A., Edler, I., Dahlback, O., Kaude, J., and Persson, S.: Left atrial myxoma diagnosed by ultrasound cardiography, Angiology 24:554, 1973.

Johnson, M. L., Seiker, H. O., Behar, V. S., and Whalen, R. E.: Echocardiographic diagnosis of a left atrial myxoma attached to the free left atrial wall, J. Clin. Ultrasound 1:75, 1973.

Popp, R. L., and Levine, R.: Left atrial mass simulating cardiomyopathy, J. Clin. Ultrasound 1:96, 1973.

Srivastavan, T. N., and Fletecher, E.: The echocardiogram in left atrial myxoma, Am. J. Med. 54:136, 1973.

Bodenheimer, M. M., Moscovitz, H. L., Pantazopoulous, J., and Donoso, E.: Echocardiographic features of experimental left atrial tumor, Am. Heart J. 88:615-620, 1974.

Jenzer, H. R., Follath, F., and Zutter, W.: The echocardiographic diagnosis of atrial myxoma, Schweiz Med. Wochenschr. 104:1570, 1974.

Kerber, R. E., Kelly, D. H., Jr., and Gutenkauf, C. H.: Left atrial myxoma, demonstrated by stop-action cardiac ultrasonography, Am. J. Cardiol. 34:838, 1974.

Martinez, E. C., Giles, T. D., and Burch, G. E.: Echocardiographic diagnosis of left atrial myxoma, Am. J. Cardiol. 33:281, 1974.

DeMaria, A. N., Vismara, L. A., Miller, R. R., Neumann, A., and Mason, D. T.: Unusual echographic manifestations of right and left heart myxomas, Am. J. Med. 59:713-720, 1975.

Potts, J. L., Johnson, L. W., Eich, R. H., Fruehan, C. T., and Obeid, A. I.: Varied manifestations of left atrial myxoma and the relationship of echocardiographic patterns of tumor size, Chest 68:781-784, 1975.

Watts, L. E., Nomeir, A. M., and DeMelo, R. A.:

Echocardiographic findings in patients with mitral valve prolapse mimicking left atrial tumor. In White, D. N., editor: Ultrasound in medicine, vol. 1, New York, 1975, Plenum Publishing Corporation, p. 100.

Fitterer, J. D., Spicer, M. J., and Nelson, W. P.: Echocardiographic demonstration of bilateral atrial myxomas, Chest **70:**282-284, 1976.

Hirschfeld, D. S., and Emilson, B. B.: Mitral valve vegetation simulating left atrial myxoma, West. J. Med. **124:**419-423, 1976.

Petsas, A. A., Gottlieb, S., Kingsley, B., Segal, B. L., and Myerburg, R. J.: Echocardiographic diagnosis of left atrial myxoma: usefulness of suprasternal approach, Br. Heart J. **38:**627-632, 1976.

Dashcoff, N., Roberts, W., Nanda, N. C., and Gramiak, R.: Echocardiographic features of biatrial myxoma, to be published.

Left atrial thrombus

Klepacki, Z., Surlowica-Sidun, B., and Zarebska, L.: Intra-atrial thrombus detected by ultrasonocardiography, Kardiol. Pol. **17:**83, 1974.

Phillips, B. J., Friedewald, V. E., Jr., Kinard, S. A., and Diethrich, E. B.: Calcified intraatrial mass detected by M-mode echocardiography and multihead transducer scanning; a case report, J. Clin. Ultrasound **2:**245, 1974 (abstract).

Poehlmann, H. W., Basta, L. L., and Brown, R. E.: Left atrial thrombus detected by ultrasound; a case report, J. Clin. Ultrasound **3:**65, 1975.

Spangler, R. D., and Okin, J. T.: Illustrative echocardiogram; echocardiographic demonstration of a left atrial thrombus, Chest **67:**716, 1975.

Furuse, A., Mizuno, A., Inoue, H., Furuta, N., and Saigusa, M.: Echocardiography and angiocardiography for detection of left atrial thrombosis, Jpn. Heart J. **17:**163-171, 1976.

Subaortic obstruction

Laurenceau, J. L., Guay, J. M., and Gagne, S.: Echocardiography in the diagnosis of subaortic membranous stenosis, Circulation **48**(suppl. 4):46, 1973 (abstract).

Davis, R. A., Feigenbaum, H., Chang, S., Konecke, L. L., and Dillon, J. C.: Echocardiographic manifestations of discrete subaortic stenosis, Am. J. Cardiol. **33:**277, 1974.

Popp, R. L., Silverman, J. F., French, J. W., Stinson, E. B., and Harrison, D. C.: Echocardiographic findings in discrete subvalvular aortic stenosis, Circulation **49:**226, 1974.

Kronzon, I., Schloss, M., Danilowicz, D., and Singh, A.: Fixed membranous subaortic stenosis, Chest **67:** 473-474, 1975.

Chandraratna, P. A., and Cohen, L. S.: Pre- and postoperative echocardiographic features of discrete subaortic stenosis cardiology, **61:**181-188, 1976.

Krueger, S. K., Hofshire, P. J., and Forker, A. D.: Echocardiographic features of combined hypertrophic and membranous subvalvular aortic stenosis; a case report, J. Clin. Ultrasound **4:**31-34, 1976.

Weyman, A. E., Feigenbaum, H., Dillon, J. C., Chang, S., Hurwitz, R. A., and Girod, D. A.: Cross-sectional echocardiography in the diagnosis of discrete subaortic stenosis, Am. J. Cardiol. **37:**358, 1976.

Hess, P. G., Nanda, N. C., DeWeese, J. A., Reeves, W. C., and Gramiak, R.: Echocardiographic features of combined membranous subaortic stenosis and acquired calcific aortic valvulopathy—a case report, Am. Heart J. **94:**349, 1977.

Nanda, N. C., Scovil, J. S., Gramiak, R., Alexson, C., and Manning, J.: Echocardiography in discrete subaortic stenosis. In White, D. N., and Brown, R. E., editors: Ultrasound in medicine, vol. 3, New York, 1977, Plenum Publishing Corporation, p. 247.

Aortic regurgitation

Joyner, C. R., Dyrda, I., and Reid, J. M.: Behavior of the anterior leaflet of the mitral valve in patients with the Austin-Flint murmur, Clin. Res. **14:**251, 1966 (abstract).

Dillon, J. C., Haine, C. L., Chang, S., and Feigenbaum, H.: Significance of mitral fluttering in patients with aortic insufficiency, Clin. Res. **18:**304, 1970 (abstract).

Winsberg, F., Gabor, G. E., and Hernberg, J. G.: Fluttering of the mitral valve in aortic insufficiency, Circulation **41:**225, 1970 (abstract).

Pridie, R. B., Beham, R., and Oakley, C. M.: Echocardiography of the mitral valve in aortic valve disease, Br. Heart J. **33:**296, 1971.

Danford, H. G., Danford, D. A., Mielke, J. E., and Peterson, L. F.: Echocardiographic evaluation of the hemodynamic effects of chronic aortic insufficiency with observations on left ventricular performance, Circulation **48:**253, 1973.

Friedewald, V. E., Jr., Futral, J. E., Kinard, S. A., and Phillips, B.: Oscillations of the interventricular septum in aortic insufficiency, J. Clin. Ultrasound **2:** 229, 1974 (abstract).

Botvinick, E. H., Schiller, N. B., Wickramasekaran, R., Klausner, S. C. and Gertz, E.: Echocardiographic demonstration of early mitral valve closure in severe aortic insufficiency; its clinical implications, Circulation, **51:**836-847, 1975.

Cope, G. D., Kisslo, J. A., Johnson, M. L., and Myers, S.: Diastolic vibration of the interventricular septum in aortic insufficiency, Circulation **51:**589, 1975.

DeMaria, A. N., King, J. F., Salel, A. F., Caudill, C. C., Miller, R. R., and Mason, D. T.: Echography and phonography of acute aortic regurgitation in bacterial endocarditis, Ann. Intern. Med. **82:**329-335, 1975.

Gray, K. E., and Barritt, D. W.: Echocardiographic assessment of severity of aortic regurgitation, Br. Heart J. **37:**691-699, 1975.

Gray, K. E., Barritt, D. W., and Ross, F. G.: Proceedings; echocardiographic assessment of severity of aortic regurgitation, Br. Heart J. **37:**558, 1975.

Mann, T., McLaurin, L., Grossman, W., and Craige, E.: Assessing the hemodynamic severity of acute aortic regurgitation due to infective endocarditis, N. Engl. J. Med. **293**:108, 1975.

D'Cruz, I., Cohen, H. C., Prabhu, R., Ayabe, T., and Glick, G.: Flutter of left ventricular structures in patients with aortic regurgitation, with special reference to patients with associated mitral stenosis, Am. Heart J. **92**:684-691, 1976.

Glasser, S. P.: Illustrative echocardiogram; late mitral valve opening in aortic regurgitation, Chest **70**:70-71, 1976.

Tingelstad, J. B., and Robertson, L. W.: Fluttering of the interventricular septum, Chest **69**:119, 1976.

Ward, J. N., Baker, D. W., Rubenstein, S. A., and Johnson, S. L.: Detection of aortic insufficiency by pulse Doppler echocardiography, J. Clin. Ultrasound **5**:5-10, 1977.

Mitral valve (miscellaneous)

Zaky, A., Grabhorn, L., and Feigenbaum, H.: Movement of the mitral ring; a study of ultrasoundcardiography, Cardiovasc. Res. **1**:121, 1967.

Wharton, C. F., and Lopez-Bescos, L. L.: Mitral valve movement; a study using an ultrasound technique, Br. Heart J. **32**:344, 1970.

Buyukozturk, K., Kingsley, B., and Segal, B. L.: The influences of heart rate, age and sex on the movements of mitral valve, Acta Cardiol. (Brux) **27**:427, 1972.

Chakorn, S. A., Siggers, D. C., Wharton, C. F. P., and Deuchar, D. C.: Study of normal and abnormal movements of mitral valve ring using reflected ultrasound, Br. Heart J. **34**:480, 1972.

Derman, U.: Changes of the mitral echocardiogram with aging and the influence of atherosclerotic risk factors, Atherosclerosis **15**:349, 1972.

Fischer, J. C., Chang, S., Konecke, L. L., and Feigenbaum, H.: Echocardiographic determination of mitral valve flow, Am. J. Cardiol. **29**:262, 1972 (abstract).

Layton, C., Gent, G., Pridie, R., McDonald, A., and Brigden, W.: Diastolic closure rate of normal mitral valve, Br. Heart J. **35**:1066, 1973.

Allen, H. N., Jobin, G., Robinson, J. G., Kraus, R., and Harris, W. S.: Effects of venous return on mitral valve closure rate during early diastole, Circulation **52**(suppl. 2):133, 1975 (abstract).

Davia, J. F., Cheitlin, M. D., De Castro, C. M., Lawless, O., and Niemi, L.: Absence of echocardiographic abnormalities of the anterior mitral valve leaflet in rheumatoid arthritis, Ann. Intern. Med. **83**:500-502, 1975.

Gramiak, R., and Nanda, N. C.: Mitral valve, In Gramiak, R., and Waag, R. C., editors: Cardiac ultrasound, St. Louis, 1975, The C. V. Mosby Co., p. 47.

Laniado, S., Yellin, E., Kotler, M., Levy, L., Stadler, J., and Terdiman, R.: A study of the dynamic relations between the mitral valve echogram and phasic mitral flow, Circulation **51**:104, 1975.

Pohost, G. M., Dinsmore, R. E., Rubenstein, J. J., O'Keefe, D. D., Grantham, N., Scully, H. E., Beierholm, E. A., Frederiksen, J. W., Weisfeldt, M. L., and Daggest, W. M.: The echocardiogram of the anterior leaflet of the mitral valve; correlation with hemodynamic and cineroentgenographic studies in dogs, Circulation **51**:88, 1975.

Rubenstein, J. J., Pohost, G. M., Dinsmore, R. E., and Harthorne, J. W.: The echocardiographic determination of mitral valve opening and closure; correlation with hemodynamic studies in man, Circulation **51**:98, 1975.

Andy, J. J., Sheikh, M. U., Ali, N., Barnes, B. O., Fox, L. M., Curry, C. L., and Roberts, W. C.: Echocardiographic observations in opiate addicts with active infective endocarditis, Am. J. Cardiol. **40**:17, 1977.

Kalmanson, D., Veyrat, C., Bouchareine, F., and DeGroote, A.: Non-invasive recording of mitral valve flow velocity patterns using pulsed Doppler echocardiography; application to diagnosis and evaluation of mitral valve disease, Br. Heart J. **39**:517-528, 1977.

Massie, B. M., Schiller, N. B., Ratshin, R. A., Parmley, W. W.: Mitral-septal separation; new echocardiographic index of left ventricular function, Am. J. Cardiol. **39**:1008, 1977.

5 Aortic valve

STRUCTURES IN BEAM

The following are structures in the beam, beginning from the chest wall:
1. Right ventricular outflow tract
2. Aortic root and leaflets
3. Left atrial cavity
4. Beam exits into the mediastinum

NORMAL TRACING (Fig. 5-1)

- The right ventricular outflow tract, aortic root, and left atrium are normally of about equal size.
- The aortic root moves anteriorly in systole and posteriorly in diastole. The wall tracings are parallel, and there is little or no change in diameter from systole to diastole. Atrial systole may produce a small, circumscribed posterior displacement of the aortic root.
- Aortic valve leaflets are recorded as thin echo sources that occupy a central position in the aorta in diastole. With the beginning of ejection, they move rapidly toward the periphery and normally are positioned adjacent to the aortic walls throughout ejection. At end-systole they move rapidly back to closure in a midaortic position. In diastole, their motion pattern is secondary to movement of the aortic root.
- When two leaflets are recorded, boxlike configurations are produced. The anterior portion of the box is the right coronary cusp, whereas the posterior leaflet is the noncoronary cusp. The left coronary cusp is occasion-

ally seen as a linear echo that occupies a midaortic position in systole (Fig. 5-2).
- Normal leaflets contain up to three lines in diastole. The width of these echo complexes is usually less than either aortic wall.
- Supravalvular recording shows the aorta to be of the same caliber as at the valve level but placed more anteriorly. The right ventricular outflow tract and aortic leaflets are not recorded. The left atrium lies behind the supravalvular aorta.

TECHNICAL CONSIDERATIONS

- Time-varied gain should be adjusted so that the anterior and posterior aortic walls are of about equal amplitude (A-mode is useful here).
- Overall gain is set at a level that records aortic valve leaflets but not so high that the cavities are filled with small echoes.
- High recording speeds are needed to demonstrate rapid movements of aortic leaflets.
- Beam direction that is too medial shows exaggerated movement of the anterior margin of the aorta.
- A low beam direction records diastolic traces only (the valve closes low in the aortic root).
- A beam direction that is too high records the systolic position of the cusps only or produces a typical supravalvular recording.
- Complete systolic and diastolic traces of two cusps are not obtainable in all patients.

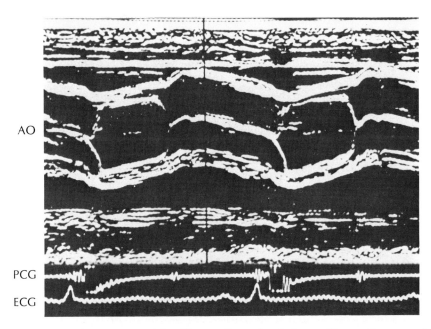

Fig. 5-1. Normal aortic root. A boxlike configuration is formed by aortic cusp echoes as they move to the periphery of the aortic lumen in systole and occupy a midaortic position in diastole. Note the parallel motion of anterior and posterior aortic walls. Ao, aortic root; PCG, phonocardiogram; ECG, electrocardiogram. (From Nanda N. C., and others: Circulation **49:**870, 1974. By permission of the American Heart Assn., Inc.)

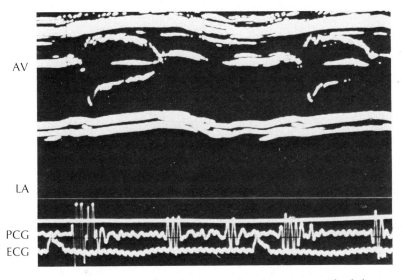

Fig. 5-2. Aortic valve (AV) recording demonstrating three cusps. The left coronary cusp appears as a linear echo between the right coronary (anterior) and the noncoronary (posterior) leaflets in systole. Its extent of movement is not recorded, since it occurs across the ultrasonic beam. The noncoronary cusp coasts toward a position of closure because of poor systolic ejection from cardiomyopathy. LA, left atrium; PCG, phonocardiogram; ECG, electrocardiogram.

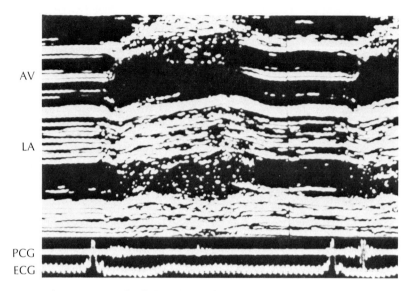

Fig. 5-3. Reverberations in the left atrium. Multiple linear echoes are seen in the left atrium (LA) moving with the aortic root and probably represent reverberations from the aortic walls. AV, aortic valve; PCG, phonocardiogram; ECG, electrocardiogram.

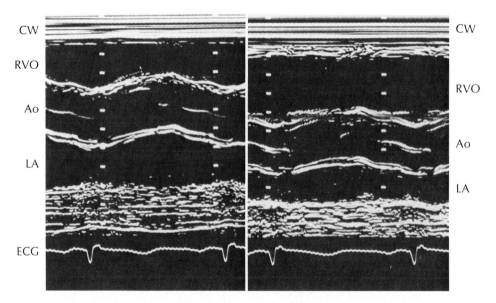

Fig. 5-4. Aortic valve recording technique. The aortic root (Ao) shown on the left is recorded from the usual left parasternal position and demonstrates nearly equal dimensions of the right ventricular outflow (RVO), left atrium (LA), and the aortic root. The recording on the right is obtained from a low chest wall transducer position (near the apex) from the same patient and shows a more posteriorly placed aortic root with a larger right ventricular outflow dimension and a smaller left atrial cavity diameter. CW, chest wall; ECG, electrocardiogram.

It is usually necessary to accept incomplete traces of cusp motion or to piece the information together from multiple recordings.

• Generally, the right coronary cusp is obtained more readily than is the noncoronary leaflet, which may require more medial angulation.

• Linear echoes may be recorded in the left atrium and are of lesser intensity than the aortic wall and move parallel to it; these may represent intracardiac reverberations (Fig. 5-3).

• Medial and superior angulation of the transducer placed low on the chest wall may also be used for recording the aortic root. In this instance the right ventricular space imaged in front may appear unduly large; this probably results from an oblique ultrasonic beam pathway that traverses the body rather than the outflow area of the ventricle (Fig. 5-4).

• Because of beam width, mitral or tricuspid valves may be superimposed on the aortic valve echo or portions of both may be recorded simultaneously.

• Inadequate suppression of reverberatory anterior echoes may affect the quality of aortic root and right ventricular outflow images.

• Both the outer (adventitial) and the inner (intimal) margins of an aortic wall may be recorded.

• In the presence of a large aortic root the left atrial dimension may appear to be miniscule; this probably results from displacement of the atrium out of the plane of the ultrasonic beam produced by a large aorta.

• The left atrial wall, recorded behind the aortic root, usually shows no motion, probably because of its nonperpendicular relationship to the ultrasonic beam in that plane and the anchoring effect of the attachment of the pulmonary veins in this region. Motion of the atrial wall, when recorded, resembles

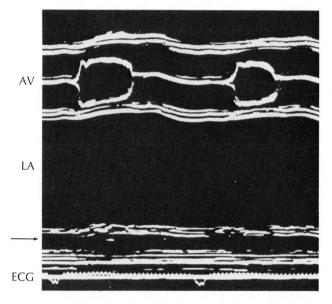

Fig. 5-5. Anatomic and functional variations in aortic valve recording. The walls of the aorta are imaged as a grouping of three linear echoes. The multiple lines probably originate from the complex shape of the walls of the sinuses of Valsalva. The early systolic rebound of the aortic leaflets (AV) toward closure may be the result of irregular systolic ejection and is shallower than those seen in subaortic membrane. The space *(arrow)* behind the enlarged left atrium (LA) most likely represents a dilated pulmonary vein. The patient presented with congestive cardiomyopathy. ECG, electrocardiogram.

a small-amplitude, rounded mitral valve echo in waveform and timing. The first peak in early diastole represents rapid decompression of the atrium; the second movement is caused by atrial systolic contraction.

• Aortic valve echoes may be more readily obtained than the mitral valve in older subjects and may be used as a landmark to obtain other cardiac structures. In these patients the aortic valve may be imaged by placing the transducer perpendicularly on the chest wall.

• One or two extra lines may be present in the aortic root lumen, near the walls, and may represent echoes from large sinuses of Valsalva (Fig. 5-5).

FINDINGS IN DISEASE
Acquired aortic stenosis and aortic regurgitation

Anatomic and functional changes. The aortic valve may be involved in a degenerative process with advancing age or as a sequel to rheumatic fever and show cusp thickening, calcification, and commissural fusion. The functional result may be isolated aortic stenosis, aortic regurgitation, or combined stenosis and regurgitation, depending on the extent of commissural fusion, the degree of irregularity of the cusp margins, and the extent of cusp deformity and stiffening. A fixed, stenotic orifice may be present when stenosis and regurgitation coexist. The left ventricle hypertrophies in pure aortic stenosis but does not show cavity dilatation unless failure, aortic regurgitation, or some other process is added.

Clinical summary. A history of acute rheumatic fever in childhood and the presence of a systolic murmur (aortic stenosis) or a blowing diastolic murmur (aortic regurgitation) suggest the clinical diagnosis of rheumatic involvement of the aortic valve. Palpation of peripheral artery pulsation in aortic regurgitation shows a collapsing impulse ("water-hammer" pulse). The carotid pulse waveform typically reveals a slow upstroke in aortic stenosis. Chest roentgenograms and fluoroscopy may reveal the presence of an enlarged left ventricle and calcification of the aortic valve. Cardiac catheterization demonstrates a pressure gradient between the left ventricle and a systemic artery in aortic stenosis.

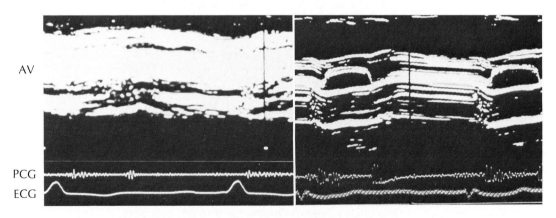

Fig. 5-6. Aortic valve disease. In the left panel, thick echoes almost filling the aortic lumen and completely obscuring cusp motion indicate an extremely heavily calcified aortic valve (AV). This patient showed evidence of severe aortic stenosis on cardiac catheterization. In the right panel, less heavy calcification is demonstrated in diastole but is probably localized, since the right coronary cusp appears of normal thickness in systole. Good cusp motion in the presence of calcification usually indicates a small or absent gradient across the valve. Frequently, aortic incompetence predominates. PCG, phonocardiogram; ECG, electrocardiogram. (From Nanda, N. C.: Am. J. Med. **62:**836, 1977.)

Left ventricular angiocardiography shows a thickened left ventricle and evidence of obstruction at the aortic valve. The leaflets may be calcified and immobile, or some upward doming in systole may occur. A jet through the stenotic orifice is often demonstrated. Aortic regurgitation is best evaluated by retrograde aortography.

Echocardiographic features

• Cusp calcification thickens the image of aortic valve leaflets so that the diastolic leaflet trace is usually wider than either aortic wall. With mild calcification the diastolic cusp echoes present a multilayered appearance while normal motion of one or both cusps can still be discerned. This finding is generally associated with minimal or no stenosis, but the valve is often regurgitant. Larger deposits of calcium result in more extensive multilayering or thick conglomerate echoes that occupy more than one third of the aortic lumen diameter (Figs. 5-6 to 5-8).

• Systolic motion of the cusps may be obliterated or restricted when stenosis is present. The image may consist of thick echo complexes that change in appearance without obvious cusp separation; limited systolic opening may be seen.

• The mitral valve flutters in the presence of aortic regurgitation.

• When aortic stenosis is present, the ven-

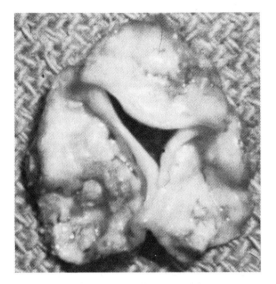

Fig. 5-7. Surgically resected calcified aortic valve. All three cusps are calcified (dense white areas) and fused at the commissures.

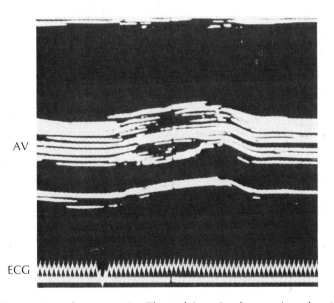

AV

ECG

Fig 5-8. Calcific aortic valve stenosis. The calcium in the aortic valve (AV) leaflets thickens their image in systole and diastole. Cusp motion in systole is markedly restricted and results in a "buttonhole" image. Generally, this pattern is associated with aortic stenosis of moderate degree. ECG, electrocardiogram.

tricular walls (including the septum) thicken symmetrically.

• In aortic regurgitation the ventricle is dilated and shows hyperdynamic contraction of the septum and posterior wall.

Comments

• The severity of aortic stenosis may be roughly estimated from the echocardiogram. Severe stenosis is generally characterized by heavy calcification that completely obscures cusp motion, whereas lightly calcified cusps showing diminished opening and closing velocities of motion and reduced excursions are associated with milder degrees of orifice obstruction (peak systolic pressure gradients below 50 to 60 mm Hg). Good cusp motion and calcification most often are not associated with the presence of a gradient, and the findings of aortic regurgitation may predominate.

• The aortic valve shows some evidence of calcification in all adults over 50 with rheu-

matic involvement of the aortic valve. Absence of calcification usually means that some other condition is present. Look for evidence of a subvalvular membrane when the clinical presentation in an adult is that of aortic valve stenosis but calcium cannot be detected echocardiographically.

• Direct measurement of aortic valve cusp separation as an indicator of the severity of aortic stenosis has not been useful in our experience. The beam may not be directed at the orifice at the angle that consistently detects a diameter that can be correlated with orifice size. In addition, when the orifice is smaller than the width of the beam, the edges will be detected and obscure the orifice. This phenomenon explains why an orifice cannot be generally imaged in patients with severe aortic stenosis.

• Calcification of the valve cusps may obscure enough of the aortic lumen that recognition of the aorta may be difficult (Fig.

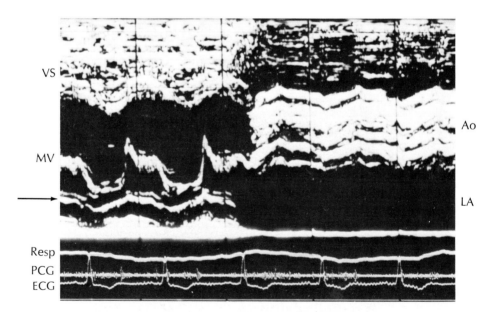

Fig. 5-9. Calcific aortic valve disease. Heavy calcification of the aortic valve virtually obscures the aortic lumen so that recognition of the aorta (Ao) is difficult. Beam scanning from the mitral valve reveals the true nature of the complex by demonstrating continuity between the ventricular septum (VS) and the anterior aortic margin and relating the mitral valve (MV) to the posterior aortic wall. The prominent echo *(arrow)* behind the mitral valve probably represents extension of calcification to the mitral annulus. LA, left atrium; Resp, respiration; PCG, phonocardiogram; and ECG, electrocardiogram.

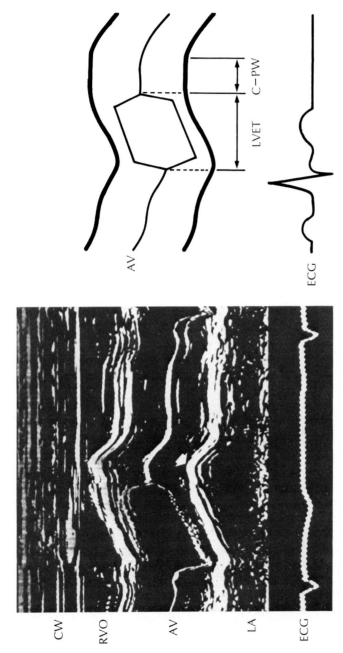

Fig. 5-10. Echocardiogram of a normal aortic root demonstrating the onset of posterior motion of the posterior aortic wall (*arrow*) well after cusp closure. When ejection is prolonged as in aortic stenosis, the interval between aortic valve closure (C) and the onset of posterior motion of posterior aortic wall (PW) motion is shortened. This also occurs when the filling and emptying patterns of the left atrium are altered. CW, chest wall; RVO, right ventricular outflow tract; AV, aortic valve; LA, left atrium; ECG, electrocardiogram; LVET, left ventricular ejection time.

5-9). In these cases, scans made into the left ventricle reveal the true nature of the echo complex by showing the expected anatomic relationships to the ventricular septum and mitral valve.

• Calcification in contiguous structures like the proximal coronary arteries or thick echoes from the atriopulmonic sulcus produced by slight lateral beam direction may mimic aortic valve calcification.

• Occasionally a patient with heavily calcified, immobile cusps may have severe aortic incompetence with practically no gradient across the aortic valve in systole.

• Calcification in the aortic walls (near cusp level) or annulus is rare in the absence of calcific aortic valve disease.

• The diastolic posterior motion of the aortic root in normal subjects begins well after cusp closure and consists of a large posterior movement followed by a further posterior

deflection coincident with atrial systole (Fig. 5-10). The factors responsible for the normal motion of the aortic root have not been well delineated. Left ventricular ejection as well as the motion of the whole heart during systole may be major determinants. Poor aortic excursions have been observed in patients with low left ventricular stroke volumes. The left atrium and the right ventricle are also in immediate contact with the aortic root, and there is some evidence to suggest that changes in aortic root posterior motion correspond to left atrial volume changes. This has led to an attempt to correlate the degree of mitral stenosis with the amplitude of posterior motion of the posterior aortic wall in diastole. Reasonable correlation was obtained. The interval between the aortic diastolic cusp closure point and the onset of aortic posterior motion is shortened in patients with nonrheumatic mitral incompetence and

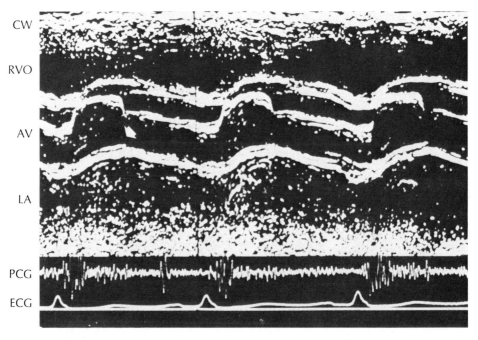

Fig. 5-11. Altered aortic root motion in mitral regurgitation. In this patient with chordae rupture the onset of posterior motion of the aortic root *(arrow)* occurs early and coincides with the time of aortic valve (AV) closure. Earlier and more rapid opening of the mitral valve with left atrial decompression may be responsible for these findings. CW, chest wall; RVO, right ventricular outflow tract; AV, aortic valve; LA, left atrium; PCG, phonocardiogram; ECG, electrocardiogram.

normal-size left atria and is prolonged in rheumatic mitral valve disease where the atria are large and baggy (Fig. 5-11). The interval is also shortened with aortic stenosis, but this appears to be related to prolonged left ventricular ejection time observed in this condition.

Paradoxical anterior motion of the aortic root in diastole with flattening or posterior motion in systole has been observed by us in two patients with congestive cardiomyopathy with grossly dilated right ventricles and pulmonary hypertension (Fig. 5-12). The abnormal motion of the aortic root in these instances may be related to the abnormal hemodynamics and enlargement of the right ventricle, influencing the motion of the contiguously located aortic root. The basal portion of the interatrial septum, whose motion is believed to be predominantly influenced by the aortic root (see p. 195), may also exhibit similar changes in its movement pattern.

Role of echocardiography. Echocardiography is a sensitive detector of aortic valve calcification. Absence of calcification in an adult over 50 means that aortic stenosis is probably not present and another cause for the clinical findings must be sought. Absence of cusp motion in an adequate echocardiographic study generally indicates severe aortic valve stenosis. Combined aortic stenosis and regurgitation can be recognized. Echocardiographic findings are coarse indicators of the severity of aortic stenosis, and exceptions to the described severity indicators are encountered.

Bicuspid aortic valve, congenital aortic stenosis and regurgitation

Anatomic and functional changes. The three commissures present in the normal three-leafed, or tricuspid, aortic valve may fail to develop normally so that a bicuspid valve with two leaflets and two commissures results. A rudimentary third commissure may occasionally be present and is called a raphe. If only one commissure develops, a

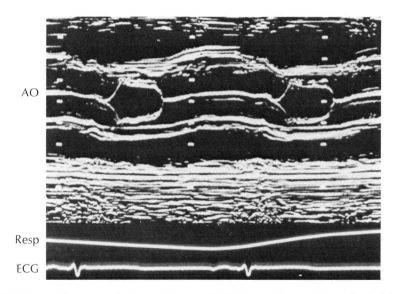

AO

Resp

ECG

Fig. 5-12. Echocardiogram of the aortic root (AO) in a patient with marked right ventricular enlargement. The vessel demonstrates paradoxical motion, moving anteriorly in diastole and somewhat posteriorly in systole. Movements of the aortic root are probably influenced by the filling and emptying patterns of adjacent cardiac chambers. In this patient an abnormal right ventricle may be responsible for the reversal of normal aortic root motion. Resp, respirations; ECG, electrocardiogram.

unicuspid valve results, but this is a rare entity, as is the quadricuspid valve, which has four cusps.

Inequality of cusp tissue in a bicuspid valve is common so that the two leaflets may be quite different in size. The orifice in bicuspid valves represents a straight line across the aortic root so that the tissues of the leaflet must be longer than the shortest distance across the aortic root to permit them to move

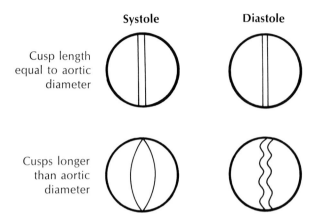

Fig. 5-13. Bicuspid aortic valves. In a bicuspid aortic valve, when cusp length is equal to the aortic diameter, there is insufficient tissue present to allow the valve to open in systole. The condition is incompatible with life. Cusps that are longer than the aortic diameter can move laterally in systole so that valve opening can occur. When the valve closes in diastole, the extra length of the valve cusps is taken up by the production of numerous folds at the line of closure. These folds are largely responsible for the echocardiographic finding of diastolic multilayering in bicuspid valves. Normal tricuspid aortic valves close smoothly without folds at the line of closure, since the length along the margins of the cusps is adequate for coaptation as well as for opening along the circumference of the aortic lumen.

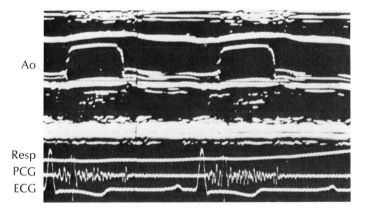

Fig. 5-14. Bicuspid aortic valve. The echocardiogram shows marked eccentricity of the aortic valve diastolic position resulting in asymmetric leaflet images in systole. The anterior cusp is large and practically occupies the whole lumen, whereas the posterior leaflet is miniscule. Ao, aortic root; Resp, respiration; PCG, phonocardiogram; ECG, electrocardiogram. (From Nanda, N. C., and others: Circulation **49**:870, 1974. By permission of the American Heart Assn., Inc.)

sideways during opening. On closure, this extra cusp length is accommodated by folding or wrinkling of the redundant leaflet tissue, present along the line of closure (Fig. 5-13).

Stenosis is often produced in a bicuspid aortic valve when insufficient cusp tissue is present to permit wide separation during systole or when the cusps fuse, forming a dome-shaped structure containing an orifice at its apex that is often asymmetrically placed in respect to the aortic root margins (congenital valvular stenosis). Systolic jets and turbulent blood flow beyond the stenosis may result in poststenotic dilatation of the aorta.

Valvular incompetence that may occur alone or in combination with stenosis is secondary to inadequate sealing, since the closure line is irregular from the folds that occur and from some thickening of leaflet margins often present in these congenitally deformed valves. Infrequently a tricuspid aortic valve may also be congenitally deformed and its leaflets fused, leading to stenosis, incompetence, or both.

Congenitally deformed valves are almost never calcified in childhood. However, they frequently calcify when adulthood is attained, so that the differentiation from an acquired disease may be difficult or impossible clinically or pathologically.

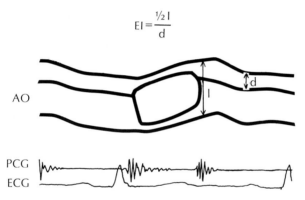

$$EI = \frac{\frac{1}{2}l}{d}$$

Fig. 5-15. Calculation of the eccentricity index. An index of 1.5 or greater is considered diagnostic of a bicuspid aortic valve. EI, eccentricity index; l, intraluminal diameter of the aortic root (AO) at end systole; d, minimum distance between the middle of the aortic cusp position in diastole and the closest aortic wall echo; PCG, phonocardiogram; ECG, electrocardiogram.

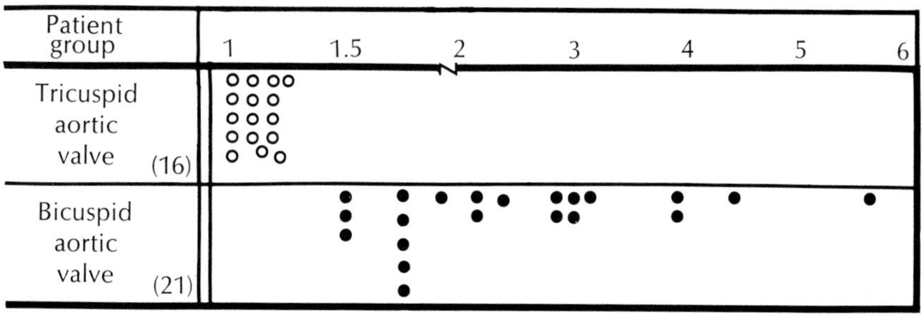

Patient group	1	1.5	2	3	4	5	6
Tricuspid aortic valve (16)	o o oo o o o o o o o o o o						
Bicuspid aortic valve (21)		•• •	• • ••	••• ••	• •	•	•

Fig. 5-16. Aortic valve eccentricity index. In this study all patients with bicuspid aortic valves showed an eccentricity index of 1.5 or greater. This differentiated them from patients with tricuspid aortic valves who demonstrated lower indices.

The left ventricle may hypertrophy if stenosis is the predominant lesion or dilate when severe incompetence is present.

Clinical summary. The bicuspid aortic valve is believed to be the most common congenital malformation of the heart or great vessels, and its incidence approaches 2% of the general population. It can be either functionally normal, stenotic, or incompetent. A soft systolic murmur, a loud early systolic ejection sound, or click, or both may be present when the valve is functioning normally. The murmur becomes harsh and long when significant stenosis develops, and the ejection click may disappear. Aortic incompetence can be recognized when an early diastolic blowing murmur is present.

Chest roentgenograms may be normal or show evidence of left ventricular enlargement. Cardiac catheterization reveals a gradient across the aortic valve when stenosis is present. Angiocardiography demonstrates systolic doming of the stenotic valve, jet formation, and poststenotic dilatation of the aorta. Retrograde aortography is useful to define the number of cusps in the aortic valve and to estimate the degree of aortic regurgitation, if present.

Echocardiographic features. Echocardiographic findings in the bicuspid aortic valve are as follows:

- In bicuspid valves, marked eccentricity

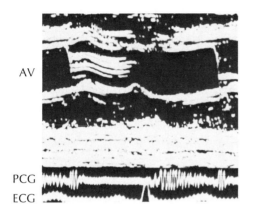

Fig. 5-17. Bicuspid aortic valve. Diastolic multilayering is a dynamic event and shows considerable beat-to-beat variation. The calculation of the eccentricity index is best performed in a beat in which a clear dominant diastolic echo is present *(right).* AV, aortic valve; PCG, phonocardiogram; ECG, electrocardiogram.

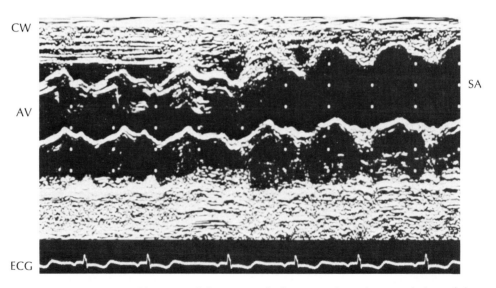

Fig. 5-18. Poststenotic dilatation of the supravalvular aorta. Superior angulation of the transducer from the aortic valve (AV) position demonstrates the supravalvular portion of the aorta (SA), which is much larger than the aortic root and is located just beneath the chest wall (CW). The patient, who was in his teens, had severe aortic stenosis documented by cardiac catheterization. ECG, electrocardiogram.

of the position of the cusps in the aortic root in diastole is present (Fig. 5-14). The ratio of one half the inner aortic diameter divided by the shortest distance from the inner aortic wall to the middle of the diastolic cusp position (eccentricity index) is usually 1.5 or greater (Figs. 5-15 and 5-16). The eccentric diastolic position results in asymmetry of the systolic images of the aortic valve so that one leaflet appears to be larger than the other.

• In systole the cusp motion appears normal.

• Multiple linear echoes are often seen in diastole, creating a "paintbrush" effect (Fig. 5-17). The folds produced on closure are the probable echo sources responsible for this pattern. They are not present during systole.

Echocardiographic findings in congenital stenosis/incompetence are as follows:

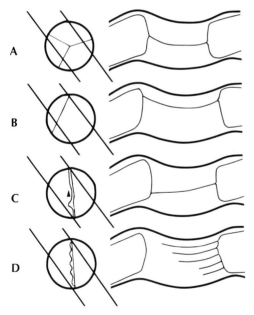

Fig. 5-19. Schematic representation of the ultrasonic beam passing through a tricuspid aortic valve **(A)**, a bicuspid aortic valve with unequal cusp size **(B)**, a bicuspid aortic valve with equal cusp size **(C)**, and a bicuspid aortic valve with multiple redundant folds **(D).** The arrow in **C** denotes the direction of movement of a redundant fold in diastole. (From Nanda, N. C., and others: Circulation **49:**870, 1974. By permission of the American Heart Assn., Inc.)

• The aortic valve cusps may appear entirely normal in valvular stenosis.

• The supravalvular portion of the aorta is frequently dilated (poststenotic dilatation; Fig. 5-18).

• The left ventricle and the mitral valve may show secondary changes from aortic valve disease.

Comments

• The eccentricity found in bicuspid valves may be due to anatomic asymmetry of the cusps or to a dominant fold that generates the diastolic echo. Since this is a dynamic phenomenon, the diastolic echo may be central or it may shift to an eccentric position from beat to beat or even during one diastolic interval with small changes in transducer angulation. Long recordings and varied transducer positions are useful in eliciting the true findings (Fig. 5-19). A midline aortic valve diastolic cusp position obtained from a single transducer position or angulation does not therefore rule out the presence of a bicuspid aortic valve.

• Variable eccentric positions of the diastolic cusp echo are present in over 50% of patients with bicuspid aortic valves. Complete reversal of the eccentricity may be seen in up to 6% of patients (Fig. 5-20).

• Diastolic eccentricity may occur in the presence of bicuspid aortic valve stenosis even though the orifice is centrally placed.

• In the presence of diastolic multilayering a markedly eccentric dominant echo can usually be detected by examining the aortic valve from various transducer positions and can be used to calculate the eccentricity index. In children, diastolic multilayering is not seen with a nonstenotic tricuspid aortic valve but may be observed in a small proportion of patients (under 15%) when the valve is stenosed. The condition is probably related to nodular, fibrotic thickening.

Interestingly, the bicuspid nature of the aortic valve can sometimes be correctly identified by echocardiography even in older patients with calcific aortic valve disease so long as the cusps retain some motion and are clearly seen in both systole and diastole.

• When aortic valve recordings are incom-

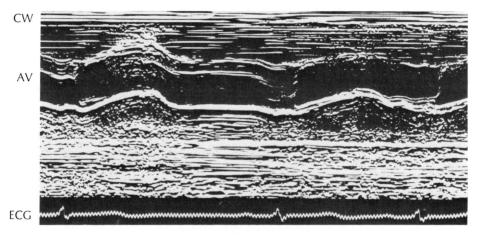

Fig. 5-20. Bicuspid aortic valve demonstrating reversal of eccentricity. The aortic valve (AV) image on the left shows an anterior eccentric position with a small anterior cusp. The recording on the right demonstrates a markedly posterior location of the cusp diastolic echo with a large anterior leaflet. ECG, electrocardiogram; CW, chest wall.

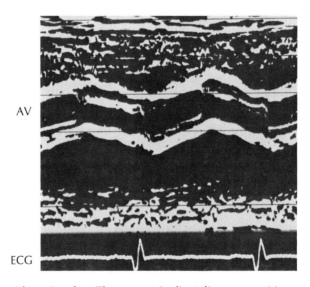

Fig. 5-21. Unicuspid aortic valve. The eccentric diastolic cusp position and images from what appear to be two leaflets are indistinguishable from a bicuspid aortic valve. These findings result from the ultrasonic beam striking the anterior and posterior margins of the unicuspid valve as it moves in the cardiac cycle. AV, aortic valve; ECG, electrocardiogram.

plete, superimposed echoes from the mitral valve or the ventricular septum may be mistaken for diastolic cusp echoes. The intimal echo or peripherally located echoes from a rather large sinus of Valsalva may also be confused with an eccentric diastolic cusp position. Demonstration of continuity of a linear diastolic echo with the systolic image of the aortic cusp is therefore necessary for establishing its origin from the aortic valve and can then be used for calculation of an eccentricity index.

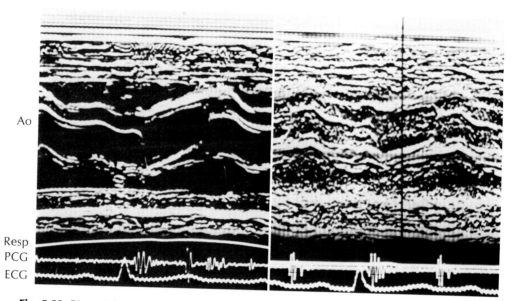

Ao

Resp
PCG
ECG

Fig. 5-22. Bicuspid aortic valve with unequal cusps. The panel on the left demonstrates echoes from an apparently normally functioning asymmetric bicuspid aortic valve in a patient with coarctation of the aorta. Note the constant anterior eccentricity of the diastolic cusp position. Multilayered echoes in diastole were not observed in this patient even with high gain setting *(right)*. Ao, aortic root; Resp, respiration; PCG, phonocardiogram; ECG, electrocardiogram. (From Nanda, N. C., and others: Circulation **49**:870, 1974. By permission of the American Heart Assn., Inc.)

• In our experience, a tricuspid aortic valve may appear slightly eccentric in diastole when it is examined from a high or very low position on the chest wall, but the eccentricity index does not reach or exceed 1.5.

• False-positive diagnoses of bicuspid aortic valves are uncommon. They have been observed in conditions with abnormal position or distortion of the aortic root, such as sinus of Valsalva aneurysm or tetralogy of Fallot, and in isolated ventricular septal defects. Caution should therefore be exercised in making the diagnosis in the presence of these conditions. The morphology of the aortic valve may also be difficult to deduce in the presence of bacterial endocarditis in which the vegetation, a strong reflector of ultrasound, may be mistaken for the diastolic cusp. In the presence of a tricuspid aortic valve, almost complete destruction or rupture of one cusp by bacterial endocarditis or trauma results in only two functioning cusps and the echocardiographic picture is that of a bicuspid aortic valve. In our experience, patients with myxomatous degeneration of the aortic valve have had correct echocardiographic interpretation of the valve structure. It is conceivable, however, that advanced myxomatous degeneration of a tricuspid aortic valve could result in marked redundancy of valvular tissue, giving rise to an elevated eccentricity index. A bicuspid aortic valve may be missed in the presence of a subaortic membrane, which may produce central dominant echoes in the aortic root in diastole.

• Complete rheumatic fusion of one commissure of a tricuspid aortic valve results in a valve that functions as a bicuspid valve. This type of acquired bicuspid aortic valve may be echocardiographically or pathologically indistinguishable from the congenital variety.

• The echocardiographic findings in two cases of unicuspid aortic valves studied by us

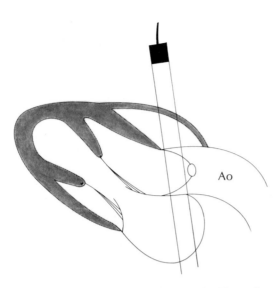

Fig. 5-23. Congenital aortic stenosis. There is fusion of the cusps forming a dome-shaped structure that contains a narrow orifice at its apex. Echocardiographic examination of the aortic valve may be normal when the beam passes through the base of the dome so that the systolic cusp position is recorded at the aortic margins. Ao, aorta.

were similar to bicuspid valves (Fig. 5-21). In a single case studied by us, a quadricuspid aortic valve looked like a tricuspid valve.

• Bicuspid aortic valves are commonly observed in patients with coarctation of the aorta (an incidence of 53% in 36 patients studied by us). Diastolic multilayering is rare in these cases, probably because the high pressures associated with aortic hypertension tend to obliterate the multiple folds present in a bicuspid aortic valve (Fig. 5-22).

• The normal systolic cusp positions seen in valvular stenosis probably result from examining the aortic valve near the base of the dome so that the systolic cusp position is at the aortic margins (Fig. 5-23). Higher beam direction may elicit echoes from the stenotic orifice that appear as parallel lines.

• Be sure to scan the supravalvular portion of the aorta. A poststenotic dilatation may identify valvular aortic stenosis even though the valve itself appears normal. In addition, a supravalvular stenosis of the aorta might be discovered and be responsible for the clinical findings of aortic stenosis (Fig. 5-24).

• IHSS can coexist with aortic stenosis.

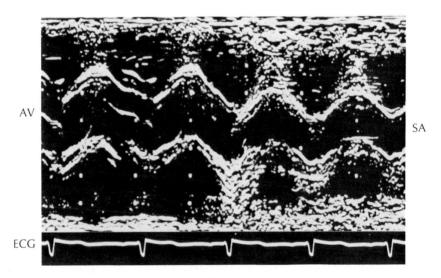

Fig. 5-24. Supravalvular aortic stenosis. Minimal superior angulation of the transducer from the aortic valve (AV) position exhibits significant narrowing of the caliber of the aorta. At surgery a constriction was present immediately above the valve level. SA, supravalvular aorta; ECG, electrocardiogram.

The septum is thick and the left ventricular outflow tract narrowed. SAMs are present and may be typical or partial. Use interventions carefully when examining any patient for associated left ventricular outflow obstruction.

• Subaortic stenosis has been described in the section dealing with the mitral valve. The typical early systolic rebound toward closure often followed by leaflet fluttering is useful to differentiate this condition from primary aortic valve disease. It is useful when the patient presents with the clinical picture suggestive of aortic stenosis.

• Good recordings of the mitral valve as well as septal and posterior wall thickness help to identify aortic regurgitation and to assess the degree of left ventricular hypertrophy resulting from the obstruction.

Role of echocardiography

• Recognition of a congenital bicuspid aortic valve by echocardiography is of clinical importance, since it is highly susceptible to bacterial endocarditis and has a special tendency to develop both stenosis and incompetence, constituting over 50% of all cases of aortic valve disease. From the surgical point of view, it is important in patients undergoing valvotomy not to incise the third rudimentary commissure or raphe present in one of the leaflets, since severe incompetence may result from improper suspension of the unsupported parts of the leaflet. Echocardiography is useful in confirming or ruling out the presence of a bicuspid aortic valve in a young subject with the so-called "functional" systolic murmur or in a patient with a loud aortic ejection sound who has no other manifestations of aortic valve disease.

• Echocardiography is of limited value in the evaluation of congenital aortic valve stenosis in children or adults in whom valvular calcification is not present.

Aortic aneurysms

Aneurysms are dilatations of the aorta that occur as a result of weakening of the wall, which permits the vessel to dilate from the high pressure. The cause of the aortic wall weakening may be atherosclerosis, endocarditis, tissue degeneration, chest trauma, or dissection. Complications include rupture into the body cavities with sudden death or slow leakage at the rupture site, aortic incompetence from dilatation of the aortic ring, or intracardiac fistula formation when the sinuses of Valsalva are involved. Left ventricular failure may develop when aortic incompetence is severe.

Aortic root dissection

Anatomic and clinical summary. This condition probably begins with rupture of a small vessel in the muscular layer or media of the aorta. The blood under high pressure

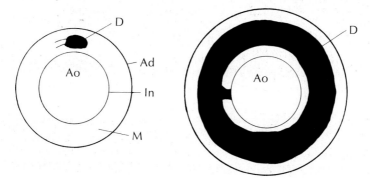

Fig. 5-25. Aortic dissection. A small vessel in the media (M) of the aorta (Ao) ruptures and begins to strip the inner wall (intima, In) away from the outer wall (adventitia, Ad), resulting in enlargement of the aorta and widening of its walls. The dissection (D) communicates with the inner lumen by producing a tear in the intima.

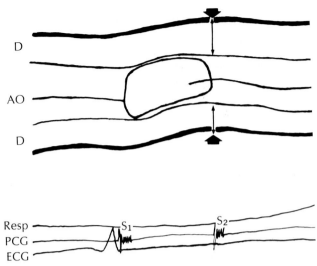

Fig. 5-26. Schematic representation of an aortic root echocardiogram in a patient with aortic root dissection. The small double-headed arrows indicate the thickness of the dissecting hematoma; the large arrows show the width of the aortic root image measured at end systole. D, width of the dissecting hematoma; AO, aorta; Resp, respirations; PCG, phonocardiogram; ECG, electrocardiogram; S_1, first heart sound; S_2, second heart sound. (From Nanda, N. C., and others: Circulation **48**:506, 1973. By permission of the American Heart Assn., Inc.)

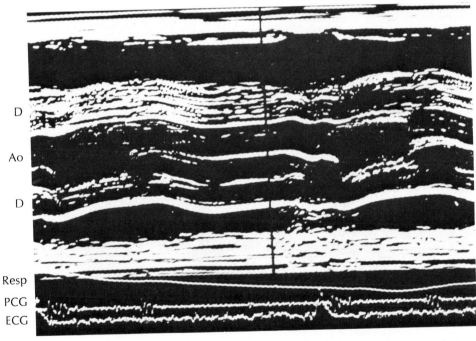

Fig. 5-27. Aortic root echogram reveals marked parallel widening of anterior and posterior walls. Aortic valve cusps are slender and show normal motion pattern. D, width of the dissecting hematoma; Ao, aorta; Resp, respirations; PCG, phonocardiogram; ECG, electrocardiogram. (From Nanda, N. C., and others: Circulation **48**:506, 1973. By permission of the American Heart Assn., Inc.)

then strips the inner wall away from the outer wall for variable distances from the original site of rupture and communicates with the inner lumen by producing a tear in the intima. A false channel is thereby created in addition to the true lumen, which carries the circulating blood (Fig. 5-25). The dissection usually begins in the ascending aorta a few centimeters above the aortic valve and then extends proximally to involve the aortic root. When the dissection process reaches branch vessels, it commonly produces occlusions. Leaks at the dissection site are common, and bleeding into the pericardial sac frequently occurs and can compress the heart, producing tamponade. Dissections can occur anywhere in the aorta, but for echocardiographic purposes this discussion concerns only with those that involve the root of the aorta.

When the dissection is acute, there is intense chest pain, and sudden collapse and death may follow. More chronic dissections produce less dramatic symptoms or rarely are asymptomatic and may be first recognized by the development of a murmur of aortic regurgitation (from aortic dilatation and distortion) in a patient with no history of underlying heart disease. A chest roentgenogram may show a localized bulge in the ascending aorta. Aortic root angiography is diagnostic and reveals the false and true lumens. Aortic regurgitation is demonstrated.

Echocardiographic features (Figs. 5-26 and 5-27)

• The aortic root is dilated and measures 42 mm or greater.

• The aortic wall is widened to at least 16 mm when the anterior wall is involved and 10 mm for posterior wall dissection (normal width up to 7 mm). Both the anterior and posterior walls are frequently involved.

• The intimal echo is usually thinner than the outer margin and generally moves parallel or nearly parallel to it throughout the cardiac cycle.

• Valve cusp echoes are normal and contained in the true lumen.

• The dissection space is usually sonolucent but may contain echo sources.

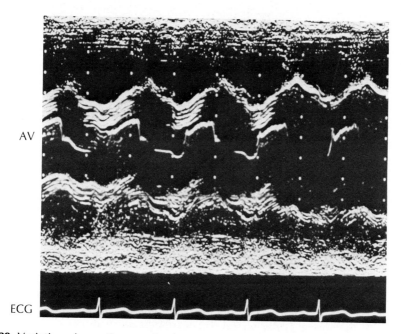

Fig. 5-28. Variations in aortic root size in aortic root dissection. The width of the aortic root recorded on the right is significantly greater as compared to the left. The anterior dissection space is incompletely recorded, but typical findings of dissection were present in other portions of the record. AV, aortic valve; ECG, electrocardiogram.

Comments

• Although aortic valve cusps show normal motion pattern, a slight tendency toward transient early systolic closure is not uncommon. Marked variations in the width of the aortic root image with slight changes in transducer angulation have also been observed and are probably related to the nonuniform thickness of the dissecting hematoma (Fig. 5-28). An intimal flap (present at the site of entry into the true lumen) may be imaged as an undulating echo in the aorta (Fig. 5-29). Associated findings on the echocardiogram may be of value. Demonstration of pericardial fluid collection by echocardiography may indicate that the dissection has ruptured into the pericardial sac. Appearance of mitral diastolic flutter indicative of aortic incompetence is another clue of aortic root involvement.

In the presence of a very large dissection (32 mm wide), the outer margin of a dissected wall may show complete loss of parallelism with the inner margin, which moves normally. In one patient studied by us, a prominent posteriorly directed movement of the outer margin was observed at the beginning of ventricular systole, probably related to systolic expansion of the unsupported margin produced by egress of blood into the aneurysm (Fig. 5-30).

• False-positives have been reported. Some originate in diseases such as atherosclerosis, which thicken the aortic wall. In other instances, a low beam position may superimpose the interventricular septum on the anterior aortic image. Simultaneous recording of the mitral ring with the posterior aortic wall has also been reported to simulate dissection.

• Calcification of the aortic valve, which produces multilayered echoes within the aor-

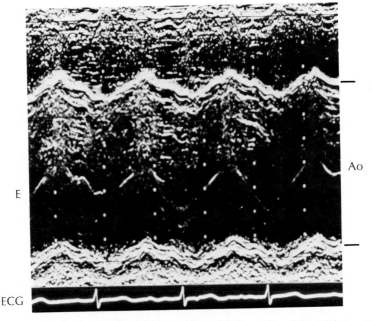

Fig. 5-29. Supravalvular aorta in a patient with aortic root dissection. The aorta (Ao) is markedly dilated and contains an abnormal undulating echo (E) within the lumen. The angiocardiogram demonstrated a large anterior dissection and intima that appeared to float freely in the supravalvular region. Echocardiograms recorded at the valve level showed parallelism between the intima and the outer aortic wall. The flapping seen in the supravalvular portion may arise from less complete anchoring of the intima or from recording near the site of the intimal tear. ECG, electrocardiogram.

tic lumen, may result in an appearance that simulates dissection. Lack of normal cusp echoes alerts the examiner, who should be very cautious in diagnosing dissection under these circumstances (Fig. 5-31).

• The number of false-positives can be reduced by eliminating those cases in which parallelism or near parallelism of the separated components of an aortic wall is not present (except when widening is very marked) or when aortic leaflets cross what appears to be the intimal echo in systole.

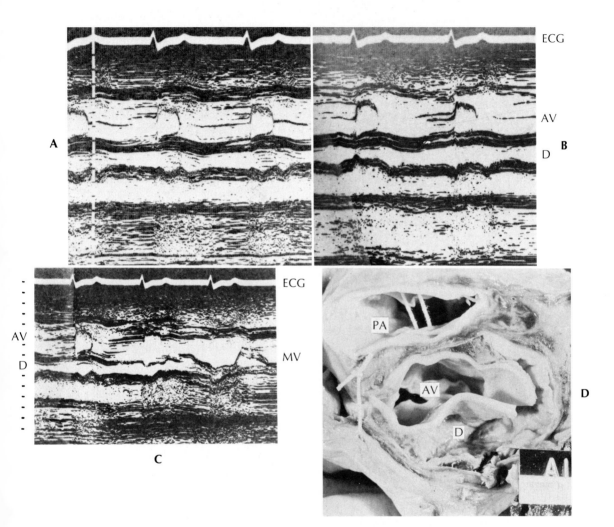

Fig. 5-30. Atypical echocardiographic findings in a patient with aortic root dissection. In **A** marked widening (32 mm) of the posterior aortic wall as well as nonparallelism of the separated margins is observed. The outer margin of the dissection cavity (D) moves posteriorly with the onset of ventricular systole. In **B,** atrial systole produces anterior movement of the outer margin of the dissected posterior aortic wall. **C** demonstrates continuity between the inner component of the dissected posterior aortic wall and the mitral valve (MV) during ultrasonic beam angulation from the aortic (AV) to the mitral valve. The autopsy specimen **(D)** shows a large dissection involving the posterior and lateral walls of the aortic root. The aortic cusps are intact. PA, pulmonary artery; ECG, electrocardiogram. (From Nanda, N. C., and others: Ann. Intern. Med. **85:**79, 1976.)

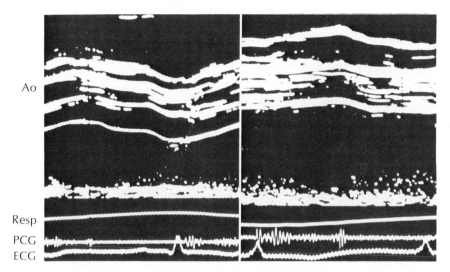

Fig. 5-31. Echocardiograms from two patients with extensive calcific aortic valve disease and no evidence of dissection. The presence of thick multilayered echoes within the aortic root (Ao) may simulate widening of the aortic walls. Resp, respiration; PCG, phonocardiogram; ECG, electrocardiogram. (From Nanda, N. C., and others: Circulation **48:**506, 1973. By permission of the American Heart Assn., Inc.)

When both walls are widened to over 16 mm (in addition to the above criteria), false-positives are virtually eliminated. Widening of the posterior aortic wall to 13 mm or less, by itself, appears to be an unreliable sign of dissecting aneurysm.

Careful attention to technical details also reduces the number of false-positive diagnoses. Occasionally, the finite width of the ultrasonic beam may result in simultaneous recording of the aortic valve cusps and thick multiple echoes from the atriopulmonic sulcus when moving the transducer toward the pulmonary valve from the aortic root position. Although this may mimic dissection, more medial transducer angulation results in disappearance of these artifactual echoes and recording of normal walls of the aortic root.

• Confusing images can be produced when a catheter is echoed in the right ventricular outflow tract or when pericardial effusion in the transverse sinus (see p. 274) widens the image of the posterior wall echo. Lack of parallelism of the echo sources plus other echocardiographic characteristics usually identify these conditions.

• Aortic valve endocarditis can be complicated by an abscess in the aortic wall. Though the involved wall may resemble dissection, the involvement of the leaflets and the localization in one aortic wall are useful in differentiating this condition from true dissection.

• False-negatives are rare, and a completely normal aortic root virtually excludes aortic root dissection, although theoretically, dissection confined to the lateral aspects of the aortic walls would be missed echocardiographically.

• Open heart surgery in which the aorta is opened may result in hematoma formation or in a localized dissection in the aortic walls and produce widened images of the walls of the aortic root in the postoperative echocardiograms.

• We have so far studied 17 cases of proved aortic root dissection. The diagnosis was made successfully in 14 of them on the basis of anterior or posterior aortic wall widening of 16 mm or more (12 patients) and isolated posterior aortic wall widening of 10 and 11 mm in the remaining two patients. The diagnosis was missed in three patients,

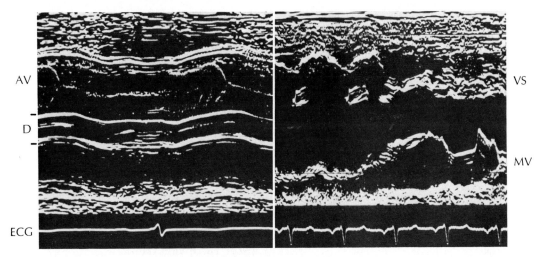

Fig. 5-32. Aortic aneurysms. An acute dissecting aneurysm *(left)* widens the aortic root and produces a dissection space (D) in the posterior aortic wall. Aortic valve leaflets (AV) are contained in the true lumen of the aorta, whose anterior wall is uninvolved in the dissection. An aneurysm of the ascending aorta, believed secondary to cystic medial necrosis, is shown on the right. The aortic root is markedly dilated and contains fragmentary images of valve leaflets. The aorta is approximately twice as wide as the left ventricular outflow tract, which lies between the ventricular septum (VS) and the mitral valve (MV) as demonstrated by beam scanning. ECG, electrocardiogram.

one because of inadequate and incomplete aortic root scanning (the beam was aimed too low and missed the dissection space), and the other two were related to extensive dissections presenting atypical echocardiographic findings.

Early in our experience, we also made three proved false-positive diagnoses of dissection. In two of them, dissection was simulated by mild fibrocalcific aortic valve disease that did not significantly affect cusp motion characteristics and hence was not recognized. In the other patient the findings of old bacterial endocarditis confused the picture.

• Mild thickening of the aortic walls (<10 mm) has been observed with rheumatoid arthritis and in systemic lupus erythematosis with Libman-Sacks endocarditis.

• Suprasternal echocardiography may be used to identify dissections in the aortic arch, away from the valve.

Role of echocardiography

• It should be reemphasized that the echocardiographic diagnosis of dissection depends on a combination of suggestive features and meticulous attention to technical details rather than on any single specific observation.

• Echocardiography is useful in ruling out dissection in patients with chest pain of unknown cause or in those with recent onset of aortic incompetence. It is also useful in clinically typical patients, since a rapid bedside diagnosis is possible. The demonstration of pericardial fluid helps to define a leaking dissection. Verification of the diagnosis of dissection by angiography is required before surgical correction is undertaken.

Nondissecting aneurysms. These cases simply show a dilatation of the aorta at the valve level and above it. The valve cusps are not thickened. Aortic regurgitation occurs when the aortic diameter exceeds 45 mm (Fig. 5-32). A beginning echocardiographer may be unable to identify the aorta when it is markedly dilated. Scanning the beam from the mitral valve through the aortic cusp echoes (they are usually seen) shows an aortic root much wider than the left ventricular outflow tract. We have seen aortic root aneurysms that measure 10 cm in diameter.

Aneurysms of the sinus of Valsalva. These aneurysms occur at the base of the aorta and most often involve the right sinus of Valsalva, which bulges into the right ventricular outflow tract. Leakage with communication to other cardiac chambers is common and produces a murmur that may be continuous

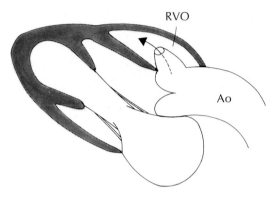

Fig. 5-33. Aneurysm of the right sinus of Valsalva. The right sinus of Valsalva is dilated and bulges into the right ventricular outflow tract (RVO). The protruding tip of the aneurysm has ruptured resulting in a shunt from the aorta (Ao) to the right ventricle.

through systole and diastole. Echocardiographic findings vary, depending on the site of the aneurysm and the direction of the fistula that may form. When the right sinus of Valsalva is involved, the right coronary cusp may appear to open to a position that crosses the anterior aortic wall and protrudes into the right ventricular outflow tract. A separate echo from the aneurysmal sac may also be seen in the right ventricular outflow tract (Figs. 5-33 and 5-34). Tricuspid and pulmonic valve motion may be altered. Experience with these uncommon lesions is too limited to permit further description.

Aortic valve vegetations

Bacterial or fungal vegetations are prone to develop on the leaflets of abnormal aortic valves, though they may also be found occasionally on previously normal cusps. They may result in regurgitant murmurs, arterial embolization, and systemic signs of infection with positive blood cultures. Cardiac catheterization and angiocardiography are usually avoided, since portions of the infected mass may be dislodged into the circulation. Echo-

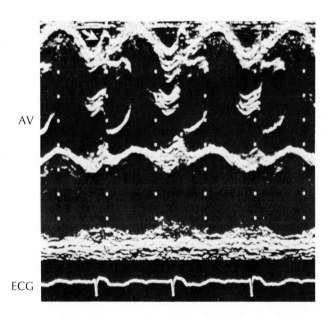

Fig. 5-34. Aneurysm of the right sinus of Valsalva. The abnormal echo *(arrow)* seen in the right ventricular outflow imaged in front of the dilated aortic root probably represents systolic protrusion of the aneurysm. AV, aortic valve; ECG, electrocardiogram.

cardiographic diagnosis depends on the size of the vegetation (large fungal masses are more readily detected than smaller bacterial vegetations), position of vegetation in the cusp and its accessibility to the ultrasonic beam, presence of calcification in it (calcium is a strong reflector), and its mobility characteristics. The echocardiogram generally shows a fuzzy thickening of the involved leaflet in systole, diastole or both (Fig. 5-35). When there is sufficient destruction of leaflet tissue to render the cusp unstable, the mass echoes may appear in the left ventricular outflow tract in front of the mitral valve in diastole and be swept into the aortic orifice in systole. Scans from the mitral valve to the supravalvular portion of the aorta are useful to document the entire systole-diastole motion of the mass (Fig. 5-36). The presence of the mass in the left ventricular outflow tract in diastole may deflect the regurgitant jet away from the mitral valve so that echocardiographic findings of aortic regurgitation may not be present. Associated widening of

the aortic wall from the infection has been seen and may simulate localized aortic root dissection.

Unsupported aortic leaflets

Aortic leaflets that have lost their normal attachment to the aortic wall as the result of chest injury or previous endocarditis become incompetent. In a few reported cases, rapid diastolic fluttering of the aortic valve has been demonstrated (Fig. 5-37). Similar findings have been seen in the so-called floppy aortic valve, in which the leaflets undergo myxomatous degeneration. In the presence of high ventricular septal defects the right coronary cusp of the aortic valve often prolapses into the right ventricle as the result of loss of support. We have been unable to recognize this condition echocardiographically.

FUNCTIONAL CHANGES

Fine, high-frequency and low-amplitude fluttering of the aortic valve in systole occurs

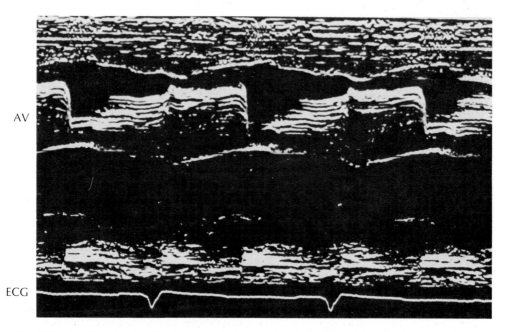

AV

ECG

Fig. 5-35. Aortic valve involvement with bacterial endocarditis. A wide echo complex is present in diastole and systole and suggests a large vegetation. At surgery scattered 1-mm calcified vegetations were present on all cusps. Their echoes summate to produce this appearance. AV, aortic valve; ECG, electrocardiogram.

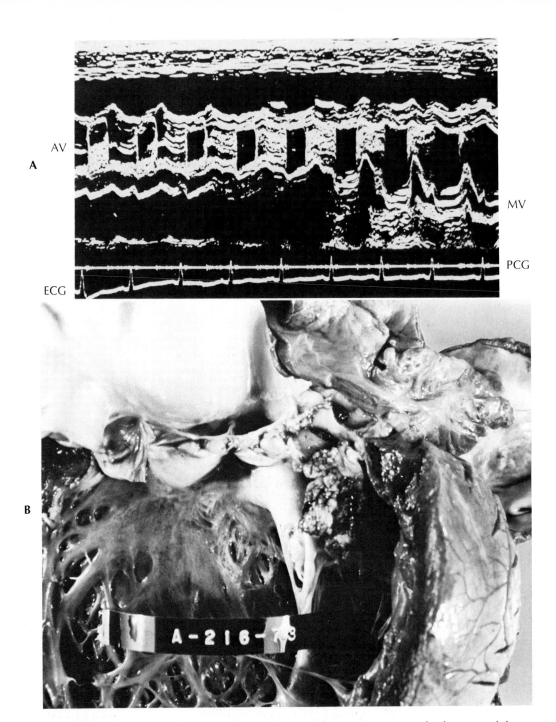

Fig. 5-36. Aortic valve vegetation. **A,** A large fungal vegetation is attached to one of the aortic valve cusps and prolapses into the left ventricle in diastole to produce the clusters of echoes seen in front of the mitral valve (MV). In systole, it is swept into the aortic orifice and appears as dense echoes that fill the lower portion of the image of the opened aortic valve (AV). Variable diastolic filling of the aortic lumen is present between the extremes of the scan, which extended from the aortic to the mitral valves. The widening of the posterior wall image resembles aortic root dissection and was produced by a sinus tract that involved the posterior aortic wall at autopsy. **B,** the pathologic specimen. ECG, electrocardiogram; PCG, phonocardiogram.

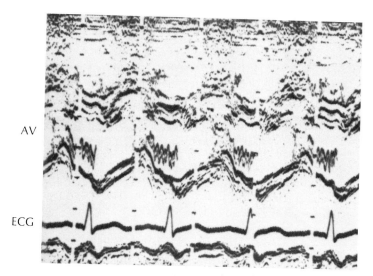

Fig. 5-37. Diastolic fluttering of the aortic valve from bacterial endocarditis. The rapid diastolic flutter results from loss of support of the aortic valve leaflets (AV) secondary to tissue destruction. In most severe cases, these vibrations may appear in the left ventricular outflow tract when aortic valve tissue prolapses in diastole. ECG, electrocardiogram.

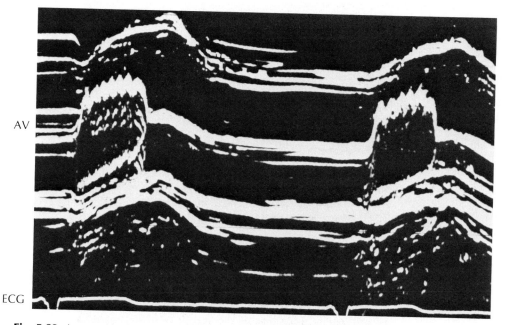

Fig. 5-38. A magnified recording of the aortic valve (AV) demonstrating high-frequency systolic fluttering of the right coronary cusp. The noncoronary leaflet also shows a subtle flutter. This is a nonspecific finding that may be seen in apparently normal individuals from the high velocities achieved during ejection. Coarser flutter results from turbulence and nonuniform ejection produced by a variety of lesions involving the left ventricle and left ventricular outflow tract as well as the proximal supravalvular region. ECG, electrocardiogram.

in normal patients and has no diagnostic significance (Fig. 5-38).

In IHSS the valve opens normally and then may close in midsystole when flow diminishes from the left ventricular outflow tract obstruction. It reopens in late systole and closes normally at end systole. The right coronary cusp has an M-shaped pattern, whereas the noncoronary cusp looks like a W. Combined recording of both cusps produces a double diamond configuration. These findings are seen in about 10% of patients with IHSS. More commonly, the aortic leaflets exhibit a coarse rolling flutter pattern probably related to turbulent flow through the valve. Flutter frequencies are usually low (5 to 50 flutters per second) with amplitudes of 3 to 4 mm (Fig. 4-39).

The aortic valve may flutter in the presence of a left ventricular leak such as mitral regurgitation or ventricular septal defect. Flutter amplitude is higher than in normal patients, though frequency is usually high. The shape of the systolic box may also change. After maximal opening is achieved, the reduction of forward flow (from regurgitation or shunt) allows the aortic leaflet to move obliquely downward in a gradual fashion to its closure at the end of ejection (Fig. 5-39) rather than crisply downward in end-systole as seen in normal patients. Similar findings have been observed in congestive cardiomyopathies without mitral regurgitation, probably from poor ejection by the left ventricle. Abnormal ejection, due to the presence of a left ventricular aneurysm, may also result in the production of coarse systolic flutter. Turbulence from abnormal flow may be another contributing factor. Systolic motion abnormalities of the aortic valve indicate that blood flow through the aortic valve is abnormal and are clues to the presence of an abnormality elsewhere.

Aortic valve systolic fluttering is found in

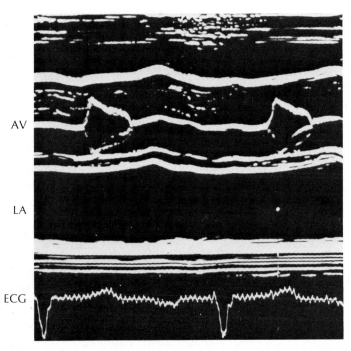

AV

LA

ECG

Fig. 5-39. Aortic valve echocardiogram in mitral incompetence. The aortic valve (AV) opens normally, but the leaflets show a gradual movement toward closure and do not maintain the normal position parallel to the aortic walls throughout systole. The abnormal movement pattern probably results from decreased forward flow from mitral regurgitation. LA, left atrium; ECG, electrocardiogram.

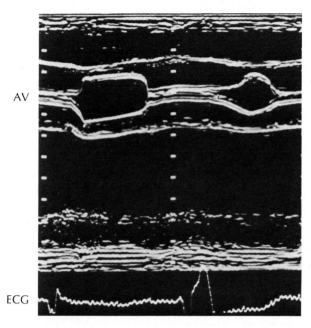

AV

ECG

Fig. 5-40. Effect of a premature ventricular contraction on aortic valve motion. The velocities of opening and closing movements of the aortic valve (AV) and the duration of ejection are reduced following a premature ventricular contraction *(right)* as compared to a normally conducted beat *(left)*. This results from a low stroke volume produced by the ventricle contracting prematurely before completion of diastolic filling. ECG, electrocardiogram.

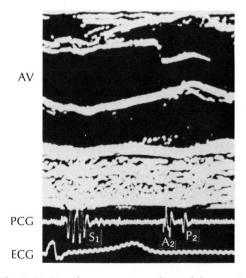

AV

PCG

ECG

Fig. 5-41. Simultaneous recording of the aortic valve (AV) and heart sounds. Aortic valve closure is closely related to the aortic component (A₂) of the second heart sound. PCG, phonocardiogram; S₁, first heart sound; P₂, pulmonic component of the second heart sound; ECG, electrocardiogram.

a wide variety of other clinical conditions in which the cause is not clear.

Disorders of cardiac rhythm that result in decreased systolic ejection (rapid atrial fibrillation, premature supraventricular or ventricular contractions) alter the waveform of the aortic valve. When the volume of ejected blood is normal, a typical square "box" is produced. When the ventricle contracts before diastolic filling is complete, the opening amplitude and the duration of opening are reduced (Fig. 5-40). In some cases the aortic valve may not open at all, or an early systolic abortive opening takes place and produces a peaked tracing or one that mimics aortic valve preclosure seen in subaortic membranous stenosis.

Diastolic opening of the aortic valve leaflets has been documented when aortic regurgitation raises the pressure in the left ventricle to a point where it is greater than aortic diastolic pressure. This is a rare finding and indicates very severe aortic regurgitation. Attempts to diagnose aortic regurgitation based on apparent leaflet separation during diastole should not be made, since it is commonly seen in patients who have competent aortic valves. This is probably an artifact occurring as a result of a low beam position that does not detect the level of leaflet closure.

The early systolic peak that occurs in sub-aortic stenosis has been described previously.

A phonocardiogram may be recorded with the aortic valve to relate the heart sounds with aortic valve opening and closing movements (Fig. 5-41).

BIBLIOGRAPHY
Aortic valve and aortic root (general)

Gramiak, R., and Shah, P. M.: Echocardiography of the aortic root, Invest. Radiol. **3:**356, 1968.

Gramiak, R., and Shah, P. M.: Echocardiography of the normal and diseased aortic valve, Radiology **96:**1, 1970.

Hernberg, J., Weiss, B., and Keegan, A.: The ultrasonic recording of aortic valve motion, Radiology **94:**361, 1970.

Francis, G. S., Hagan, A. D., Oury, J., and O'Rourke, R. A.: Accuracy of echocardiography for assessing aortic root diameter, Br. Heart J. **37:**376, 1975.

Pratt, R. C., Parisi, A. F., Harrington, J. J., and Sasahara, A. A.: The influence of left ventricular stoke volume on aortic root motion, Circulation **53:**947, 1976.

Reeves, W., Ettinger, U., Nanda, N. C., Gramiak, R., and DeWeese, J. A.: Assessment of aortic prosthesis size and valve calcification by echocardiography, Clin. Res. **24:**237A, 1976.

Scovil, J. A., Nanda, N. C., Gross, C. M., Lombardi, A. C., Gramiak, R., Lipchick, E. O., and Manning, J. A.: Echocardiographic studies of abnormalities associated with coarctation of the aorta, Circulation **53:**953-956, 1976.

Atsuchi, Y., Nagai, Y., Komatsu, Y., Nakamura, K., Shibuya, M., and Hirosawa, K.: Echocardiographic manifestations of annuloaortic ectasis; its "paradoxical" motion of the aorta and premature systolic closure of the aortic valve, Am. Heart J. **93:**428-433, 1977.

Hess, P. G., Nanda, N. C., Thomson, K. R., Schwartz, R. G., Ross, A., and Gramiak, R.: Systolic motion patterns of the aortic valve; clinical echo correlates, Circulation **56:**50, 1977.

Reeves, W. C., Nanda, N. C., and Gramiak, R.: Relation of aortic valve closure to aortic root motion, Clin. Res. **25:**248A, 1977.

Aortic aneurysms

Millward, D. K., Robinson, N. J., and Craige, E.: Dis-

secting aortic aneurysm diagnosed by echocardiography in a patient with rupture of the aneurysm into the right atrium, Am. J. Cardiol. **30:**427, 1972.

Nanda, N. C., Gramiak, R., and Shah, P. M.: Diagnosis of aortic root dissection by echocardiography, Circulation **48:**506, 1973.

Cooperberg, P., Mercer, E. N., Mulder, D. S., and Winsberg, F.: Rupture of a sinus Valsalva aneurysm; report of a case diagnosed preoperatively by echocardiography, Radiology **113:**171, 1974.

Kronzon, I., and Mehta, S. S.: Illustrative echocardiogram; aortic root dissection, Chest **65:**88, 1974.

Rothbaum, D. A., Dillon, J. C., Chang, S., and Feigenbaum, H.: Echocardiographic manifestation of right sinus of Valsalva aneurysm, Circulation **49:**768, 1974.

Warren, S. G., Waugh, R. A., Kisslo, J., and Johnson, M. L.: Echocardiographic abnormalities in ruptured right coronary sinus of Valsalva aneurysm, Circulation **50**(suppl. 3):249, 1974 (abstract).

Weill, F., Kraehenbuhl, J. R., Ricatte, J. P., Aucant, D., Gillet, M., and Makridis, D.: Ultrasonic diagnosis of aortic dissections and aneurysmal fissurations, Ann. Radiol. (Paris) **17:**49, 1974.

Yuste, P., Aza, V., Minguez, I., Cerezo, L., and Martinez-Bardiu, C.: Dissecting aortic aneurysm diagnosed by echocardiography, Br. Heart J. **36:**111, 1974.

Brown, O. R., Popp, R. L., and Kloster, F. E.: Echocardiographic criteria for aortic root dissection, Am. J. Cardiol. **36:**17, 1975.

Krueger, S. K., Starke, H., Forker, A. D., and Eliot, R. S.: Echocardiographic mimics of aortic root dissection, Chest **67:**441, 1975.

Moothart, R. W., Spangler, R. D., and Blout, S. G., Jr.: Echocardiography in aortic root dissection and dilatation, Am. J. Cardiol. **36:**11, 1975.

Hirschfeld, D. S., Rodriguez, H. J., and Schiller, N. B.: Duplication of aortic wall seen by echocardiography, Br. Heart J. **38:**843-850, 1976.

Matsumoto, M., Matsuo, H., Beppu, S., Yoshioka, Y., Kawashima, Y., Nimura, Y., and Abe, H.: Echocardiographic diagnosis of ruptured aneurysm of sinus of Valsalva, report of two cases, Circulation **53:**382, 1976.

Nanda, N. C., Ong, L. S., and Barold, S. S.: Unusual echocardiographic motion pattern in aortic root dissection, Ann. Intern. Med. **85:**79, 1976.

Nanda, N. C., Lever, H., Gramiak, R., Ross, A., Reeves, W., Hess, P., Zesk, J., and Combs, R.: Reliability of echocardiography in the diagnosis of aortic root dissection, Circulation **56:**68, 1977.

Aortic stenosis

Yeh, H. C., Winsberg, F., and Mercer, E. M.: Echocardiographic aortic valve orifice dimension; its use in evaluating aortic stenosis and cardiac output, J. Clin. Ultrasound **1:**182, 1973.

Feizi, O., Symons, C., and Yacoub, M.: Echocardiography of the aortic valve, I. Studies of normal aortic valve, aortic stenosis, aortic regurgitation and mixed aortic valve disease, Br. Heart J. **36:**341, 1974.

Bennett, D. H., Evans, D. W., and Raj, M. V.: Proceedings; echocardiographic estimation of the systolic pressure gradient in aortic stenosis, Br. Heart J. **37:**557, 1975.

Weyman, A. E., Feigenbaum, H., Dillon, J. C., and Chang, S.: Cross-sectional echocardiography in assessing the severity of valvular aortic stenosis, Circulation, **52:**828-834, 1975.

Glanz, S., Hellenbrand, W. E., Berman, M. A., and Talner, N. S.: Echocardiographic assessment of the severity of aortic stenosis in children and adolescents, Am. J. Cardiol. **38:**620-625, 1976.

Hurwitz, R. A., Weyman, A. B., Feigenbaum, H., Girod, D. A., and Dillon, J. C.: Cross-sectional echocardiographic assessment of severity of aortic stenosis in children, Am. J. Cardiol. **37:**144, 1976 (abstract).

Johnson, G. L., Meyer, R. A., Schwartz, D. C., Korfhagen, J., and Kaplan, S.: Left ventricular function by echocardiography in children with fixed aortic stenosis, Am. J. Cardiol. **38:**611-619, 1976.

Talano, J., Frazin, L., Stephanides, L., Croke, R., Loeb, H., and Gunnar, R.: Echocardiographic index for estimating the severity of aortic stenosis, Circulation 54(suppl. 2):233, 1976.

Chang, S., Clements, S., Chang, J.: Aortic stenosis; echocardiographic cusp separation and surgical description of aortic valve in 22 patients, Am. J. Cardiol. **39:**499, 1977.

Supravalvular aortic stenosis

Usher, B. W., Goulden, D., and Murgo, J. P.: Echocardiographic detection of supravalvular aortic stenosis, Circulation **49:**1257, 1974.

Bolen, J. L., Popp, R. L., and French, J. W.: Echocardiographic features of supravalvular aortic stenosis, Circulation **52:**817, 1975.

Nasrallah, A. T., and Nihill, M.: Supravalvular aortic stenosis; echocardiographic features, Br. Heart J. **37:** 662, 1975.

Bicuspid aortic valve

Nanda, N. C., Gramiak, R., Manning, J., Mahoney, E. B., Lipchik, E. O., and DeWeese, J. A.: Echocardiographic recognition of the congenital bicuspid aortic valve, Circulation **49:**870, 1974.

Nanda, N. C., and Gramiak, R.: Echocardiographic studies in unicommissural aortic stenosis, Clin. Res. **24:**232A, 1976.

Radford, D. J., Bloom, K. R., Izukawa, R., Moes, C. A. F., and Rowe, R. D.: Echocardiographic assessment of bicuspid aortic valves, Circulation **53:** 80, 1976.

Scovil, J. A., Nanda, N. C., Gramiak, R., and Lipchik, E. O.: Echocardiographic assessment of aortic valve morphology, Circulation 54(suppl. 2):112, 1976 (abstract).

Aortic valve vegetations

Gottlieb, S., Khuddus, S. A., Balooki, H., Dominguez, A. E., and Myerburg, R. J.: Echocardiographic diagnosis of aortic valve vegetations in Candida endocarditis, Circulation **50:**826-830, 1974.

Martinez, E. C., Burch, G. E., and Files, T. D.: Echocardiographic diagnosis of vegetative aortic bacterial endocarditis, Am. J. Cardiol. **34:**845, 1974.

DeMaria, A. N., King, J. F., Salel, A. F., Caudill, C. C., Miller, R. R., and Mason, D. T.: Echography and phonography of acute aortic regurgitation in bacterial endocarditis, Ann. Intern. Med. **82:**329, 1975.

Wray, T. M.: The variable echocardiographic features in aortic valve endocarditis, Circulation **52:**658-663, 1975.

Arvan, S., Cagin, N., Levitt, B., and Kleid, J. J.: Echocardiographic findings in a patient with Candida endocarditis of the aortic valve, Chest **70:**300-302, 1976.

Hirschfeld, D. S., and Schiller, N.: Localization of aortic valve vegetations by echocardiography, Circulation **53:**280, 1976.

Yoshikawa, J., Tanaka, K., Owaki, T., and Kato, H.: Cord-like aortic valve vegetation in bacterial endocarditis; demonstration by cardiac ultrasonography, report of a case, Circulation **53:**911-914, 1976.

Fox, S., Kotler, M. N., Segal, B. L., and Parry, W.: Echocardiographic diagnosis of acute aortic valve endocarditis and its complications, Arch. Intern. Med. **137:**85-89, 1977.

Moorthy, K., Prakash, R., Aronow, W. S.: Echocardiographic appearance of aortic valve vegetations in bacterial endocarditis due to Actinobacillus actinomycetemcomitans, J. Clin. Ultrasound **5:**49-51, 1977.

Flail aortic leaflets

Lee, C. C., Das, G., and Weissler, A. M.: Characteristic echocardiographic manifestations in ruptured aortic valve leaflet, Circulation 50(suppl. 3):144, 1974 (abstract).

Chandraratna, P. A., Samet, P., Robinson, M. J., and Byrd, C.: Echocardiography of the "floppy" aortic valve; report of a case, Circulation **52:**959-962, 1975.

Wray, T. M.: Echocardiography manifestations of flail aortic valve leaflets in bacterial endocarditis, Circulation **51:**832-835, 1975.

Corrigall, D., Strunk, B. L., and Popp, R. L.: Phonocardiographic and echocardiographic features of ruptured aortic valvular cusp, Chest **69:**669-671, 1976.

Estevez, C. N., Dillon, J. C., Walker, P. D., Feigenbaum, H., and Chang, S.: Echocardiographic manifestations of aortic cusp rupture in a case of myxomatous degeneration of the aortic valve, Chest **69:** 544, 1976.

Rolston, W. A., Hirschfeld, D. S., Emilson, B. B., and Cheitlin, M. D.: Echocardiographic appearance of ruptured aortic cusp, Am. J. Med. **62:**133-138, 1977.

6 Tricuspid valve

STRUCTURES IN BEAM

During tricuspid valve recording the ultrasonic beam generally passes through the following structures:

1. Chest wall
2. Anterior wall of the right ventricle
3. Right ventricular cavity
4. Anterior leaflet of the tricuspid valve
5. Right atrial cavity
6. Right atrial posterior wall

Occasionally, the interatrial septum may be identified behind the tricuspid valve, and in this instance the ultrasonic beam traverses through the following structures in an anteroposterior direction:

1. Chest wall
2. Anterior right ventricular wall
3. Right ventricular cavity
4. Anterior tricuspid valve leaflet
5. Right atrium (represents the space between the closed position of the tricuspid valve and the interatrial septum)
6. Interatrial septum
7. Left atrial cavity
8. Left atrial posterior wall

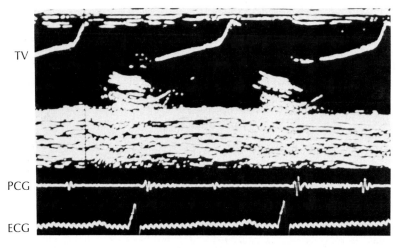

Fig. 6-1. Tricuspid valve (TV) recording in a normal adult. Only the systolic segment and the diastolic opening movement are recorded, producing a "gull-wing" appearance. PCG, phonocardiogram; ECG, electrocardiogram.

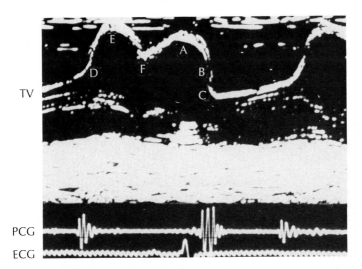

Fig. 6-2. Complete recording of the tricuspid valve (TV) demonstrating functional events labeled by the same convention as that used for the mitral valve. PCG, phonocardiogram; ECG, electrocardiogram.

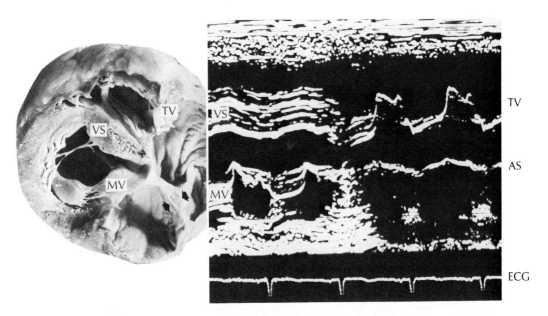

Fig. 6-3. Identification of the atrial septum. The atrial septum (AS) is recorded during ultrasonic beam scanning from the mitral to the tricuspid valve (TV) and is continuous with the mitral valve (MV). The specimen of the heart, on the left, demonstrates the anatomic continuity between the atrial septum *(black arrows)* and the mitral valve. VS, ventricular septum; ECG, electrocardiogram. (From Nanda, N. C., and others: Ultrasound Med. **2:**1, 1976.)

NORMAL TRACING

In the normal adult, only the systolic segment and the diastolic opening movement of the anterior leaflet are generally recorded (Fig. 6-1). With cardiac rotation or right ventricular enlargement the tricuspid valve is displaced laterally and becomes more accessible to the ultrasonic beam, resulting in complete recordings (Fig. 6-2). The contour of the tracing resembles the mitral valve. With the onset of diastole (D), the tricuspid valve opens briskly and inscribes a large anterior movement that is associated with rapid blood flow into the right ventricle. The maxi-

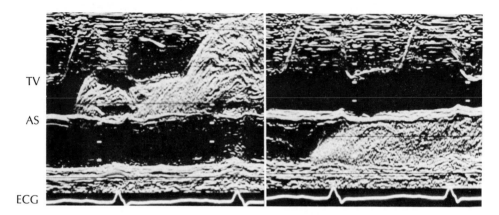

Fig. 6-4. Identification of the atrial septum using contrast injections. Injection of indocyanine green into the right atrium (via a catheter inserted at surgery) demonstrates echoes in the region of the tricuspid valve (TV) and limited by the atrial septum (AS). On the right, contrast injection into the left atrial cavity reveals dense echoes behind the atrial septum. No echoes are present in the right atrial cavity in front of the atrial septum. ECG, electrocardiogram.

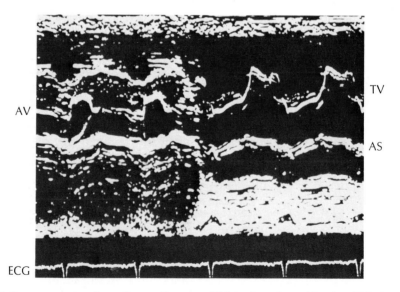

Fig. 6-5. Beam scanning from the aortic valve (AV) to the tricuspid valve (TV) shows the close proximity of the atrial septum (AS) to the posterior aortic wall. ECG, electrocardiogram. (From Nanda, N. C., and others: Ultrasound Med. **2:**1, 1976.)

mal opening position is designated E. Thereafter, the pressure gradient across the valve decreases, and the tricuspid valve moves toward a position of semiclosure, F. The valve remains stationary in this position until atrial systole, which results in a large excursion (A wave). With ventricular systole the tricuspid valve moves posteriorly as it closes (C). Occasionally, a small hump may be observed on the A-C segment and is termed B. The closed tricuspid valve, like the mitral, should show no intrinsic motion during systole, but a gradual anterior movement is frequently observed and is related to ventricular systole as it affects tricuspid annulus motion (Fig. 6-2).

During ultrasonic beam sweeping from the mitral to the tricuspid valve, the mitral valve can be shown frequently to end in a linear structure that moves anteriorly in systole and posteriorly in diastole. This represents the interatrial septum, and the tricuspid valve is recorded in front of it (Figs. 6-3 and 6-4). The basal portion of the interatrial septum is recorded during this maneuver. Moving the ultrasonic beam from the tricuspid to the aortic valve also reveals the interatrial septum to be close to the posterior wall of the aorta, which is probably largely responsible for its motion pattern (Fig. 6-5).

Complete recordings of the anterior tricuspid leaflet are commonly seen in normal infants and children, since the sternum is relatively unossified and does not constitute a barrier to the passage of the ultrasonic beam.

With right ventricular enlargement the tricuspid valve may be recorded in front of the ventricular septum and occasionally in front of the aortic root recording. In the presence of gross right ventricular enlargement the right ventricular posterior wall may be recorded behind the tricuspid valve. It has the same motion characteristics as the left ventricular posterior wall (Fig. 6-6).

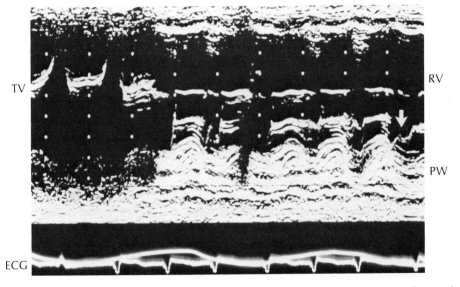

Fig. 6-6. Beam scanning from tricuspid valve to the right ventricular cavity. The study begins in the usual tricuspid valve (TV) position and shows the beam leaving the heart through the right atrial wall. Scanning over the body of the enlarged right ventricle (RV) demonstrates linear chordae echoes at the level of the anterior tricuspid leaflet as well as the more deeply situated posterior (inferior) tricuspid leaflet *(arrow)*. The posterior right ventricular wall (PW) resembles that of the left ventricle, which could be seen in a different beam position. ECG, electrocardiogram.

Septal and posterior leaflets

In normal children and in adults with right heart enlargement, a second leaflet of the tricuspid valve can be recorded moving in an opposite direction to the anterior leaflet in diastole and coapting with it at the beginning of systole. Correlation with anatomic specimens indicates that the ultrasonic beam traversing the anterior tricuspid leaflet and the ventricular or atrial septum would traverse the septal leaflet of the tricuspid valve (Fig. 6-7). Thus, echocardiographic recordings of two leaflets of the tricuspid valve together with simultaneous imaging of the ventricular or atrial septum identify the posteriorly moving leaflet as the septal cusp of the tricuspid valve. The posterior (or inferior) leaflet of the tricuspid valve lies deeper to the ultrasonic plane required for simultaneous imaging of valve leaflets and septa. It can be identified when the ultrasonic beam is angled off the anterior leaflet of the tricuspid valve inferiorly to image the right ventricular posterior wall. In this projection the posteriorly moving leaflet recorded in front of the right ventricular posterior wall represents the posterior or the inferior leaflet (Fig. 6-6).

TECHNICAL CONSIDERATIONS

- Since the tricuspid valve is situated behind the sternum, its detection requires a long sound pathway and, consequently, high gain settings.
- For optimal recordings, it is frequently necessary to suppress reverberatory echoes from the chest wall that clutter the anterior region. This may be accomplished using anterior gain suppression or time-varied gain. One should be careful, though, not to use excessive time-varied gain, since it may accentuate posterior reverberations and mask abnormalities in that region (Fig. 6-8).
- When the cardiac window is small, placing the transducer in the subxiphoid region may help detect the tricuspid valve with superior and medial beam angulation.
- With right ventricular enlargement the tricuspid valve may be recorded more posteriorly in relation to the chest wall and may be misidentified as the mitral valve (Fig. 6-9). In such cases, more lateral angulation reveals a mitral valve located more posteriorly.
- An undulating linear echo is sometimes recorded in the right atrial cavity behind the

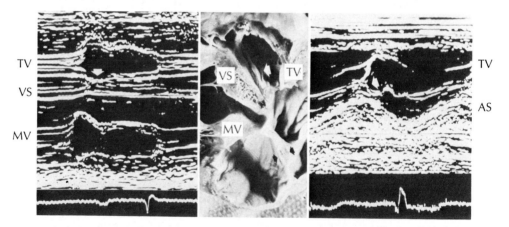

Fig. 6-7. Identification of the septal leaflet of the tricuspid valve. Correlation with the anatomic specimen identifies the posteriorly moving cusp of the tricuspid valve (TV) as the septal leaflet *(white arrows)* when it is recorded simultaneously with the ventricular septum *(left)* or the atrial septum *(right)*. The posterior or the inferior cusp of the tricuspid valve is not recorded, since it is located deeper to the ultrasonic plane required for simultaneous imaging of these structures. MV, mitral valve; VS, ventricular septum; AS, atrial septum. The black arrows on the anatomic specimen denote the atrial septum. (From Nanda, N. C., and others: Ultrasound Med. **2:**1, 1976.)

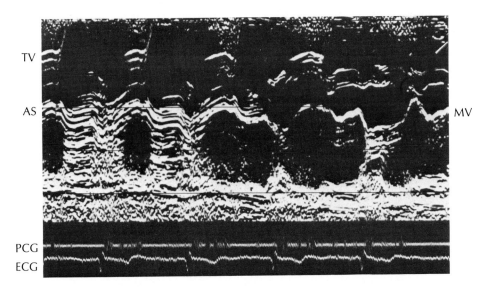

Fig. 6-8. Reverberations behind the atrial septum. Multiple linear reverberatory echoes are visible posterior to the atrial septum. Changes in beam angulation and a decrease in the time-varied gain proved effective in eliminating them. TV, tricuspid valve; AS, atrial septum; MV, mitral valve; PCG, phonocardiogram; ECG, electrocardiogram.

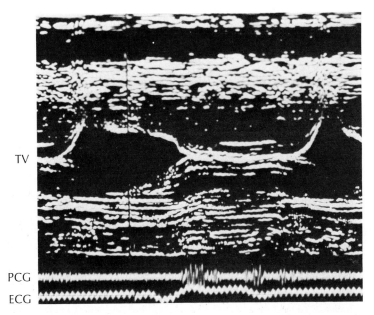

Fig. 6-9. Tricuspid valve recording in a patient with a large right ventricle. The tricuspid valve is recorded more posteriorly in relation to the chest wall and may be misidentified as the mitral valve. Anterior suppression has given a bandlike appearance to the reverberatory echoes, which may be mistaken for the ventricular septum. In this patient, more lateral angulation revealed a more posteriorly located mitral valve. TV, tricuspid valve; PCG, phonocardiogram; ECG, electrocardiogram.

tricuspid valve, and this may represent the flap normally present at the opening of the inferior vena cava (Eustachian valve). (Figs. 6-10 and 6-11). This should not be confused with the atrial septal echo, which has a char-

acteristic motion pattern and can be shown to be continuous with the mitral valve.

• If the transducer is angled too medially, a prominent linear echo with a large-amplitude excursion and moving anteriorly in

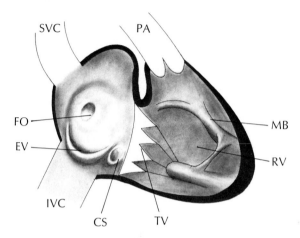

Fig. 6-10. Right heart anatomy. The inflow and outflow portions of the right ventricle are shown along with the muscle bands (MB) present in the wall at the junction of the two segments. The transverse band just beneath the pulmonary valve is the crista supraventricularis. The various venous orifices and their valves are demonstrated. SVC, superior vena cava; FO, fossa ovalis; EV, eustachian valve, which is present at the mouth of the inferior vena cava (IVC); CS, opening of the coronary sinus, which is partially covered by a flap called the Thebesian valve; TV, tricuspid valve; PA, pulmonary artery; RV, right ventricle.

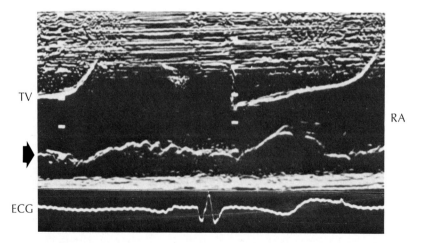

Fig. 6-11. Tricuspid valve recording with the ultrasonic beam exiting through the right atrium. The echo-free space behind the tricuspid valve (TV) represents the right atrial cavity (RA). The origin of the undulating echo *(arrow)* in the right atrium is obscure but may represent the flap at the mouth of the inferior vena cava or coronary sinus. ECG, electrocardiogram.

systole and posteriorly in diastole may be observed anteriorly and probably represents the anterior right atrial wall. In this instance, minimal lateral angulation should result in detection of the tricuspid valve.

FINDINGS IN DISEASE
Tricuspid stenosis

Anatomic and functional changes

• In this entity, there is fusion of the commissures of the tricuspid leaflets, resulting in a stenotic or obstructed tricuspid orifice. The valve may rarely develop calcification.

• The condition is uncommon and may be rheumatic or congenital in nature. Frequently, it coexists with rheumatic mitral stenosis.

• The stenosed orifice results in enlargement of the right atrium and increased right atrial pressure to propel blood through the narrow orifice in diastole.

Clinical summary. Clinically, the prominent A wave on the jugular venous pulse and a middiastolic rumble, which becomes louder during inspiration, suggests the presence of tricuspid stenosis. The diagnosis may be difficult in the presence of coexisting mitral stenosis, which also produces a middiastolic murmur. Cardiac catheterization reveals a diastolic gradient across the tricuspid valve. Angiocardiogram may show a thickened and immobile tricuspid valve.

Echocardiographic features

• The tricuspid valve shows a slow diastolic slope under 35 mm/sec (Fig. 6-12). This results from slow right atrial emptying.

• The A wave may be attenuated or obliterated in patients retaining sinus rhythm.

• The posterior leaflet has been reported moving in the same direction as the anterior cusp (since the fused cusps form a "funnel"), and valvular calcifications have been detected. Tricuspid stenosis is sufficiently rare that we have not observed either of these findings.

Comments

• A normal diastolic slope of the tricuspid valve (greater than 35 mm/sec) excludes the presence of tricuspid stenosis.

• Slow diastolic slopes may be seen with restrictive processes involving the right ven-

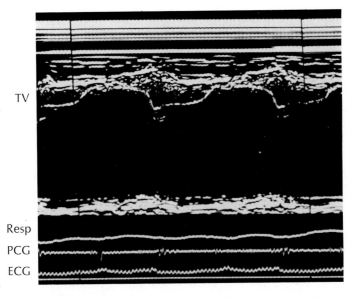

Fig. 6-12. Tricuspid valve stenosis. This patient has rheumatic heart disease with mitral and tricuspid valve stenosis. Echocardiogram shows a noncalcified tricuspid valve (TV) with a flat diastolic slope. At surgery, valve orifice would admit only one fingertip. Resp, respiration; PCG, phonocardiogram; ECG, electrocardiogram. (From Gramiak, R., and Waag, R. C.: Cardiac ultrasound, St. Louis, 1975, The C. V. Mosby Co.)

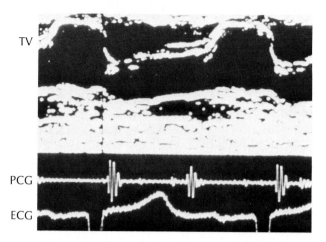

Fig. 6-13. Flat diastolic slopes of the tricuspid valve (TV) in a patient with right ventricular hypertrophy. There was no evidence for tricuspid valve stenosis. PCG, phonocardiogram; ECG, electrocardiogram.

tricle or other conditions associated with reduced right ventricular compliance (Fig. 6-13).

Role of echocardiography. Echocardiography is of limited usefulness in the diagnosis of tricuspid valve stenosis, since slow diastolic slopes are commonly seen with other right ventricular problems. The technique is useful in excluding the presence of tricuspid stenosis in patients with rheumatic heart disease.

Tricuspid valve prolapse

Anatomic and functional changes
• This condition is characterized by a myxomatous change in the tricuspid valve with evidence of leaflet redundancy. The chordae tendineae are often elongated, and this results in buckling or prolapse of the valve into the right atrium in mid to late systole.
• It frequently coexists with mitral valve prolapse.

Clinical summary. A loud midsystolic click followed by a late systolic murmur of tricuspid incompetence may be heard. These findings resemble those seen in mitral valve prolapse. The existence of this anomaly is difficult to prove during cardiac catheterization and angiography, since the passage of the right heart catheter through the tri-

cuspid valve orifice may normally prevent proper coaptation of the valve leaflets and makes it difficult to visualize the valve anatomy.

Echocardiographic features
• Large mid to late posterior displacement of the tricuspid valve below the closure point during systole (Fig. 6-14).

Comments
• The echocardiographic finding in this entity is similar to that observed in the mitral valve echocardiograms of patients with prolapsing mitral valves.
• Systolic sagging and straight downhill motion of the tricuspid valve throughout systole appear to be less specific, since they have been observed with right ventricular enlargement or tricuspid incompetence in the absence of evidence for valve prolapse (Fig. 6-14).
• The diagnosis of tricuspid valve prolapse should be advanced with caution in patients with large pericardial effusions, since cardiac swinging may produce motion artifacts that simulate tricuspid valve prolapse.
• A prolonged PR interval may result in preclosure of the tricuspid valve in diastole, and the tricuspid valve trace may thereafter show posterior motion with the onset of systole. This may be misdiagnosed as tricuspid

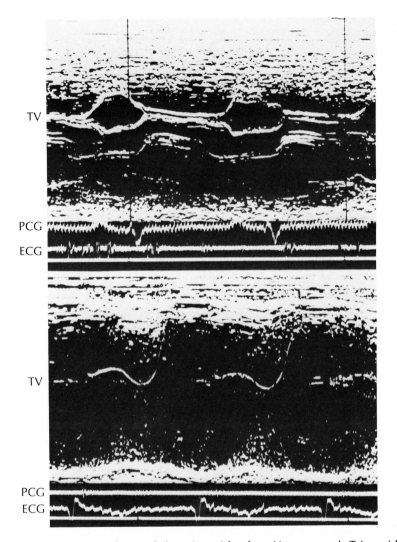

Fig. 6-14. Systolic abnormalities of the tricuspid valve. *Upper panel,* Tricuspid valve echocardiogram in a patient with tricuspid incompetence due to right heart dilatation. The systolic segments show straight downhill slopes. *Lower panel,* Tricuspid valve echocardiogram from a patient with typical echocardiographic features of mitral valve prolapse. The tricuspid valve executes a sharp posterior movement in midsystole, raising the possibility of associated tricuspid valve prolapse. TV, tricuspid valve; PCG, phonocardiogram; ECG, electrocardiogram. (From Nanda, N. C., and others; Circulation **51:**268, 1975. By permission of the American Heart Assn., Inc.)

valve prolapse if the simultaneously recorded electrocardiogram is not carefully inspected.

• A premature ventricular contraction may be followed by a systolic interval during which the valve sags in normal patients.

Role of echocardiography. The sensitivity and specificity of echocardiography in evaluating tricuspid valve prolapse have not been defined so far. Unlike the mitral valve the tricuspid valve cannot be easily examined from various transducer positions in most cases, and tricuspid valve prolapse may go undetected.

Right atrial myxomas

Anatomic and functional changes

• Myxomas occur less commonly in the right atrium as compared to the left atrial cavity. They usually consist of jellylike masses attached to the atrial septum by a stalk.

• A myxoma may obstruct right ventricular inflow, since it frequently prolapses into the right ventricle following the opening of the tricuspid valve in diastole. During systole it moves back into the right atrial cavity.

• Portions of the tumor may be detached and embolize into the pulmonary circulation. Hemorrhage may occur into the tumor, and rarely it may get infected.

• Tumor may spread by contiguity, and satellite tumors may be found in the vicinity of the primary tumor. A left atrial myxoma may coexist with the right atrial tumor.

• Surgical resection is feasible and curative, although recurrence has been reported.

Clinical summary

• Myxomas have varied manifestations and can mimic any cardiovascular disorder.

• Obstruction to right ventricular inflow frequently produces a diastolic murmur not unlike that heard in tricuspid stenosis. Typically, the murmur may change in character with alteration in body position.

• A right atrial angiogram with a catheter positioned in the superior or inferior vena cava outlines the mass.

Echocardiographic features

• A mass or abnormal grouping of linear, wavy, or punctate echoes is observed behind the tricuspid valve in diastole (Figs. 6-15 and 6-16).

• Since tumor echoes follow the opening movement of the tricuspid valve by a short interval, a small echo-free space may be recorded between the tricuspid valve opening movement and the initial appearance of tumor echoes.

• The diastolic slope of the tricuspid valve may be decreased because of slow right atrial emptying resulting from tricuspid valve orifice obstruction produced by the tumor.

• If the tumor is large or the stalk is short

with attachment near the outflow portion of the right atrium, tumor echoes may also be recorded behind the tricuspid valve systolic position.

• The prolapsing portion of the tumor may be detected during diastole in the right ventricular cavity recorded in front of the ventricular septum (Fig. 4-50). Occasionally, it may be identified in the right ventricular outflow anterior to aortic root recording.

• Examination of the right atrial cavity from various transducer positions may reveal tumor echoes in systole. In diastole they move anteriorly towards the tricuspid valve, producing echo-free spaces posteriorly.

Comments

• A right atrial myxoma may be missed if the tricuspid valve region is not examined using both high- and low-gain settings. Very high gain may make it difficult to differentiate tumor echoes from the reverberatory clutter present normally in the anterior region. A very low gain, on the other hand, may result in poor display of the echoes from the myxoma.

• Multilayered echoes are occasionally detected behind the tricuspid valve systolic segment in normal patients and probably represent intracardiac reverberations. Changes in ultrasonic beam angulation often result in their disappearance and clarify their nature.

• Reverberations from a myxoma located in the right ventricular cavity (and detected in front of the tricuspid valve recording) may be recorded posteriorly in the region of the tricuspid valve and right atrium, simulating a right atrial tumor. Ultrasonic scanning of the right atrial cavity is negative for a myxoma originating in that chamber (see Fig. 7-21).

• The echocardiographic features of a right atrial myxoma are not specific, and similar findings may be produced by other types of tumors, such as an invasion by a hypernephroma and a right atrial extension of a calcified clot originating in the inferior vena cava. Atrial septal aneurysm or redundant tissue attached to the eustachian valve (hamartoma) may move into the tricuspid orifice with

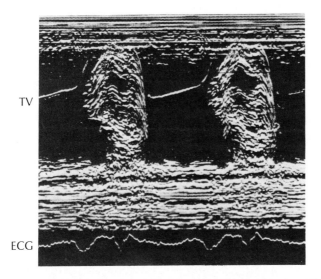

Fig. 6-15. Right atrial myxoma. Slender images of the tricuspid valve (TV) are seen in systole and as the valve opens anteriorly in early diastole. The dense multilinear echo pattern that appears in diastole, a short interval after tricuspid valve opening, arises in a right atrial myxoma as it prolapses into the tricuspid orifice. In systole the mass is displaced into a portion of the right atrium not in the examining beam. ECG, electrocardiogram.

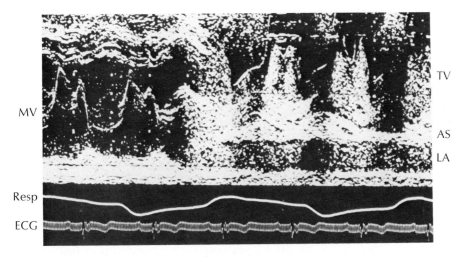

Fig. 6-16. Right atrial myxoma. A scan from the mitral valve (MV) to the tricuspid valve (TV) reveals a mass of echoes behind the tricuspid valve in diastole from a right atrial myxoma. At surgery a portion of the myxoma protruded into the left atrial cavity through a patent foramen ovale and was believed to be responsible for the transient stroke (produced by a myxoma embolus) that necessitated hospital admission. The clusters of echoes in the left atrial cavity (LA) behind the atrial septum (AS) probably arise from this portion of the mass. The thickening of the atrial septum may be due to the presence of the stalk that attached in this area. This patient is the father of a young girl whose right ventricular outflow myxoma is shown in Figs. 7-19 and 7-20. The presence of mitral valve prolapse in the father is an incidental finding. Resp, respiration; ECG, electrocardiogram.

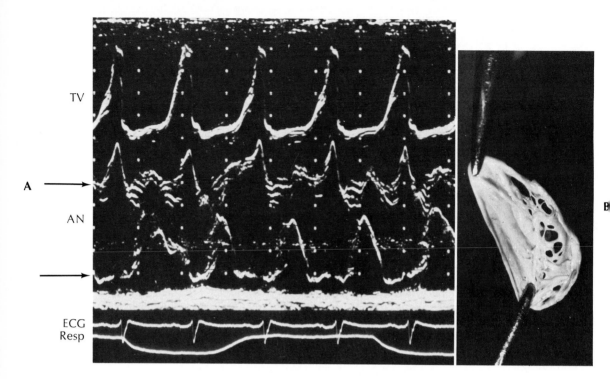

Fig. 6-17. Aneurysm of interatrial septum. **A,** The undulating pattern behind the tricuspid valve (TV) arises in an aneurysm (AN) of the atrial septum whose anterior and posterior limits are shown by the arrows. The phasic differences in motion between the anterior and posterior limits as well as the changes in waveform related to respiration suggest the presence of an undulating membranelike structure rather than a solid mass. **B,** The surgical specimen shows the thin-walled fenestrated aneurysmal sac, whose complex wall is probably responsible for the multilayered echoes recorded anteriorly. ECG, electrocardiogram; Resp, respiration.

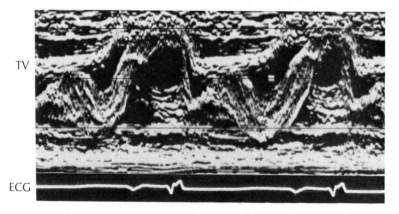

Fig. 6-18. Tricuspid valve recording in an infant with a membrane in the right atrium. A dense mass of echoes with a large amplitude of motion is observed behind the tricuspid valve in systole and diastole, mimicking a right atrial myxoma. The patient had a large membrane attached to the eustachian valve of the interior vena cava and encroaching on the tricuspid valve orifice. TV, tricuspid valve; ECG, electrocardiogram.

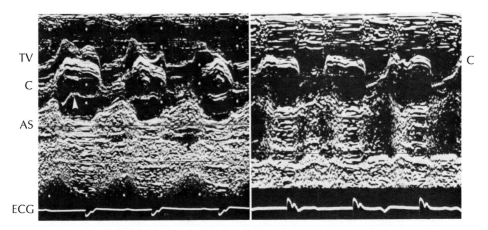

Fig. 6-19. Pacing catheters. *Left,* Multilayered echoes (C) from a pervenous right ventricular pacing catheter recorded behind the anterior tricuspid leaflet (TV) mimic those produced by a right atrial myxoma. The arrow denotes the septal leaflet of the tricuspid valve. *Right,* The thick echo complex (C) produced by a pacing catheter simulates a calcified tricuspid valve. AS, atrial septum; ECG, electrocardiogram.

blood flow and mimic a right atrial myxoma (Figs. 6-17 to 6-18).

• Multiple or thick echoes from right ventricular pacing catheters may be recorded behind the tricuspid valve and simulate a myxoma (Fig. 6-19).

• Examine other cardiac chambers, especially the left atrial cavity, for the presence of sister myxomas. Recordings of the interatrial septum may be useful in this regard (Fig. 6-20).

• Myxomas may be familial and examination of other family members of a patient with a myxoma may be indicated.

• It is unpardonable for an echocardiographer to miss an atrial tumor; hence the detailed coverage of a rare lesion.

Role of echocardiography. Echocardiography probably is the best technique for the diagnosis of a right atrial myxoma. Right heart catheterization is dangerous, since it may dislodge a portion of the tumor or produce hemorrhage in it. Therefore, it is mandatory to perform an echocardiogram in all suspected cases before cardiac catheterization.

Tricuspid valve endocarditis

Anatomic and functional changes

• The tricuspid valve may get infected by a bacterial or fungal organism, although this is uncommon.

• Organisms may enter the bloodstream through a venous injection (common in drug addicts) or may simply extend from left-sided cardiac valves through a communication such as a ventricular septal defect.

• Endocarditis results in the formation of small friable vegetations with tissue destruction, and gross valvular incompetence may follow. Fungal vegetations are much larger than bacterial vegetations.

Clinical summary

• Clinically, the patient may present with a systolic murmur of tricuspid incompetence. Signs of right heart failure may be present. The liver, as well as the jugular venous pulse, may show a prominent systolic pulsation (V wave). Constitutional symptoms, such as fever and malaise, are also present.

• Blood cultures are positive for the causative organism.

Echocardiographic features

• The tricuspid valve shows thick, shaggy, or fuzzy multilayered echoes (Fig. 6-21), which may be present throughout the cardiac cycle. Coarse or fine undulations may be present.

• Generally, the diastolic slope of the tricuspid valve is not reduced.

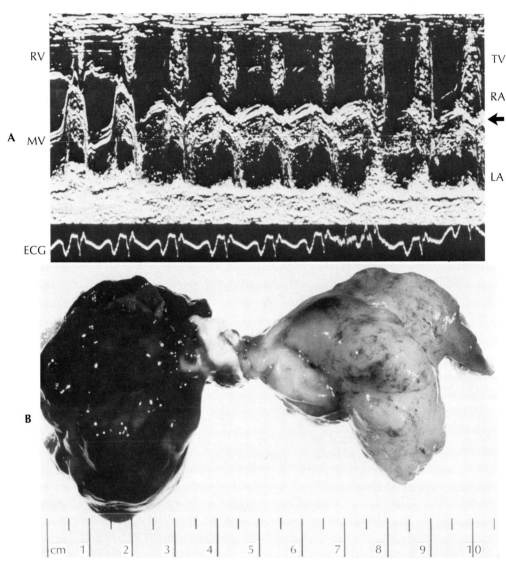

Fig. 6-20. A, Interatrial septal recording in a patient with biatrial myxomas. As the beam is moved from the mitral (MV) to the tricuspid valve (TV), tumor echoes are observed behind both valves in diastole as the myxomas prolapse into the ventricles. Tumor echoes are also present in the atria on either side of the interatrial septum *(arrow).* The left atrial tumor is seen in contact with the interatrial septum throughout the cardiac cycle, whereas the right atrial tumor is recorded mainly in diastole. **B,** At surgery the two tumors were connected by a common stalk that passed through the atrial septum *(bottom).* RV, right ventricle; RA, right atrium; LA, left atrium; ECG, electrocardiogram. (From Dashcoff, N., and others: Am. J. Med., in press.)

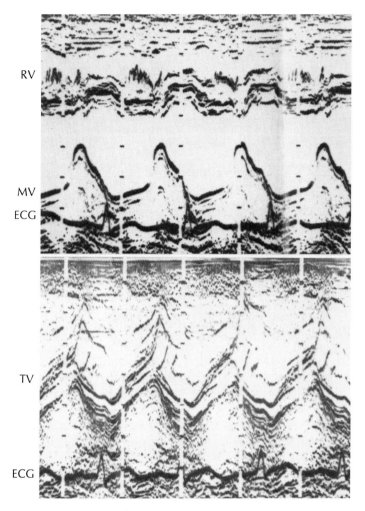

RV

MV

ECG

TV

ECG

Fig. 6-21. Tricuspid valve vegetation. Portions of the septal leaflet of the tricuspid valve are recorded in the right ventricle (RV) adjacent to the ventricular septum and show coarse and fine undulations in systole *(upper panel)*. The anterior leaflet of the tricuspid valve (TV) seen in the lower panel demonstrates nonspecific multilayering with hints of coarse diastolic fluttering. MV, mitral valve; ECG, electrocardiogram.

Comments

• Fungal vegetations are readily detected since they are large. Bacterial vegetations, on the other hand, tend to be smaller and may be missed. It is essential to scan as much of the leaflet surface as possible, using different beam directions. An attempt should also be made to examine the septal and inferior leaflets of the tricuspid valve in suspected cases (Fig. 6-21).

• A large tricuspid valve vegetation may produce an echocardiographic picture indistinguishable from that of a myxoma.

Role of echocardiography. Positive echocardiographic findings are generally thought to signify the presence of a large vegetation with fairly extensive tissue destruction. Diagnostic right heart catheterization is dangerous because of the risk of embolization. A normal tricuspid valve does not exclude the presence of a vegetation.

Right heart catheters (pacing wires)

Clinical summary. Catheters may be temporarily inserted in the right heart for monitoring pressures and cardiac output. A Swan-Ganz catheter with an inflatable balloon at the tip is commonly advanced into the right atrium through a peripheral vein and then floats into the pulmonary circulation. More permanent wires are often inserted pervenously into either the coronary sinus or lodged at the apex of the right ventricle to electrically stimulate the atrium or the ventricle.

With right ventricular pacing catheters the

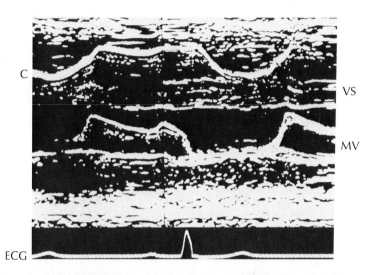

Fig. 6-22. Demonstration of right ventricular pacing catheter (C) in the right ventricular cavity during mitral valve (MV) recording. VS, ventricular septum; ECG, electrocardiogram. (From Nanda, N. C., and others: Ultrasound Med. **2:**1, 1976.)

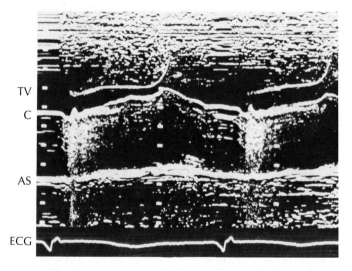

Fig. 6-23. Right ventricular pacing catheter. The catheter (C) is visualized just behind the tricuspid valve (TV). Note the presence of multiple reverberations from the catheter. AS, atrial septum; ECG, electrocardiogram.

electrocardiogram shows a vertical spike just before the onset of the QRS complex, which is widened because of abnormal activation of the ventricle. The pacing spike is seen before the P wave, and the QRS complex is not widened in patients with coronary sinus catheters. Fluoroscopy or chest roentgenograms are useful in outlining the course of the catheter in the heart and demonstrating the position of the tip.

Echocardiographic features

Echocardiographic features of transvenous right ventricular pacing catheters are as follows:

• They often present as prominent single-layered or multilayered thick echo complexes recorded in front of the tricuspid valve, immediately posterior to it, or superimposed on it. The catheter echo generally moves anteriorly with the onset of diastole, remains flat thereafter, and then moves posteriorly with the beginning of systole (Figs. 6-22 and 6-23). It exhibits no motion or gradual ante-

rior motion during the remainder of systole. Thus, its motion pattern resembles that of an atrioventricular valve, except that the posterior motion tends to occur later in systole as compared to the tricuspid or mitral valve and is probably related to catheter inertia.

• The right atrial portion of the catheter may be visualized as a thick echo complex just in front of the posterior right atrial wall recorded deep to the tricuspid valve.

• The tricuspid valve may show a prominent systolic anterior movement in the presence of complete atrioventricular block. This occurs only when atrial systole coincides with ventricular systole and is not observed when the P wave falls in diastole (Fig. 6-24). A small-amplitude systolic anterior motion of the tricuspid valve may also be observed in patients with complete heart block who do not have pacing catheters when the P wave falls in systole. The abnormal motion of the tricuspid valve is probably due to altered movement of the tricuspid annulus resulting

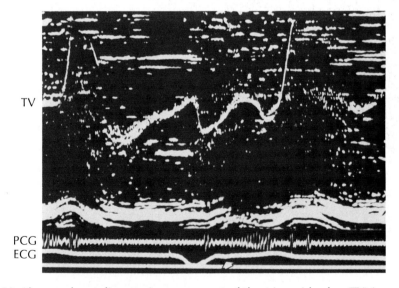

Fig. 6-24. Abnormal systolic anterior movement of the tricuspid valve (TV) in a patient with complete heart block and transvenous right ventricular pacemaker. Abnormal motion was observed only when atrial contraction occurred simultaneously with ventricular systole. This may result from altered motion of the tricuspid annulus produced by atrial systole and augmented by the presence of a catheter in the tricuspid orifice. PCG, phonocardiogram. The arrow denotes the P wave of the electrocardiogram (ECG). (From Nanda, N. C., and others: Ultrasound Med. **3A:**113, 1977.)

from simultaneous contractions of both atria and ventricles and augmented by the presence of a catheter in the tricuspid orifice.

Echocardiographic features of transvenous pulmonary artery catheters are as follows:

• They may present all the echocardiographic features detailed above.

• They may be differentiated from transvenous right ventricular pacing catheters since they are readily detected in the right ventricular outflow imaged in front of the aortic root and pulmonary valve recordings (Fig. 6-25).

Coronary sinus catheters have the following echocardiographic features:

• They are identified further posterior to the tricuspid valve in the region of the atrial septum (Fig. 6-26). In general, they present as multilayered complexes that resemble the atrial septum in motion pattern apart from

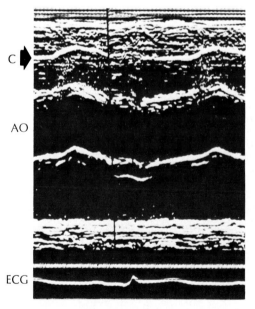

Fig. 6-25. Right ventricular outflow catheter. The Swan-Ganz catheter presents as a prominent linear echo (C) in the right ventricular outflow tract recorded in front of the aortic root (Ao). The tip of the catheter was lodged in a distal pulmonary artery branch. ECG, electrocardiogram. (From Nanda, N. C., and others: Circulation **48**:506, 1973. By permission of the American Heart Assn., Inc.)

the presence of small, circumscribed humps in late diastole or early systole. In some instances, catheter echoes may mask the atrial septal image.

• They may be detected in the right atrial cavity but are not visualized in the right ventricle in front of the tricuspid valve recording.

Comments

• Occasionally, the catheter echo has been mistaken for tricuspid valve recording since the stronger echoes from the catheter may mask the relatively weak echoes from the normal tricuspid valve.

• Multilayered catheter echoes behind the tricuspid valve in diastole and occasionally in systole may mimic those produced by a right atrial myxoma or tricuspid valve vegetation.

• Transvenous right ventricular pacing catheters may be detected in the right ventricle in front of the ventricular septum during mitral valve or left ventricular cavity recordings. This is not common, however, since the catheter generally does not traverse the plane of the right ventricular cavity imaged during this examination.

• The catheter may form a large loop, which projects into the right ventricular outflow and may be detected in front of the aortic root or pulmonary valve recordings. A redundant loop of this type may be commonly found when a temporary pacing wire is lodged at the apex of the right ventricle through a saphenous vein.

• Catheter echoes in the vicinity of the ventricular septum may be mistaken for portions of the septal complex, and an erroneous diagnosis of a thickened ventricular septum may be made.

• The space between the catheter echo and the chest wall may be mistaken for pericardial effusion when the anterior right ventricular wall is suppressed by low-gain settings.

• Reverberations from a right ventricular catheter may be imaged in the left ventricular cavity and may erroneously point to the presence of a catheter in that chamber (Fig. 6-27). Reverberations may be present even

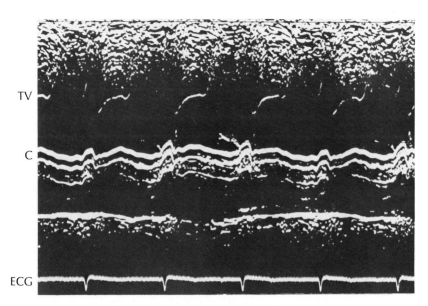

Fig. 6-26. Coronary sinus pacing catheter. Multiple linear echoes from the coronary sinus pacing catheter (C) are observed deep to the tricuspid valve (TV) in the region of the atrial septum and show prominent humps whose onset occurs just before the beginning of the QRS complex. The atrial septal image has been masked by the catheter echoes. ECG, electrocardiogram. (From Nanda, N. C., and others: Ultrasound Med. **2:**1, 1976.)

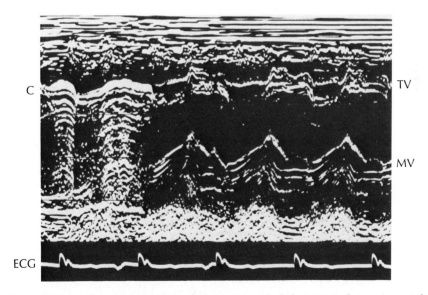

Fig. 6-27. Right ventricular catheter reverberations in left ventricular cavity. Multiple reverberations from a right ventricular pacing catheter (C) are imaged posteriorly over the left ventricle and obscure local landmarks. With beam angulation, the catheter image is recorded behind the tricuspid valve (TV), the reverberation artifacts disappear, but the ventricular septum is still not well seen. MV, mitral valve; ECG, electrocardiogram. (From Nanda, N. C., and others: Ultrasound Med. **2:**1, 1976.)

though the catheter itself is not imaged in the right ventricular cavity.

• Catheters in the coronary sinus may also be detected in the vicinity of the posterior wall of the aorta during ultrasonic beam scanning from the tricuspid valve to the aortic valve.

• A catheter located in the right ventricular apex may produce a characteristic change in the motion of the ventricular septum. This

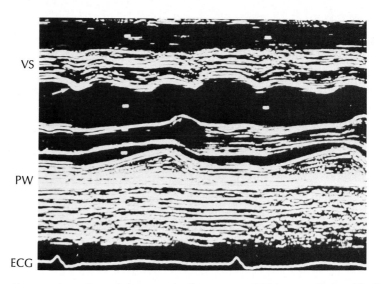

Fig. 6-28. Abnormal motion of the ventricular septum (VS) in a patient with right ventricular endocardial pacing catheter. The ventricular septum exhibits a prominent but brief posterior movement *(arrow)* following the onset of the QRS complex. Thereafter, the septum moves briefly anteriorly and then shows a normal motion pattern. PW, left ventricular posterior wall; ECG, electrocardiogram.

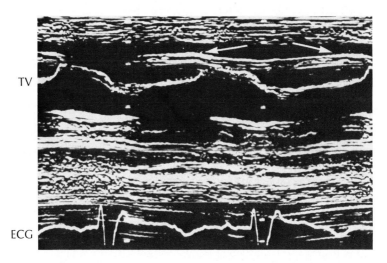

Fig. 6-29. Tricuspid valve recording in a patient with double outlet right ventricle following surgical repair. The patch *(arrows)* used to close the defect is recorded in the right ventricle in front of the tricuspid valve (TV), simulating a right ventricular catheter. ECG, electrocardiogram.

consists of a prominent brief posterior motion occurring 40 to 100 msec after the pacing spike and followed by a short, rapid anterior movement. The septal motion thereafter remains normal (Fig. 6-28). Absence of this movement may denote improper pacemaker positioning. Patients with left bundle branch block (without pacemakers) may also show a similar posterior septal deflection, but it is followed by abnormal septal motion during the remainder of systole. We have also observed a delay in the onset of the posterior motion of the anterior right ventricular wall during systole in some patients with right ventricular pacemakers.

• Transient expansion of the left ventricular cavity produced normally during atrial systole appears more prominent in patients with coronary sinus pacemakers.

• The patch used in the surgical closure of a large ventricular septal defect (as in double outlet right ventricle) may be imaged in front of the tricuspid valve or in contact with it in diastole, simulating a right ventricular catheter (Fig. 6-29).

Role of echocardiography

• The echocardiographic technique may be used to differentiate a coronary sinus from a transvenous right ventricular pacing catheter in an occasional patient in whom the location of the pacemaker cannot be determined confidently electrocardiographically or fluoroscopically. The usefulness of the echocardiographic method is limited, since the tip of a catheter is not visualized in most instances.

• Catheter echoes may mimic cardiac structural echoes and result in misdiagnosis if they are not recognized during echocardiographic examinations.

Tricuspid valve diastolic flutter

The various conditions associated with tricuspid valve diastolic flutter are listed in Table 6.

Comments

• Tricuspid valve diastolic flutter may be absent in patients with mild pulmonary valve incompetence, since the tricuspid valve is not situated directly below the pulmonary

Table 6. Tricuspid valve diastolic flutter

Condition	Type	Etiology
Normal infants	High frequency	Thin, small cusps
Pulmonary valve incompetence	High frequency	Regurgitant jet striking the open leaflets
Truncal insufficiency	High frequency	Regurgitant jet striking the open leaflets
Atrial septal defect	High frequency	Increased flow through the tricuspid valve in diastole
Sinus of Valsalva—right atrial communication	High frequency	Increased flow through the tricuspid valve in diastole
Sinus of Valsalva—right ventricular fistula	High frequency	Diastolic jet striking the open leaflets
Dextrotransposition of great vessels following balloon septostomy	High frequency	Bidirectional shunting at atrial level
Dextrotransposition of great vessels following Mustard procedure	High and low frequency	Abnormal blood flow pathways and turbulence produced by the intra-atrial baffle
Chordae-papillary muscle rupture	High and low frequency	Unsupported leaflets
Atrial flutter/fibrillation	Coarse undulations; not true flutter	

valve and the right ventricular crista tends to divert the regurgitant jet away from it. It is more commonly observed with severe pulmonary incompetence, which results in enlargement of the right ventricular cavity and permits the tricuspid valve to come in more direct contact with the regurgitant jet. In patients with atrial septal defects the flutter tends to occur in patients with large left-to-right shunts with pulmonary-to-systemic blood flow ratios of 2.3:1 or more (Fig. 6-30). The flutter usually disappears following surgical closure of the defect. Diastolic flutter of the septal leaflet of the tricuspid valve (Fig. 6-31) is especially common in the ostium primum type of defect, probably because of its proximity to the site of the defect, which is situated in the basal portion of the atrial septum.

• Chordae rupture of the tricuspid valve

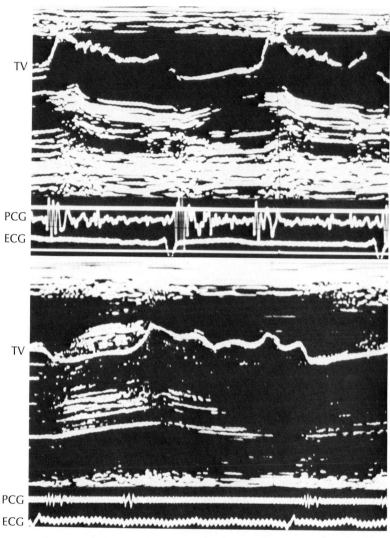

Fig. 6-30. *Upper panel,* Tricuspid valve diastolic flutter in a patient with a large atrial septal defect of the secundum type. *Lower panel,* Coarse diastolic undulations of the tricuspid valve produced by atrial fibrillation. The recording speed is 125/mm sec. TV, tricuspid valve; PCG, phonocardiogram; ECG, electrocardiogram. (From Nanda, N. C., and others: Ultrasound Med. **1:**11, 1975.)

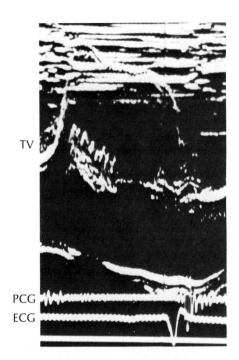

Fig. 6-31. Tricuspid valve echocardiogram (×2) from a patient with ostium primum septal defect showing prominent flutter of the septal cusp in diastole. The anterior leaflet appears to be relatively stable. TV, tricuspid valve; PCG, phonocardiogram; ECG, electrocardiogram. (From Nanda, N. C., and others: Ultrasound Med. **1:**11, 1975.)

is rare but may produce bizarre, erratic diastolic fluttering of the unsupported tricuspid leaflets.

• Expansion of the tricuspid valve image is of considerable value in the detection of tricuspid valve diastolic fluttering, especially when it is subtle and of small amplitude. Higher recording speeds in the range of 100 to 150 mm/sec are useful in distinguishing diastolic flutter from coarse undulations observed in atrial flutter or fibrillation.

Congenital left ventricular–right atrial shunt

Anatomy and functional changes

• This is an unusual type of ventricular septal defect that opens directly into the right atrium above the tricuspid valve or opens first into the right ventricle and then into the right atrium through a second deficiency in the tricuspid septal leaflet, which is partially adherent to the edges of the defect. The shunt may thus be either solely from the left ventricle to the right atrium or at both ventricular and atrial levels (Figs. 6-32 and 6-33).

• This entity is associated with enlargement of the right heart.

Clinical summary. The constant systolic flow of blood from the left ventricle to the right side of the heart produces a pansys-

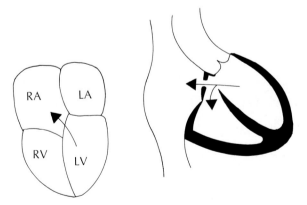

Fig. 6-32. Left ventricular–right atrial communication. A defect is present in the upper portion of the membranous ventricular septum so that the left ventricular blood enters the right atrium (RA) without traversing the right ventricle (RV) *(left).* When the septal leaflet of the tricuspid valve is deficient and partially adherent to the edges of the ventricular septal defect, the left ventricle (LV) communicates with both the right atrium and the right ventricle *(right).* LA, left atrium.

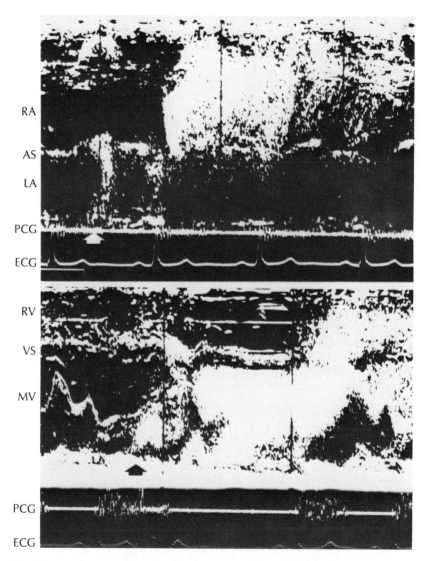

Fig. 6-33. Ultrasonic contrast injections using indocyanine green. *Upper panel,* Contrast injection into the left atrium in diastole *(arrow)* produces dense echoes in the right atrium during the subsequent ventricular systole consistent with left ventricular–right atrial communication. No contrast material in the right atrium during the preceding diastole indicates absence of an atrial septal defect. *Lower panel,* Contrast injection into the left ventricle in diastole *(arrow)* shows filling of the left ventricular outflow tract with subsequent leakage into the right ventricle during ventricular systole indicative of a ventricular septal defect. RA, right atrium; AS, atrial septum; LA, left atrium; RV, right ventricle; VS, ventricular septum; MV, mitral valve; PCG, phonocardiogram; ECG, electrocardiogram. (From Nanda, N. C., and others: Circulation **51:** 268, 1975. By permission of the American Heart Assn. Inc.)

tolic murmur. Cardiac catheterization would show an increase in oxygen saturation at the level of the right atrium and upper right ventricle. Left ventricular angiography accurately categorizes the site of the defect.

Echocardiographic features

- The prominent finding is a high-frequency, low-amplitude flutter of the tricuspid valve in systole (Fig. 6-34).
- The right ventricle is enlarged.

Comments

- Tricuspid valve systolic fluttering is observed only when the shunt is through the tricuspid valve and is probably related to the passage of the left ventricular jet of blood through deformed leaflets, the margins of which are fused to the defect. The flutter disappears following surgical closure of the defect. Fluttering is not observed when the defect is above the level of the tricuspid valve.
- Infective vegetations present on the tricuspid valve may also show prominent systolic flutter, but the association of shaggy or fuzzy-appearing echoes characteristic of endocarditis distinguishes it from that produced by the left ventricular–right atrial shunt.

Role of echocardiography. Echocardiographic findings appear to be highly specific in this type of defect, which is clinically difficult to distinguish from a garden variety ventricular septal defect.

Abnormal systolic anterior movements of tricuspid valve

Abnormal systolic anterior movements of the tricuspid valve have been occasionally observed, but their etiology is not always clear. Systolic bulges superimposed on the tricuspid valve region have been observed in patients with aneurysms of the membranous ventricular septum and probably represent images of the aneurysm itself. We have recently observed early and midsystolic localized bulging of the tricuspid valve in patients

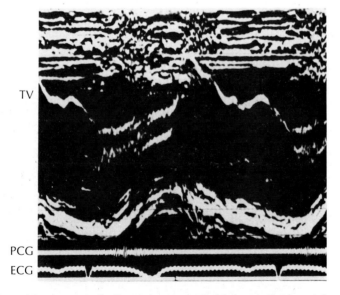

Fig. 6-34. Tricuspid valve systolic flutter in congenital left ventricular–right atrial shunt. The tricuspid valve echocardiogram shows a low-amplitude, high-frequency systolic flutter and an undulating movement in diastole (average frequency of systolic flutter 65 cycles/sec; average amplitude 3.5 mm). The structure posterior to the tricuspid valve is the interatrial septum. TV, tricuspid valve; PCG, phonocardiogram; ECG, electrocardiogram. (From Nanda, N. C., and others: Circulation **51**:268, 1975. By permission of the American Heart Assn., Inc.)

with restrictive ventricular septal defects and right ventricular outflow obstruction when the right ventricular systolic pressure exceeded that in the left ventricle. The mechanism for this systolic protrusion of the tricuspid valve into the right ventricular cavity may be related to a Bernoulli or Venturi phenomenon. In one patient there was redundant tricuspid valve tissue, which may have contributed to the restrictive nature of the defect.

As mentioned earlier, the tricuspid valve

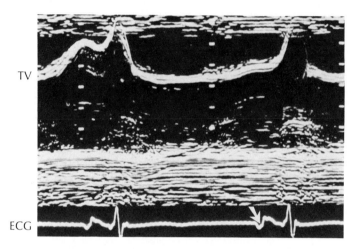

Fig. 6-35. Late opening tricuspid valve in a patient with congestive cardiomyopathy. The tricuspid valve (TV) on the right does not open until the occurrence of atrial systole *(arrow)*, whereas the recording on the left shows a relatively normal timing of the opening movement that is small in amplitude. A more effective opening of the valve occurs later with atrial systole. ECG, electrocardiogram.

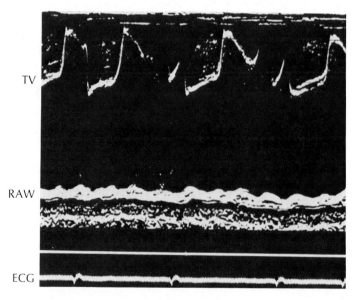

Fig. 6-36. The posterior right atrial wall (RAW) exhibits coarse undulations in this patient with atrial flutter–fibrillation. TV, tricuspid valve; ECG, electrocardiogram.

may show a prominent systolic anterior movement in patients with transvenous right ventricular pacing catheters and complete atrioventricular block.

Exaggerated motion of the heart in patients with large pericardial effusions has been known to produce motion artifacts that mimic abnormal systolic anterior movements of the tricuspid valve.

FUNCTIONAL OBSERVATIONS

Alterations in the tricuspid valve or atrial septal movement patterns may be produced by changes in right heart hemodynamics.

• Prolongation of the A-C segment with a prominent B point of the tricuspid valve is frequently observed in patients with increased right ventricular end-diastolic pressures.

• Some patients with congestive cardiomyopathy may show a marked delay in the opening of the tricuspid valve as compared to the mitral; occasionally the valve opens only during atrial systole (Fig. 6-35).

• The interatrial septum may show poor motion in low cardiac output states.

• Coarse undulations of the tricuspid valve may be seen in patients with atrial flutter or fibrillation. The posterior right atrial wall may also show similar undulations (Fig. 6-36).

• The tricuspid valve may show a prominent A wave in patients with cardiomyopathy, severe pulmonary valve stenosis and severe pulmonary hypertension. This probably reflects vigorous contraction of the right atrium in the face of increased right ventricular diastolic pressure.

• The EF slope of the tricuspid valve may be reduced during a short R-R interval in patients with atrial fibrillation (Fig. 6-37).

• Complete heart block may result in

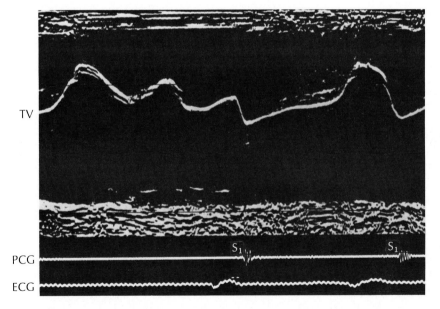

Fig. 6-37. The tricuspid valve in atrial fibrillation. The cycle on the left is prolonged, and the diastolic contour shows three prominent peaks. The first results from valve opening; the latter two are probably caused by continual right atrial filling and emptying from uncoordinated atrial movements during a long diastolic interval. The third peak, which resembles an A wave, is produced by ventricular systole, which abruptly terminates the undulating motion of the valve. In the second cycle the EF slope is flattened. The rapid downstroke thereafter is produced by ventricular systole and should not be confused with the true EF slope. S_1, first heart sound; PCG, phonocardiogram; TV, tricuspid valve; ECG, electrocardiogram.

changes in the motion pattern of the tricuspid valve.

• Patients with tricuspid valve incompetence do not show characteristic echocardiographic features. The right ventricle may be enlarged and in adults two leaflets of the tricuspid valve may be fully recorded.

• Echocardiographic studies during cardiac catheterization may be useful in delineating the presence and severity of tricuspid incompetence. Injections of indocyanine green in the upper portion of the right atrium take a significantly longer time (20 to 40 cardiac cycles) to clear from the area of the tricuspid valve (as observed on the tricuspid valve echocardiogram) in patients with tricuspid incompetence than they do in normal patients. Patients with low cardiac output may also show a delayed clearance.

BIBLIOGRAPHY
Tricuspid valve stenosis

Joyner, C. R., Hey, B. E., Jr., Johnson, J., and Reid, J. M.: Reflected ultrasound in the diagnosis of tricuspid stenosis, Am. J. Cardiol. **19:**66, 1967.

Schloss, M., and Kronzon, I.: The echocardiographic diagnosis of "concealed" tricuspid stenosis, Cathet. Cardiovasc. Diagn. **1:**405-408, 1975.

Tricuspid valve prolapse and tricuspid regurgitation

Chandraratna, P. A. N., Lopez, J. M., Fernandez, J. J., and Cohen, L. S.: Echocardiographic detection of tricuspid valve prolapse, Circulation **51:**823, 1975.

Horgan, J. H., Beachley, M. C., and Robinson, F. D.: Tricuspid valve prolapse diagnosed by echocardiogram, Chest **68:**822-824, 1975.

Seides, S. F., DeJoseph, R. L., Brown, A. E., and Damato, A. N.: Echocardiographic findings in isolated surgically created tricuspid insufficiency, Am. J. Cardiol. **35:**679-682, 1975.

Nanda, N. C., Shah, P. M., and Gramiak, R.: Echocardiographic evaluation of tricuspid valve incompetence by contrast injections, Clin. Res. **24:**233A, 1976.

Right atrial tumor

Harbold, N. B., Jr., and Gau, G. T.: Echocardiographic diagnosis of right atrial myxoma, Mayo Clin. Proc. **48:**284, 1973.

Farooki, Z. O., Henry, J. G., and Green, E. W.: Echocardiographic diagnosis of right atrial extension of Wilms' tumor, Am. J. Cardiol. **36:**363-365, 1975.

Atsuchi, Y., Nagai, Y., Nakamura, K., Komatsu, Y.

and Osamura, Y.: Echocardiographic diagnosis of prolapsing right atrial myxoma, Jpn. Heart J. **17:**798-803, 1976.

Farooki, Z. Q., Green, E. W., and Arciniegas, E.: Echocardiographic pattern of right atrial tumor motion, Br. Heart J. **38:**580-583, 1976.

Yuste, P., Asin, E., Cerdan, F. J., and delaFuente, A.: Illustrative echocardiogram; echocardiogram in right atrial myxoma, Chest **69:**94, 1976.

Dashcoff, N., Boersma, R. B., Nanda, N. C., Gramiak, R., Andersen, M. N., and Subramanian, S.: Bilateral atrial myxomas; echocardiographic considerations, in press.

Tricuspid valve endocarditis

Lee, C. C., Ganguly, S. N., Magnisalis, K., and Robin, E.: Detection of tricuspid valve vegetations by echocardiography, Chest **66:**432-433, 1974.

Kisslo, J., Von Ramm, O. T., Haney, R., Jones, R., Juk, S. S., and Behar, V. S.: Echocardiographic evaluation of tricuspid valve endocarditis; an M mode and two dimensional study, Am. J. Cardiol. **38:**502-507, 1976.

Right heart catheters

Charuzi, Y., and Kraus, R.: Echocardiographic visualization of right heart catheters. In White, D. N., and Brown, R. E., editors: Ultrasound in medicine, vol. 3, New York, 1977, Plenum Publishing Corp., p. 265.

Nanda, N. C., Reeves, W. C., Gramiak, R., and Barold, S.: Echocardiography of pacing catheters, Clin. Res. **25:**241A, 1977.

Nanda, N. C., Reeves, W. C., and Gramiak, R.: Abnormal systolic anterior motion of atrio-ventricular valves in complete heart block, Ultrasound Med. **3A:**113, 1977.

Tricuspid valve diastolic flutter

Nanda, N. C., Gramiak, R., and Manning, J. A.: Echocardiographic studies of the tricuspid valve in atrial septal defect. In White, D., editor: Ultrasound in medicine, vol. 1, New York, 1975, Plenum Publishing Corp., p. 11.

Congenital left ventricular–right atrial shunt

Nanda, N. C., Gramiak, R., and Manning, J. A.: Echocardiography of the tricuspid valve in congenital left ventricular–right atrial communication, Circulation **51:**268-272, 1975.

Tricuspid valve (general; including atrial septum)

Nimura, Y., Matsuo, H., Matsumoto, M., Kitabatake, A., and Abe, H.: Interatrial septum in ultrasonocardiotomogram and ultrasoundcardiogram, Med. Ultrason. **9:**58, 1971.

Matsumoto, M.: Ultrasonic features of interatrial septum; its motion analysis and detection of its defect, Jpn. Circ. J. **37**:1383, 1973.

Kawai, N., Gewitz, M., Eshaghpour, E., and Linhart, J. W.: Echocardiographic determination of right atrial dimensions and volume, Circulation **50**(suppl. 3):28, 1974 (abstract).

Nanda, N. C., Gramiak, R., Manning, J., and Gross, C. M.: Echocardiographic identification of the interatrial septum; clinical usefulness, Circulation **52** (suppl. 2):221, 1975.

Nanda, N. C., Gramiak, R., Viles, P., Manning, J., and Gross, C.: Echocardiographic identification of the inter-atrial septum behind the tricuspid valve Circulation **52**(suppl. 2):221, 1975.

Nanda, N. C., Gramiak, R., Viles, P., Manning, J., Gross, C.: Echocardiography of the inter-atrial septum. In White, D. N., and Barnes, R., editors: Ultrasound in medicine, vol. 2, New York, 1976, Plenum Publishing Corp., p. 1.

Matsumoto, M., Nimura, Y., Matsuo, H., Nagata, S., Mochizuki, S., Sakakibara, H., and Abe, H.: Interatrial septum in B-mode and conventional echocardiograms—clue for the diagnosis of congenital heart diseases, J. Clin. Ultrasound, **3**:29-37, 1975.

Dillon, J. C., Weyman, A. E., and Feigenbaum, H.: Cross-sectional echocardiographic examination of the interatrial septum, Am. J. Cardiol. **37**:132, 1976.

Arcilla, R. A., Mathew, R., Sodt, P., Lester, L., Cahill, N., and Thilenius, O. G.: Right ventricular mass estimation by angioechocardiography, Cathet. Cardiovasc. Diagn. **2**:125-136, 1976.

Gewitz, M., Eshaghpour, E., Holsclaw, D. S., Miller, H. A., and Kawai, N.: Echocardiography in cystic fibrosis, Am. J. Dis. Child, **131**:275-280, 1977.

7 Pulmonary valve

STRUCTURES IN BEAM

In the adult an oblique beam angulation is required to detect the pulmonary valve, and the following structures are imaged in anteroposterior direction.

1. Chest wall
2. Anterior right ventricular wall (may not be well seen)
3. Right ventricular outflow
4. Left (posterior) pulmonary valve cusp
5. Posterior pulmonary artery wall and adjacent to it a thick echo complex representing the atriopulmonic sulcus
6. Left atrial cavity
7. Left atrial posterior wall

In normal infants and rarely in young adults with very large pulmonary arteries the ultrasonic beam traverses the pulmonary root more transversely, and the following structures are recorded:

1. Chest wall
2. Anterior and posterior walls of the pulmonary root. Within the lumen both anterior and posterior cusps of the pulmonary valve may be recorded.
3. Left atrial cavity
4. Left atrial posterior wall

NORMAL TRACING (Figs. 7-1 and 7-2)

In the normal adult the left or posterior cusp of the pulmonic valve demonstrates gradual early diastolic posterior motion. The rate of this movement generally decreases until atrial systole, which produces a transient, circumscribed posterior motion (A dip). The magnitude of the A dip varies with respiration, being maximum during the inspiratory phase. In our experience the maximum depth of the A dip averages 4.4 mm (range 3 to 12 mm). With the onset of ventricular systole the valve cusp opens and moves to a posterior position. The rate of this opening is relatively slow in the range of 100 to 300 mm/sec. The systolic segment of the pulmonary valve is generally incompletely recorded but may show gradual anterior motion; this is followed by a rapid anterior deflection as the valve closes in diastole.

Hemodynamic correlations

The pulmonary circuit is a low pressure system as compared to the systemic circulation. In the normal patient the right ventricular diastolic pressure (average 4 mm Hg) is only slightly lower than the pulmonary artery diastolic pressure (average 9 mm Hg), and therefore the diastolic gradient across the pulmonary valve is low (about 5 mm Hg). The gradient is probably lower during atrial systole, and this permits a transient upward motion of the pulmonary valve cusp, producing an A dip. During the inspiratory phase of respiration the augmented venous return produces an increase in the right ventricular diastolic pressure and lowers the diastolic gradient across the pulmonary valve, especially during atrial systole, resulting in an increase in the size of the A dip. Thus, the pulmonary valve tracing appears to be in-

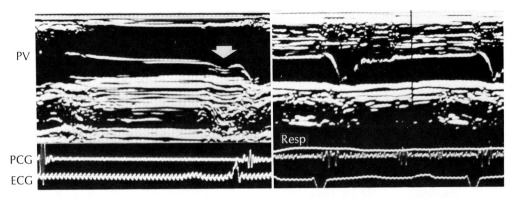

Fig. 7-1. *Left,* Normal pulmonary valve (PV) showing oblique position of the cusp echo in diastole, a large A dip *(arrow)* following atrial systole, and a slow valve opening slope characteristic of normal pulmonary artery pressure. *Right,* Pulmonary hypertension. The pulmonary valve shows no displacement following atrial systole and a general straightening of the diastolic cusp image with steeper valve opening slopes. Resp, respirations; PCG, phonocardiogram; ECG, electrocardiogram. (From Nanda, N.C., and others: Circulation **50**:575, 1974.)

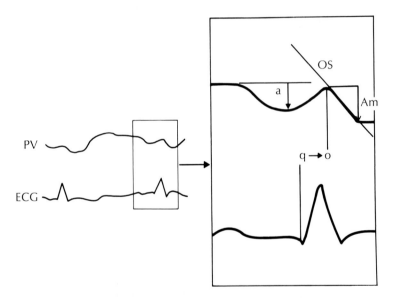

Fig. 7-2. Pulmonary valve measurement technique. A representative tracing of the pulmonary valve echo through the cardiac cycle illustrates the parameters commonly studied. PV, pulmonary valve echo; ECG, electrocardiogram; OS, maximal opening slope of the pulmonary valve; a, posterior displacement observed following atrial systole; qo, pre-ejection period of the right ventricle; Am, amplitude of the valve opening movement. (From Nanda, N. C., and others: Circulation **50**:575, 1974.)

fluenced by changing hemodynamic events in the right ventricle.

It is possible that the early diastolic posterior motion of the pulmonary valve results from slight upward movement of the cusp due to rapid right ventricular filling in early diastole. Other factors such as posterior motion of the entire pulmonary artery in diastole may also be playing a role in generating this motion pattern.

The opening of the pulmonary valve occurs during the early portion of right ventricular contraction when the pressure is not rising rapidly, and hence the valve opening movements are relatively slow.

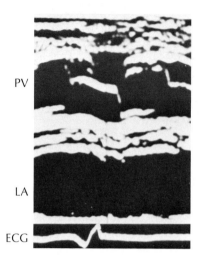

Fig. 7-3. Pulmonary valve (PV) recording demonstrating anterior and posterior *(left)* cusps. The anterior and posterior walls of the pulmonary artery move anteriorly in systole and posteriorly in diastole. The thick complex behind the posterior wall represents the atriopulmonic sulcus and separates the pulmonary artery from the left atrium (LA). ECG, electrocardiogram.

In normal infants the anterior cusp of the pulmonary valve can also be recorded. It moves anteriorly with the beginning of systole and coapts with the posterior (left) leaflet in diastole, forming a boxlike configuration. The cusps are contained within the margins of the pulmonary root, which moves anteriorly in systole and posteriorly in diastole (Figs. 7-3 and 7-4).

TECHNICAL CONSIDERATIONS

• Relatively high-gain settings are required for the detection of the pulmonary valve. Generally, maximum time-varied gain is needed to suppress the reverberatory echoes from the chest wall that clutter the anterior region. The proximity of lung tissue requires a long and upwardly oblique beam direction so that usually only a single, posterior valve cusp is detected. Elevation of valve cusp during opening therefore produces a posterior deflection on the echocardiogram, whereas the downward closing motion is imaged as an anterior deflection.

• Successful detection of the pulmonary valve depends on finding a thick linear echo complex, which represents the atriopulmonic sulcus. Small adjustments of the transducer in this region frequently result in the recording of a thin, linear moving echo from the posterior or left cusp of the pulmonary valve

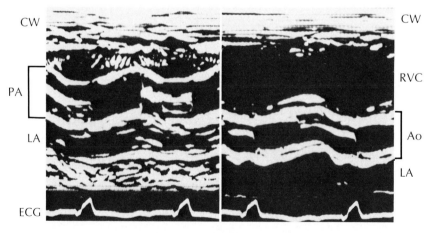

Fig. 7-4. Pulmonary and aortic root recordings in a neonate. The pulmonary artery (PA) is larger than the aortic root (Ao) and is located more anteriorly. CW, chest wall; RVO, right ventricular outflow; LA, left atrium; ECG, electrocardiogram.

in the clear space observed in front of the sulcus (Fig. 7-5).

• Turning the patient's head to the left side and placing the patient in the left lateral decubitus (at an angle of approximately 30 to 45 degrees) may be necessary to obtain adequate images of the pulmonary valve.

• Aortic valve echoes may be misdiagnosed as pulmonary valve echoes during patient examination when the anterior wall of the aorta is not well visualized and only the noncoronary cusp is imaged.

• In case gradual angulation of the transducer toward the left shoulder from the aortic root position fails to record the pulmonary valve, placing the transducer an interspace higher than that used for imaging the aortic valve and directing the beam laterally may be helpful. Pulmonary valve detection may also be attempted by displacing the transducer superiorly from the mitral valve recording position.

• The larger acoustic windows in neonates and younger children permit adequate images of both walls of the pulmonary artery as well as both anterior and posterior valve cusps, since the pulmonary root can be ex-

amined from a higher position on the chest wall.

• In the adult the ultrasonic beam passes through the right ventricular outflow, and hence the pulmonary valve is viewed from its right ventricular surface (Fig. 7-6). The anterior wall of the pulmonary artery is not recorded, and the first moving echo adjacent to the chest wall represents the anterior right ventricular wall. The space in front of the diastolic position of the pulmonary valve cusp represents the right ventricular outflow area immediately beneath the pulmonary valve. The space behind the valve cusps denotes the posterior portion of the lumen of the pulmonary artery immediately above the valve level.

• One must remember that the size of the A dip changes with transducer position (beam angulation) as well as with respiration. The maximum depth of the A dip obtained in a given patient should therefore be taken. Care should also be taken to obtain the A dips during the inspiratory phase of respiration, since they may be very small or even absent in an occasional normal patient during expiration.

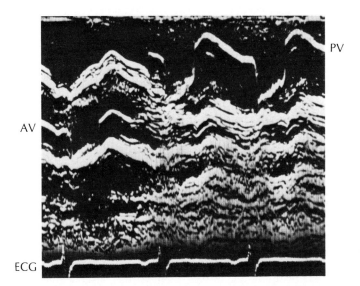

Fig. 7-5. Beam scanning from the aortic to the pulmonary valve. Note the more anterior position of the pulmonary valve. The echo complex posterior to it represents the atriopulmonic sulcus. AV, aortic valve; PV, pulmonary valve; ECG, electrocardiogram.

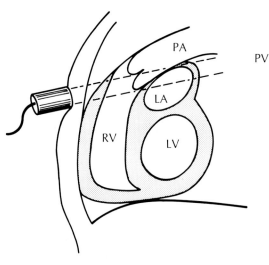

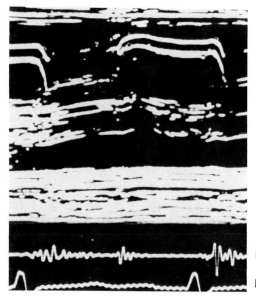

Fig. 7-6. Schematic representation of the pathway of the ultrasonic beam as it obliquely traverses the right ventricular outflow–pulmonary artery area during pulmonic valve detection. The upward oblique beam direction explains why usually only a single posterior valve cusp is detected and illustrates how elevation of the valve cusp toward opening produces a posterior deflection on the echogram. PA, pulmonary artery; RV, right ventricle; LA, left atrium; LV, left ventricle. (From Nanda, N.C., and others: Circulation **50:**575, 1974.)

Fig. 7-7. Variations in pulmonary valve contour. The posterior cusp of the pulmonary valve (PV) in this patient shows a double contour in diastole and systole probably related to the ultrasonic beam imaging contiguous portions of the same leaflet. PCG, phonocardiogram; ECG, electrocardiogram.

- The most common reason for failure to detect pulmonary valve cusp echoes is a beam direction that is not angled sufficiently upward and laterally. Excessive lateral angulation should be avoided, since the pulmonary valve lies in close proximity to the aortic valve.
- In infants, when the beam is directed across the pulmonary artery walls, the wall motion is similar to that of the aortic root and includes a posterior dip associated with atrial systole. In these instances, A dips of the valve cusps mainly reflect the motion of the entire vessel. If the beam is somewhat oblique in relation to the vessel walls, the A dip of the valve cusp represents a combination of displacement of the entire structure complex plus intrinsic valve cusp elevation from atrial systole.
- The pulmonary valve tracing may show a

double contour, especially when the pulmonary artery is enlarged (Fig. 7-7).
- Remember, the pulmonary valve is the most difficult valve to detect and your elation will be great when you first find it! It marks an early step in the attainment of technical expertise so dear to the heart of every echocardiographer.

FINDINGS IN DISEASE
Pulmonary hypertension

Anatomic and functional changes
- In this entity there is an increase in the vascular resistance of the pulmonary circulation resulting from narrowing of the pulmonary arteries produced by hypertrophy of the wall muscle. This may be either primary, when the cause is not known, or secondary to increased pulmonary blood flow (as may occur with an atrial septal defect) or to increased pressure in the left atrium and pulmonary veins (as may occur in mitral stenosis).
- Elevation of the pulmonary artery dia-

Table 7. Pulmonary valve echocardiographic findings in pulmonary normotensive and hypertensive patients

Mean pulmonary artery pressure	Diastolic position	Opening slope mm/sec (mean)	A dip mm (mean) (NSR only)	PEP/$\sqrt{}$ R-R msec (mean) (NSR only)	Opening amplitude mm (mean)
≤20 mm Hg (22 patients)	Oblique	211 SE 12.7	4.4 SE 0.46	85.07 SE 4.36	8.68 SE 0.92
>20 mm Hg (41 patients)	Straight	420 SE 15.8	0.92 SE 0.34	110.3 SE 4.00	11.15 SE 0.47
Level of significance of *t* value*		$P < 0.001$	$P < 0.001$	$P < 0.001$	$P < 0.05$

Abbreviations: NSR, normal sinus rhythm; PEP, right ventricular pre-ejection period; $\sqrt{}$ R-R, square root of the interval (in sec) between two consecutive QRS complexes of the electrocardiogram; SE, standard error. *Derived using unpaired *t*-test with unequal number of observations. (From Nanda, N. C., and others: Circulation **50**:575, 1974. By permission of the American Heart Assn., Inc.)

Table 8. Relation of A dip to pulmonary artery pressure

Mean pulmonary artery pressure (mm Hg)	A dip		
	>2 mm	≤2 mm	Absent
≤20 (22 patients)	21	1	0
21-40 (10 patients)	1	8	1
>40 (15 patients)	2*	0	13

*Severe right heart failure. (From Nanda, N. C., and others: Circulation **50**:575, 1974. By permission of the American Heart Assn., Inc.)

stolic pressure reflects the increased vascular resistance in the pulmonary circuit. The systolic pressures in the right ventricle and the pulmonary artery are also raised, since the right ventricle has to contract more forcefully to open the pulmonary valve and propel blood through the pulmonary circuit. The degree of elevation of the pulmonary artery diastolic pressure depends upon the severity of the disease process. The right atrial pressure as well as the diastolic pressure of the right ventricle may remain within normal limits. Eventually the right ventricle fails with elevation of its diastolic pressure. The right atrial pressure is then also elevated.

• Pulmonary and tricuspid valve incompetence may supervene as a result of dilatation of the pulmonary artery and the right-sided chambers.

Clinical summary. Clinically, there is evidence for right heart enlargement, and the pulmonic component of the second heart sound is loud. A loud, early systolic ejection sound, or click, may be heard. Signs of underlying etiology (for instance, mitral stenosis) may be present. In severe cases, there is evidence for right heart failure and pulmonary valve incompetence resulting from dilatation of the annulus. The chest roentgenogram may show an enlarged pulmonary artery with a decrease in the perfusion of peripheral lung fields. Cardiac catheterization and angiocardiography assess the severity of the disease process as well as outline the underlying etiologic entity.

Echocardiographic features. Adults with uncomplicated pulmonary hypertension show a characteristic echocardiographic pattern (see Tables 7 and 8).

• There is a general straightening of the diastolic cusp image with attenuation or obliteration of the early diastolic posterior motion and the A dip.

• The valve opening images exhibit steeper slopes as compared to the normal, generally in the range of 450 mm/sec (Fig. 7-8).

• The opening movement of the pulmonary valve occurs late, resulting in prolongation of the right ventricular pre-ejection period (measured from the beginning of the QRS complex of the electrocardiogram to the onset of pulmonary valve opening movement).

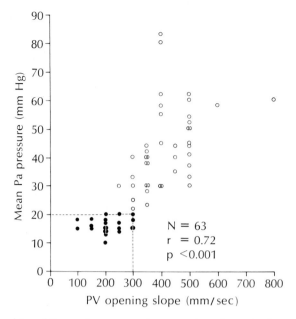

Fig. 7-8. Relationship of the pulmonary valve opening slope to the mean pulmonary artery pressure. The correlation coefficient (r value) is 0.72. The solid circles represent patients with normal pulmonary artery pressure (mean pulmonary artery pressure <20 mm Hg), whereas the open circles denote pulmonary hypertensive patients. (From Nanda, N. C., and others: Circulation **50:**575, 1974.)

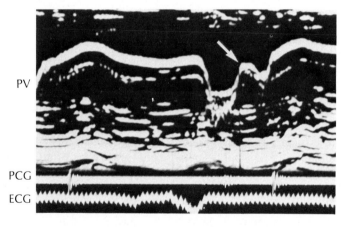

Fig. 7-9. Recording of the pulmonary valve (PV) in pulmonary hypertension demonstrates a prominent notch *(arrow)* and fine fluttering in systole. PCG, phonocardiogram; ECG, electrocardiogram.

- There is an increase in the amplitude of the opening movement of the pulmonary valve.
- In patients maintaining sinus rhythm the A dip can be used to assess the severity of pulmonary hypertension. With mean pulmonary artery pressures between 21 and 40 mm Hg, the A dip shows decreased amplitude of motion (under 2 mm), whereas more severe pulmonary hypertension with mean

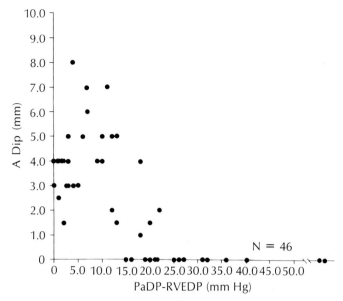

Fig. 7-10. Relationship of the A dip to the diastolic pressure gradient across the pulmonary valve. When the difference between the pulmonary artery diastolic pressure (PaDP) and the right ventricular end-diastolic pressure (RVEDP) reaches 25 mm Hg, the pulmonary valve A dip is regularly absent. This occurs in moderately severe to severe pulmonary hypertension.

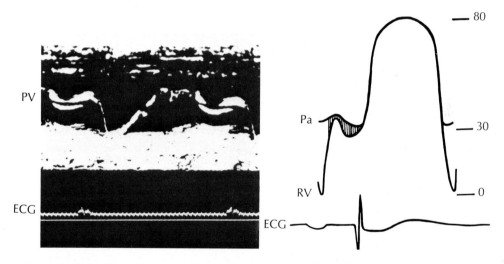

Fig. 7-11. Right heart failure and pulmonary hypertension. The pulmonary valve echo is from a patient with severe pulmonary hypertension complicated by severe right heart failure. A large A dip is observed. The valve opens rapidly, and the amplitude of the opening movement is large. The representation of the right ventricular and pulmonary artery pressure tracings was obtained at cardiac catheterization in this patient. The high right ventricular end-diastolic pressure (38 mm) results in a low gradient (4 mm) across the pulmonary valve in diastole (shaded). PV, pulmonary valve echo tracing; ECG, electrocardiogram; Pa, pulmonary artery pressure tracing; RV, right ventricular pressure tracing. The scale represents pressures in millimeters of mercury. (From Nanda, N. C., and others: Circulation **50:**575, 1974.)

pressures exceeding 40 to 50 mm Hg generally results in complete obliteration of the A dip.

• Systolic notching or fluttering of the pulmonary valve may be observed (Fig. 7-9).

Comments

• In uncomplicated pulmonary hypertension, there is a selective increase in the pulmonary artery diastolic pressure without an appreciable increase in the right ventricular diastolic pressure. The resulting high diastolic pressure gradient minimizes the effect of diastolic right ventricular hemodynamic events on the tense pulmonary valve so that the early diastolic posterior displacement and the A dip are attenuated or obliterated, depending upon the degree of elevation of the pulmonary artery diastolic pressure. No A dips are generally seen when the diastolic gradient exceeds 20 to 25 mm Hg (Fig. 7-10). When severe right heart failure supervenes, the diastolic pressure in the right ventricle may be markedly elevated. This results in a decrease in the pressure gradient across the pulmonary valve (Fig. 7-11), and the A dips may again appear or become prominent. In this situation the pulmonary valve echocardiogram may be misinterpreted as indicative of normal pulmonary artery pressure and resistance. An awareness that the patient has right heart failure clinically in addition to a prominent B point on the tricuspid valve tracing and other echocardiographic features of pulmonary hypertension, such as rapid valve opening slopes, straight valve images in early diastole, and increased right ventricular pre-ejection period, should prevent misdiagnosis.

• In pulmonary hypertension, accentuated valve opening slopes result from the rapidly rising pressure in the right ventricle. The increased amplitude of the opening movement of the pulmonary valve may be an indicator of accompanying pulmonary artery dilatation.

• The increased right ventricular pre-ejection period in pulmonary hypertension reflects the late opening of the pulmonary valve resulting from the longer time taken by the right ventricle to generate enough pressure

to overcome the pulmonary vascular resistance and force open the pulmonary valve. The pre-ejection period may also be increased in the presence of an abnormality of the conduction system, such as right bundle branch block.

• That the A dip of the pulmonary valve is a hemodynamic event and not merely the reflection of posterior motion of the whole pulmonary root induced by atrial contraction is supported by observations in patients with transposition of the great vessels complex. In this entity, due to abnormal position of the pulmonary artery, both walls of the vessel, as well as anterior and posterior cusps of the pulmonary valve, can be easily recorded. It can be clearly shown that the magnitude of the A dip is significantly larger than the corresponding posterior motion of the pulmonary artery walls occurring during this period (Fig. 7-12). Also, both cusps of the pulmonary valve can be shown to move in opposite directions following atrial systole and resulting in prominent separation of the leaflets (Fig. 7-13). The occasional recording of a small A dip in patients with severe uncomplicated pulmonary hypertension may be entirely related to posterior motion of the whole pulmonary root secondary to atrial contraction. In a given patient, therefore, comparison of the size of the A dip with the corresponding motion of the posterior pulmonary artery wall from atrial systole may provide a clue to the true nature of the A dip.

• Cessation of effective right ventricular flow in midsystole and pulmonary artery annular dilatation permitting the pulmonary leaflets to remain partially open in the bloodstream have been invoked as factors that may be responsible for the finding of systolic notching or fluttering of the pulmonary valve in pulmonary hypertension. The reliability of this finding as an indicator of pulmonary hypertension has not yet been fully evaluated, and we have occasionally seen it in apparently normal patients.

• The interval between tricuspid valve closure and the opening of the pulmonary valve increases with elevated pulmonary artery diastolic pressure.

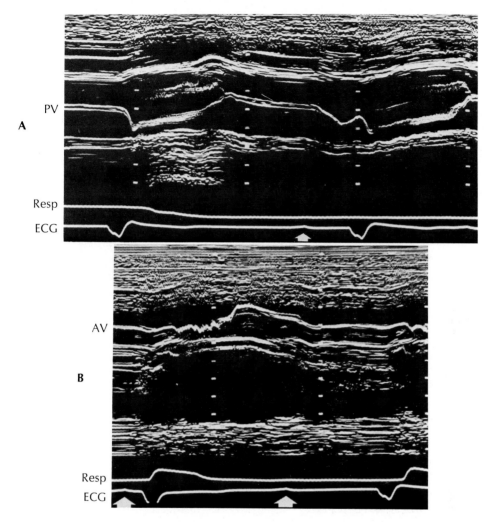

Fig. 7-12. A, Echocardiogram of the pulmonary artery in a patient with transposition of great arteries. Atrial systole results in a large posterior deflection of the pulmonary valve (PV) cusp, whereas the walls of the pulmonary artery show relatively small displacements during the same period. Resp, respiration. The arrow shows the P wave of the electrocardiogram (ECG). (The patient had complete heart block.) **B,** Echocardiogram of the aortic root from the same patient. During atrial systole the valve cusp image as well as the aortic walls show small circumscribed posterior displacements of equal magnitude. AV, aortic valve; Resp, respiration. The arrows denote the P waves of the electrocardiogram (ECG). (From Nanda, N. C., and others: Ultrasound Med. **3A:**159, 1977.)

• Some of the echocardiographic features of pulmonary hypertension in adults have been extended to pediatric patients. A good correlation between the ventricular pre-ejection period and pulmonary vascular resistance has been shown in children with normally related great vessels, as well as in those with dextrotransposition complexes. The pulmonary systolic notch occurs earlier in systole when pulmonary hypertension is associated with a right-to-left shunt through a ventricular septal defect.

• The thickness of the anterior right ventricular wall can be measured at end-diastole

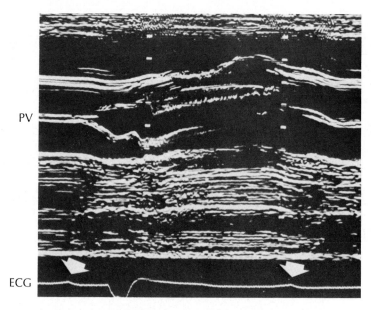

Fig. 7-13. Echocardiogram of the pulmonary artery in a patient with transposition of great arteries. During atrial systole the anterior cusp executes an anterior deflection; the posterior cusp moves posteriorly, resulting in prominent separation of the two leaflets. The pulmonary valve also shows a tendency toward early systolic closure, probably related to some subpulmonic obstruction. PV, pulmonary valve. The arrows denote the P waves of the electrocardiogram (ECG), which also showed complete heart block. (From Nanda, N. C., and others: Ultrasound Med. **3A:**159, 1977.)

using high-frequency transducers (3.5 or 5.0 MHz) and is useful in following the degree of right ventricular hypertrophy resulting from pulmonary hypertension.

• The left ventricle and the mitral valve may appear abnormal in the presence of pulmonary hypertension, even though no disease involves the left heart. The left ventricular cavity may appear small, the opening rate of the mitral valve and the EF slope may be reduced, and prolonged mitral-septal apposition in diastole is frequent. These findings are probably the result of compression of the left ventricle by the enlarged right ventricle with some compliance changes arising in a stiff ventricular septum.

• High-speed recordings (100 to 150 mm/sec) are required for accurate measurement of the pulmonary valve opening slopes.

Role of echocardiography. Echocardiography is useful not only in the detection of pulmonary hypertension but also in assessing its severity in a semiquantitative manner in patients retaining sinus rhythm. The reliability is enhanced if the clinical findings are correlated with the echocardiographic features and if careful attention is paid to the various technical pitfalls. Echocardiographic studies of other cardiac valves and chambers may shed light on the underlying cause (such as mitral stenosis or atrial septal defect). Serial echocardiographic studies of the pulmonary valve may be useful in following cases of pulmonary embolism or after surgery for correction of the condition leading to pulmonary hypertension. A dramatic decrease in the pulmonary artery pressure may result in the normalization of the pulmonary valve echocardiogram (Fig. 7-14).

Pulmonary valve stenosis

Anatomic and functional changes

• The leaflets are thickened and fused to varying degrees with a small central or eccentric orifice.

• During ventricular systole the fused leaf-

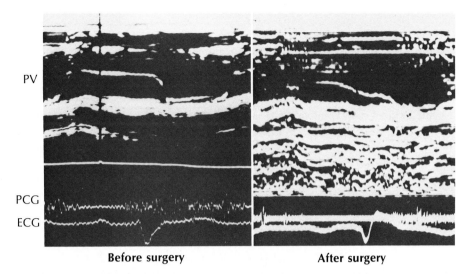

Before surgery   **After surgery**

Fig. 7-14. Pulmonary hypertension. The pulmonary valve (PV) echocardiogram shown on the left was obtained from a patient with a ventricular septal defect and moderately severe pulmonary hypertension. The pulmonary valve image is straight in diastole with no A dip and the valve opening movement is rapid. Following surgical repair of the defect *(right),* the valve image in diastole has become oblique and the A dip has reappeared. The valve opening slope is also relatively slow. Postoperative cardiac catheterization revealed pulmonary artery pressures in the normal range. PCG, phonocardiogram; ECG, electrocardiogram.

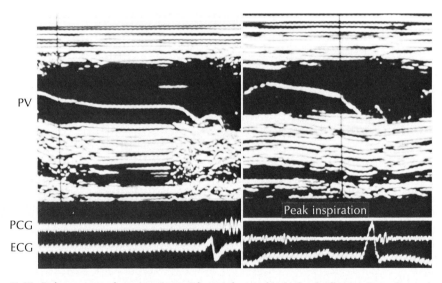

Fig. 7-15. Pulmonary valve opening with atrial systole. In both illustrations the pulmonary valve makes a strong movement toward opening following atrial systole and before the onset of the QRS complex. The cusp rebounds toward closure and then reopens with ventricular systole. Left panel was obtained from a patient with valvular pulmonary stenosis (gradient 40 mm Hg). Right panel obtained from a pulmonary normotensive subject (mean pulmonary artery pressure 20 mm Hg) and at peak inspiration. PV, pulmonary valve echo tracing; PCG, phonocardiogram; ECG, electrocardiogram. (From Nanda, N. C., and others: Circulation **50:**575, 1974.)

lets move upward, forming a dome (as the right ventricle forces blood through the narrow orifice at its tip) and descend in diastole. The pulmonary valve may be bicuspid.

• The right ventricular systolic pressure is elevated to propel blood through the obstructed valve orifice. The right ventricular diastolic pressure is also elevated, especially when failure ensues. Both the systolic and the diastolic pressures in the pulmonary artery are, on the other hand, reduced.

Clinical summary. Turbulence from the obstructed orifice produces a harsh systolic murmur. In patients with mild-to-moderate stenosis, a loud ejection sound, or click, may be heard in early systole. There is evidence for right ventricular hypertrophy. Eventually signs of heart failure may be present. The chest roentgenogram may show evidence of right ventricular enlargement and diminished perfusion of the peripheral lung fields. Cardiac catheterization reveals a pressure gradient across the pulmonary valve and angiocardiography outlines systolic doming of the valve and demonstrates a jet through the stenotic orifice.

Echocardiographic features

• A large A dip or even full "opening" of the pulmonary valve with atrial systole has been observed in patients with moderate and severe pulmonary valve stenosis (Figs. 7-15 and 7-16). A positive gradient across the pulmonary valve resulting from reduced pulmonary artery pressure and increased right ventricular end-diastolic pressure is responsible for this phenomenon.

• A marked delay in pulmonary valve opening and closure as compared to the aortic valve may be observed with severe pulmonic valve stenosis. Lesser degrees of delay are seen in milder forms of pulmonary valve stenosis.

• Some patients may show a tendency towards full opening of the pulmonary valve in early to middiastole.

Comments

• Full "opening" of the pulmonary valve with atrial systole has occasionally been demonstrated in normal subjects at peak inspiration (Fig. 7-15). Diastolic opening of the pulmonary valve has also been noted in an occasional patient with constrictive pericarditis

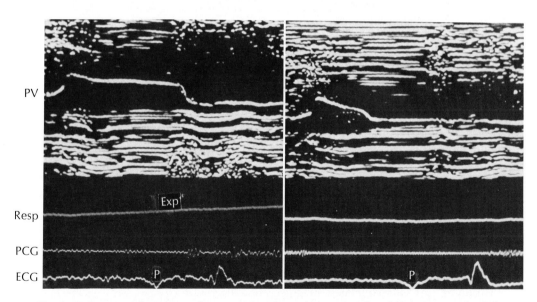

Fig. 7-16. Severe pulmonary valve stenosis. The pulmonary valve (PV) image on the left shows "full" opening following atrial systole during the expiratory phase (Exp) of respiration (Resp). The tracing on the right is obtained during inspiration and shows the valve in a fully opened position in middiastole before the onset of the P wave. PCG, phonocardiogram, ECG, electrocardiogram.

(Fig. 7-17), rupture of the sinus of Valsalva aneurysm into the right atrium, tricuspid incompetence, and Ebstein's anomaly and appears to be related to rapid elevation of the right ventricular diastolic pressure in the presence of essentially normal pulmonary artery pressure. The specific diagnostic value of this finding in patients with pulmonary valve stenosis is therefore limited.

• Recent work from our laboratory has suggested that pulmonary valve preopening is not detected in a significant number of patients with severe isolated pulmonary valve stenosis, presumably because the thickened and deformed leaflets do not respond to the small positive pressure gradient produced by atrial systole. Diastolic opening of the pulmonary valve is also not generally observed in the presence of coexistent infundibular stenosis.

• Estimation of cusp mobility of the stenotic pulmonary valve cannot be obtained by echocardiography since the opening movements merely represent the upward motion or doming of the fused cusps.

• In patients with severe pulmonary valve stenosis the tricuspid valve may show a large A wave. The ventricular septum may be hypertrophied, and the left ventricular cavity appears to be small. The left ventricular posterior wall thickness is within normal limits.

• Delayed closure of the pulmonary valve relative to that of the aortic valve may also be seen in other conditions like atrial septal defects and Ebstein's anomaly.

Role of echocardiography. Echocardiography is of limited value in the diagnosis of this entity. Many patients with mild pulmonary valve stenosis and a significant number with severe orifice obstruction may show normal pulmonary valve echocardiograms. Pulmonary valve stenosis should be suspected if a large A dip is present during expiration. In our experience, echocardio-

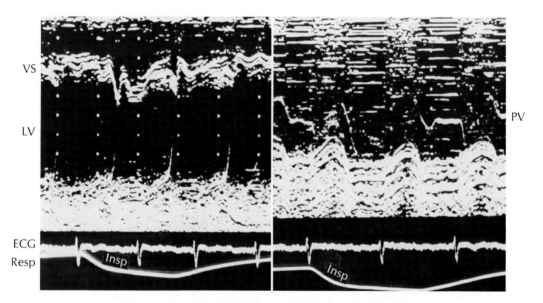

Fig. 7-17. Constrictive pericarditis. *Left,* The ventricular septum (VS) shows a bulge into the left ventricle (LV), which is localized to diastole during the inspiratory phase of respiration. The normal augmentation of the systemic venous return during inspiration (Insp) and the impaired ability of the right ventricular walls to distend in diastole from constrictive pericarditis may result in a transient increase in the right ventricular diastolic pressure, producing a septal bulge into the left ventricle. *Right,* The inspiratory rise in the right ventricular diastolic pressure also results in the pulmonary valve (PV) showing a large movement toward opening in early diastole. This is confined to the inspiratory phase of respiration (Insp). ECG, electrocardiogram.

graphic demonstration of full "opening" of the pulmonary valve with atrial systole in all phases of respiration (Fig. 7-16) and marked delay in pulmonary valve closure as compared to the aortic valve is diagnostic of severe pulmonic valve stenosis.

Infundibular stenosis

Anatomic and functional changes. Obstruction in the outflow portion of the right ventricle (or the infundibulum) may be caused by a discrete fibrous ring just below the pulmonary valve or, more commonly, by thickened, elongated muscle tissue, forming a tunnellike narrow segment. Right ventricular pressures are elevated, whereas the pulmonary artery pressure is reduced. Infundibular stenosis may be associated with pulmonary valve stenosis.

Clinical summary. Clinical findings are generally similar to those in pulmonary valve stenosis with the exception that the pulmonary component of the second heart sound may not be diminished in intensity. Cardiac catheterization shows markedly elevated pressures in the body of the right ventricle, the presence of a low-pressure infundibular chamber between the area of narrowing and the pulmonary valve, and low pressure in the pulmonary artery. Angiocardiography outlines the level of the obstruction and differentiates this entity from pulmonary valvular stenosis.

Echocardiographic features. The pulmonary valve may show coarse systolic flutter (Fig. 7-18), which may overlap into diastole. The turbulence induced by blood flowing through a narrow chamber may account for this finding. The A dips have also been reported to be small in these subjects. It has been suggested that in patients with severe infundibular stenosis, A dips would be absent, since stenosis protects the valve leaflets from diastolic hemodynamic events in the right ventricle.

Comments. In our experience the systolic segments of the pulmonary valve may be normal in some patients with this entity.

Role of echocardiography. The role of echocardiography in the diagnosis of this

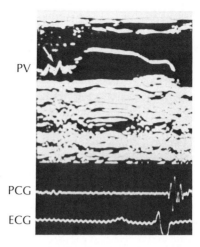

Fig. 7-18. Infundibular pulmonary stenosis. The pulmonary valve cusp (PV) shows a coarse flutter pattern during mid to late systole *(arrow)* and a normal diastolic configuration. PCG, phonocardiogram; ECG, electrocardiogram.

condition has not yet been established, and additional work is required to elucidate the sensitivity and specificity of the echocardiographic findings.

Right ventricular outflow myxoma

Anatomic and functional changes
• This is a rare lesion.
• When large, the tumor may produce right ventricular outflow obstruction. Complications such as embolization or tumor infection may occur.

Clinical summary. A harsh systolic murmur simulating pulmonary valve stenosis may be present when the tumor produces right ventricular outflow obstruction. An angiocardiogram performed with a catheter in the superior or inferior vena cava outlines the tumor mass in the right ventricle.

Echocardiographic features
• An abnormal mass of echoes may be recorded in the right ventricular outflow area in front of the pulmonary valve image throughout the cardiac cycle (Fig. 7-19).
• Prolapse of the tumor segment into the main pulmonary artery is indicated by the presence of abnormal echoes following the

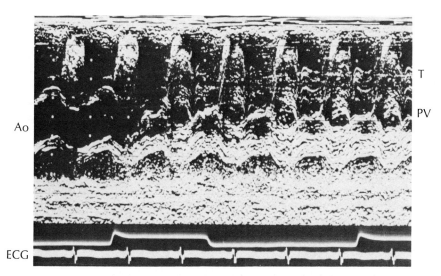

Fig. 7-19. Right ventricular outflow myxoma. Examination of the right ventricular outflow by ultrasonic beam scanning from the aortic to the pulmonic valve (PV). Tumor echoes (T) are observed throughout the cardiac cycle in front of the pulmonary valve while they are confined to diastole in front of aortic root (Ao) recording. ECG, electrocardiogram.

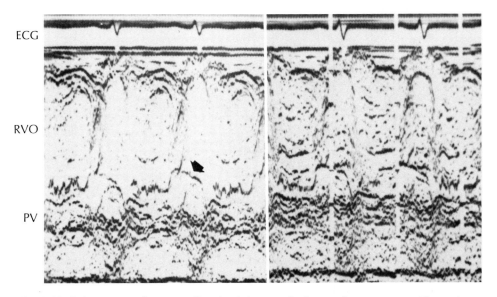

Fig. 7-20. Pulmonary valve recording in right ventricular outflow myxoma. The pulmonary valve *(arrow)* lies posteriorly in a widened outflow space (RVO) and appears structurally normal. Tumor echoes are present in the RVO and demonstrate wide excursions with the cardiac cycle. With increased gain *(right)* tumor echoes follow the pulmonary leaflet in systole suggesting that a portion of the main mass passes into the pulmonary artery. PV, pulmonary valve; ECG, electrocardiogram. (From Nanda, N. C., and others: Am. J. Cardiol. **40:**272, 1977.)

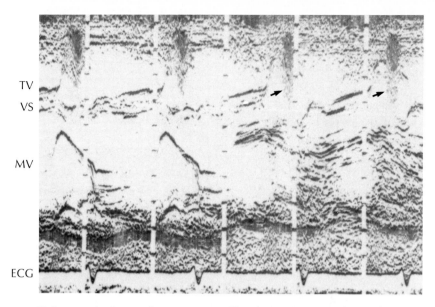

Fig. 7-21. Right ventricular outflow myxoma. The tumor mass produces dense echoes in front of the tricuspid valve (TV). Less prominent reverberations *(arrows)* extend posteriorly to the level of the closed position of the tricuspid valve and may erroneously suggest that a portion of the tumor extends into the tricuspid orifice or the right atrium. VS, ventricular septum; MV, mitral valve; ECG, electrocardiogram.

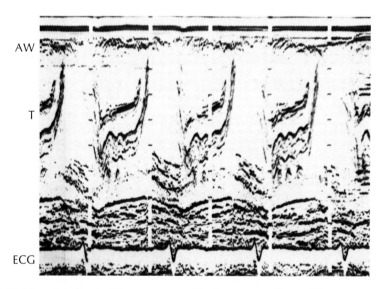

Fig. 7-22. Right ventricular outflow myxoma. The beam was directed in a manner similar to that used for pulmonary valve recording. The wide bands of echoes seen partially in diastole and more completely in systole simulate the motion pattern of an atrioventricular valve as they move toward the transducer at the onset of diastole from a relatively stationary systolic position. These probably arise in the main tumor mass, whereas the rapidly moving components with large excursions may represent the proved polypoid extensions from the main mass. The systolic undulations of the main mass may be an indication of the gelatinous nature of the tumor, which would permit quivering during the phase of most rapid blood flow. AW, anterior right ventricular wall; T, tumor echoes; ECG, electrocardiogram. (From Nanda, N.C., and others: Am. J. Cardiol. **40:** 272, 1977.)

pulmonary leaflet as it opens in systole (Fig. 7-20).

• Tumor echoes may not be seen posterior to the diastolic cusp image if the prolapsing portion returns to the outflow area in diastole.

Comments

• Examination of the right ventricular outflow area recorded in front of the aortic root may fail to show the full extent of the tumor mass. The tumor may be seen in this region only in diastole, and this finding may also be seen with a right atrial myxoma, which prolapses into the right ventricular cavity in diastole.

• Tumor echoes may also be seen in the right ventricle in front of the tricuspid valve recording and anterior to the ventricular septum. Occasionally, reverberations from the tumor may be recorded more posteriorly behind the tricuspid valve diastolic position, mimicking a right atrial myxoma (Fig. 7-21).

• A tumor present in the body of the right ventricle or in the lower portion of its outflow may produce abnormal echoes throughout the cardiac cycle in front of the aortic root recording.

• Successful detection of a right ventricular tumor requires skill in the examination of the right heart as well as an awareness of the nature of reverberation artifacts. These may obscure right heart cavities or produce spurious echo patterns, which require the use of varied beam positions and careful control of instrument sensitivity for correct identification.

• When the beam is angled in the region of the pulmonary valve to detect the greatest range of motion of the tumor echoes, the pulmonary valve may not be observed and the tumor echoes may simulate the motion pattern of an atrioventricular valve as they move toward the transducer at the onset of diastole from a relatively stationary systolic position. Inspection of echocardiograms without knowledge of the transducer orientation may thus result in a false diagnosis of a thickened tricuspid valve or a tumor mass located in the right atrial cavity (Fig. 7-22).

• A prominent low-frequency systolic fluttering of the tumor echoes may be observed

with a myxoma and may reflect its soft gelatinous nature. Additional experience is required to determine the usefulness of this finding in differentiating myxomas from other cardiac tumors.

Role of echocardiography. Echocardiography may be the first diagnostic study that indicates the true nature of this lesion. Right heart catheterization for diagnostic purposes may be hazardous, since catheter manipulation may result in hemorrhage into the tumor or dislodgement of a tumor fragment, which may embolize in the pulmonary circulation. It should be emphasized that the echocardiographic findings are not distinctive enough to be regarded as evidence of a myxoma as such and may apply to other cardiac tumors and masses as well.

MISCELLANEOUS OBSERVATIONS

• Isolated diastolic flutter of the pulmonary valve is an uncommon echocardiographic finding. We have observed its appearance in a patient with both pulmonary artery branch stenosis and pulmonary valve incompetence, the latter occurring as a complication following repair of tetralogy of Fallot (Fig. 7-23). Appearance of flutter after surgery in this patient was probably related to "ventricularization" of the proximal pulmonary artery (right ventricle and the proximal pulmonary artery virtually acting as one chamber) produced by combination of the distal branch stenosis and a thickened pulmonary valve rendered incompetent by valvotomy. There was no evidence of infundibular obstruction following surgery. We have occasionally observed pulmonary valve diastolic flutter in normal neonates but not in older children.

• Pulmonary valve and heart sounds. Pulmonary valve echocardiograms have been used to delineate the relationship between heart sounds and hemodynamic events. It has been shown in normal subjects that pulmonary valve closure on the echocardiogram precedes the phonocardiographically recorded pulmonic component of the second heart sound by an interval of 30 to 75 msec (Fig. 7-23). This discrepancy suggests that valve closure is not directly responsible for

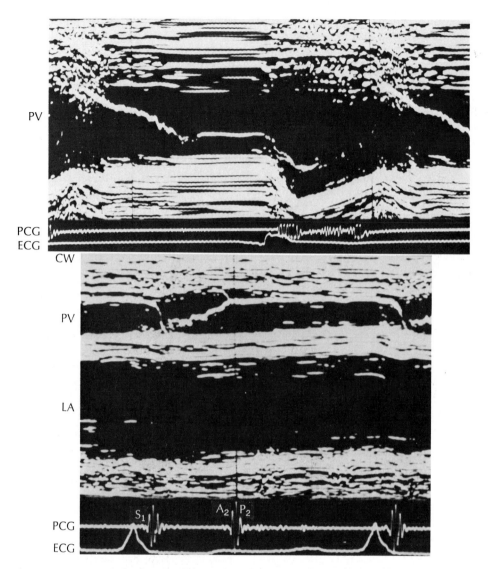

Fig. 7-23. *Top,* Diastolic flutter of the pulmonary valve. The patient presented with pulmonary artery branch stenosis and tetralogy of Fallot with pulmonary valve stenosis. Diastolic flutter of the pulmonary valve (PV) appeared after surgical repair of tetralogy and pulmonary valvotomy, which rendered the valve incompetent. The flutter is probably related to "ventricularization" of the proximal pulmonary artery produced by branch stenosis and an incompetent pulmonary valve. PCG, phonocardiogram; ECG, electrocardiogram. (From Nanda, N. C., and others: Ultrasound Med. **3A:**163, 1977.) *Bottom,* Simultaneous recording of pulmonary valve and heart sounds. Pulmonary valve (PV) closure is represented by coaptation of anterior and posterior (left) pulmonary leaflets. The point of closure does not coincide with the pulmonic component (P₂) of the second heart sound, which occurs significantly later. The pulmonary valve tracing also shows changes typical of severe pulmonary hypertension. The patient presented with cardiomyopathy; the mean pulmonary artery pressure was 71 mm Hg. CW, chest wall; LA, left atrium; PCG, phonocardiogram; S₁, first heart sound; A₂, aortic component of second heart sound; ECG, electrocardiogram.

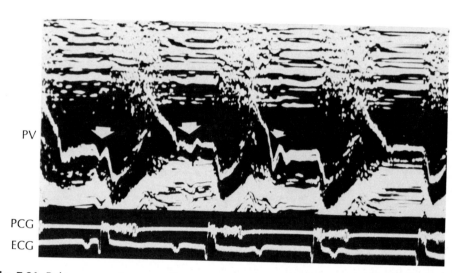

Fig. 7-24. Pulmonary valve recording in complete heart block. The A dips *(arrows)* on the pulmonary valve (PV) correspond to the P waves of the electrocardiogram (ECG), which shows complete heart block. PCG, phonocardiogram. (From Nanda, N. C., and others: Ultrasound Med. **3A:**163, 1977.)

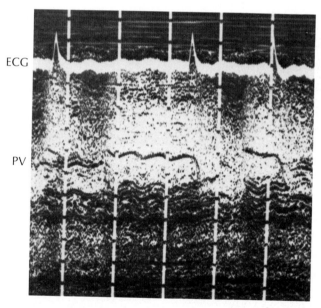

Fig. 7-25. Pulmonary valve recording in atrial flutter–fibrillation. The pulmonary valve (PV) shows coarse diastolic undulations, which are transmitted from the right atrium. They represent rapid and irregular atrial activity. ECG, electrocardiogram. (Courtesy Cardiology Division, Genesee Hospital, Rochester, N.Y.)

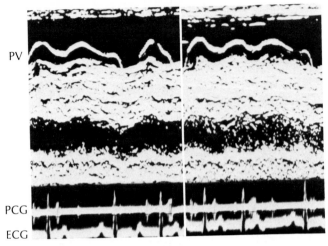

PV

PCG

ECG

Fig. 7-26. Pulmonary valve movements in cardiac arrhythmia. When the preceding R-R interval is short, the pulmonary valve may remain closed during systole from incomplete filling of the right ventricle and reduced force of contraction. On the left the first QRS complex does not result in pulmonary valve (PV) opening. On the right, two consecutive ventricular systoles do not generate enough pressure to open the valve. The third beat follows a longer diastolic interval and moves the valve to an open position. PCG, phonocardiogram; ECG, electrocardiogram.

the production of the second heart sound. These observations support the concept that the second heart sound is caused by vibrations from decelerations of columns of blood.

Right-sided ejection sounds (ejection clicks) have been shown to coincide with the position of maximal opening of the pulmonary valve cusp. This applies to both pulmonary hypertension and pulmonary valve stenosis and suggests that these sounds are valvular in origin and not related to systolic dilatation of the pulmonary artery as has been suspected in the past.

Absence or attenuation of the pulmonary ejection click during inspiration in some patients with severe pulmonic valve stenosis may be explained on the basis of premature full opening of the valve with atrial systole during this phase of respiration.

• Functional changes. In patients with complete heart block the A dips on the pulmonary valve echo tracings correspond with the randomly occurring P waves of the electrocardiogram (Fig. 7-24). A dips are not observed in patients with atrial fibrillation, but the pulmonary valve may show coarse di-

astolic undulations, transmitted from the right atrium (Fig. 7-25). In the presence of arrhythmia, the pulmonic valve may not show any opening movement during systole if the preceding diastolic interval is short and the ventricle relatively empty (Fig. 7-26).

BIBLIOGRAPHY
Pulmonary valve (general)

Gramiak, R., Nanda, N. C., and Shah, P. M.: Echocardiographic detection of pulmonary valve, Radiology **102:**153, 1972.

Weyman, A. E., Dillon, J. C., Feigenbaum, H., and Chang, S.: Pulmonary valve echo motion in pulmonary regurgitation, Br. Heart J. **37:**1184-1190, 1975.

Shaub, M., Wilson, R., and Young, G.: High frequency oscillations of the pulmonary valve leaflet in double-chamber right ventricle, J. Clin. Ultrasound **4:**115-118, 1976.

Asayama, J., Matsuura, T., Endo, N., Watanabe, T., Matsukubo, H., Furukawa, K., and Ijichi, H.: Echocardiographic findings of idiopathic dilatation of the pulmonary artery, Chest **71:**5, 1977.

Chandraratna, P. A., San Pedro, S., Elkins, R. C., and Grantham, N.: Echocardiographic, angiocardiographic and surgical correlations in right ventricular myxoma simulating valvular pulmonic stenosis, Circulation **55:**619-622, 1977.

Kramer, N. E., Gill, S. S., Patel, R., and Towne,

W. D.: Pulmonary valve vegetations detected with echocardiography, Am. J. Cardiol. **39:**1064, 1977.

Nanda, N. C., Barold, S. S., Gramiak, R., Ong, L. S., and Heinle, R. A.: Echocardiographic features of right ventricular outflow tumour prolapsing into the pulmonary artery, Am. J. Cardiol. **40:**272, 1977.

Nanda, N. C., Gramiak, R., and Manning, J.: Diastolic flutter of the pulmonary valve; echocardiographic studies, Ultrasound Med. **3A:**163, 1977.

Pulmonary hypertension

Nanda, N. C., Gramiak, R., Robinson, T., and Shah, P. M.: Evaluation of pulmonary hypertension by echocardiography, J. Clin. Ultrasound **1:**255, 1973.

Nanda, N. C., Gramiak, R., Shah, P. M., and Robinson, T.: Echocardiographic diagnosis of pulmonary hypertension, Excerpta Medica **277:**12, 1973.

Nanda, N. C., Gramiak, R., Robinson, T. I., and Shah, P. M.: Echocardiographic evaluation of pulmonary hypertension, Circulation **50:**575, 1974.

Weyman, A. E., Dillon, J. C., Feigenbaum, H., and Chang, S.: Echocardiographic patterns of pulmonary valve motion with pulmonary hypertension, Circulation **50:**905, 1974.

Hirschfeld, S., Meyer, R., Schwartz, D. C., Korfhagen, J., and Kaplan, S.: The echocardiographic assessment of pulmonary artery pressure and pulmonary vascular resistance, Circulation **52:**642, 1975.

Kerber, R. E., and Maximov, M.: Determinants of pulmonic valve opening velocity—experimental echocardiographic studies, Circulation **54**(suppl. 2): 61, 1976.

Rosenthal, A., Tucker, C. R., Williams, R. G., Khaw, K. T., Streider, D., and Shwachman, H.: Echocardiographic assessment of cor pulmonale in cystic fibrosis, Pediatr. Clin. North Am. **23:**327-344, 1976.

Johnson, G. L., Meyer, R. A., Korfhagen, J., and Kaplan, S.: Non-invasive assessment of pulmonary artery pressure in children with complete right bundle branch block, Am. J. Cardiol. **39:**265, 1977.

Nanda, N. C., Scovil, J., and Gramiak, R.: Further echocardiographic observations on the pulmonary valve "A" dip. In White, D. N., and Brown, R. E.: Ultrasound in medicine, vol. 3, 1977, Plenum Publishing Corp., p. 159.

Nixon, J. V., Haper, J., Jones, J., and Mullins, C. B.: Echocardiographic evaluation of changes in right ventricular diameter and wall thickness in chronic progressive pulmonary arterial hypertension, Clin. Res. **25:**242A, 1977.

Pulmonary valve stenosis

Weyman, A. E., Dillon, J. C., Feigenbaum, H., and Chang, S.: Echocardiographic patterns of pulmonary valve motion in valvular pulmonary stenosis, Am. J. Cardiol. **34:**644-651, 1974.

Weyman, A. E., Dillon, J. C., Feigenbaum, H., and Chang, S.: Echocardiographic differentiation of infundibular from valvular pulmonary stenosis, Am. J. Cardiol. **36:**21-26, 1975.

Nanda, N. C., Lombardi, A., and Gramiak, R.: Assessment of severity of pulmonary valve stenosis by echocardiography, Clin. Res. **24:**232A, 1976.

8 Left ventricle

STRUCTURES IN BEAM

The following structures are encountered during ultrasonic examination of the left ventricular cavity:
1. Chest wall
2. Anterior right ventricular wall
3. Right ventricular cavity
4. Ventricular septum
5. Left ventricular cavity containing the mitral apparatus
6. Left ventricular posterior wall

Recordings from the left ventricular cavity obtained just past the tip of the mitral leaflets represent the central portion or the transverse diameter of the cavity (Fig. 8-1).

Lateral and inferior direction of the beam from this position may pass through the chest wall, anterior wall of the left ventricle, left ventricular cavity, and posterior left ventricular wall. The ventricular septum and the anterior wall of the right ventricle will not be imaged in this position.

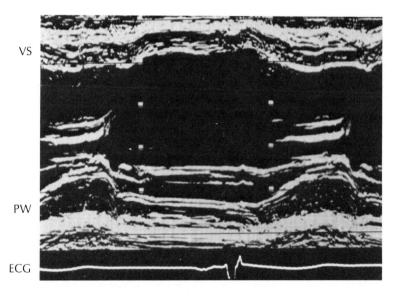

Fig. 8-1. Echocardiogram of the left ventricular cavity. The record is obtained just past the tips of the mitral leaflets, whose fragments are seen in the record. Relatively slow moving chordal echoes are present in front of the left ventricular posterior wall (PW). VS, ventricular septum; ECG, electrocardiogram.

Inferior angulation of the beam from the short axis position also results in the linear chordae echoes being replaced by thicker and more prominent echoes of the posterior papillary muscle located adjacent to the posterior left ventricular wall. Occasionally in a patient with a large cardiac window the area of the apex may be visualized by further inferior and lateral angulation of the transducer (Fig. 8-2).

NORMAL TRACING (Fig. 8-1)

At the level of the transverse or the short axis of the left ventricle the ventricular septum moves posteriorly during systole and has an anterior motion in diastole. The ventricular septum also thickens in systole as it contracts and increases its width by about 30% of the diastolic thickness. The left ventricular posterior wall generally shows greater amplitude of motion than the ventricular septum and moves anteriorly in systole and posteriorly during ventricular relaxation. The endocardial echo shows a greater amplitude and more rapid motion in both systole and diastole than does the epicardium. Atrial contraction may result in some further expansion of the ventricular cavity manifested by slight circumscribed anterior motion of the ventricular septum and corresponding posterior motion of the left ventricular posterior wall. The ventricular septum may show a small notch during the isovolumic relaxation period, probably due to twisting or rotational movement of the heart during this phase of the cardiac cycle. Fragments of the mitral valve, particularly the posterior leaflet, and thin linear echoes from the chordae are seen within the cavity of the ventricle in this projection.

Movements of the ventricular septum and the left ventricular posterior wall toward

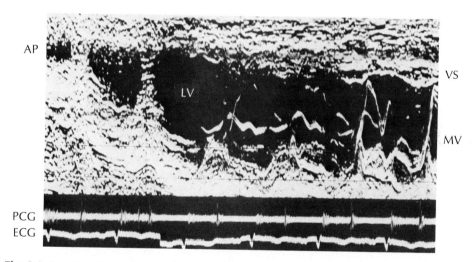

Fig. 8-2. Examination of the cardiac apex. The apex was first identified in multiple beam sweeps along the long axis of the left ventricle as the narrowest portion of the left ventricular cavity adjacent to lung. This beam sweep begins at the apex (AP) and extends into the mitral valve (MV). Note how the posterior wall angles posteriorly as the cavity widens. The character and motion of the posterior wall in the apical region are obscured by the presence of a papillary muscle, reverberation artifacts, and incomplete motion recording from a nonperpendicular orientation of the beam to the sloping left ventricular wall. The vertical bars of reverberation artifacts are probably produced by systolic retraction of the apex toward the base, bringing the muscular wall at the tip into the beam in systole. The patient has mitral valve prolapse. VS, ventricular septum; LV, left ventricular cavity; MV, mitral valve; ECG, electrocardiogram; PCG, phonocardiogram.

each other during systole represent contraction of the short axis of the ventricle. Motion of these structures away from each other during diastole denotes ventricular relaxation to permit inflow of the pulmonary venous blood from the left atrium.

TECHNICAL CONSIDERATIONS

• Ideally, the transducer should be directed almost perpendicularly to the chest surface when the mitral valve is detected, and then the beam should be angled inferiorly and laterally (less than 20 degrees) to obtain echoes from the left ventricular cavity just past the tips of the mitral leaflets. The left ventricular cavity dimensions may change significantly (as much as 25%) if the transducer is placed too high or too low on the chest wall. On the echocardiographic record, both the ventricular septum and the anterior wall of the aorta are imaged at approximately the same level from the chest wall if the transducer position is relatively perpendicular to it. The anterior wall of the aorta appears to be located more posteriorly if a low transducer position is used. With a high transducer position the anterior wall of the aorta may be recorded closer to the chest wall as compared to the ventricular septum.

• In many patients it is not possible to scan the whole of the left ventricular cavity, since the size of the cardiac window is considerably smaller than that of the left ventricular cavity. Therefore, a steep oblique direction of the ultrasonic beam is required to visualize portions of the left ventricular cavity near the region of the posterior papillary muscle and the apex so that motion amplitude of these structures may be erroneously depicted and dropouts degrade image content.

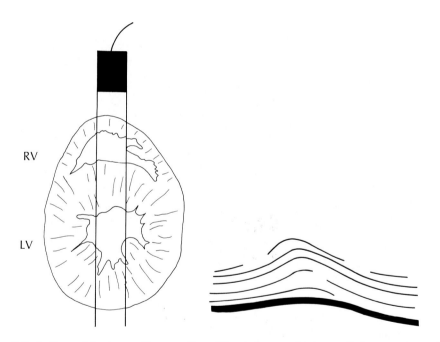

Fig. 8-3. Left ventricular wall recording. The left ventricular wall has an irregular inner aspect in which trabeculae of various sizes are present. Their projections into the cavity as well as the bases of the crypts formed between them can produce multiple echo sources, which may be confusing when assessing the thickness of the myocardium. Selection of the first echo source that is continuous throughout the cardiac cycle and that demonstrates the known motion characteristics of the left ventricular posterior wall endocardium yields the most reproducible results. RV, right ventricle; LV, left ventricle.

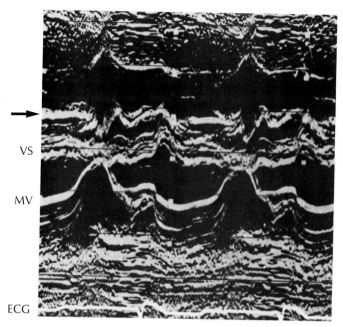

Fig. 8-4. The septal leaflet *(arrow)* of the tricuspid valve is imaged adjacent to the ventricular septum (VS) and may be mistaken as a part of the septal complex if it is not completely recorded. Portions of the anterior tricuspid leaflet are seen further anteriorly. MV, mitral valve; ECG, electrocardiogram.

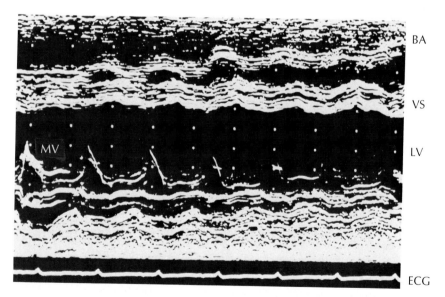

Fig. 8-5. Recording of a muscle band in the right ventricular cavity. Echoes from a right ventricular muscle band (BA) may be closely applied to the right side of the septum, resulting in an apparently thickened ventricular septal image. Alterations in beam angulation generally result in separation of the muscle band from the septum and allow accurate identification of both structures. VS, ventricular septum; MV, mitral valve; ECG, electrocardiogram.

- Echoes from posteriorly located chordae may be confused with those from the endocardium. Although they move in the same general direction as the endocardium, their slopes and amplitudes of motion are considerably smaller. Minimal angulation of the transducer with slight increase in the gain frequently enhances the endocardial echo and distinguishes it from the relatively stronger images of the chordae tendineae. Also, scanning upward into the mitral valve region usually shows the continuity of the chordal echoes with the mitral leaflets. It is possible that the extra echoes detected in front of the endocardium may actually be emanating in some instances from trabeculae of the posterior left ventricular wall and that multiple echoes are simultaneously recorded because of beam width (Fig. 8-3).

- The right side of the septum may not be well delineated in some subjects. Near-gain suppression is frequently required to obliterate the reverberatory echoes from the chest wall that frequently clutter the anterior region. Near-gain suppression should be used only after the right side of the septum can be reasonably well delineated using low-gain settings. Arbitrary introduction of the near suppression may mask the right side of the septum, or reverberatory clutter may be confused with the right side of the septum, which may then appear to be falsely thickened, depending upon the depth of the near suppression. The right side of the septum may be recognized as the anterior-most echo that moves and is parallel to the left side of the septum in diastole. Structures that may be in contact with the right side of the septum, such as the tricuspid valve (Fig. 8-4) or its supporting apparatus may be mistaken for part of the septal complex. Other structures such as a muscle band may be imaged in the right ventricular cavity and may be mistaken for the right side of the septum (Fig. 8-5). However, careful scanning may show the structural echo to be in the cavity of the right ventricle and clarify its true nature. The same problem may occur in the presence of a right heart pacing catheter. The stronger echoes from the wire may mask the true right side of the septum.

- The right side of the septum may be dif-

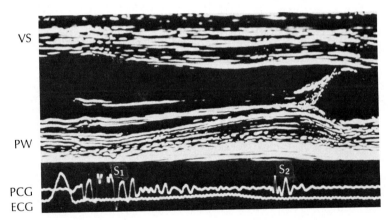

Fig. 8-6. High speed (375 mm/sec) recording of the left ventricular wall demonstrating its relationship to the heart sounds and the electrocardiogram. The first heart sound (S₁) begins before the onset of ventricular ejection, which is denoted by anterior motion of the left ventricular posterior wall (PW). The left ventricular posterior wall continues to move anteriorly for some distance even after cessation of ejection, which is indicated by the occurrence of the first or aortic component of second heart sound (S₂). The time interval between the onset of the QRS complex of the electrocardiogram (ECG) and the beginning of the anterior motion of the left ventricular posterior wall represents the pre-ejection period. VS, ventricular septum; PCG, phonocardiogram.

ficult to delineate in patients with marked septal hypertrophy, since the septum may show poor mobility so that incorrect identification may lead to underestimation of septal thickness.

• The ventricular septum is not a flat partition but is curved with its convexity toward the right ventricular cavity; areas not perpendicular to the ultrasonic beam may not be well observed and may produce image dropouts.

• The left ventricular posterior wall echo continues to make a brief movement anteriorly even after the aortic valve has closed (timed by a simultaneously recorded phonocardiogram), and this may reflect anterior motion of the whole heart during the isovolumic relaxation period, since the ventricle has ceased to contract (Fig. 8-6). The recorded motion of the ventricular septum and of the left ventricular posterior wall is influenced by the movement of the whole heart during the cardiac cycle.

• The motion of the heart walls is also affected by respiration (Fig. 8-7). With inspiration there is a slight decrease of the left ventricular cavity dimensions, and this is probably related to a slight decrease in the filling pressure of the left ventricle during this phase of respiration.

• Very slow speed scans (10 to 25 mm/sec) of the left ventricle from the aortic root level to the apical region have been used to estimate the shape of the left ventricle. Aneurysms of the apical portion can be recognized by this technique, since the normal tapering of the cavity at the apex is replaced by an area of cavity widening (Fig. 8-8). Measurement of the length of the ventricular cavity can only be accomplished if the scanning speed matches the paper speed and the beam is vertically oriented during the scan. In practice, this combination is impossible to achieve.

• In difficult patients a subxiphoid technique may be used to visualize the cavity of

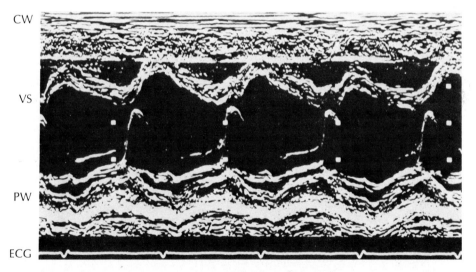

Fig. 8-7. Variations in left ventricular dimension. A recording of the left ventricular cavity obtained in a child with a ventricular septal defect shows considerable variation in apparent cavity size in a series of heart beats occurring over a two-second interval. The end-diastolic dimension varies between 3.0 and 3.3 cm, which introduces a variation of approximately 30% when volume is calculated using the cube formula. Possible explanations for the differences include cardiac displacement during respiration, different degrees of cardiac filling related to respiratory phase or unrecognized slight changes in beam position or angulation. CW, chest wall; VS, ventricular septum; PW, left ventricular posterior wall; ECG, electrocardiogram.

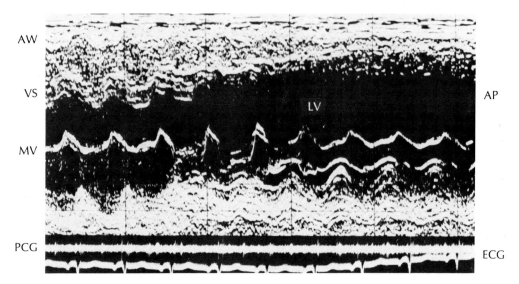

Fig. 8-8. Echocardiogram in a patient with left ventricular aneurysm involving the apex. Beam scanning demonstrates widening of the left ventricular cavity as the apex is approached in contrast to progressive narrowing seen in a normal subject. AW, anterior right ventricular wall; VS, ventricular septum; MV, mitral valve; LV, left ventricular cavity; AP, apex; PCG, phonocardiogram; ECG, electrocardiogram.

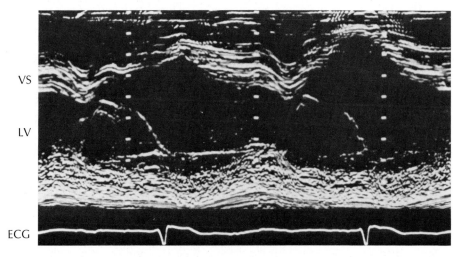

Fig. 8-9. Septal dropouts and left ventricular dimensions. An inadequate recording shows multiple dropouts of the septal image as indicated by abrupt termination of linear echoes derived from musculature of the septum. At end-systole, septal and endocardial imaging is more complete and could yield a reasonable estimate of end-systolic volume. End-diastolic volume, on the other hand, would be spuriously increased if measured from a record of this type. VS, ventricular septum; LV, left ventricle; ECG, electrocardiogram.

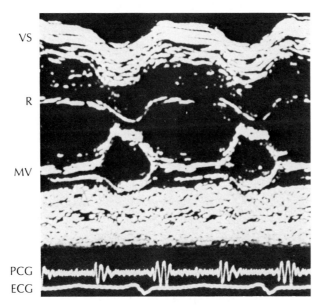

Fig. 8-10. Intracardiac reverberations. A thin, linear echo (R) with the motion pattern of the ventricular septum (VS) is recorded in the left ventricular outflow and probably represents a septal reverberation. MV, mitral valve; PCG, phonocardiogram; ECG, electrocardiogram.

the left ventricle, particularly the apical region.

• It is a common error to record only one side of the ventricular septum, usually the right, and in this way spuriously enlarge the short axis (Fig. 8-9).

• The endocardial surface of the posterior wall may not be recorded and may require the use of time-varied gain for adequate visualization.

• Linear echoes may be seen below the left side of the septum and probably represent reverberatory artifacts (Fig. 8-10).

DETERMINATION OF LEFT VENTRICULAR FUNCTION

Echocardiography has been used to determine the same parameters of left ventricular function described earlier in the section dealing with angiocardiography. However, M-mode echocardiography does not provide a full image of the left ventricular cavity at end-systole and end-diastole, so it is necessary to create a model left ventricle from a single short axis dimension by applying the relationship of this dimension to the known geometry of the normal left ventricle. In this manner, a volume is calculated based on the assumption that all ventricles fit the same geometric model and that all areas contract symmetrically.

Echocardiographic measurement technique

All measurements pertaining to the left ventricle are taken at the level of the short axis with the beam traversing the cavity just below the tip of the mitral leaflets (Fig. 8-11).

• The left ventricular end-diastolic dimension (Dd) is taken as the perpendicular distance between the left septal and left ventricular posterior wall endocardial surfaces measured at the R wave peak of a simultaneously recorded electrocardiogram.

• The left ventricular end-systolic dimension (Ds) is measured as the shortest perpendicular distance between the endocardial surfaces of the left side of the ventricular septum and the left ventricular posterior wall during systole.

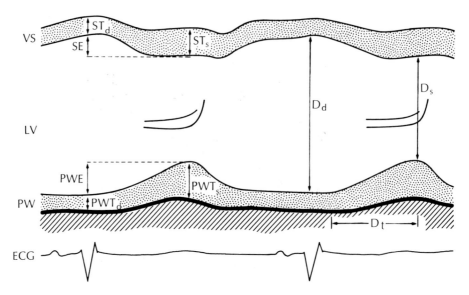

Fig. 8-11. Measurement technique for determination of left ventricular function. VS, ventricular septum; LV, left ventricle; PW, left ventricular posterior wall; ECG, electrocardiogram; D_d, end-diastolic dimension; D_s, end-systolid dimension; ST_d, ventricular septal thickness in diastole; ST_s, ventricular septal thickness in systole; SE, ventricular septal excursion; PWTD, posterior wall thickness in diastole; PWTS, posterior wall thickness in systole; PWE, posterior wall excursion; D_t, left ventricular ejection time.

- The left ventricular ejection time (Dt) is measured in seconds or milliseconds as the period from the onset of systolic anterior motion of the left ventricular posterior wall to its maximal anterior excursion. It also represents the duration of shortening of the left ventricular posterior wall.

- The excursions of the ventricular septum (SE) and left ventricular posterior wall (PWE) are measured in millimeters as the maximum perpendicular distances from the diastolic endocardial surface of the ventricular septum and left ventricular posterior wall (at the R wave of the ECG) to the level of the maximal systolic excursions.

- Ventricular septal thickness (STd) is measured in millimeters as the distance between the right and left endocardial surfaces of the ventricular septum at the time of the R wave peak of a simultaneously recorded electrocardiogram. The left ventricular posterior wall thickness (PWTd) is measured in millimeters as the distance from the left ventricular endocardial to epicardial surfaces at

the time of the R wave peak of the ECG. Maximal septal (STs) and posterior wall (PWTs) widths during systole can also be measured.

- Peak systolic or diastolic velocities of the ventricular septum and left ventricular posterior wall are measured in millimeters per second as the maximal slopes of the endocardial surfaces of the ventricular septum and left ventricular posterior wall, respectively, during systole or diastole.

Estimation of parameters

Ventricular volume. The method for the calculation of the left ventricular volumes is based on the fact that the left ventricle in the normal subject closely resembles a solid ellipse (Fig. 8-12). One also assumes that (1) the two short axes of the ellipse (D) are equal, (2) the long axis (L) is twice the short axis, (3) the echocardiographic left ventricular dimension approximates the short axis, and (4) the left ventricular walls contract uniformly.

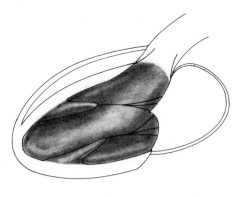

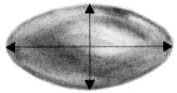

Fig. 8-12. Left ventricular volume. The assumption that the left ventricular cavity *(top)* closely resembles a solid ellipse *(bottom)* forms the basis for the echocardiographic determination of left ventricular volume. The short axis of the ellipse corresponds to the left ventricular cavity dimension obtained echocardiographically just past the tip of the mitral valve. Both the short axes of the left ventricle are also assumed to be equal and half the long axis. A cross section at the level of the short axis would be circular in configuration.

The formula for volume (V) of such a geometric model is as follows:

$$V = \frac{L}{D} \times \frac{\pi}{6} \times D^3$$

Since $L = 2D$, and $\pi \sim 3.0$,

$$V = \frac{2D}{D} \times \frac{3}{6} \times D^3$$

$$V = D^3$$

Thus, the volume of the ellipse can be calculated by cubing the short axis.

Cubing the echocardiographically obtained end-diastolic dimension of the left ventricle therefore gives an estimate of the end-diastolic volume, whereas cubing the end-systolic dimension provides an approximation of the end-systolic volume. The difference between the two volumes represents the stroke volume.

End-diastolic volume $= Dd^3$
End-systolic volume $= Ds^3$
Stroke volume (SV) $= Dd^3 - Ds^3$

Myocardial contraction
Ejection fraction. Relating the stroke volume to the end-diastolic volume gives the ejection fraction and represents an index of the extent of left ventricular fiber shortening.

$$\text{Ejection fraction (EF)} = \frac{SV}{Dd^3}$$

Fractional shortening. The extent of minor axis change (percentage change, or $\%\Delta$) correlates closely with ejection fraction and is a simpler way of estimating myocardial contractility.

$$\%\Delta = \frac{Dd - Ds}{Dd} \times 100$$

Normal subjects show values in excess of 25%.

Mean velocity of circumferential fiber shortening (mean V_{CF}). This parameter represents the change in the internal circumference of the left ventricle at its minor axis during systole divided by the duration of shortening or ejection time (Dt).

End-diastolic circumference $= \pi \times Dd$ (cm)
End-systolic circumference $= \pi \times Ds$ (cm)
Change in internal circumference (mean V_{CF})

$$\text{cm/sec} = \frac{\pi Dd - \pi Ds}{Dt(\text{sec})} = \frac{\pi(Dd - Ds)}{DT}$$

Since mean V_{CF} varies with the size of the ventricular chamber, it is convenient to normalize it by dividing it by end-diastolic circumference to permit comparison of chambers of differing sizes.

Mean VCF (normalized for heart size)

$$\text{in circumferences/sec} = \frac{\pi(Dd - Ds)}{Dt \times \pi Dd} =$$

$$\frac{Dd - Ds}{Dt \times Dd} \text{ circumferences/sec.}$$

Wall thickness. Systolic thickening of the ventricular septum and the left ventricular posterior wall can be evaluated by subtracting the end-diastolic thickness from the maximal systolic width and dividing it by the diastolic thickness and expressing it as a percentage.

$$\% \text{ septal thickening} = \frac{STs - STd}{STd} \times 100$$

$\% \text{ posterior wall thickening} =$

$$\frac{PWTs - PWTd}{PWTd} \times 100$$

Left ventricular mass. The total mass of the left ventricular (LV) myocardium can be calculated by determining the end-diastolic volume of the ventricular cavity and the end-diastolic volume of the whole ventricle, including the myocardium, and subtracting cavity volume from total volume.

End-diastolic cavity volume in cubic
$$\text{centimeters} = D_d{}^3$$

assuming the thickness of the whole LV myocardium to be uniform and equal to LV posterior wall thickness.

Total ventricular volume (cavity + wall) in cc =
$$(D_d + 2PWT_d)^3$$

Total volume of LV myocardium in cc =
$$(D_d + 2PWT_d)^3 - D_d{}^3$$

A correction factor that represents the specific gravity of cardiac muscle (1.05) converts muscle volume into weight in grams.

$$\text{LV mass (g)} = [(D_d + 2PWT_d)^3 - D_d{}^3] \times 1.05$$

Posterior wall and septal velocities. The peak as well as mean systolic and diastolic velocities of motion of the left ventricular posterior wall and the ventricular septum have also been used as measures of left ventricular function. Mean velocities are calculated by noting the excursion of the ventricular septum or left ventricular posterior wall in systole or diastole and dividing it by the duration in seconds.

Mean velocity of ventricular septum

$$\text{in systole (mm/sec)} = \frac{SE(mm)}{Dt(sec)}$$

Mean velocity of LV posterior wall

$$\text{in systole (mm/sec)} = \frac{PWE(mm)}{Dt(sec)}$$

Comments

• The use of a single dimension is the most important limitation of the echocardiographic technique for assessment of left ventricular function. The short axis determined by echocardiography may be incorrect because of improper beam position or when left ventricular trabeculae are confused with the true endocardial echo. The technique samples only a small portion of the left ventricular muscle mass, and it is necessary to assume that the same thickness and motion patterns are present throughout. Wall motion may be erroneously depicted when the beam is not truly perpendicular to the axis of motion. Finally, the assumptions regarding cavity geometry have been shown to be incorrect when cardiac enlargement is present.

• In dilated hearts the ratio of the long axis to the short axis of the ventricle may be reduced to 1.5 or less, since the ventricle becomes more spherical with increasing size. In such instances the cube formula is highly inaccurate for volume calculations, and the following formula may be more useful: volume = 7 ÷ (2.4 + diastolic dimension) × cube of diastolic dimension.

• Since there is a good correlation between the left ventricular echocardiographic dimensions and the angiographically determined volumes, a regression equation can be computed and also used for volume estimations: End-diastolic volume = 59 × diastolic dimension − 153; end-systolic volume = 47 × systolic dimension − 120.

• Various other methods have been suggested for measuring the diastolic dimension of the left ventricle. Some workers take the maximum dimension in diastole; others take it at the **Q** wave of the ECG to avoid slight distortion of wall motion occurring during the isovolumic relaxation phase of the left ventricle. More recently it has been suggested that the cavity dimension should be taken before the peak of the P wave, since the ventricular cavity expands slightly (1 to 2 mm) with atrial contraction. In general the differences between various measurement techniques in adults are small—on the order of 1 to 2 mm. In children, however, these differences may result in significant changes in the calculated ventricular volumes, since the cavity dimensions are small.

• Echocardiographic dimensions have been recorded simultaneously with left ventricular pressures in patients undergoing cardiac catheterization. Using these data, a pressure-dimension curve or derived pressure volume loop for each cardiac cycle can be constructed, allowing calculation of total ventricular work and separation of volume and pressure work. Analysis of the diastolic portion of this curve allows quantitation of the diastolic properties or compliance (stiffness) of the ventricle. Note that this technique avoids contrast medium injection (during angiography), which by itself may alter left ventricular function. Peak systolic wall stress may also be measured, and this is an important determinant of myocardial oxygen consumption.

• A severe proximal lesion of the left coronary artery may result in extensive ischemia or damage, which is most severe in the apical region of the left ventricle. Therefore, localized akinetic areas and aneurysms are commonly present in the distal left ventricle. Reduced contraction of the posterior left ventricular wall usually indicates severe disease of the circumflex branch of the left coronary artery and also of the right coronary artery (both of which supply this area) and hence is not commonly seen. Usually, inability to record adequate echoes from this region probably stems from the nonperpendicular relationship of the walls to the ultrasonic beam.

• Measurement of the left ventricular ejection time using the posterior wall echo may not be accurate. The exact point of onset of anterior motion may be difficult to determine accurately. Also, maximum anterior motion may occur well after the cessation of ejection. A more accurate measurement may be obtained from a simultaneously recorded carotid pulse or from an aortic valve echocardiogram (measuring the interval between cusp opening and cusp closure from a beat with an exactly similar R-R interval).

• In the presence of a conduction defect of the left ventricle, such as left bundle branch block, the ventricular septum may show transient rapid posterior motion with the beginning of the QRS complex, followed by an abnormal anterior motion during the remainder of systole. Abnormal anterior motion of the ventricular septum during systole may also occur with conditions producing right-sided volume overload, such as an atrial septal defect. The effect of these changes on the calculation of ventricular volumes has not been adequately evaluated so far.

• In patients with poor left ventricular function the velocity of the opening movement of the mitral valve as well as the EF slope may be reduced, although these are not constant findings. The amplitude of motion of the mitral valve may also be decreased. The area subtended by the open mitral leaflets in diastole also provides a measure of the left atrial output, whereas the area enclosed by the aortic leaflets in systole gives an estimate of the left ventricular forward flow.

• Prolongation of the AC segment with a prominent plateau or prominent B point on the mitral valve echocardiogram has been reported to be associated with increased left ventricular end-diastolic pressure. This probably results from a markedly elevated atrial component of left ventricular and left atrial pressures secondary to changes in the compliance of the left ventricle. The delay may also result from the left ventricle taking a longer time to generate sufficient pressure to reverse the gradient across the mitral orifice and close the mitral valve.

ROLE OF ECHOCARDIOGRAPHY

• Assessment of left ventricular function by echocardiography is useful in entities such as cardiomyopathies and valvular heart disease in which the ventricle is affected uniformly. In these categories the echocardiographically determined parameters have correlated very well with angiographic measurements of left ventricular function.

• Using the mitral valve as a reference point and recording the left ventricular dimensions just below its tip have been found to be highly reproducible on different occasions in the same subject, even when measured by different observers. Serial echocardiographic studies in the same patient during physiologic or pharmacologic interventions are useful in determining their effects on cardiac function. They are also useful in following the natural history of a disease process, evaluating the effect of various cardiac therapies on ventricular function, and assessing the beneficial effect of surgical procedures such as valve replacement. Serial studies may also result in the early detection of development of left ventricular dysfunction produced by certain cardiotoxic pharmacologic agents such as doxorubicin (Adriamycin) (Fig. 8-13).

• In pre-excitation or WPW syndrome, small transient humps have been observed on the left side of the ventricular septum and the endocardial echo before onset of ventricular ejection, and these may provide useful information regarding the abnormal activation pathways.

• Echocardiographic assessment of left ventricular function is unreliable in the presence of segmental wall abnormalities often seen with coronary artery disease.

• M-mode echocardiography is generally not useful in detecting clots that may form

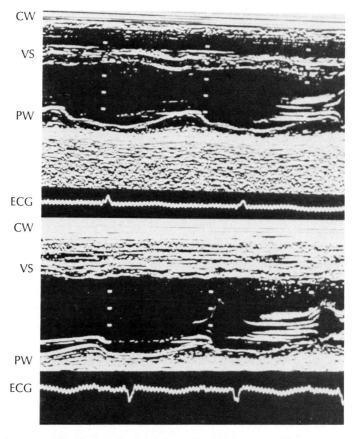

Fig. 8-13. Left ventricular dysfunction produced by Adriamycin. The upper panel shows a control left ventricular cavity recording from a patient suffering from carcinoma. The ventricular septum (VS) and the left ventricular posterior wall (PW) show normal amplitude of motion. The lower panel was obtained following a course of Adriamycin therapy and shows increased left ventricular cavity diameter as well as reduction in the amplitudes of the ventricular septum and posterior wall motion. Fractional shortening (%Δ) reduced to 18% from a control value of 35% and the mean V_{CF} decreased to 0.48 from the pretherapy value of 1.16. CW, chest wall; ECG, electrocardiogram.

in dilated left ventricular cavities or in association with a ventricular aneurysm. In an occasional patient they have presented as multilayered echoes in the left ventricular cavity. In one instance, dense moving echoes that simulated a myxomatous mass were present in the left ventricular cavity and originated from a large organized thrombus.

• Echocardiography is useful in detecting a left ventricular tumor or myxoma, a rare lesion with echocardiographic features similar to those of tumors present in other cardiac chambers (Fig. 8-14).

CORONARY ARTERY DISEASE

Anatomic and functional changes

• The two coronary arteries, which arise from the base of the aorta, course over the surface of the heart, giving branches that penetrate to supply the heart muscle. The left main coronary artery branches into the circumflex vessel and the left anterior main descending artery (LAD) shortly after its origin from the aorta.

• The LAD system supplies the anterior wall of the ventricle, the apex, and upper two thirds of the ventricular septum (through various septal perforating branches). The lower portion of the septum is supplied generally by the right coronary artery through its posterior descending branch. In approximately 10% of patients, the lower third of the ventricular septum is supplied by a dominant circumflex artery. The posterior wall of the left ventricle and the right ventricle are supplied by both the right coronary artery and the circumflex branch of the left main vessel.

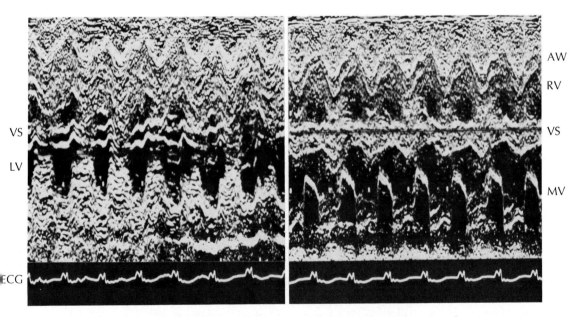

Fig. 8-14. Ventricular fibromas. A large intramural fibroma (5.5 by 3 by 4.5 cm) arose from the left ventricular wall at the apex without involvement of the papillary muscles, chordae, or mitral valve. A portion of the mass that protruded into the left ventricular cavity (LV) presents as an intermittent mass of echoes best seen in systole. When the mitral valve (MV) was studied, an unusually wide echo-containing region was seen in front of the anterior wall (AW) of the right ventricle. This probably represents a second fibroma (3.5 by 2.5 by 2.5 cm) growing outwardly from the anterior right ventricular wall. These tumors were present at autopsy in a 2½-year-old child with multiple congenital anomalies and a brain tumor (medulloblastoma). VS, ventricular septum; ECG, electrocardiogram.

• Atherosclerotic plaques produce significant obstruction to the blood supply and lead to underperfusion and ischemia or infarction of the myocardial segment supplied by the affected vessel. Myocardial infarction may result in thinning of the ventricular wall with hypokinesia, akinesia, or dyskinesia of the muscle. Myocardial infarction may also produce a pericardial reaction. Other complications include rupture of the ventricular wall, papillary muscle dysfunction, and rupture and perforation of the ventricular septum.

Clinical summary. Anginal pains suggest the presence of myocardial ischemia, whereas prolonged chest pain heralds myocardial infarction. Electrocardiographic changes as well as high blood concentrations of cardiac enzymes (leakage from damaged heart muscle) are valuable in the diagnosis. Coronary arteriograms outline the extent and severity of lesions, and the left ventricular angiogram demonstrates underperfused areas of muscle as wall motion abnormalities.

Echocardiographic features

• Decreased excursion (less than 3 mm) or paradoxical systolic anterior motion of the ventricular septum may be observed, especially when there is an obstructing lesion in the proximal left anterior descending vessel, which supplies the upper two thirds of the ventricular septum (Fig. 8-15). In our experience, this finding is a reliable indicator of significant disease (more than 75% narrowing) in both the proximal left anterior descending and posterior descending vessels and is uncommon in isolated proximal left anterior descending disease. Although this echocardiographic feature has a high degree of specificity, its sensitivity is limited. Exaggerated motion of the left ventricular posterior wall may occur in association with decreased septal motion as a compensatory phenomenon. Decreased septal motion may

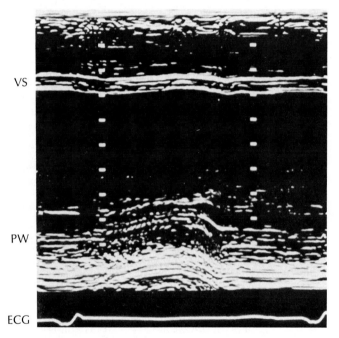

Fig. 8-15. Left ventricular cavity recording in coronary artery disease. The ventricular septum (VS) is thin and shows paradoxical anterior motion as well as absence of significant thickening during systole. The left ventricular cavity is dilated. The patient had severe disease involving the proximal left anterior descending vessel. PW, left ventricular posterior wall; ECG, electrocardiogram.

be evident only during myocardial ischemia, which may be brought on by sustained hand grip during the echocardiographic examination.

• The left ventricular posterior wall may show poor motion in patients with posterior wall ischemia or infarction.

• Additional evidence of scarred or ischemic myocardium is the presence of inadequate systolic thickening of the left ventricular posterior wall or ventricular septum. Systolic thickening may even be absent (Fig. 8-15). The ventricular septum may be very thin in patients with anteroseptal infarction.

• The anterior wall of the left ventricle may show paradoxical motion when it is involved.

• As noted earlier, an increase in the size of the left ventricular cavity during slow speed scanning to the apex suggests the presence of an aneurysm in that area. Paradoxical motion of the apical region may be present. Coarse, large-amplitude systolic flutter of the aortic valve has also been noted and probably results from asymmetric contraction of the left ventricle, producing an abnormal jet effect and excessive turbulence.

• In advanced stages of the disease the left ventricular end-diastolic pressure may be elevated, and this may result in prolongation of the A-C interval with a prominent B point on the mitral valve echocardiogram.

• Echocardiographic findings of a flail mitral valve may be present when there is disruption of the subvalvular apparatus. Acute volume overload of the left ventricle from mitral regurgitation may produce hyperkinetic septal motion. Holosystolic sagging of the mitral valve with a decreased EF slope has occasionally been noted in patients with papillary muscle dysfunction. The sensitivity of these findings is limited.

• Dilatation of the right ventricle may be observed in patients with ventricular septal rupture.

• Pericardial effusion may be present.
Comments

• Despite the presence of segmental abnormalities in coronary artery disease, the echocardiographically determined end-diastolic volume correlates fairly well with that obtained by angiography according to some workers.

• Newer techniques like cross-sectional echocardiography and ECG-gated B-scans appear more useful in demonstrating segmental abnormalities of the ventricular wall as well as in visualizing narrowing and aneurysm formation near the origin of the left main vessel. Attempts have also been made to utilize the Doppler technique to assess the patency of saphenous vein grafts.

• Abnormal systolic anterior movement of the mitral valve has occasionally been observed in patients with myocardial infarction as well as in those with ventricular aneurysms. The reason for this is not known.
Role of echocardiography

• The value of echocardiography in the diagnosis of coronary artery disease is limited as far as the assessment of left ventricular function is concerned.

• Wall motion abnormalities may provide a clue to the extent of damage to the ventricular muscle. Serial echocardiographic studies have also been useful in following up patients with angina as well as those with myocardial infarction. Large end-diastolic volumes together with evidence for increased left ventricular end-diastolic pressure are indicators of poor prognosis. Surgical revascularization procedures also carry an increased risk in this group of patients.

• Spatial visualization of the left ventricular cavity using two-dimensional echocardiographic techniques may provide additional information regarding the status of left ventricular function in coronary artery disease.

BIBLIOGRAPHY
Left ventricular function

Edler, I., and Hertz, C. H.: Use of ultrasonic reflectoscope for continuous recording of movements of heart walls, Kung. Fysiograf. Sallsk. Lund. Fordhandl. **24:**40, 1954.

Feigenbaum, H., Zaky, A., and Nasser, W. K.: Use of ultrasound to measure left ventricular stroke volume, Circulation **35:**1092, 1967.

Bowyer, A. F., Jutzy, R. V., Coggin, J., Crawford, R. B.,

and Johns, V. J.: Contributions of ultrasound to the study of upright exercising man, Am. J. Cardiol. **21:** 92, 1968.

Feigenbaum, H., Popp, R. L., Chip, J. N., and Haine, C. L.: Left ventricular wall thickness measured by ultrasound, Arch. Intern. Med. **121:**391, 1968.

Feigenbaum, H., Wolfe, S. B., Popp, R. L., Haine, C. L., and Dodge, H. T.: Correlation of ultrasound with angiocardiography in measuring left ventricular diastolic volume, Am. J. Cardiol. **23:**111, 1969 (abstract).

Popp, R. L., Wolfe, S. B., Hirata, T., and Feigenbaum, H.: Estimation of right and left ventricular size by ultrasound; a study of the echoes from the interventricular septum, Am. J. Cardiol. **24:**523, 1969.

Stone, J. M., Haine, C. L., Chang, S., and Feigenbaum, H.: The use of ultrasound to detect volume overloads of the left ventricle, Circulation **40**(suppl. 3):196, 1969 (abstract).

Winsberg, F., and Goldman, H. S.: Echo patterns of cardiac posterior wall, Invest. Radiol. **4:**173, 1969.

Askanas, A., Rajszys, R., and Sandowski, Z.: Measurement of the thickness of the left ventricular wall in man using the ultrasound technique, Pol. Med. J. **9:**62, 1970.

Eggleton, R. C., Townsend, C., Herrick, J., Templeton, G., and Mitchell, J. H.: Ultrasonic visualization of left ventricular dynamics, IEEE Transactions of Sonics and Ultrasonics, SU-17, 1970.

Feigenbaum, H., Dillon, J. C., Haine, C. L., and Chang, S.: Effect of elevated atrial component of left ventricular pressure on mitral valve closure, Am. J. Cardiol. **25:**95, 1970 (abstract).

Feigenbaum, H., Stone, J. M., Lee, D. A., Nasser, W. K., and Chang, S.: Identification of ultrasound echoes from the left ventricle using intracardiac injections of indocyanine green, Circulation **41:**615, 1970.

Kraunz, R. F., and Kennedy, J. W.: An ultrasonic determination of left ventricular wall motion in normal man; studies at rest and after exercise, Am. Heart J. **79:**36, 1970.

Murray, J. A., Johnston, W., and Reid, J. M.: Echocardiographic determination of left ventricular performance, Ann. Intern. Med. **72:**777, 1970.

Pennock, R., Kingsley, B., Kawai, N., Kimbiris, D., and Segal, B. L.: Stroke volume and cardiac output measured by echocardiography, Am. J. Cardiol. **25:** 121, 1970 (abstract).

Popp, R. L., and Harrison, D. C.: Ultrasonic cardiac echography for determining stroke volume and valvular regurgitation, Circulation **41:**493, 1970.

Sjogren, A. L., Hytonen, I., and Frick, M. H.: Ultrasonic measurements of left ventricular wall thickness, Chest **57:**37, 1970.

Wirth, J., and Wenzelides, K.: Heart muscle thickening measurement with ultrasound, Cor Vasa **12:**112, 1970.

Fortuin, N. J., Hood, W. P., Jr., Sherman, E., and Craige, E.: Determinations of left ventricular volumes by ultrasound, Circulation **44:**575, 1971.

Gibson, D. G.: Measurement of left ventricular volumes in man by echocardiography and comparison with biplane angiographs, Br. Heart J. **33:**614, 1971.

Kraunz, R. F., and Ryan, T. J.: Ultrasound measurements of ventricular wall motion following administration of vasoactive drugs, Am. J. Cardiol. **27:**464, 1971.

Paraskos, J. A., Grossman, W., Saltz, S., Dalen, J. E., and Dexter, L.: A noninvasive technique for the determination of circumferential fiber shortening in man, Circ. Res. **29:**610, 1971.

Pombo, J. F., Troy, B. L., and Russell, R. O., Jr.: Left ventricular volumes and ejection fraction by echocardiography, Circulation **43:**480, 1971.

Popp, R. L., Schroeder, J. S., Stinson, E. B., Shumway, N. E., and Harrison, D. C.: Ultrasonic studies for the early detection of acute cardiac rejection, Transplantation **11:**543, 1971.

Cooper, R., Karliner, J. S., O'Rourke, R. A., Peterson, K. L., and Leopold, G. R.: Ultrasound determinations of mean fiber-shortening rate in man, Am. J. Cardiol. **29:**257, 1972.

Cooper, R. H., O'Rourke, R. A., Karliner, J. S., Peterson, K. L., and Leopold, G. R.: Comparison of ultrasound and cineangiographic measurements of the mean rate of circumferential shortening in man, Circulation **46:**914, 1972.

Feigenbaum, H., Popp, R. L., Wolfe, S. B., Troy, B. L., Pombo, J. R., Haine, C. L., and Dodge, H. T.: Ultrasound measurements of the left ventricle; a correlative study with angiocardiography, Arch. Intern. Med. **129:**461, 1972.

Fortuin, N. J., Hood, W. P., Jr., and Craige, E.: Evaluation of left ventricular function by echocardiography, Circulation **46:**26, 1972.

King, D. L., Jaffee, C. O., Schmidt, D. H., and others: Left ventricular volume determination by cross-sectional cardiac ultrasonography, Radiology **104:**201, 1972.

McDonald, I. G., Feigenbaum, H., and Chang, S.: Analysis of left ventricular wall motion by reflected ultrasound; application to assessment of myocardial function, Circulation **46:**14, 1972.

Murray, J. A., Johnston, W., and Reed, J.: echocardiographic determination of left ventricular dimensions, volumes and performance, Am. J. Cardiol. **30:**252, 1972.

Orlando, E., D'Antuono, G., Cipolla, C., and others: Analysis of left ventricular wall motion by means of ultrasound, G. Ital. Cardiol. **2:**234, 1972.

Teichholz, L. E., Kreulen, T. H., Herman, M. V., and Gorlin, R.: Problems in echocardiographic volume determinations; echo-angiographic correlations, Circulation **46**(suppl. 2):75, 1972 (abstract).

Troy, B. L., Pombo, J., and Rackley, C. E.: Measurement of left ventricular wall thickness and mass by echocardiography, Circulation **45:**602, 1972.

Abbasi, A. S., MacAlpin, R. N., Eber, L. M., and Pearce, M. L.: Left ventricular hypertrophy diagnosed by echocardiography, N. Engl. J. Med. **289:** 118, 1973.

Belenkie, I., Nutter, D. O., Clark, D. W., McCraw,

D. B., and Raizner, A. E.: Assessment of left ventricular dimensions and function by echocardiography, Am. J. Cardiol. **31**:755, 1973.

Follath, F., Schmitt, H. E., and Burkart, F.: Echocardiographic evaluation of left ventricular function, Schweiz Med. Wochenschr. **103**:1776, 1973.

Gibson, D. G.: Estimation of left ventricular size by echocardiography, Br. Heart J. **35**:128, 1973.

Gibson, D. G., and Brown, D. J.: Measurement of instantaneous left ventricular dimension and filling rate in man using echocardiography, Br. Heart J. **35**:1141, 1973.

Konecke, L. L., Feigenbaum, H., Chang, S., Corya, B. C., and Fischer, J. C.: Abnormal mitral valve motion in patients with elevated left ventricular diastolic pressures, Circulation **47**:989, 1973.

Levitsky, S., and Merchani, F. J.: Noninvasive methods of measuring myocardial contractility, Surg. Ann. **5**: 205, 1973.

Ludbrook, P., Karliner, J. S., Peterson, K., Leopold, G., and O'Rourke, R. A.: Comparison of ultrasound and cineangiographic measurements of left ventricular performance in patients with and without wall motion abnormalities, Br. Heart J. **35**:1026, 1973.

Orlando, E., D'Antuono, G., Cascella, D., Petralia, S., and Degli Esposti, G. C.: Echocardiographic study of left ventricular function, G. Ital. Cardiol. **3**:414, 1973.

Pernod, J., Terdjman, M., Kermarec, J., and Haguenauer, G.: Myocardial contraction; study by ultrasonic echography (results in 200 normal patients), Nouv. Presse Med. **2**:2393, 1973.

Popp, R. L., Alderman, E. L., Brown, O. R., and Harrison, D. C.: Sources of error in calculation of left ventricular volumes by echography, Am. J. Cardiol. **31**: 152, 1973.

Altobelli, S. A., and Murgo, J. P.: A simple technique for obtaining continuous left ventricular diameter and derived indices from strip chart echocardiography, Circulation **50**(suppl. 3):28, 1974 (abstract).

Bennett, D. H., and Evans, D. W.: Correlation of left ventricular mass determined by echocardiography with vectorcardiographic and electrocardiographic voltage measurements, Br. Heart J. **36**:981, 1974.

Benzing, G., Stockert, J., Nave, E., and Kaplan, S.: Evaluation of left ventricular performance; circumferential fiber shortening and tension, Circulation **49**:925, 1974.

Bowyer, A. F., Jain, A. C., and Marshall, R. J.: Left ventricular function curves by ultrasound in normal and cardiomyopathy subjects, Circulation **50**(suppl. 3):217, 1974 (abstract).

Chapelle, M.: A new technique: study by echography of the contractile function of the myocardium, Arch. Mal. Coeur, **67**:721, 1974.

Demaria, A. N., Vismara, L. A., Auditore, K., Amsterdam, E. A., Zelis, R., and Mason, D. T.: Effects of nitroglycerin on left ventricular cavitary size and cardiac performance determined by ultrasound in man, Am. J. Med. **57**:754-760, 1974.

Frishman, W., Smithen, C., Befler, B. Kligfield, P., and Killip, T.: Noninvasive assessment of clinical response to oral propranolol therapy, Am. J. Cardiol. **35**:635, 1974.

Gibson, D. G., and Brown, D. J.: Measurement of peak rates of left ventricular wall movement in man; comparison of echocardiography with angiography, Br. Heart J. **37**:677, 1974.

Gibson, D. G., and Brown, D. J.: Relation between diastolic left ventricular wall stress and strain in man, Br. Heart J. **36**:1066, 1974.

Gibson, D. G., and Brown, D. J.: Use of echocardiography in the evaluation of left ventricular function, Proc. R. Soc. Med. **67**:140, 1974.

Grossman, W., McLaurin, L. P., Moos, S. P., Stefadouros, M. A., and Young, D. I.: Wall thickness and diastolic properties of the left ventricle, Circulation **49**:129, 1974.

Ludbrook, P., Karliner, J. S., London, A., Peterson, K. L., Leopold, G. R., and O'Rourke, R. A.: Posterior wall velocity; an unreliable index of total left ventricular performance in patients with coronary artery disease, Am. J. Cardiol. **33**:475, 1974.

Madeira, H. C., Ziady, G., Oakley, C. M., and Pridie, R. B.: Echocardiographic assessment of left ventricular volume overload, Br. Heart J. **36**:1175, 1974.

McDonald, I. G.: Assessment of myocardial function by echocardiography, Adv. Cardiol. **12**:221, 1974.

McDonald, I. G., and Hobson, E. R.: A comparison of the relative value of noninvasive techniques—echocardiography, systolic time intervals and apexcardiography, Am. Heart J. **88**:454, 1974.

Nimura, Y., Kunori, S., and Beppo, S.: UCG Ultrasoundcardiogram and left ventricular function, Jpn. J. Clin. Med. **32**:297, 1974.

Quinones, M. A., Gaasch, W. H., and Alexander, J. K.: Echocardiographic assessment of left ventricular function; with special reference to normalized velocities, Circulation **50**:42, 1974.

Roelandt, J., TenCate, F., VanDorp, W., Bom, N., and Hugenholtz, P. G.: Limitations of quantitative determination of left ventricular volume by multiscan echocardiography, Circulation **50**(suppl. 3):28, 1974 (abstract).

Teichholz, L. E., Cohen, M. V., Sonnenblick, B. M., and Gorlin, R.: Study of left ventricular geometry and function by B-scan ultrasonography in patients with and without asynergy, N. Engl. J. Med. **291**: 1220, 1974.

Alpert, J. S., Franics, G. S., Vieweg, W. V. R., Johnson, A. D., and Hagan, A. D.: Echocardiographic assessment of left ventricular function in aortic insufficiency, Circulation **52**(suppl. 2):69, 1975 (abstract).

Boughner, D. R., Nolan, J. P., and Rechnitzer, P.: Usefulness of echocardiographic peak velocity of circumferential fibre shortening. Presented at 1975 American Institute of Ultrasound in Medicine meeting, Winston-Salem, N.C., Oct., 1975 (abstract).

Burggraf, G. W., and Craige, E.: Echocardiographic studies of left ventricular wall motion and dimensions after valvular heart surgery, Am. J. Cardiol. **35**:473, 1975.

Chandra, M. S., Kerber, R. E., Brown, D. D., and Funk, D. C.: Echocardiography in Wolff-Parkinson-White syndrome, Circulation 52(suppl. 2):49, 1975.

Chang, S., Feigenbaum, H., and Dillon, J.: Condensed M-mode echocardiographic scan of the symmetrical left ventricle, Chest 68:93, 1975.

DeMaria, A. N., Lies, J. E., King, J. F., Miller, R. R., Amsterdam, E. A., and Mason, D. T.: Echographic assessment of atrial transport, mitral movement, and ventricular performance following electroversion of supra-ventricular arrhythmias, Circulation 51:273, 1975.

Dillon, J. C.: Evaluation of drug therapy in heart disease employing echocardiography. In Dengler, H. J., editor: Assessment of pharmacodynamic effects in human pharmacology, Stuttgart, 1975, F. K. Schattauer.

Dohmen, H., Roelandt, J., Durrer, D., Wellens, H.: Wall motion abnormalities in WPW syndrome studied with echo, Circulation 52(suppl. 2):34, 1975 (abstract).

Dumesnil, J. G., Laurenceau, J. I., Labatut, A., and Gagne, S.: Echocardiographic study of changes in regional ventricular function following nitroglycerine and surgical correlation, Circulation 52(suppl. 2): 134, 1975 (abstract).

Feigenbaum, H.: Echocardiographic examination of the left ventricle, Circulation 51:1-7, 1975.

Frishman, W., Smithen, C., Befler, B., Kligfield, P., and Killip, T.: Noninvasive assessment of clinical response to oral propranolol therapy, Am. J. Cardiol. 35:635-644, 1975.

Gehrke, J., Leeman, S., Raphael, M., and Pridie, R. B.: Non-invasive left ventricular volume determination by two-dimensional echocardiography, Br. Heart J. 37:911, 1975.

Hirschfeld, S., Meyer, R., Schwartz, D. C., Korfhagen, J., and Kaplan, S.: Measurement of right and left ventricular systolic time intervals by echocardiography, Circulation 51:304, 1975.

Hunter, S., Mortera, C., Sheridan, D., and Tynan, M.: Age related changes in left ventricular size and performance; an echocardiographic study, Circulation 52(suppl. 2):198, 1975.

Kanakis, C., Wyndham, C. R. C., Younce, C., Miller, R., and Rosen, K.: Echocardiographic findings in the Wolff-Parkinson-White syndrome, Circulation 52 (suppl. 2):200, 1975.

Karliner, J. S., and O'Rourke, R. A.: Usefulness and limitations of assessment of internal shortening velocity by ultrasound in man, Chest 63:361-364, 1975.

Kaye, H. H., Tynan, M., and Hunter, S.: Validity of echocardiographic estimates of left ventricular size and performance in infants and children, Br. Heart J. 37:371-375, 1975.

Linhart, J. W., Mintz, G. S., Segal, B. L., Kawai, N., and Kotler, M. N.: Left ventricular volume measurement by echocardiography; fact or fiction? Am. J. Cardiol. 36:114, 1975.

Mashiro, I., Kinoshita, M., Tomonaga, G., Hoshino, T., and Kusukawa, R.: Comparison of measurements

of left ventricle by echography and cineangiography, Jpn. Circ. J. 39:23-35, 1975.

Popp, R. L., Filly, K., Brown, O. R., and Harrison, D. C.: Effect of transducer placement on echocardiographic measurement of left ventricular dimensions, Am. J. Cardiol. 35:537, 1975.

Quinones, M. A., Gaasch, W. H., Cole, J. S., and Alexander, J. K.: Echocardiographic determination of left ventricular stress-velocity relations, Circulation 51: 689-700, 1975.

Quinones, M. A., Gaasch, W. H., Cole, J. S., and Alexander, J. K.: Determination of the time course of left ventricular wall stress and velocity of fiber shortening in man by simultaneous left ventricular pressure and echocardiographic recording; preliminary report, Cardiovasc. Res. Cent. Bull. 13:63-77, 1975.

Ratshin, R. A., Rackley, C. E., and Russell, R. O., Jr.: Quantitative echocardiography; accuracy of ventricular volume analysis by area-length, linear regression and quadratic regression formulae, Am. J. Cardiol. 35:165, 1975 (abstract).

Roelandt, J., Brand, M., Vletter, W. B., Nauta, J., and Hugenholtz, P. G.: Echocardiographic diagnosis of pseudoaneurysm of the left ventricle, Circulation 52:466-472, 1975.

Shors, C. M.: Cardiac function determined by echocardiogram, Crit. Care Med. 3:5-7, 1975.

Teichholz, L. E.: Echocardiography in valvular heart disease, Prog. Cardiovasc. Dis. 17:283-302, 1975.

Theroux, P., Francis, G., Hagan, A., Johnson, A., and O'Rourke, R.: Echocardiographic study of interventricular septal motion in the Wolff-Parkinson-White syndrome, Circulation 52(suppl. 2):70, 1975 (abstract).

Vincent, G. M., Davis, D., Ziter, F., Wilson, D. E., and Richards, K.: Echocardiography in Duchenne dystrophy, Circulation 52(suppl. 2):253, 1975.

Yow, M. V., and Reichek, N.: Left ventricular end-diastolic pressure and echocardiographic mitral valve closure, Circulation 52(suppl. 2):51, 1975 (abstract).

Andrias, C. W., Deane, L. V., Bornstein, A. B., and Gaasch, W. H.: Relative sensitivity of systolic time intervals and echocardiography in the assessment of a positive inotropic intervention in normal subjects, Circulation 54(suppl. 2):59, 1976.

Brenner, J. I., and Waugh, R. A.: The effect of phasic respiration and atrial systole on the echocardiographic determination of left ventricular function. In White, D. N., and Barnes, R., editors: Ultrasound in medicine, vol. 2, New York, 1976, Plenum Publishing Corp., p. 103.

Chandra, M. S., Kerber, R. E., Brown, D. D., and Funk, D. C.: Echocardiography in Wolff-Parkinson-White syndrome, Circulation 53:943, 1976.

Demaria, A. N., Neumann, A., Tonkon, M. J., and Mason, D. T.: Clinical superiority of systolic time intervals compared to echographic fiber shortening rate determined by digitalis-induced increase in contractility, Circulation 54(suppl. 2):214, 1976.

DeMaria, A. N., Vera, Z., Neumann, A., and Mason,

D. T.: Alterations in ventricular contraction pattern in the Wolff-Parkinson-White syndrome, Circulation 53:249, 1976.

DeMaria, A. N., Miller, R. R., Amsterdan, E. A., Markson, W., and Mason, D. T.: Mitral valve early diastolic closing velocity in the echocardiogram; relation to sequential diastolic flow and ventricular compliance, Am. J. Cardiol. 37:693-700, 1976.

Johnson, A. D., Alpert, J. S., Francis, G. S., Vieweg, V. R., Ockene, I., and Hagan, A. D.: Assessment of left ventricular function in severe aortic regurgitation, Circulation 54:975-979, 1976.

Mashiba, H., Fujino, T., Ito, M., and Kanaya, S.: Detection of the pre-excitation sites in WPW syndrome by echocardiography, Am. J. Cardiol. 37:154, 1976.

Massie, B., Schiller, N., and Parmley, W.: Mitral-septal separation; a new echocardiographic index of left ventricular function, Circulation 54(suppl. 2):190, 1976.

Mathews, E. C., Jr., Henry, W. L., DelNegro, A. A., Flitcher, R. O., Snow, J. A., and Epstein, S. E.: Echocardiographic abnormalities in asymptomatic chronic alcoholics, Clin. Res. 24:229A, 1976.

McDonald, I. G.: Echocardiographic assessment of left ventricular function in aortic valve disease, Circulation 53:860-864, 1976.

McDonald, I. G.: Echocardiographic assessment of left ventricular function in mitral valve disease, Circulation 53:865-871, 1976.

Morcerf, F. P., Duarte, E. P., Salcedo, E. E., and Siege, W.: Echocardiographic findings in false aneurysm of the left ventricle, Cleve. Clin. Q. 43:71-76, 1976.

Nanda, N. C., and Yu, P. N.: Effect of Tolamolol on cardiac arrhythmias and left ventricular function; clinical and echocardiographic studies, Tolamolol Symposium, Excerpta Medica, 1976.

Upton, M. T., Gibson, D. G., and Brown, D. J.: Echocardiographic assessment of abnormal left ventricular relaxation in man, Br. Heart J. 38:1001-1009, 1976.

Wanderman, K. L., Goldberg, M. J., Stack, R. S., and Weissler, A. M.: Left ventricular performance in mitral regurgitation assessed with systolic time intervals and echocardiography, Am. J. Cardiol. 38:831-835, 1976.

Wharton, T. P., Jr., Sloss, L. T., and Cohn, P. F.: Can echocardiographic parameters reliably predict generalized left ventricular dysfunction? Circulation 54 (suppl 2):111, 1976.

Bahler, A. S., Teichholz, L. E., Gorlin, R., and Herman, M. V.: Correlations of electrocardiography and echocardiography in determination of left ventricular wall thickness; study of apparently normal subjects, Am. J. Cardiol. 39:189-195, 1977.

Barr, S., DeMaria, A. N., Neuman, A., Weinnert, L., Miller, R. R., and Mason, D. T.: Left ventricular mass in valvular heart deiase; echocardiographic-electrocardiographic correlations, Clin. Res. 25:207A, 1977.

Cohn, P. F., Angoff, G. H., Zoll, P. M., Braunwald, E., Markis, J. E., Graboys, T. B., Green, L. H., and Sloss, L. J.: Echocardiographic evaluation of left ventricular function using non-invasively-induced post-extrasystolic potentiation, Clin. Res. 25:213A, 1977.

Davidson, K. H., Parisi, A. F., Harrington, J. J., Barsamian, E. M., and Fishbein, M. C.: Pseudoaneurysm of the left ventricle; an unusual echocardiographic presentation, Ann. Intern. Med. 86:430-433, 1977.

Devereux, R. B., and Reichek, N.: Echocardiographic determination of left ventricular mass in man; anatomic validation of the method, Circulation 55:613-618, 1977.

Dunn, F. G., Chandraratna, P., deCarvalho, J. G. R., Basta, L. L., and Frohlich, E. D.: Pathophysiologic assessment of hypertensive heart disease with echocardiography, Am. J. Cardiol. 39:789, 1977.

Horton, J. D., Sherber, H. S., and Lakatta, E. G.: Distance correction for precordial electrocardiographic voltage in estimating left ventricular mass; an echocardiographic study, Circulation 55:509-512, 1977.

Reeves, W., Nanda, N. C., and Gramiak, R.: Echocardiography in chronic alcoholism following prolonged periods of abstinence. In White, D. N., and Brown, R. E., editors: Ultrasound in medicine, vol. 3, New York, 1977, Plenum Publishing Corp., p. 169.

Ross, A. M., and Michaelson, S.: Left ventricular contraction patterns by mechanical, two dimensional real time echocardiography, Clin. Res. 25:250A, 1977.

Stefadouros, M. A., and Canedo, M. I.: Reproducibility of echocardiographic estimates of left ventricular dimensions, Br. Heart J. 39:390-398, 1977.

Sze, K., Nanda, N. C., Chacko, A., O'Mara, R., Gordon, D., and Bennett, J.: Echocardiography and Tc-99 pyrophosphate myocardial scanning in patients undergoing adriamycin therapy (abstract). Submitted for publication.

Ventricular septum

McCann, W. D., Harbold, N. B., and Giuliani, B. R.: The echocardiogram in right ventricular overload, J. A. M. A. 221:1243, 1972.

Meyer, R. A., Schwartz, D. C., Benzing, G., and Kaplan, S.: Ventricular septum in right ventricular volume overload; an echocardiographic study, Am. J. Cardiol. 30:349, 1972.

Tajik, A. J., Gau, G. T., Schattenberg, T. T., and Ritter, D. G.: Normal ventricular septal motion in atrial septal defect, Mayo Clin. Proc. 47:635, 1972.

Brown, O. R., Popp, R. L., and Harrison, D. C.: Abnormal interventricular septal motion in patients with significant disease of the left anterior descending coronary artery or other conditions of septal failure, Am. J. Cardiol. 31:123, 1973 (abstract).

Kerber, R. E., Dippel, W. F., and Abboud, F. M.: Abnormal motion of the interventricular septum in right ventricular volume overload; experimental and clinical echocardiographic studies, Circulation 48:86, 1973.

McDonald, I. G.: Echocardiographic demonstration of

abnormal motion of the interventricular septum in left bundle branch block, Circulation 48:272, 1973.

Abbasi, A. S., Eber, L. M., MacAplin, R. N., and Kattus, A. A.: Paradoxical motion of interventricular septum in left bundle branch block, Circulation 49: 423, 1974.

Adams, N., McFadden, R. B., Chambers, J., Cornish, D., and Vogel, J. H. K.: Acquired paradoxic septal motion following successful coronary artery bypass surgery, J. Clin. Ultrasound 2:221, 1974 (abstract).

Assad-Morell, J. L., Tajik, A. J., and Guiliani, E. R.: Aneurysm of membranous interventricular septum; echocardiographic features, Mayo Clin. Proc. 49:164, 1974.

Assad-Morell, J. L., Tajik, A. J., and Giuliani, E. R.: Echocardiographic analysis of the ventricular septum, Prog. Cardiovasc. Dis. 17:219, 1974.

Burch, G. E., Giles, T. D., and Martinez, E. C.: Echocardiographic abnormalities of interventricular septum associated with absent Q syndrome, J. A. M. A. 228:1665, 1974.

Burch, G. E., Giles, T. D., and Martinez, E.: Echocardiographic detection of abnormal motion of the interventricular septum in ischemic cardiomyopathy, Am. J. Med. 57:293, 1974.

Dillon, J. C., Chang, S., and Feigenbaum, H.: Echocardiographic manifestations of left bundle branch block, Circulation 49:876, 1974.

Hagan, A. D., Francis, G. S., Sahn, D. J., Karliner, J., Friedman, W. F., and O'Rourke, R.: Ultrasound evaluation of systolic anterior septal motion in patients with and without right ventricular volume overload, Circulation 50:248, 1974.

Sayaya, J., Longo, M. R., and Schlant, R. C.: Echocardiographic interventricular septal wall motion and thickness; a study in health and disease, Am. Heart J. 87:681, 1974.

Seagren, S. C., and Pool, P. E.: Effects of abnormal septal motion of surgery for constrictive pericarditis, J. Clin. Ultrasound 2:248, 1974 (abstract).

Weiss, N., Chaval, S., and Ludbrook, P. A.: Echocardiographic recognition of paradoxical interventricular septal motion associated with right ventricular premature beats, Circulation 50(suppl. 3):250, 1974 (abstract).

Yoshikawa, J., Owaki, T., Kato, H., and Tanaka, K.: Abnormal motion of interventricular septum of patients with prosthetic valves, J. Clin. Ultrasound 2:265, 1974.

Beaver, B. M., Khullar, S., Kolush, A. J., Fulkerson, P. K., and Leighton, R. F.: Relationship between left ventricular septal motion (echocardiography) and perfusion (isotope scan) in coronary artery disease, Circulation 52(suppl. 2):134, 1975 (abstract).

Sapire, D. W., and Black, I. F.: Echocardiographic detection of aneurysms of the interventricular septum associated with ventricular septal defect; a method of noninvasive diagnosis and follow-up, Am. J. Cardiol. 36:797-801, 1975.

Yoshikawa, J., Owaki, T., Kato, H., and Tanaka, K.: Ul-

trasonic diagnosis of ventricular aneurysm, Jpn. Heart J. 16:394-403, 1975.

Zoneraich, S., Zoneraich, O., and Rhee, J. J.: Echocardiographic evaluation of septal motion in patients with artificial pacemakers, vectorcardiographic correlations, Circulation 52(suppl. 2):135, 1975 (abstract).

Gibson, T. C., Grossman, W., McLaurin, L. P., Moos, S., and Craige, E.: An echocardiographic study of the interventricular system in constrictive pericarditis, Br. Heart J. 38:738, 1976.

Gomes, J. A., Damato, A. N., Ticzon, A. R., Dhatt, M. S., and Moran, H. E.: Echocardiographic patterns of interventricular septal motion and dimensional changes during right ventricular pacing from different sites, Clin. Res. 24:219A, 1976.

Hearne, M. J., Sherber, H. S., and Deleon, A. C., Jr.: Paradoxical motion of the interventricular septum in a patient with normal right heart hemodynamics, Chest 69:125-127, 1976.

Kerin, N. Z., Edelstein, J., and Derue, R. G.: Ventricular septal defect complicating acute myocardial infarction; echocardiographic demonstration confirmed by angiocardiograms and surgery, Chest 70:560-563, 1976.

Payvandi, M. N., and Kerber, R. E.: Echocardiography in congenital and acquired absence of the pericardium, Circulation 53:86, 1976 (abstract).

Pearlman, A. S., Clark, C. E., Henry, W. L., Morganroth, J., Itscoitz, S. B., and Epstein, S. E.: Determinants of ventricular septal motion; influence of relative right and left ventricular size, Circulation 54:83, 1976.

Shapiro, J., Boxer, R., and Krongrad, E.: Echocardiographic observations in patients with postoperative right bundle branch block pattern, Circulation 54 (suppl. 2):46, 1976.

Weyman, A. E., Wann, S., Feigenbaum, H., and Dillin, J. C.: Mechanism of abnormal septal motion in patients with right ventricular volume overload; a crosssectional echocardiographic study, Circulation 54: 179, 1976.

Wilson, R. L., Shaub, M. S., and Young, G.: The echocardiographic appearance of a partially disrupted ventricular septal defect repair; a case report, J. Clin. Ultrasound 4:41-43, 1976.

Fujii, J., Watanabe, H., Kuboki, M., and Kato, K.: Echocardiographic assessment of VCG and ECG criteria for ventricular septal hypertrophy, Clin. Res. 25:223A, 1977.

Gordon, M. J., and Kerber, R. E.: Interventricular septal motion in patients with proximal and distal left anterior descending coronary artery lesions, Circulation 55:338-341, 1977.

Mueller, T., Kerber, R., and Marcus, M.: Comparison of interventricular septal motion by ventriculography and echocardiography in right ventricular volume overload, Clin. Res. 25:240A, 1977.

Righetti, A., Crawford, M. N., O'Rourke, R. A., Schelbert, H., Daily, P. O., and Ross, J.: Interventricular septal motion and left ventricular function after coronary bypass surgery; evaluation with echocardiography and radionuclide angiography, Am. J. Cardiol. 39:372, 1977.

Stickley, L. P., Wang, P. N., Dwyer, J. C., Ring, E. M., Hamilton, W. P., Stickley, L. P., and Mueller, H. S.: Echocardiographic analysis of septal motion in pacemaker patients, Clin. Res. 25:261A, 1977.

Bowles, D., Ross, A., Hess, P., Nanda, N. C., and Combs, R. C.: Ventricular septal excursion and thickening; a non-specific echocardiographic measurement (abstract). Submitted for publication.

Ross, A., Gramiak, R., Waag, R., and Nanda, N. C.: Maximum ventricular septal velocity measurements obtained by computer; a new mode of measurement (abstract). Submitted for publication.

Left ventricular masses

Farooki, Z. Q., Henry, J. G., Arciniegas, E., and Green, E. W.: Ultrasonic pattern of ventricular rhabdomyoma in two infants, Am. J. Cardiol. 34:842-844, 1974.

Levisman, J. A., Macalpin, R. N., Arbasi, A. S., Ellis, N., and Eber, L. M.: Echocardiographic diagnosis of a mobile, pedunculated tumor in the left ventricular cavity, Am. J. Cardiol. 36:957-959, 1975.

Horgan, J. H., O'M Shiel, F., and Goodman, A. C.: Tumor invasion of the interventricular septum detected by conventional echocardiography, J. Clin. Ultrasound 4:133-134, 1976.

Orsmond, G. S., Knight, L., Dehner, L. P., Nicoloff, D. M., Nesbitt, M., and Bessinger, F. B., Jr.: Alveolar rhabdomyosarcoma involving the heart; an echocardiographic angiographic and pathologic study, Circulation 54:837-843, 1976.

Tomoike, H., Kawaguchi, K., Takeshita, A., Hirata, T., and Nakamura, M.: Echocardiographic recognition of the cardiac mural tumor, Jpn. Heart J. 17:106-113, 1976.

DeJoseph, R. L., Shiroff, R. A., Levenson, L. W., Martin, C. E., and Zelis, R. F.: Echocardiographic diagnosis of intraventricular clot, Chest 71:417, 1977.

Farooki, Q. Z., Adelman, S., and Green, E. W.: Echocardiographic differentiation of a cystic and a solid tumor of the heart, Am. J. Cardiol. 39:107-111, 1977.

Coronary artery disease

Inoue, K., Smulyan, H., Mookherjee, S., and Eich, R. H.: Ultrasonic measurement of left ventricular wall motion in acute myocardial infarction, Circulation 43:778, 1971.

Wharton, C. F., Smithen, C. S., and Sowton, E.: Changes in left ventricular movement after acute myocardial infarction measured by reflected ultrasound, Br. Med. J. 4:75, 1971.

Feigenbaum, H., Corya, B. C., Chang, S., Konecke, L. L., and Fischer, J. C.: Echocardiographic detection of dyskinetic and akinetic segments of the left ventricle, J. Clin. Invest. 51:28a, 1972 (abstract).

Fogelman, A. M., Abbasi, A. S., Pearce, M. L., and Kattus, A. A.: Echocardiographic study of the abnormal motion of the posterior left ventricular wall during angina pectoris, Circulation 46:905, 1972.

Petersen, J. L., Johnston, W., Hessel, E. A., and Murray, J. A.: Echocardiographic recognition of left ventricular aneurysm, Am. Heart J. 83:244, 1972.

Ratshin, R. A., Rackley, C. E., and Russell, R. O.: Serial evaluation of left ventricular volumes and posterior wall movement in the acute phase of myocardial infarction using diagnostic ultrasound, Am. J. Cardiol. 29:286, 1972.

Stefan, G., and Bing, R. J.: Echocardiographic findings in experimental myocardial infarction of the posterior left ventricular wall, Am. J. Cardiol. 30:629, 1972.

Jacobs, J. J., Feigenbaum, H., Corya, B. C., and Phillips, J. F.: Detection of left ventricular asynergy by echocardiography, Circulation 48:263, 1973.

Kerber, R. E., and Abboud, F. M.: Echocardiographic detection of regional myocardial infarction, Circulation 47:997, 1973.

Kreamer, R., Kerber, R. E., and Abboud, F. M.: Ventricular aneurysm; use of echocardiography, J. Clin. Ultrasound 1:60, 1973.

Cahill, N. S., and Falicov, R.: Echocardiographic and angiocardiographic correlation of left ventricular segmental wall motion abnormalities, Circulation 50 (suppl. 3):218, 1974 (abstract).

Corya, B. C., Feigenbaum, H., Rasmussen, S., and Knoebel, S. B.: Echocardiographic findings predicting mortality in acute myocardial infarction, Circulation 50(suppl. 3):29, 1974 (abstract).

Corya, B. C., Feigenbaum, H., Rasmussen, S., and Black, M. J.: Anterior left ventricular wall echoes in coronary artery disease; linear scanning with a single element transducer, Am. J. Cardiol. 34:652, 1974.

Corya, B. C., Feigenbaum, H., Rasmussen, S., Black, M. J.: Echocardiographic features of congestive cardiomyopathy compared with normal subjects and patients with coronary artery disease, Circulation 49: 1153, 1974.

Goldstein, S., and Willem de Jong, J.: Changes in left ventricular wall dimension during regional myocardial ischemia, Am. J. Cardiol. 34:56, 1974.

Ratshin, R. A., Boyd, C. N., Rackley, C. E., and Russell, R. O.: The accuracy of ventricular volume analysis by quantitative echocardiography in patients with coronary artery disease with and without wall motion abnormalities, Am. J. Cardiol. 33:164, 1974 (abstract).

Sjogran, A. L.: Left ventricular wall thickness measured ultrasonically in patients with recent myocardial infarction, Ann. Clin. Res. 6:177-186, 1974.

Teichholz, L. E., Cohen, M. V., Sonnenblick, E. H., and Gorlin, R.: Study of left ventricular geometry and function by B-scan ultrasonography in patients with and without asynergy, N. Engl. J. Med. 291:1220-1226, 1974.

Bergeron, G. A., Cohen, M. V., Teichholz, L. E., and Gorlin, R.: Echocardiographic analysis of mitral valve motion after acute myocardial infarction, Circulation 51:82, 1975.

Chandraratna, P. A. N., Balachandran, P. K., Shah, P. M., and Hodges, M.: Echocardiographic observations on ventricular septal rupture complicating acute myocardial infarction, Circulation 51:506, 1975.

Corya, B. C.: Applications of echocardiography in acute myocardial infarction. In Brest, A. N., editor-in-chief: Cardiovascular clinics, Philadelphia, 1975, F. A. Davis Co., pp. 113-127.

Corya, B. C., Rasmussen, S., Knoebel, S. B., Black, M. J., and Feigenbaum, H.: Echocardiographic left ventricular function related to coronary bypass mortality, Circulation 52(suppl. 2):133, 1975 (abstract).

Corya, B. C., Rasmussen, S., Knoebel, S. B., and Feigenbaum, H.: Echocardiography in acute myocardial infarction, Am. J. Cardiol. 36:1975.

Decoodt, P. R., Mathey, D. G., and Swan, J. H. C.: Abnormal left ventricular filling in coronary artery disease by automated analysis of echocardiograms, Circulation 52(suppl. 2): 133, 1975 (abstract).

DeJoseph, R. L., Seides, S. F., Lindner, A., and Demato, A. N.: Echocardiographic findings of ventricular septal rupture in acute myocardial infarction, Am. J. Cardiol. 36:346, 1975.

Franklin, D., Sasayama, S., McKown, D., Kemper, S., and Ross, J., Jr.: Ventricular wall thickness during acute coronary artery occlusion in conscious dogs, Circulation 52(suppl. 2):65, 1975 (abstract).

Heikkil, J., and Nieminen, M.: Echoventriculographic detection, localization, and quantification of left ventricular asynergy in acute myocardial infarction; a correlative echo and electrocardiographic study, Br. Heart J. 37:46, 1975.

Henning, H., Schelbert, H., Crawford, M. H., Karliner, J. S., Ashburn, W., and O'Rourke, R. A.: Left ventricular performance assessed by radionuclide angiocardiography and echocardiography in patients with previous myocardial infarction, Circulation 52:1069, 1975.

Joffe, C. D., Brik, H., Herman, M., and Teichholz, L.: Echocardiographic diagnosis of left anterior descending coronary artery disease, Am. J. Cardiol. 35:146, 1975 (abstract).

Kerber, R. F., Marcus, M. L., Ehrhard, J., Wilson, R., and Abboud, F. M.: Correlation between echocardiographically demonstrated segmental dyskinesis and regional myocardial perfusion, Circulation 52:1097, 1975.

Parisi, A. F., and Sasahara, A. A.: Echocardiography; its application to coronary artery disease, Compr. Ther. 1:25-32, 1975.

Roelandt, J., Van Den Brand, M., Vletter, W. B., Nauta, J., and Hugenholtz, P. G.: Echocardiographic diagnosis of pseudoaneurysm of the left ventricle, Circulation 52:466, 1975.

Sweet, R. L., Moraski, R. E., Russel, R. O., Jr., and Rackley, C. E.: Relationship between echocardiography, cardiac output, and abnormally contracting segments in patients with ischemic heart disease, Circulation 52:634, 1975.

Weyman, A., Feigenbaum, H., Dillon, J., and Champ, S.: Evaluation of left ventricular apical aneurysms by real-time cross sectional echocardiography, Circulation 52(suppl. 2):33, 1975.

Widlansky, S., McHenry, P. L., Corya, B. C., and Phillips, J. F.: Coronary angiography, echocardiographic and electrocardiographic studies on a patient with variant angina due to coronary artery spasm, Am. Heart J. 90:631, 1975.

Yoshikawa, J., Owaki, T., Kato, H., and Tanaka, K.: Ultrasonic diagnosis of ventricular aneurysm, Jpn. Heart J. 16:394, 1975.

Corya, B. C., Rasmussen, S., Feigenbaum, H., Black, M. J., and Knoebel, S. B.: Echocardiographic detection of scar tissue in patients with coronary artery disease, Am. J. Cardiol. 37:129, 1976 (abstract).

Dillon, J. C., Feigenbaum, H., Weyman, A. E., Corya, B. C., Peskoe, S., and Chang, S.: M-mode echocardiography in the evaluation of patients for aneurysmectomy, Circulation 53:657, 1976.

Dortimer, A. C., DeJoseph, R. L., Shiroff, R. A., Liedtke, A. J., and Zelis, R.: Distribution of coronary artery disease; prediction by echocardiography, Circulation 54:724-729, 1976.

Feigenbaum, H., Corya, B. C., Dillon, J. C., Weyman, A. E., Rasmussen, S., Black, M. J., and Chang, S.: Role of echocardiography in patients with coronary artery disease, Am. J. Cardiol. 37:775, 1976.

Fujii, J., Watanabe, H., and Kato, K.: Detection of the site and extent of the left ventricular asynergy in myocardial infarction by echocardiography and B-scan imaging, Jpn. Heart J. 17:630-648, 1976.

Gabor, G., Lengyel, M., Rev, J., and Polak, G. Y.: Echocardiographic study of left ventricular posterior wall motion in angina pectoris, Cor Vasa 18:169-178, 1976.

Johnson, M. L.: Echocardiographic evaluation of left ventricular size and function and its application in coronary artery disease, Adv. Cardiol. 17:105-122, 1976.

Kerber, R. E., Marcus, M. L., Wilson, R., and Ehrhardt, J.: Echocardiographic assessment of "compensatory hyperactivity" of opposing cardiac wall motion in acute experimental myocardial ischemia, Am. J. Cardiol. 37:147, 1976.

Kerber, R. E., Marcus, M. L., Ehrhardt, J., and Abboud, F. M.: Effect of intra-aortic balloon counterpulsation on the motion and perfusion of acutely ischemic myocardium; an experimental echocardiographic study, Circulation 53:853-859, 1976.

Kramer, N., Chawla, K., Patel, R., and Towne, W.: Differentiation of right ventricular hypertrophy from true posterior wall myocardial infarction by echocardiography, Circulation 54(suppl. 2): 235, 1976.

Nieminen, M., and Heikkila, J.: Echoventriculography in acute myocardial infarction, III. Clinical correlations and implications of the noninfarcted myocardium, Am. J. Cardiol. 38:1-8, 1976.

Stack, R. S., Lee, C. C., Reddy, B. P., Taylor, M. L., and Weissler, A. M.: Left ventricular performance in coronary artery disease evaluated with systolic time intervals and echocardiography, Am. J. Cardiol. 37: 331-339, 1976.

Teichholz, L. E., Kreulen, T., Herman, M. V., and Gorlin, R.: Problems in echocardiographic volume determinations; echocardiographic-angiographic correlations in the presence of absence of asynergy, Am. J. Cardiol. **37:**7-11, 1976.

Weissler, A. M., Stack, R. S., Lee, C. C., and Reddy, B. P.: Systolic time intervals and echocardiography in coronary artery disease. In Russek, H. I., editor: Cardiovascular problems; perspectives and progress, Baltimore, 1976, University Park Press, pp. 39-48.

Weissler, A. M., Stack, R. S., Lee, C. C., Reddy, B. P., and Taylor, M. L.: Left ventricular performance in coronary artery disease by systolic time intervals and echocardiography, Trans. Am. Clin. Climatol. Assoc. **87:**36-47, 1976.

Weyman, A. E., Feigenbaum, H., Dillon, J. C., Johnston, K. W., and Eggleton, R. C.: Non-invasive visualization of the left main coronary artery by cross-sectional echocardiography, Circulation **54:**169, 1976.

Joffe, C. D., Brik, H., Teichholz, L. E., Herman, M. V., Gorlin, R.: Echocardiographic diagnosis of left anterior descending coronary artery disease, Am. J. Cardiol. **40:**11, 1977.

Sylvester, L., Combs, R., Popio, K., Nanda, N., and Ross, A.: Use of echocardiography to predict patterns of coronary artery obstruction (abstract). Submitted for publication.

9 Pericardial effusion

ANATOMIC SUMMARY

The pericardium normally contains a small amount of fluid (<25 ml), which separates the visceral layer (epicardium) from the parietal layer, which is applied to mediastinal structures and the lung. The pericardium is attached superiorly to the ascending aorta, the pulmonary artery, and the superior vena cava. Attachment is also present at the inferior vena cava and at the point where the pulmonary veins enter the left atrium. These attachments tend to divide the pericardial sac into sinuses. The transverse sinus lies between the aorta and the left atrium and crosses the heart from right to left (Fig. 9-1). The oblique sinus lies between the pulmonary veins and extends downward behind the left atrium (Fig. 9-2). Between these two sinuses is a narrow portion of the left atrium that has no pericardial covering.

Pericarditis can be secondary to infection, tumor implants, or injury. Pericardial effu-

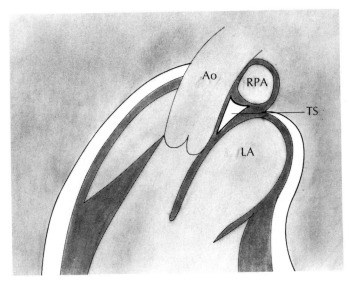

Fig. 9-1. Transverse sinus of the pericardium. A large pericardial effusion is shown as a clear area extending over the heart walls. It has also filled the transverse sinus (TS) situated between the aorta (Ao) and left atrium (LA) and beneath the right pulmonary artery (RPA). The transverse sinus can be detected frequently during ultrasonic examination of the aorta and left atrium in the presence of large pericardial effusions.

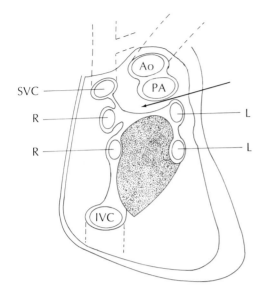

Fig. 9-2. Oblique sinus of the pericardium. The heart has been removed and the posterior pericardium and sites of pericardial attachment to various vessels are shown. The oblique sinus *(stippled)* lies mainly behind the left atrium between the entrance of the pulmonary veins (L, R) and extends downward over the right atrium as well. In the areas where the pericardium extends from vessel to vessel the pericardial space is obliterated. The transverse sinus *(arrow)* lies between the great vessels (Ao, PA) and the pericardial reflections that extend between the right and left superior pulmonic veins. SVC, superior vena cava; IVC, inferior vena cava.

sion also results from heart failure, kidney disease, bleeding diathesis, cardiac puncture, or abnormalities of metabolism such as hypothyroidism. A relatively small amount of fluid may produce tamponade if it accumulates rapidly. With slower buildup of fluid the pericardium stretches, and there may be little or no functional loss, even with large effusions.

The distribution of pericardial fluid is of interest to echocardiographers. Most of the fluid is located around the left ventricle, and small effusions tend to accumulate behind the posterior wall. As the effusion increases, fluid appears anteriorly over the right ventricle, and the extension beyond the apex may be very large (Fig. 9-3). Under these circumstances, fluid can also be detected in the transverse sinus of the pericardium and behind the left atrial wall. The narrow bare area between the superior pulmonary veins never contains fluid and is often recorded behind the left atrium on scans made from the mitral to the aortic valves. This fact is responsible for the often quoted statement that pericardial effusion never occurs behind the left atrium. Scans made from the mitral to the tricuspid valve examine a lower portion of the

Fig. 9-3. Pericardial effusion. Schematic representation of the heart demonstrating the presence of pericardial effusion. Note the large extension beyond the apex.

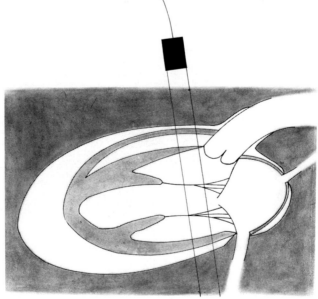

left atrium where pericardial fluid can be seen frequently in the presence of large effusions.

CLINICAL SUMMARY

The patient may be asymptomatic or may present with chest pain and signs of infection, history of chest injury, previous malignant tumor, thyroid malfunction, or kidney disease. Clinical findings include distant, faint heart sounds, a low-voltage ECG, and evidence of cardiac enlargement. A friction rub may be present over the heart if portions of the inflamed and roughened pericardium grate against each other during the cardiac cycle. Pulsus paradoxus may be present. With cardiac tamponade the systemic venous pressure increases while the arterial pressure decreases. The chest roentgenogram shows enlargement of the cardiac silhouette with noncongested pulmonary vasculature. Fluoroscopy will show either absent or diminished pulsation of the cardiac margins.

Angiocardiography may show an apparent widening of the ventricular wall. CO_2 injected into the right atrium shows thickening of the right atrial wall image as a sign of fluid applied to the heart wall.

EXAMINATION TECHNIQUE

The examination technique begins with location of the mitral valve followed by direction of the beam beyond the tip of the leaflets

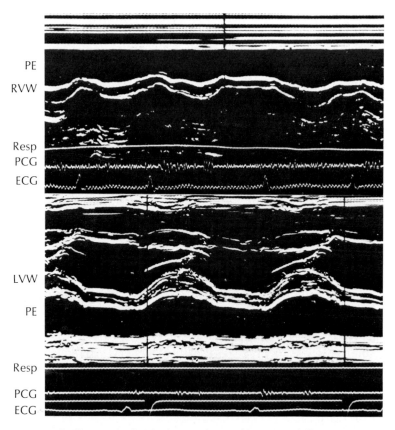

Fig. 9-4. Pericardial effusion. Individual recordings of anterior wall motion *(upper panel)* and posterior wall motion *(lower panel)* are shown. The pericardial effusion spaces (PE) are identified. Identification of both margins of the right ventricular wall (RVW) and left ventricular wall (LVW) helps to minimize diagnostic errors. Resp, respiration; PCG, phonocardiogram; ECG, electrocardiogram. (From King, D. L.: Diagnostic ultrasound, St. Louis, 1974, The C. V. Mosby Co.)

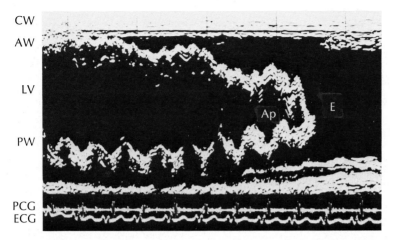

Fig. 9-5. Large pericardial effusion shown by beam scanning technique. When the beam is initially directed through the left ventricular cavity (LV), no significant anterior space is present, though a prominent posterior space is observed. As the beam is moved toward the apex (Ap) of the heart, the anterior space widens dramatically. Further angulation of the beam reveals a large fluid-filled pericardial space with no image of the heart. The slow undulations of the anterior heart wall during the scanning interval are produced by respirations and probably represent a shifting of the heart in the beam and not a true cavity diameter change. CW, chest wall; AW, anterior right ventricular wall; PW, left ventricular posterior wall; E, pericardial effusion; PCG, phonocardiogram; ECG, electrocardiogram.

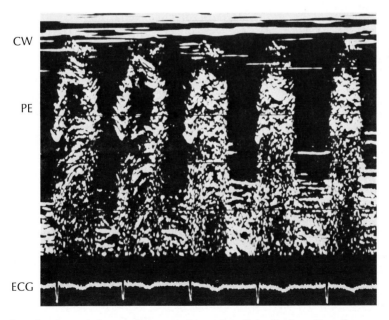

Fig. 9-6. Examination of the cardiac apex in pericardial effusion. Peculiar grouping of echoes is recorded intermittently during ventricular systole and represents the excessive movement of the cardiac apex as it moves in and out of the ultrasonic beam during examination. CW, chest wall; PE, pericardial effusion space; ECG, electrocardiogram.

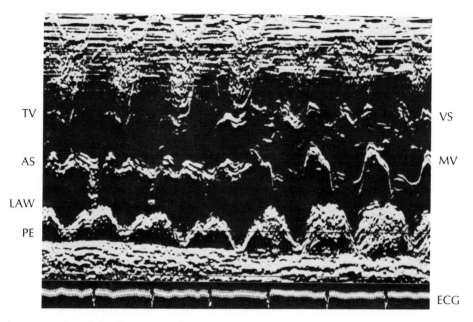

Fig. 9-7. Pericardial effusion (PE) behind the left atrial wall. Ultrasonic beam scanning from the tricuspid (TV) to the mitral valve (MV) demonstrates the presence of pericardial effusion space behind the left atrial wall (LAW) recorded posterior to the atrial septum (AS). VS, ventricular septum; ECG, electrocardiogram. (From Nanda, N. C., and others: Circulation **54:**500, 1976.)

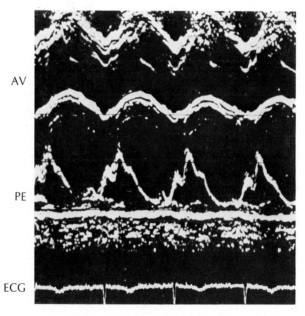

Fig. 9-8. Pericardial effusion behind the left atrium. Left atrial wall recorded behind the aortic root demonstrates hyperdynamic motion and a pericardial effusion space (PE) posteriorly. AV, aortic valve; ECG, electrocardiogram.

where the posterior left ventricular wall is recognized by its rhythmic movements during the cardiac cycle. Instrument gain should be adjusted to provide clear images of the heart walls but not so high that pericardial effusion spaces might be masked. It is sometimes easier and simpler to examine the anterior and posterior heart walls separately, adjusting instrument sensitivity for optimal recording in each area (Fig. 9-4). The use of a step attenuator, present on all modern equipment, simplifies rapid sampling of a variety of gains and is particularly helpful in identifying the pericardium behind the left ventricle by its high echo intensity, which disappears last as attenuation is increased. Beam scanning is a useful maneuver when evaluating echo-free spaces around the heart

and should be used in all cases. A complete echocardiographic examination, of course, must be carried out routinely.

ECHOCARDIOGRAPHIC FINDINGS
(Fig. 9-4)

- In the absence of pericardial effusion the moving heart walls are closely placed against tissues that appear solid (contain many non-moving echoes).
- Small pericardial fluid collections produce an echo-free space behind the left ventricular posterior wall in systole, but in diastole there may be no space. The depth of a systolic space is seldom more than 5 mm. The volume of fluid in the pericardial sac is around 50 to 75 ml.
- Moderate effusions produce posterior

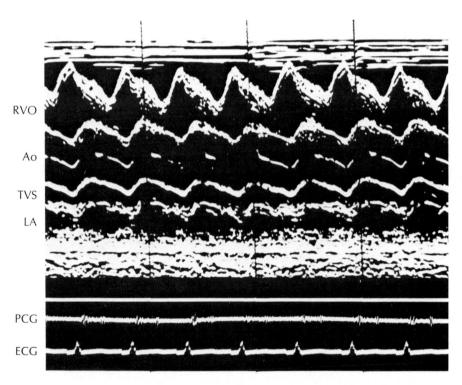

Fig. 9-9. The transverse sinus of the pericardium. This patient has a large pericardial effusion, which is clearly seen in front of the right ventricular outflow tract (RVO). The transverse sinus (TVS) is seen behind the posterior aortic wall and in front of the left atrial cavity (LA). The transverse sinus characteristically shows a changing width during the cardiac cycle and has a pattern of aortic motion rather than left atrial. Ao, aorta; PCG, phonocardiogram; ECG, electrocardiogram. (From King, D. L.: Diagnostic ultrasound, St. Louis, 1974, The C. V. Mosby Co.)

spaces in systole and diastole. The posterior systolic depth is around 10 mm, and an anterior space of about 5 to 10 mm is present. The volume of fluid in the pericardial sac is about 200 to 300 ml.

• Very large effusions show wide anterior and posterior spaces of 15 to 20 mm or more. Beam scanning to the apex may reveal a fluid-filled pericardial space with no image of the heart (Fig. 9-5) or an intermittent appearance of multiple echoes produced by the apex of the heart moving into the beam (Fig. 9-6). Effusions of this size are generally in the 1000 to 1500 ml range.

• With very large effusions, fluid can be demonstrated behind the left atrium (in the oblique sinus) by scanning the beam from the mitral to the tricuspid valve (Fig. 9-7) or, rarely, behind the aortic root recordings (Fig. 9-8).

• The image of the posterior aortic wall is widened when fluid fills the transverse sinus.

Unlike aortic wall dissection the margins of the widened wall do not usually move parallel to each other, and the outer margin is thinner than the inner (Figs. 9-9 and 9-10).

COMMENTS

• Gain that is excessive may image reverberations that mask pericardial effusion spaces. Vary the gain or use a step attenuator to image the pericardium clearly and to show pericardial effusion spaces or other spaces surrounding the heart without clutter (Fig. 9-11).

• Quantitation of the size of the pericardial effusion is difficult, and we have found the qualitative estimates described above to be sufficient in clinical practice. Some workers have used the difference between the diameters of the pericardium (pericardial volume) and epicardium (heart volume) at end-diastole for a quantitative estimate of the volume of pericardial fluid. It is, however, not very

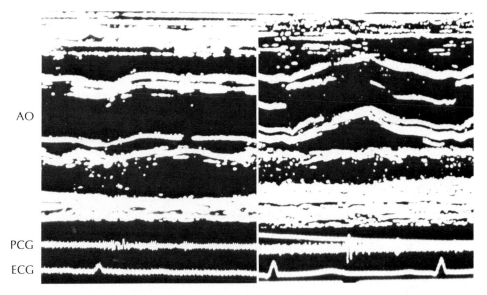

Fig. 9-10. *Left,* Echocardiogram from a patient with a large pericardial effusion demonstrating nonparallel widening of the posterior margin of the aortic root (AO), due to fluid in the transverse sinus of the pericardium. *Right,* A linear nonmoving echo is imaged behind the aortic root in a patient with no evidence of pericardial effusion. This probably represents the left atrial posterior wall, and the space behind is the left inferior pulmonary vein. Total absence of motion of this structure indicates that it is not anatomically related to the aortic root. PCG, phonocardiogram; ECG, electrocardiogram.

accurate since it does not take into account the distribution of the fluid.

• Remember, a homogeneous material that separates the chest wall from the pericardium or the pericardium from the heart wall, whether fluid, tumor, or thrombus, may produce echo-free spaces.

• The nature of the pericardial fluid cannot be determined from echocardiographic examination. Hemorrhage-, infection-, or tumor-produced effusions may have the same appearance as clear fluid. Blood clots in the pericardium may echo and result in a false-negative study.

• Fluid collection occurs preferentially toward the apex of the heart (Fig. 9-12) rather than at the base, since the heart does not freely float in effusion but is suspended at the base by the attachment of the great vessels and the large veins. Alterations in body position therefore may not produce significant changes in the width of the spaces.

• The fluid distribution can be variable but is especially altered when the pericardium is bound to the heart wall and results in loculation of fluid. This is commonly present in patients who have had previous cardiac surgery and in whom the anterior space is obliterated while a large posterior effusion space is present. Tumor involvement of the pericardium or other causes of adhesion (for instance, following radiation) may produce bizarre distributions.

• Occasionally an extra pulsating echo can be seen anteriorly just beneath the chest wall (in front of the anterior right ventricular wall) in some transducer positions, and it may represent signals from a rather prominent internal mammary artery.

Anterior echo-free spaces

• Subepicardial fat may be responsible for anterior echo-free spaces (up to 15 mm wide, surgical proof) that mimic pericardial effu-

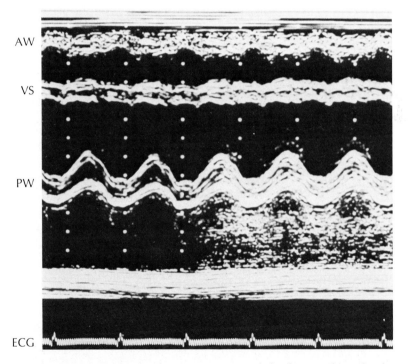

Fig. 9-11. Gain settings and echo-free spaces around the heart. The echo-free space behind the left ventricular posterior wall (PW) shown on the left is obscured by increasing the sensitivity of the instrument *(right)*. AW, anterior right ventricular wall; VS, ventricular septum; ECG, electrocardiogram.

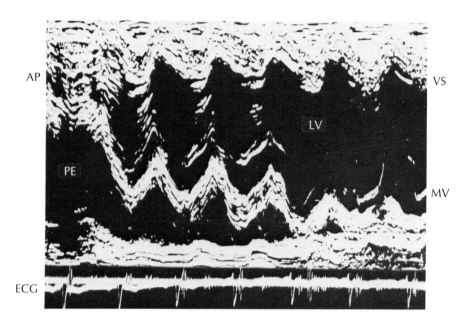

Fig. 9-12. Examination of the cardiac apex in pericardial effusion. Beam scanning from the left ventricular apex (AP) to the mitral valve (MV) demonstrates marked widening of the pericardial effusion (PE) space in the region of the apex where pericardial effusions tend to collect preferentially. LV, left ventricle; VS, ventricular septum; ECG, electrocardiogram.

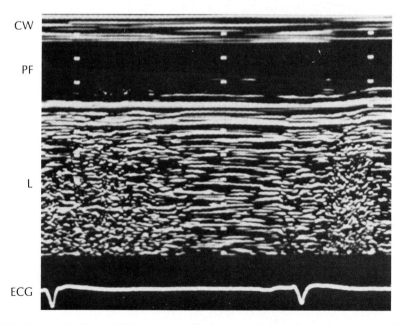

Fig. 9-13. Demonstration of left pleural effusion by placing the transducer in the left posterior axillary line. Pleural fluid (PF) is represented by an echo-free space that separates the chest wall (CW) from the lung (L) posteriorly. ECG, electrocardiogram.

sions. Beam scanning toward the apex of the heart usually shows that the echo-free space caused by fat becomes smaller as the apex is approached. Pericardial effusions, on the other hand, generally become wider at the apex.

• A pericardial cyst may show a large anterior echo-free space without evidence of sonolucent areas posteriorly. Fluoroscopy may be helpful in differentiating it from pericardial effusion.

• The interventricular septum may be mistaken for the anterior right ventricular wall when excessive near suppression is used or when the septum is studied near its junction with the left ventricular wall (the small size of the right ventricular cavity in this region results in the septum being imaged in close proximity to the anterior right ventricular wall).

• The presence of a catheter in the right ventricle (often in the setting of the coronary care unit) may mask echoes from the anterior right ventricular wall, and the sonolucent space in front of it may simulate pericardial effusion.

Posterior echo-free spaces

• A large left pleural effusion produces an echo-free space behind the left ventricular posterior wall that resembles a posterior pericardial effusion. There is never an anterior space over the heart, and the fluid never extends behind the left atrium since this chamber lies in the mediastinum and pleural fluid is excluded from this region by the anatomy of the pleural sacs. It is useful to place the transducer far laterally in the axilla to show pleural fluid (which is interposed between the chest wall and the lung) away from the heart as a confirmatory step (Fig. 9-13).

• Posterior echo-free spaces may also be produced by collapsed lung, consolidation (when extensive and occurring on the left

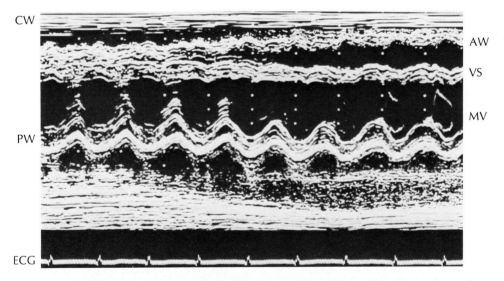

Fig. 9-14. Echo-free spaces resulting from left pneumonectomy. A beam scan from the distal portion of the left ventricle to the region of mitral valve (MV) reveals anterior and posterior echo-free spaces that represent fluidlike material that fills the pleural space after the lung is removed. The more solid-appearing echoes deep to the posterior wall (PW) may originate in normal thoracic structures that have been displaced to the left. The intensity of the epicardial echo suggests that the pericardium is closely applied and that no pericardial effusion space is present. Note that beam scanning demonstrates the junction of the anterior right ventricular wall (AW) and the ventricular septum (VS) and results in a thick echo complex. CW, chest wall; ECG, electrocardiogram.

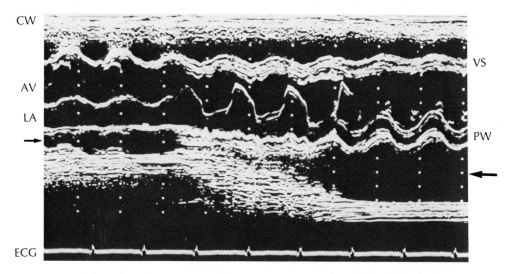

Fig. 9-15. Beam scanning from the aortic valve (AV) to the left ventricular cavity in a patient following left pneumonectomy. The echo-free space *(large arrow)* behind the left ventricular posterior wall (PW) represents fluid that fills the pleural space when the lung is removed. The smaller echo-free space *(small arrow)* behind the left atrium (LA) is not continuous with the pleural fluid and probably represents sonolucent tissues in the mediastinum. CW, chest wall; VS, ventricular septum; ECG, electrocardiogram.

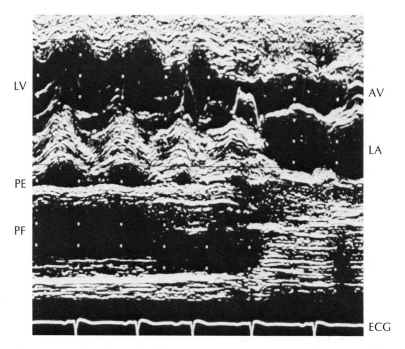

Fig. 9-16. Beam scanning from the left ventricular cavity to the aortic valve in a patient with both pericardial and pleural effusions. The pericardium separates pericardial effusion (PE) from the large left pleural fluid collection (PF). The pleural effusion does not extend behind the left atrial cavity (LA) recorded behind the aortic valve (AV), since the pleural space does not reach into the posterior mediastinum. LV, left ventricle; ECG, electrocardiogram.

side), and following a left pneumonectomy, (fluidlike fibrinous material and adhesions fill the space previously occupied by lung tissue; Figs. 9-14 and 9-15).

• When pleural and pericardial effusions coexist, the typical findings of pericardial effusion are present, but a second echo-free space may be recorded behind a relatively thin pericardial echo (Fig. 9-16).

• The inferior left pulmonic vein may produce a false-positive diagnosis of effusion posteriorly. This structure is usually located behind the posterior wall at a level where the mitral valve is imaged. Beam sweeps reveal its localized nature, and the space disappears when the beam leaves the mitral valve area (Fig. 9-17). A large coronary sinus may also produce an echo-free space behind the mitral valve (Fig. 9-18).

• Chordae echoes may mimic endocardial echoes, and the space between the true endocardial echo and the epicardial echo may be misdiagnosed as effusion. When calcifica-

tion is present in the mitral annulus, it may be thought to be the epicardial echo and the space behind it mistaken for pericardial fluid collection. Positive identification of the chordae, endocardial, and epicardial echoes at the level past the tip of the mitral valve should be achieved by observing their relationship to the mitral valve.

• The epicardium-lung interface appears thick because the difference in acoustic impedance is greater between air and solid than between solid and liquid. In the presence of a large effusion, this interface generally loses its prominence, since lung is no longer present behind it and the acoustic mismatch is not excessive (Fig. 9-19).

• The parietal pericardium does not move as much as the visceral pericardium during ventricular ejection since it is anchored to the mediastinum posteriorly. As the pericardial fluid volume increases, the movement of the parietal pericardium decreases in relation to the epicardium and usually becomes flat.

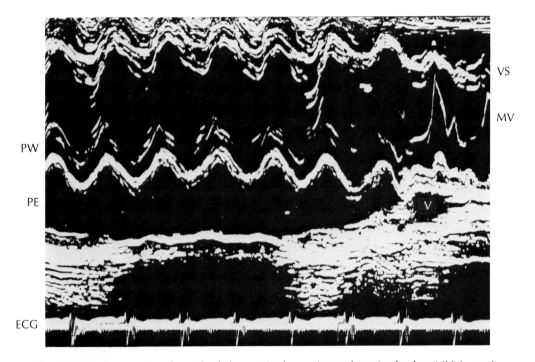

Fig. 9-17. Beam scanning from the left ventricular cavity to the mitral valve (MV) in pericardial effusion. The localized space (V) behind the mitral valve represents the left inferior pulmonic vein as it enters the heart and is clearly separated from the pericardial effusion (PE), which is identified behind the left ventricular posterior wall (PW). VS, ventricular septum; ECG, electrocardiogram.

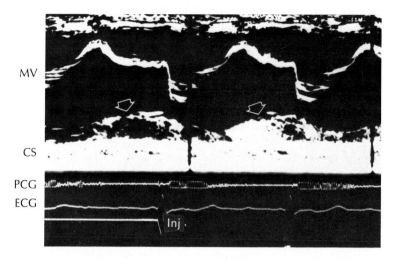

Fig. 9-18. Ultrasonic identification of the coronary sinus. This patient was shown to have a persistent left superior vena cava that drained into an enlarged coronary sinus. Contrast injection into the left superior vena cava filled a space behind the mitral valve (MV) identifying it as the coronary sinus (CS, *arrows*). PCG, phonocardiogram; ECG, electrocardiogram.

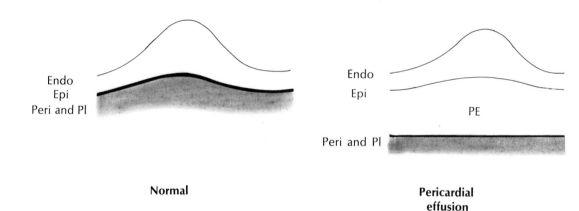

Normal

Pericardial effusion

Fig. 9-19. Left ventricular posterior wall recording in pericardial effusion. In the normal subject *(left)* the epicardial-pericardial-lung interface is a thick linear echo complex produced by a large acoustic mismatch resulting from the presence of air in the lung, which is situated posteriorly. When a large pericardial effusion (PE) develops, the epicardial echo is usually seen as a thinner line since the acoustic impedance of the heart muscle is not so markedly different from that of the fluid that has collected posteriorly. Endo, endocardium; Epi, epicardium or visceral pericardium; Peri, parietal pericardium; Pl, pleura.

However, some pericardial movement can be observed, especially as the apex is approached.

• In the presence of smaller effusions the rhythmic motion of the parietal pericardium may be mistaken for that produced by epicardium and the fluid collection missed.

• Normally, reverberatory clutter is present for some distance behind the thick pericardium-lung interface. No echoes are re-

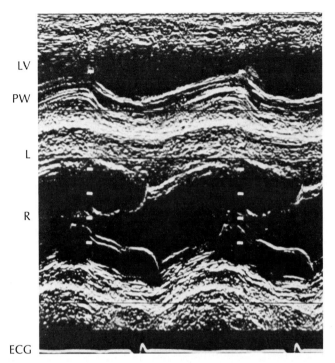

LV

PW

L

R

ECG

Fig. 9-20. Shadowing, reverberations and false retrocardiac spaces. Passage of the ultrasonic beam through the posterior wall (PW) of the left ventricle (LV) produces a band of reverberations that arises in the heart-lung interface (L). Since there is no significant penetration of lung tissue by ultrasound an acoustic shadow is produced. Long-range reverberations can project apparent structural echoes in the shadowed region and create the impression of a bounded echo-free space. In this illustration prominent motion of valve leaflet and heart wall reverberations (R) preclude an erroneous diagnosis of pericardial effusion or left pleural effusion. Motionless reverberations, on the other hand, could create the false impression of an effusion. ECG, electrocardiogram.

corded in the space beyond as a result of acoustic shadowing produced by nonpenetration of lung by ultrasound. However, linear echoes that represent reverberation artifacts from a cardiac structure may be positioned in this empty region and the space in front of it misdiagnosed as effusion (Fig. 9-20). This occurs frequently when the sensitivity is very low so that the thick interface with its adjacent band of clutter loses its prominence. A false-positive diagnosis of effusion is avoided by utilizing graded changes in sensitivity or damping, which will identify the true nature of the echoes imaged. Also, no pericardial effusion space is detected anteriorly.

• As mentioned earlier, it is useful to examine the cardiac apex for effusions since effusion spaces tend to be larger in this area. Also, an effusion may be predominantly localized to the apical region (Fig. 9-21). The oblique relation of the ultrasonic beam to the posterior left ventricular wall that curves anteriorly to form the apex, however, may result in its nonrecognition since it may show attenuated motion or may even become flat. The papillary muscle components, on the other hand, may retain a good amplitude of motion because of their more favorable orientation to the ultrasonic beam and may mimic posterior left ventricular wall motion; the segment of the left ventricular cavity imaged behind may be mistaken for pericardial effusion. Beam scanning toward the mitral valve establishes continuity of the

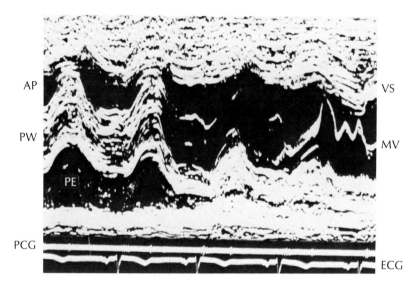

Fig. 9-21. Pericardial effusion at the cardiac apex. Beam scanning from the left ventricular cavity to the mitral valve (MV) reveals a large pericardial effusion (PE) predominantly located in the apical region (AP) with a relatively small space behind the left ventricular posterior wall (PW) at the level of the short axis. No effusion space was present anteriorly in this patient, who was studied following open heart surgery. VS, ventricular septum; PCG, phonocardiogram; ECG, electrocardiogram.

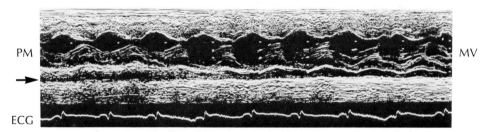

Fig. 9-22. Beam scanning of the left ventricular cavity in pericardial effusion. At the level of the short axis of the left ventricle just past the tip of the mitral valve (MV) a pericardial effusion space is detected posteriorly. Near the left ventricular apex, prominent echoes from the posterior papillary muscle (PM) appear and may be mistaken for the left ventricular posterior wall, since they have a similar motion pattern. In this instance, the echo-free space between the papillary muscle and the true posterior wall, which shows a relatively flat movement pattern from an oblique ultrasonic beam direction, may be misdiagnosed as pericardial effusion and the space *(arrow)* behind the true left ventricular posterior wall misinterpreted as a left pleural effusion. An erroneous diagnosis can be avoided by following the epicardial echo from the base of the heart to the apex and by relating papillary muscle echoes to chordae and to the mitral valve. ECG, electrocardiogram.

papillary muscle with the chordae and the mitral valve and confirms the identity of the posterior ventricular wall. Attention to this detail should avoid false-positive diagnosis of pericardial effusion or an erroneous diagnosis of coexisting left pleural effusion (Fig. 9-22).

Cardiac swinging

• Increased mobility of the ventricular and atrial walls is often seen with pericardial ef-

fusion and provides a clue to its presence during patient examination. The reason for this is not well understood, but it may be related to the abolition of the normal restrictive effect of the pericardium on the heart. Attenuation of motion may occur when tamponade supervenes or when clotted blood dominates the picture, as may be seen with chronic rupture of an aortic dissecting aneurysm into the pericardial sac.

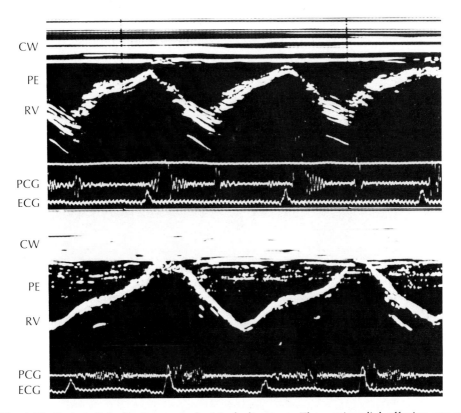

Fig. 9-23. Pericardial effusion and electrical alternans. The pericardial effusion space (PE) is shown between the stationary echoes of the chest wall (CW), which include the pericardium and the moving echoes arising in the anterior wall of the right ventricle (RV). In the upper panel the right ventricle moves posteriorly in systole and anteriorly in diastole on every cardiac cycle, and there is no variation in the height of the QRS complexes of the ECG. In the lower panel the heart is swinging in the large effusion space so that it moves posteriorly during an entire cardiac cycle and returns anteriorly on the next cardiac cycle. The height of the QRS complexes of the electrocardiogram (ECG) changes in an alternating manner (electrical alternans) so that the taller QRS complexes correspond to a more anterior location of the heart as compared to the smaller ones. When the heart is displaced posteriorly, the relative increase in the distance between the ECG electrode on the chest wall and the heart results in a smaller QRS voltage. Electrical alternans occurs when the frequency of swinging is approximately one half the heart rate and the size of the effusion is large. PCG, phonocardiogram.

• The heart may swing in the pericardial effusion space with a resultant change in the pattern of wall motion. Normally, the right ventricular wall moves posteriorly in systole and anteriorly in diastole. When the heart swings, it may move posteriorly in one cardiac cycle and anteriorly on the next so that the heart is physically nearer to the chest wall with every alternate beat. This form of cardiac swinging is associated with electrical alternans (Fig. 9-23).

• Another form of cardiac swinging that does not show a beat-to-beat variation alters the recorded motion patterns of cardiac valves during systole. The AV valves show SAMs or valve prolapse patterns (Fig. 9-24), whereas the semilunar valves show late systolic collapse of the aortic valve or systolic notching of the pulmonic valve (Figs. 9-25 and 9-26). The aortic root may show paradoxical anterior motion in diastole (Fig. 9-27), and the ventricular septum may exhibit an abnormal anterior movement in systole. Beat-to-beat changes in the mitral valve wave form may also be observed (Fig. 9-28). The left ventricular posterior wall may show attenuated amplitude of motion in systole or even reversal of its normal pattern so that it

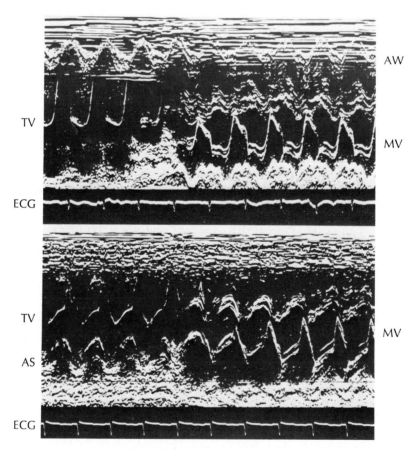

Fig. 9-24. Tricuspid and mitral valve prolapse patterns associated with pericardial effusion. The upper panel was recorded in the presence of a large effusion; the lower panel shows the same patient after resolution of fluid and return of normal valve motion patterns. AW, anterior right ventricular wall; TV, tricuspid valve; MV, mitral valve; AS, atrial septum; ECG, electrocardiogram. (From Nanda, N. C., Gramiak, R., and Gross, C. M.: Circulation **54:**500, 1976.)

resembles the left atrial wall. Occasionally, the anterior right ventricular wall may reverse its movement pattern during the cardiac cycle (Fig. 9-29). The abnormal or reversed motion patterns of the heart walls make their identification difficult for the beginning echocardiographer who is looking for typical motion. It may be erroneously concluded that the left ventricular posterior wall is unrecordable in that patient.

• The abnormal valve or wall tracings seen with cardiac swinging appear to represent a vectorial summation of the magnitude and direction of various factors—intrinsic valve or wall motion, movement of adjacent structures, cardiac displacement due to ven-

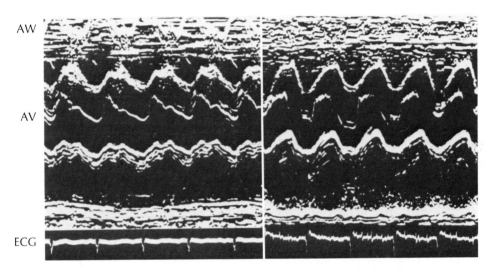

Fig. 9-25. Early systolic movement of the aortic valve toward closure with attenuation of aortic root motion in the presence of large pericardial effusion *(left)*. Normal structure motion, following resolution of pericardial fluid, is demonstrated on the right. AW, anterior right ventricular wall; AV, aortic valve; ECG, electrocardiogram. (From Nanda, N. C., Gramiak, R., and Gross, C. M.: Circulation **54**:500, 1976.)

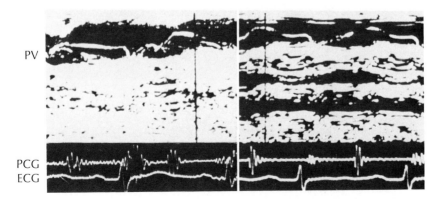

Fig. 9-26. Systolic notching of the pulmonary valve (PV) observed with large pericardial effusion *(left)*. Normal systolic pattern obtained following reduction of fluid is illustrated in the right panel. PCG, phonocardiogram. ECG, electrocardiogram. (From Nanda, N. C., Gramiak, R., and Gross, C. M.: Circulation **54**:500, 1976.)

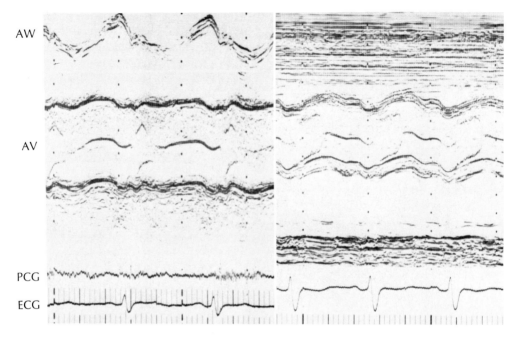

Fig. 9-27. Abnormal aortic root motion in pericardial effusion. *Left,* Paradoxical anterior motion of the aortic root is noted in diastole with a large pericardial effusion. *Right,* Normal aortic root motion pattern is seen following resolution of fluid. AW, anterior right ventricular wall; AV, aortic valve; PCG, phonocardiogram; ECG, electrocardiogram. (From Nanda, N. C., Gramiak, R., and Gross, C. M.: Circulation **54:**500, 1976.)

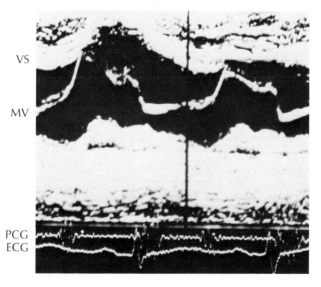

Fig. 9-28. Mitral valve recording in a patient with a large pericardial effusion. The amplitude and EF slope of the mitral valve change from beat to beat, even though the transducer is kept stationary, probably because of cardiac swinging. VS, ventricular septum; MV, mitral valve; PCG, phonocardiogram; ECG, electrocardiogram.

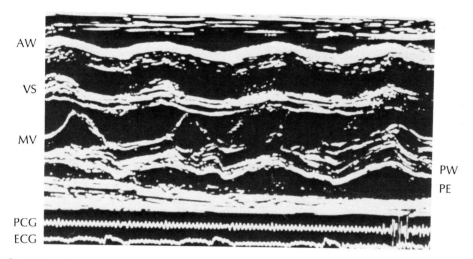

Fig. 9-29. Altered anterior right ventricular wall motion in pericardial effusion (PE). Complete reversal of the normal motion pattern is observed. The anterior wall (AW) moves anteriorly in systole and posteriorly in diastole. The left ventricular posterior wall (PW) moves normally. VS, ventricular septum; MV, mitral valve; PCG, phonocardiogram; ECG, electrocardiogram. (From Nanda, N. C., Gramiak, R., and Gross, C. M.: Circulation **54:**500, 1976.)

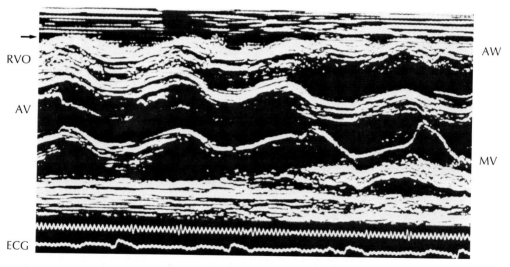

Fig. 9-30. Beam scanning from the aortic to the mitral valve in pericardial effusion. A large pericardial effusion *(arrow)* has reversed the motion of the anterior right ventricular wall (AW) and has distorted the outflow space (RVO), apparently thickening the image of the anterior aortic wall. The beam scan relates this finding to the right ventricular outflow tract and eliminates aortic root dissection as a possible cause. AV, aortic valve; MV, mitral valve; ECG, electrocardiogram.

tricular contraction, and a rocking or rotary motion of the heart about its attachment to the great vessels. These changes disappear when the pericardial fluid is removed or resolves with therapy. Do not attempt to diagnose conditions that feature systolic motion abnormalities of the heart valves in the presence of pericardial effusion. The final determination regarding the true nature of the observed valve motion abnormality should be made only after a repeat echocardiogram is obtained following resolution of fluid accumulation.

• Pericardial fluid may "compress" the right ventricular outflow tract in front of the aortic root and reverse the motion of the anterior right ventricular wall so that the picture may mimic aortic root dissection (Fig. 9-30). Beam sweeping maneuvers to the mitral valve demonstrate the true nature of the findings. A narrow right ventricular outflow has also been observed by us in the presence of a solid tumor mass involving the chest wall and encroaching on the right ventricular wall (Fig. 9-31).

• Peculiar circular echoes may be imaged in the region of the right ventricular outflow recorded in front of the aortic root in patients with pericardial effusion (Fig. 9-32). These represent echoes from the right ventricular outflow, which moves excessively and passes in and out of the beam during the cardiac cycle to produce this peculiar configuration. Similar echoes may rarely be seen in patients without pericardial effusion.

Cardiac tamponade

• The serious complication of tamponade is not diagnosable by echocardiography. Changes in the EF slopes of the mitral valve, abnormal septal motion, alteration of chamber size with respiration, and premature opening of the pulmonic valve have been observed but require clinical testing before reliability can be established. We have observed in tamponade a straightening of the diastolic trace of the aortic valve with loss of the posterior motion associated with atrial systole (which is usually prominent in large effusions as a result of cardiac swinging, Fig. 9-33). This also requires clinical substantiation.

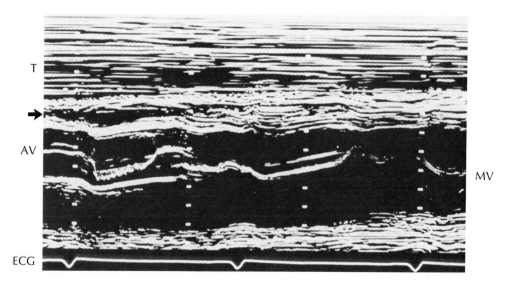

Fig. 9-31. Beam scanning from the aortic to the mitral valve in a patient with a mediastinal tumor. The tumor (T) encroaches on the right ventricle, compressing it. The right ventricular cavity in front of the mitral valve is practically obliterated while the size of the right ventricular outflow tract *(arrow)* is markedly diminished. AV, aortic valve; MV, mitral valve; ECG, electrocardiogram.

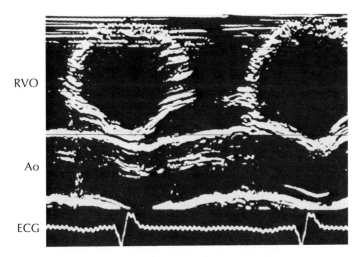

Fig. 9-32. Right ventricular outflow tract in pericardial effusion. The pericardium attaches superiorly to the pulmonary artery so that effusion may be demonstrated adjacent to the right ventricular outflow tract. In this illustration, excessive rotary movements of the heart pass the right ventricular outflow tract (RVO) across the examining beam with each cardiac cycle and result in circular images produced by its walls with intervening clear spaces, which represent pericardial effusion. In some patients with no effusion, excessive epicardial fat may mimic this appearance. Ao, aortic root; ECG, electrocardiogram.

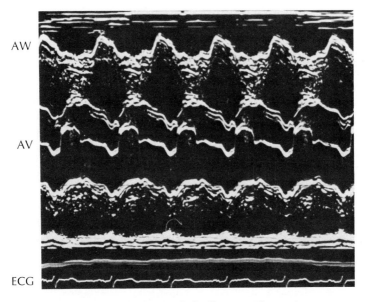

Fig. 9-33. Aortic root recording in pericardial effusion. The patient presented with a large pericardial effusion. The aortic root and valve (AV) show a large circumscribed posterior displacement following atrial systole, probably related to cardiac swinging. Complete obliteration of this movement has been noted when cardiac tamponade supervenes. AW, anterior right ventricular wall; ECG, electrocardiogram.

Constrictive pericarditis

• Constrictive pericarditis is produced by an adherent pericardium, which restricts diastolic expansion of the ventricles. Flattening of the diastolic trace of the left ventricular posterior wall may occur (Fig. 9-34), and the transient posterior motion produced by atrial systole may be lost. Septal motion may be abnormal. These findings are not specific for pericardial constriction and may be produced by other restrictive processes of the myocardium. Normal traces may also be found when the pericardial constriction is unevenly distributed and an uninvolved portion of the heart is examined.

In our experience, constrictive pericarditis with thickened and calcified pericardium does not produce an echo-free space, but multiple posterior reverberations are common. A calcified pericardium anteriorly may present a formidable barrier to the ultrasonic beam, making it difficult to identify any cardiac structures.

Pericardial thickening

• Pericardial thickening is rarely recognized echocardiographically. Carefully recorded images of the pericardium made with various sensitivity or damping changes may demonstrate apparent thickening. This is also a new technique that requires further evaluation.

Surgical or congenital absence of the pericardium

• Absence of the pericardium is usually associated with increased motion of the left ventricular posterior wall.

Miscellaneous

• Pericardial effusion usually improves access to cardiac structures, since the presence of fluid anteriorly tends to minimize chest wall reverberations. However, remember that anterior structures like the tricuspid and pulmonary valves are imaged more posteriorly than in normal subjects.

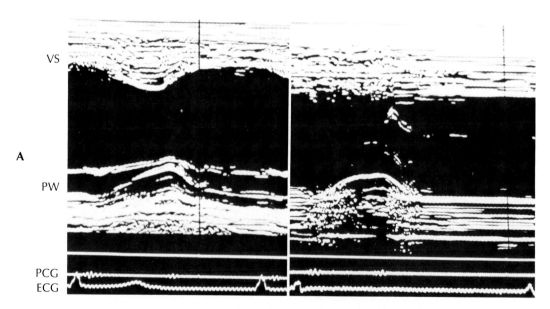

Fig. 9-34. Left ventricular wall motion in constrictive pericarditis. In a normal subject **(A)** a gradual expansion of the left ventricular cavity occurs throughout diastole. **B,** In constrictive pericarditis, the ventricular septum (VS) and the left ventricular posterior wall (PW) remain parallel during diastole, and diastolic expansion is limited to a brief period following the generation of the second heart sound. PCG, phonocardiogram; ECG, electrocardiogram.

• An enthusiastic trainee echocardiographer, during his initiation into the mystique of the technique, remarked on the ease by which pericardial effusions could be diagnosed, but by the time he received his "diploma" (considerably later and much wiser, no doubt) was heard to say that the diagnosis, like the road of life, was tricky and fraught with many traps for the unwary.

ROLE OF ECHOCARDIOGRAPHY

• Echocardiography is the best available clinical technique for the detection of pericardial effusion and has replaced invasive study such as contrast or CO_2 angiography. Accuracy is high if the factors that produce false-positive and false-negative results are understood and controlled. In general, problems may arise with the diagnosis of small effusions, especially if they are loculated, but larger fluid collections around the anterior and posterior heart walls should be readily detected. With increasing experience the number of false-positive and false-negative diagnoses should be small.

• Cardiac enlargement can be differentiated from pericardial effusion, and areas of loculation may be determined, particularly in postoperative patients. Unsuspected cases of pericardial effusion are often detected in patients with heart disease and heart failure. Pericardial effusion that coexists with pleural effusion may be diagnosed. Echocardiography is particularly useful to follow the course of pericardial effusion with serial studies. This is especially true in renal failure, where marked changes in the total amount of fluid may occur with repeated dialysis due to body fluid shifts.

• In the presence of purulent effusions, when adhesions result in loculation of fluid, pericardiocentesis may be carried out over areas where the echo-free spaces are wide so that a good yield can be obtained and puncture of heart walls avoided.

• A specially constructed transducer with a hole in the center to allow passage of a needle may be used for pericardiocentesis. The needle is advanced under echocardiographic control so that the tip can be seen to enter the anterior echo-free space. This potentially useful method may significantly reduce the risks of the procedure. Echocardiography is of limited usefulness in diagnosing tamponade, pericardial thickening, and constrictive pericarditis.

BIBLIOGRAPHY

Feigenbaum, H., Waldhausen, J. A., and Hyde, L. P.: Ultrasound diagnosis of pericardial effusion, J.A.M.A. 191:107, 1965.

Feigenbaum, H., Zaky, A., and Waldhausen, J. A.: Use of ultrasound in the diagnosis of pericardial effusion, Ann. Intern. Med. 65:443, 1966.

Feigenbaum, H., Zaky, A., and Grabhorn, L.: Cardiac motion in patients with pericardial effusion; a study using ultrasound cardiography, Circulation 34:611, 1966.

Moss, A., and Bruhn, F.: The echocardiogram; an ultrasound technic for the detection of pericardial effusion, N. Engl. J. Med. 274:380, 1966.

Feigenbaum, H., Zaky, A., and Waldhausen, J. A.: Use of reflected ultrasound in detecting pericardial effusion, Am. J. Cardiol. 19:84, 1967.

Goldberg, B. B., Ostrum, B. J., and Isard, J. J.: Ultrasonic determination of pericardial effusion, J.A.M.A. 202:103, 1967.

Pate, J. W., Gardner, H. C., and Norman, R. S.: Diagnosis of pericardial effusion by echocardiography, Ann. Surg. 165:826, 1967.

Rothman, J., Chase, N. E., and Kricheff, I. I.: Ultrasonic diagnosis of pericardial effusion, Circulation 35:358, 1967.

Klein, J. J., and Segal, B. L.: Pericardial effusion diagnosed by reflected ultrasound, Am. J. Cardiol. 22:57, 1968.

Feigenbaum, H.: Diagnostic ultrasound as an aid to the management of patients with pericardial effusion, Chest 55:59, 1969.

Bilek, J., Lukas, D., and Hula, J.: Echocardiography in pericardial effusion; case report, Vnitrni Lek. 16:428, 1970.

Feigenbaum, H.: Echocardiographic diagnosis of pericardial effusion, Am. J. Cardiol. 26:475, 1970.

Gabor, G. E., Winsberg, F., and Bloom, H. S.: Electrical and mechanical alternation in pericardial effusion, Chest 59:341, 1971.

Werning, C.: Ultrasound diagnostics of pericardial effusion, Dtsch. Med. Wochenschr. 97:816, 1972.

Abbasi, A. S., Ellis, N., and Flynn, J. U.: Echocardiographic M-scan technique in the diagnosis of pericardial effusion, J. Clin. Ultrasound 1:300, 1973.

Ellis, K., and King, D. L.: Pericarditis and pericardial effusion; radiologic and echocardiographic diagnosis, Radiol. Clin. North Am. 11:393-413, 1973.

Ultrasound in the diagnosis of pericardial effusion, China Med. J. 7:411, 1973.

Follath, F., and Heierli, B.: Echocardiography in pericardial effusion, Schweiz Med. Wochenschr. **104:** 1572, 1974.

Horowitz, M. S., Rossen, R. M., Harrison, D. C., and Popp, R. L.: Ultrasonic evaluation of constrictive pericardial disease, Circulation **50**(suppl. 3):87, 1974 (abstract).

Horowitz, M. S., Schultz, C. S., Stinson, E. B., Harrison, D. C., and Popp, R. L.: Sensitivity and specificity of echocardiographic diagnosis of pericardial effusion, Circulation **50:**239, 1974.

Pedersen, J. F.: Multitransducer scanning in pericardial effusion; diagnosis and aid in puncture, J. Clin. Ultrasound **2:**244, 1974 (abstract).

Ratshin, R. A., Smith, M. K., and Hood, W. P., Jr.: Possible false-positive diagnosis of pericardial effusion by echocardiography in presence of large left atrium, Chest **65:**112, 1974.

D'Cruz, I. A., Cohen, H. C., Prabhu, R., and Glick, G.: Diagnosis of cardiac tamponade by echocardiography; changes in mitral valve motion and ventricular dimensions, with special reference to paradoxical pulse, Circulation **52:**460-465, 1975.

Kerber, R. E., and Sherman, B.: Echocardiographic evaluation of pericardial effusion in myxedema; incidence and biochemical and clinical correlations, Circulation **52:**823-827, 1975.

Nanda, N. C., Gramiak, R., and Gross, C. M.: Altered systolic motion of cardiac valves in pericardial effusion; echocardiographic studies, Circulation **52**(suppl. 2):134, 1975 (abstract).

Schloss, M., Kronzon, I., Gelber, P. M., Reed, G. E., and Berger, A.: Cystic thymoma simulating constrictive pericarditis; the role of echocardiography in the differential diagnosis, J. Thorac. Cardiovasc. Surg. **70:**143-146, 1975.

Yuste, P., Torres, Carballada, M. A., and Miguel Alonso, J. L.: Mechanism of electric alternans in pericardial effusion; study with ultrasonics, Arch. Inst. Cardiol. Mex. **45:**197, 1975.

D'Cruz, I., Cohen, H. C., Prarhu, R., and Glick, G.: Echocardiography in mechanical alternans; with a note on the findings in discordant alternans within the left ventricle, Circulation **54:**97-102, 1976.

Elkayam, U., Kotler, M. N., Segal, B., and Parry, W.: Echocardiographic findings in constrictive pericarditis; a case report, Isr. J. Med. Sci. **12:**1308-1312, 1976.

Krueger, S. K., Zucker, R. P., Dzindzio, B. S., and Forker, A. D.: Swinging heart syndrome with predominant anterior pericardial effusion, J. Clin. Ultrasound **4:**113-114, 1976.

Lemire, F., Tajik, A. J., Giuliani, E. R., Gau, G. T., and Schattenberg, T. T.: Further echocardiographic observations in pericardial effusion, Mayo Clin. Proc. **51:**13-18, 1976.

Levisman, J. A., and Abbasi, A. A.: Abnormal motion of the mitral valve with pericardial effusion; pseudoprolapse of the mitral valve, Am. Heart J. **91:**18, 1976.

Nanda, N. C., Reeves, W., and Gramiak, R.: Echocardiographic demonstration of pericardial effusion behind the left atrium, Clin. Res. **24:**232A, 1976.

Nanda, N. C., Gramiak, R., and Gross, C. M.: Echocardiography of cardiac valves in pericardial effusion, Circulation **54:**500-504, 1976.

Payvandi, M. N., and Kerber, R. E.: Echocardiography in congenital and acquired absence of the pericardium; an echocardiographic mimic of right ventricular volume overload, Circulation **53:**86-92, 1976.

Prakash, R., Moorthy, K., Del Vicario, M., and Aronow, W. S.: Reliability of echocardiography in quantitating pericardial effusion; a prospective study, Clin. Res. **24:**236A, 1976.

Riba, A. L., and Morganroth, J.: Unsuspected substantial pericardial effusions detected by echocardiography, J.A.M.A. **236:**2623-2625, 1976.

Schiller, N. B., and Botvinick, E.: Right ventricular compression; a reliable echocardiographic sign of cardiac tamponade. In White, D. N., and Barnes, R., editors: Ultrasound in medicine, vol. 2, New York, 1976, Plenum Publishing Corp., p. 91.

Shah, P. M., and Nanda, N. C.: Echocardiography in the diagnosis of pericardial effusion, Cardiovasc. Clin. **7:**125-130, 1976.

Vignola, P. A., Pohost, G. M., Curfman, G. D., and Myers, G. S.: Correlation of echocardiographic and clinical findings in patients with pericardial effusion, Am. J. Cardiol. **37:**701-707, 1976.

Zoneraich, S., Zoneraich, O., and Rhef, J. J.: New, poorly recognized echocardiographic findings; occurrence in patients with pericardial effusion, J.A.M.A. **236:**1954-1957, 1976.

Allen, J. W., Harrison, E. L., Camp, J. C., Borsari, A., Turnier, E., and Lau, F. Y. K.: The role of serial echocardiography in the evaluation and differential diagnosis of pericardial disease, Am. Heart J. **93:** 560, 1977.

D'Cruz, I., Prabhu, R., Cohen, H. C., and Glick, G.: Potential pitfalls in quantification of pericardial effusions by echocardiography, Br. Heart J. **39:**529, 1977.

Foote, W. C., Jefferson, C. M., and Price, H. L.: False positive echocardiographic diagnosis of pericardial effusion; result of tumor encasement of the heart simulating constrictive pericarditis, Chest **71:**546, 1977.

Greene, D. A., Kleid, J. J., and Naidu, S.: Unusual echocardiographic manifestation of pericardial effusion, Am. J. Cardiol. **39:**112-115, 1977.

10 Prosthetic valves

Diseased cardiac valves are frequently excised at surgery and replaced by prosthetic devices. They are generally used in the left side of the heart (mitral or aortic position) but have been occasionally required in the tricuspid orifice. During surgery the size of the valve ring is measured by insertion of a calibrated occluder so that a prosthesis of an appropriate size can be selected.

TYPES OF PROSTHETIC VALVES
Ball valves (Fig. 10-1)

Ball valves consist of a round poppet (ball) enclosed in a cage. The ball sits in the sewing ring during closure and prevents regurgitation. When open, the poppet moves to the apex of the cage. The earliest models of a commonly used prosthesis (Starr-Edwards) consisted of a silicone rubber (silastic) ball and a cage made of metallic alloy. Newer models have a hollow metal poppet, and the whole prosthesis is cloth covered except for a metallic track on which the ball can move in the cage (Model 7400). In situ cloth becomes covered with endothelium, which prevents wear and clot formation. Smeloff-Cutter is another type of ball valve that resembles the Starr-Edwards prosthesis.

Central disc valves (Fig. 10-2)

In the central disc valve prosthesis the ball is replaced by a flat disc, and the cage is short or low profile. The Cross-Jones variety has an open-ended titanium cage with a silastic disc; the Starr-Edwards model 6500 uses a hollow metallic disc. The Beall valve has a pyrolite carbon disc and the Kay-Shiley device has a silastic disc.

Eccentric disc valves (Fig. 10-2)

Eccentric disc valves are valves in which the disc tilts open in the manner of a toilet seat to approximately 50 to 80 degrees. Both the Bjork-Shiley and the Lillehei-Kaster valves use pyrolite carbon discs within a low-profile metallic cage.

Bioprostheses

Recently, porcine as well as human aortic valves mounted on metallic frame stents have been used in the mitral and aortic positions. Tissue valves have also been constructed from fascia lata.

SELECTION OF PROSTHESIS

The availability and widespread usage of various types of prosthetic devices testify to the fact that a perfect prosthetic valve has not yet been designed.

Caged ball prostheses

Advantages. More experience has been gained with this valve than with other types. In general the incidence of complications like thrombosis is low.

Disadvantages. The valve is bulky, projects significantly into the left ventricular outflow tract, and may lead to outflow obstruction. It may impinge on the ventricular

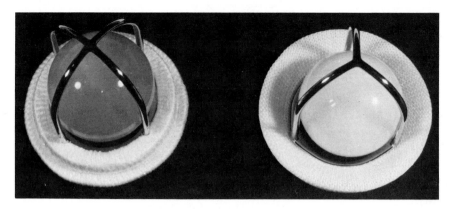

Fig. 10-1. Ball valves. A mitral *(left)* and an aortic *(right)* Starr-Edwards caged ball prostheses are shown. They consist of a round poppet (ball) enclosed in a metallic cage. The ball sits in the suture ring during closure and prevents incompetence. When open, the ball moves to the apex of the cage.

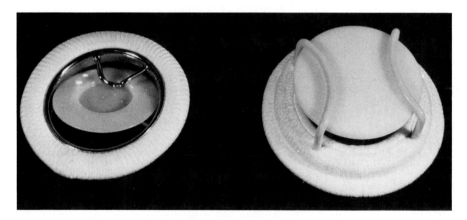

Fig. 10-2. Disc valves. In a central disc prosthesis (Beall valve; *right*) the ball is replaced by a flat disc, and the cage is short or low profile. An eccentric disc prosthesis (Bjork-Shiley valve; *left*) is a newer type of disc valve wherein the disc tilts open in the manner of a toilet seat to approximately 50 to 85 degrees during diastole.

wall, and produce arrhythmias. Diastolic pressure gradients across the valve have been noted.

Disc valves

Advantages. Disc valves do not project significantly into the left ventricular outflow area and do not impinge on the ventricular septum or walls. Therefore, the incidence of arrhythmias is lower. Also, they do not produce a low cardiac output state by mechanical obstruction.

Disadvantages. In general these valves have higher incidence of malfunction than other types since stress and wear are less evenly distributed.

Bioprostheses

Advantages. Bioprostheses have a very low incidence of thromboembolism.

Disadvantages. There has been limited experience with this type of valve, which shows increased incidence of valvular leaks and a tendency to calcify.

COMPLICATIONS OF PROSTHESES
Ball or disc variance

Ball or disc variance denotes development of abnormal changes in the silastic poppets or discs. It is not seen with metallic prostheses. There may be an increase in the size and distortion of shape of the ball or disc, probably from absorption of lipids from blood. Mechanical wear and tear may result in grooving, cracking, or decrease in the size of the ball, which may lead to complete extrusion of the ball or trapping in the apex or the inflow area. There may be intermittent jamming of the disc, or it may get caught in a fixed position.

Thrombosis and vegetations

Formation of excessive thrombus on the cage or ring prevents complete opening or closure of the poppet. It may produce obstruction to the blood flow and sticking of the ball, as may the presence of vegetations on the prosthesis. Vegetations or thrombi may embolize distally.

Perivalvular leak and dehiscence of suture ring

Presence of infection or thrombus on the prosthesis may loosen or disintegrate the surgical attachment of the prosthesis to the valve ring, resulting in paravalvular leaking and rocking of the prosthesis.

Low cardiac output

If the prosthesis is too large for the left ventricle or the aorta, it may impede blood flow, resulting in a low cardiac output state. A large mitral prosthesis may also distort the aorta and misalign the aortic leaflets, producing aortic incompetence, or exert undue tension on its suture line, resulting in the development of a periprosthetic leak. Incorporation of the large prosthetic cage in a ventricular wall may result in cardiac arrhythmias.

Hemolysis

Movements of the ball and cage may damage red blood cells or platelets.

CLINICAL ASSESSMENT OF PROSTHETIC FUNCTION

During diastole the ball or disc (in the mitral or tricuspid position) is pushed towards the apex of the cage as blood flows from the atrium to the ventricle. In systole, it is thrown against the base of the prosthesis (sewing ring area), effectively preventing regurgitation into the atrium. With an aortic prosthesis the poppet moves toward the apex of the cage in systole, allowing forward flow into the aorta, and coapts with the base of the cage in diastole, preventing regurgitation into the ventricle. The impact of the poppet or disc against the apex or base of the cage in the opening or closing position produces audible sounds (clicks). Since small pressure gradients are frequently present across the prosthesis, low-intensity murmurs are often heard. Multiple opening clicks may be present, especially with an aortic prosthesis, and result from the poppet bouncing and striking the apex of the cage several times during systole. With prosthetic dysfunction the clicks may get muffled or even disappear intermittently, although occasionally a low-intensity mitral closing click may be heard normally when the ball has drifted toward the base of the cage in late diastole. Opening and closing clicks are frequently inaudible or faint with disc prosthesis, especially the eccentric valves. Paravalvular leaks may produce significant murmurs, although they may become soft or even disappear when the insufficiency is severe and the cardiac output low.

Phonocardiography may be used to document the audible sounds and murmurs. Cinefluoroscopy is useful in detecting rocking of the prosthesis and in trapping or sticking of the radiopaque poppets and discs. Cardiac catheterization and angiography may be used to assess the degree of insufficiency.

STRUCTURES IN BEAM
Mitral prosthesis

1. Chest wall
2. Anterior right ventricular wall
3. Right ventricle
4. Ventricular septum
5. Mitral prosthesis

6. Left atrial or left ventricular cavity
7. Posterior left atrial or ventricular wall

Aortic prosthesis

1. Chest wall
2. Right ventricular outflow
3. Aortic root and prosthesis
4. Left atrium
5. Posterior left atrial wall

Tricuspid prosthesis

1. Chest wall
2. Anterior right ventricular wall
3. Right ventricle
4. Tricuspid prosthesis
5. Right atrial cavity
6. Posterior right atrial wall

ECHOCARDIOGRAPHIC EXAMINATION

• A mitral prosthesis is usually best located by placing the transducer near the cardiac apex and directing it toward the head and medially (Figs. 10-3 and 10-4). Multiple tracings should be obtained from various positions and angles to determine variations in poppet movements, since maximal slopes and amplitudes are taken for measurement.

• An aortic prosthesis may be best detected by placing the transducer in the suprasternal region or in the right clavicular fossa and directing the beam inferiorly and medially (Fig. 10-5). It may also be detected from the cardiac apex or, occasionally, by placing the transducer in a high right parasternal region.

• A prosthesis in the tricuspid position (Fig. 10-6) can be examined by angling the ultrasonic beam medially and inferiorly from the mitral or the aortic position, but experience so far with the prosthesis in this position is too limited to make any definitive statements.

• In a few patients, excellent prosthetic echoes may be detected from the third or fourth left parasternal space. This particularly applies to the tilting disc valves in the mitral and aortic positions.

• A phonocardiogram should be recorded simultaneously with prosthetic echoes and is useful in assessing its functional status.

NORMAL TRACINGS

In a caged ball prosthesis in the mitral or tricuspid position (hollow poppet), the anteriormost prosthetic echo is usually from the apex of the cage and is represented by a prominent linear signal exhibiting gradual anterior motion in systole and posterior movement in diastole. The movement of the cage reflects the motion of the ring or annulus to which it is attached. At the onset of diastole the poppet echo makes a large anterior excursion to join that from the cage and usually remains in contact with it throughout diastole. As systole begins, the poppet echo moves sharply to the sewing ring and then remains parallel to the cage echo throughout the period of ventricular contraction. The slow diastolic slope of the ball echo and the absence of the A wave may be related to inertia of the ball as well as to persistence of a mild diastolic pressure gradient across the valve. The echo from the sewing ring is thick, moves like the annulus (and hence the cage echo), and is generally

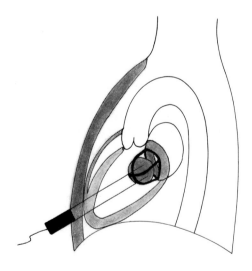

Fig. 10-3. Mitral prosthesis examination technique. A mitral prosthesis is generally best detected by placing the transducer low on the chest wall and directing the beam superiorly and medially. This passes the beam along the long axis of the valve and results in optimal recordings of the cage and ball motion.

recorded posterior to the poppet echo. Beam scanning maneuvers from the aortic valve to the mitral valve demonstrate continuity between the ring echo and the posterior wall of the aortic root. Multiple reverberatory echoes may be seen behind the poppet. Acoustic shadowing may be observed, since ultrasound does not penetrate the hollow metallic poppets. In the systolic closed position the left atrial component of the pop-

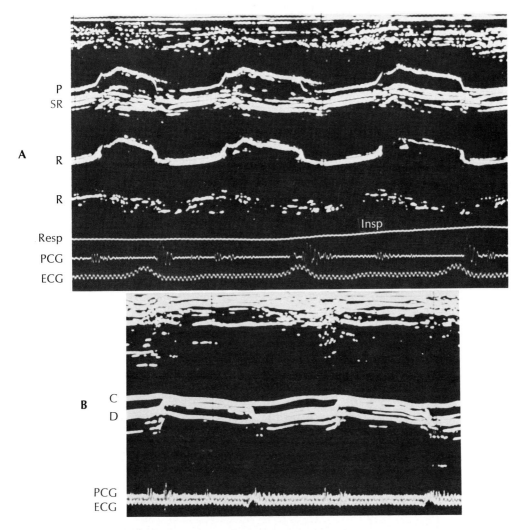

Fig. 10-4. Mitral prostheses. A typical echo pattern from a caged ball mitral prosthesis with a metallic ball is shown in **A.** The echo arising from the poppet (P) shows a shallow, early diastolic, posterior dip, which is a normal rebound from the cage that is partially imaged adjacent to the poppet in early systole. The thick echo complex behind the anterior image of the ball arises in sewing (suture) ring (SR). Reverberation artifacts (R) from the poppet and sewing ring are imaged posteriorly. A disc prosthesis is shown in **B.** Shallow excursions of the disc (D) are demonstrated as the valve closes and opens, contacting the struts of the cage (C). The sewing ring is seen behind the disc echo in diastole; in systole it merges with the disc echo. Resp, respiratory excursions; PCG, phonocardiogram; ECG, electrocardiogram.

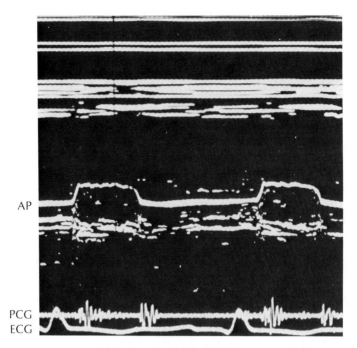

Fig. 10-5. Aortic prosthesis imaged from a suprasternal transducer position. The poppet moves toward the transducer at the beginning of systole. With diastole, it moves inferiorly (away from the transducer) to its closure position. Note the fine undulations of the poppet in systole. The aortic prosthesis lies relatively deep when imaged from a suprasternal position. AP, aortic prosthesis; PCG, phonocardiogram; ECG, electrocardiogram.

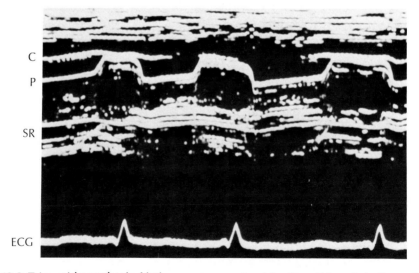

Fig. 10-6. Tricuspid prosthesis. Various components of the Starr-Edwards ball prosthesis are shown. The anterior position of the prosthesis, the absence of a ventricular septal echo, and partial demonstration of atrial septal echoes behind the sewing ring (SR) identifies the location in the tricuspid position. C, cage; P, poppet; ECG, electrocardiogram.

pet may be observed in the left atrial cavity recorded behind the aortic root.

Echoes obtained from the disc valve prosthesis generally resemble those recorded from a caged ball prosthesis.

The echocardiographic pattern may be different if a Silastic ball is used, since ultrasound can penetrate silicone rubber (Fig. 10-7). In this situation the posterior surface of the ball may also produce signals that mimic those from the anterior portion but are located behind the ring echo. This is related to the slower speed of sound in Silastic (960 m/sec versus 1540 m/sec in tissue), which re-

sults in the width of the ball echo (distance between the anterior and posterior portions of the ball) appearing greater than its actual dimension. Occasionally, the sound traveling through the Silastic ball reaches the sewing ring, since the ball is in its open position; an echo from the sewing ring then appears behind the posterior ball echo in diastole. A correction factor (0.64) has been determined for measurements made through Silastic rubber, and accurate measurement of ball diameter may be obtained by multiplying the actual measurement with this number.

With a bioprosthesis, prominent linear

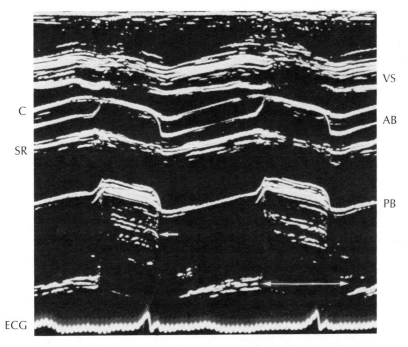

Fig. 10-7. Silastic mitral prosthesis. The various components of the prosthesis are identified. The anterior portion of the poppet or ball (AB) makes a sharp anterior movement at the beginning of diastole to reach the cage (C) and remains in contact with it throughout diastole. With the onset of systole it shows a rapid posterior movement toward the sewing ring (SR) as it closes. During systole the cage, poppet, and sewing ring exhibit gradual anterior motion, reflecting annular movement produced by left ventricular contraction. Attenuation of the speed of sound as it passes through the Silastic poppet results in the recording of the posterior portion of the ball (PB) deep in the left atrial cavity and produces an apparent increase in the ball diameter. For similar reasons, additional echoes *(horizontal arrow)* from the sewing ring may be recorded behind the posterior ball in diastole. Acoustic shadowing *(double-headed arrow)* may be observed, since the prosthesis is a strong attenuator of ultrasound. VS, ventricular septum; ECG, electrocardiogram.

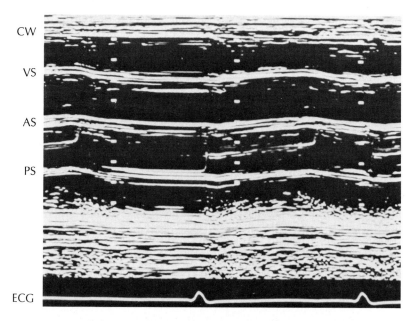

Fig. 10-8. Porcine aortic heterograft in the mitral valve position. The stent on which the porcine valve is supported is imaged as its anterior (AS) and posterior (PS) components. The valve leaflets within the stent show boxlike opening toward the periphery in diastole and are in midposition in systole as they coapt during closure. The ventricular septum (VS) moves paradoxically, a common finding after valve replacement. CW, chest wall; ECG, electrocardiogram.

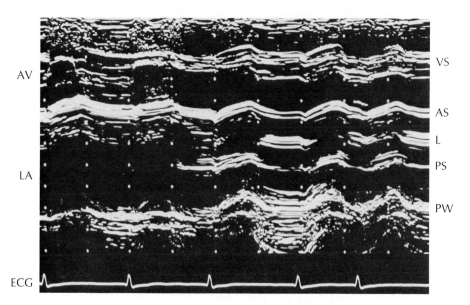

Fig. 10-9. Porcine aortic heterograft in the mitral position. Beam scanning from the aortic valve (AV) demonstrates continuity of the anterior stent (AS) of the porcine heterograft with the posterior aortic wall. Diastolic multilayering of the porcine leaflets (L) is present, probably related to valve cusp redundancy. VS, ventricular septum; PS, posterior stent; LA, left atrium; PW, left ventricular posterior wall; ECG, electrocardiogram.

echoes arise from the anterior and posterior portions of the stent; within these echoes thin signals from the leaflets can be observed (Fig. 10-8). Two cusps are usually seen, and they separate as they open in diastole. The cusps coapt with each other following ventricular systole. Echoes from stents exhibit gradual anterior motion in systole and posterior movement during diastole and reflect the movement of the mitral annulus. The anterior portion of the stent can be seen to be in continuity with the posterior wall of the aorta. Occasionally multiple lines may be seen in systole and are probably related to the redundancy of the porcine aortic leaflets (Fig. 10-9).

As mentioned earlier, a prosthesis in the *aortic position* usually requires examination from a suprasternal or apical position of the transducer to place the beam into the axis of poppet or disc motion. In the suprasternal position the ball or disc echo can be seen to move anteriorly in systole as it opens, remain in contact with the cage echo, and then move posteriorly in diastole. Echoes from the sewing ring parallel those from the cage throughout the cardiac cycle. During diastole the echo from the poppet or disc (in its closed position) follows the cage and sewing ring echo. In systole the poppet may show coarse flutter related to turbulent flow.

The apex examining position shows identical timing of events, but poppet and cage motion are opposite those obtained from a suprasternal position.

Movements of an aortic prosthesis studied from a parasternal beam position do not record the excursion of the poppet faithfully, since the direction of motion is essentially across the beam and not in its axis (Fig. 10-10).

MEASUREMENT TECHNIQUE

The following echocardiographic measurements may be useful in assessing mitral prosthetic valve function.

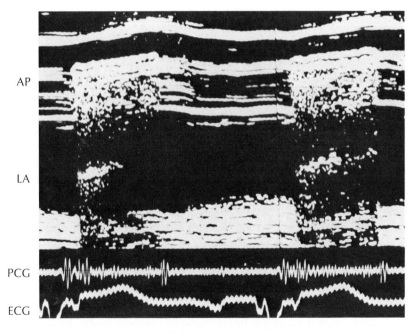

Fig. 10-10. Aortic prosthesis imaged from a parasternal transducer position. Dense echoes from the poppet are observed in systole. However, its motion is not recorded since the direction of its movement is across the ultrasonic beam. The linear echoes probably emanate from the components of the cage of the prosthesis. Note poppet reverberations in the left atrium and the shadowing effect posteriorly. AP, aortic prosthesis; LA, left atrium; PCG, phonocardiogram; ECG, electrocardiogram.

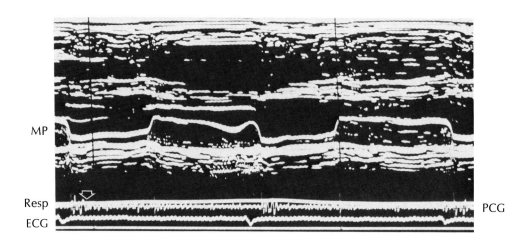

MP

Resp

ECG

PCG

Fig. 10-11. Echocardiogram from a patient with Starr-Edwards caged-ball prosthesis. At peak inspiration *(left)* the poppet shows a large A dip, which disappears during expiration *(right)*. MP, mitral prosthesis; Resp, respiratory tracing. The arrow represents the onset of inspiration. PCG, phonocardiogram; ECG, electrocardiogram. (From Nanda, N. C., and others: Ultrasound Med. **3A;**109, 1977.)

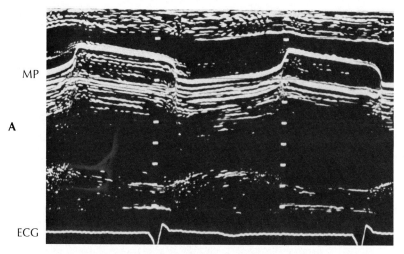

MP

A

ECG

Fig. 10-12. A, Recordings of a mitral prosthesis (MP). The slow diastolic slopes with linear reverberations mimic a calcified mitral valve. ECG, electrocardiogram. **B,** Low-gain recordings of a mitral prosthesis (MP) mimic a stenotic noncalcified mitral valve. The other components of the prosthesis are not recorded. CW, chest wall; PCG, phonocardiogram; ECG, electrocardiogram. **C,** Low-gain echoes from a mitral disc prosthesis. Various components of the cage as well as reverberations from a disc prosthesis are effectively masked, and the tracing may be mistaken for that of a normal mitral valve. CW, chest wall; MP, mitral prosthesis; PCG, phonocardiogram; ECG, electrocardiogram.

• Both average and maximum opening and closing velocities of the poppet or disc echo.

• Maximal excursion of the poppet echo, measured as the distance traveled by the ball or disc echo at the beginning of diastole. Since the expected ball or disc excursion for a given prosthesis can be obtained from the manufacturer, it is useful to determine prosthetic valve type, model number and size from the hospital chart or the surgeon.

• The interval between the aortic component of the second heart sound (which can be determined from a simultaneously recorded phonocardiogram) and the opening click of the ball or disc (A2-OM interval). For a Silastic caged ball mitral prosthesis, the normal intervals range from 70 to 170 msec

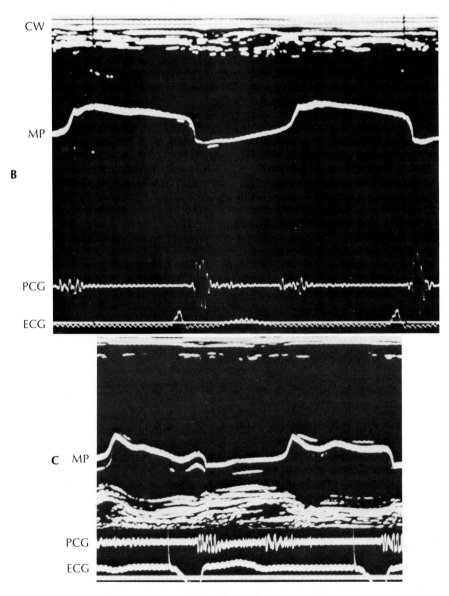

Fig. 10-12, cont'd. For legend see opposite page.

(mean, 100 msec), with a maximum beat to beat variation of 20 msec for patients in normal sinus rhythm. For atrial fibrillation the range is 70 to 140 msec, mean, 103 msec, maximum beat-to-beat variation, 30 msec.

• As mentioned earlier, the diameter of a Silastic ball can be determined by measuring the distance between the anterior and posterior echoes of the ball and multiplying it by 0.64.

COMMENTS

• During a long diastolic period the mitral poppet or the disc may transiently float back toward the closed position in late diastole. We find this circumscribed posterior motion becomes more prominent during inspiration and is attenuated or even disappears during the expiratory phase (Fig. 10-11). This is probably related to lowering of the left atrial pressure during inspiration. It is frequently seen in the early postoperative period and occurs with both normal sinus rhythm and atrial fibrillation. Occasionally, the ball echo may also show a small notch in early diastole.

• All components of a mitral prosthesis may not be seen in a tracing. When low gain is used, the ball echo has the appearance of a stenotic or normal mitral valve and may be mistaken for it (Fig. 10-12). Echoes from the anterior or posterior portions of the stent of a tissue valve may also mimic classic mitral stenosis. A long PR interval may result in premature closure of a normally functioning poppet. This is a rare finding.

• The ventricular septum may show paradoxical motion following insertion of a mitral or aortic prosthesis. The reason for this is poorly understood.

• Multiple reverberations and artifacts from beam width appear more common and more severe when prosthetic heart valves are examined. The intense reflections resulting from the large acoustic mismatch present between blood and metal interfaces act in a manner analogous to high sensitivity in emphasizing the width of the beam. Commonly, images of a mitral prosthesis may be recorded simultaneously with the aortic valve (Figs. 10-13 and 10-14). In one patient studied by us recently, multiple reverberations from a

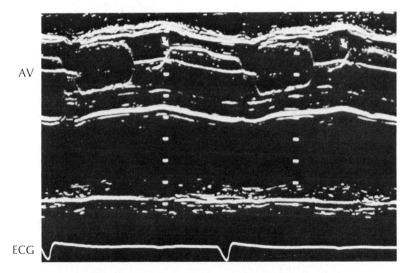

Fig. 10-13. Beam width artifact. Echoes from a mitral prosthesis *(arrows)* are seen superimposed on the aortic valve (AV) because of a relatively wide beam that passes through both structures. Since the mitral prosthesis was detected by the low intensity portion of the periphery of the beam, only the most intense reflections from the poppet are imaged. ECG, electrocardiogram.

Lillehei-Kaster aortic prosthesis were recorded in the left atrial cavity and simulated structural echoes.

ECHOCARDIOGRAPHIC FINDINGS
Mitral prosthetic dysfunction

• A significant change in the diameter of a silastic ball indicates the presence of ball variance or thrombosis.

• Absence of ball motion (concluded after careful examination from various transducer positions) points to poppet immobilization, which is frequently caused by massive thrombus or vegetation formation.

• Absence of the normal diastolic coaptation of the ball or disc echo with the cage echo indicates the presence of an obstructing mass such as vegetations or a large thrombus within the cage. Transient sticking of the ball in the partially open position or failure of the ball to open at all in one cardiac cycle may be seen. Delayed opening of the poppet due to sticking may be suggested by a prolonged interval between the aortic component of the second heart sound and the poppet opening movement (A2-OM interval). In these cases, inspection of the echocardiographic tracing alone may be sufficient, since the poppet echo contacts the cage echo well after the onset of posterior movement of the cage in diastole (Fig. 10-15).

• Reduction in the poppet or disc excursion, opening and closing velocities, and the EF slope also denote prosthetic malfunction. However, remember that these parameters are also affected by other factors, such as low cardiac output, changes in heart rate, and the force of ventricular contraction, and hence are of limited value in recognizing prosthetic dysfunction.

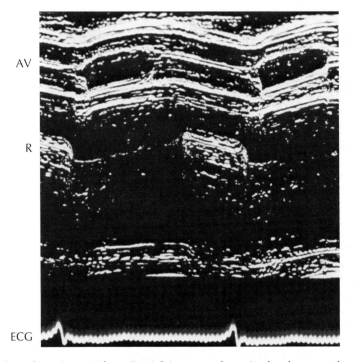

Fig. 10-14. Reverberation artifact. Partial images of a mitral valve prosthesis (R) are demonstrated in the left atrial cavity behind the aortic root in diastole in a position somewhat deeper than when recorded directly. A portion of the beam was probably deflected onto the prosthesis early in its passage to produce some path length elongation and to image the prosthesis deeper than normal and in the axis of aortic root and left atrium recording. AV, aortic valve; ECG, electrocardiogram.

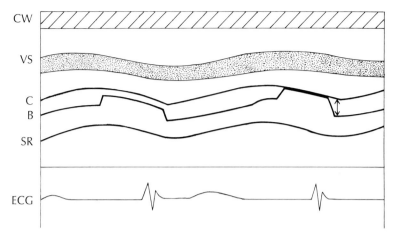

Fig. 10-15. Mitral prosthetic dysfunction. A schematic representation of the mitral prosthesis demonstrates on the left absence of contact between the cage (C) and the ball (B) in diastole, indicating the presence of a large obstructing thrombus or vegetations within the cage. *Right,* the opening movement of the ball is delayed so that it strikes the cage well after the onset of the posterior movement of the cage in diastole. *Double-headed arrow* denotes the distance between the ball and cage at the onset of systole and represents the maximal excursion of the poppet. CW, chest wall; VS, ventricular septum; SR, sewing ring; ECG, electrocardiogram.

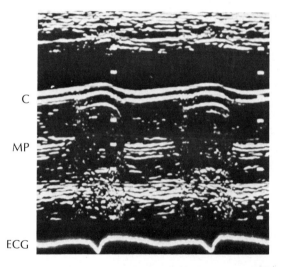

Fig. 10-16. Mitral prosthesis dysfunction. The cage (C) of the disc prosthesis (MP) shows an abnormal anterior motion in diastole as well as noncontact of the disc echo with the cage. At surgery a large thrombus involved the cage with partial dehiscence of the sewing ring. ECG, electrocardiogram.

• With dehiscence of the sewing ring, partial detachment of the prosthesis from the annulus may result in an abrupt step or notch in the cage or ring echo. With excessive rocking of the cage, intermittent echoes may be obtained from the cage, since it moves in and out of the ultrasonic beam. In our experience the cage may also show an abnormal anterior motion in diastole (Fig. 10-16).

• Prosthetic leak into the left atrium may result in a decrease in the A2-OM interval because of an elevated left atrial pressure. Normalization of the septal motion may also occur and is probably related to the need to eject the increased blood volume in the left ventricle that results from the paravalvular leak.

• Left ventricular intracavitary echoes are occasionally seen in patients with mitral prostheses. Their origin and significance are not yet clear, but they may represent minute pieces of cloth, fibrin deposits detached from the prosthesis, or hemolysis of red cells in a dysfunctioning prosthesis (Fig. 10-17).

• It is not yet clear whether the disappearance of the late diastolic circumscribed,

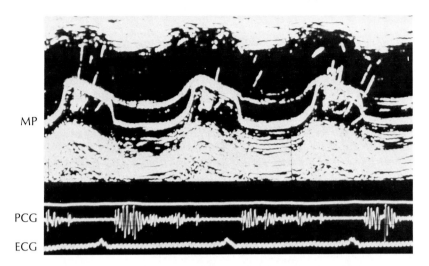

Fig. 10-17. Spontaneous contrast effects in a patient with malfunctioning mitral prosthesis (MP). This patient was actively hemolyzing during the study. The echocardiogram showed clusters of echoes closely associated with prosthesis in diastole and floating anteriorly in the left ventricular outflow tract. These echoes strongly resemble a dilute contrast injection, although there is no invasion during this examination. PCG, phonocardiogram; ECG, electrocardiogram.

posterior motion of the mitral disc or poppet (seen in the early postoperative period) represents prosthetic dysfunction.

Aortic prosthetic dysfunction

• Massive thrombosis on the ball or disc prosthesis may be associated with a large mass of echoes obscuring its motion. In one patient studied by us, massive vegetations on a Starr-Edwards prosthesis that formed an abscess around the annulus and protruded into the left ventricular outflow tract, obstructing it, were imaged as dense echoes in the left ventricular outflow area and in the region of the aortic annulus (Fig. 10-18).

• Severe paraprosthetic leak into the left ventricle may result in preclosure of the mitral valve. Mitral diastolic flutter also points to the presence of aortic regurgitation. Mild aortic incompetence may be seen normally with homograft aortic prostheses.

ROLE OF ECHOCARDIOGRAPHY

• The overall usefulness of echocardiography in the evaluation of prosthetic dysfunction is limited, although many investigators

have demonstrated its value in individual cases. Serial studies may prove useful in the early detection of malfunction before telltale clinical changes. Baseline tracings should be obtained in the immediate postoperative period and should be compared with regular follow-up examinations. Although positive echocardiographic findings are helpful in the diagnosis of prosthetic malfunction (beware low cardiac output state), no conclusions can be drawn when the echocardiographic record appears to be normal. We have had several cases where significant prosthetic dysfunction was present, but the echocardiograms obtained painstakingly from various transducer angulations were absolutely normal.

• A simultaneously recorded phonocardiogram is often useful in assessing prosthetic malfunction since the acoustic events can be timed with the motion of the prosthesis. This has been shown to be useful in evaluating patients with multiple prosthetic valves, since it is often difficult to know which valve is producing which sound.

• Echocardiography may prove to be particularly useful for early detection of mal-

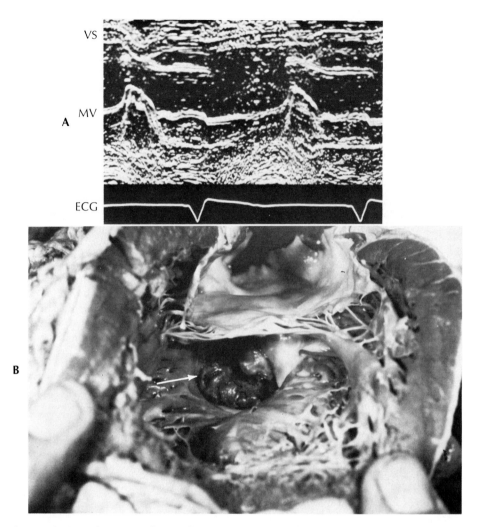

Fig. 10-18. A, Left ventricular outflow in a patient with aortic prosthesis endocarditis. Abnormal, linear moving echoes are present in the left ventricular outflow in diastole and represent a mass of vegetations protruding into the outflow tract from the aortic prosthesis. VS, ventricular septum; MV, mitral valve; ECG, electrocardiogram. **B,** Autopsy specimen of the patient whose echocardiogram is shown in **A.** Large vegetations (fungal) are observed protruding into the left ventricle.

function of tissue valves, since development of restriction of cusp motion or calcification would be expected to be recognized readily.

• In general, large thrombi or bacterial vegetations on a prosthesis are not detected by ultrasound since the stronger echoes from the prosthetic components tend to obscure relatively weak signals from abnormal tissues.

• There is very little data regarding echocardiographic recognition of aortic and tricuspid prosthesis dysfunction.

• A significant contribution of echocardiography to patient care is in the selection of a prosthesis that can be easily accommodated in the cavity of the left ventricle. In the presence of a narrow left ventricular outflow tract (less than 20 mm), a low-profile disc valve rather than a bulky caged ball prosthesis is recommended in the mitral po-

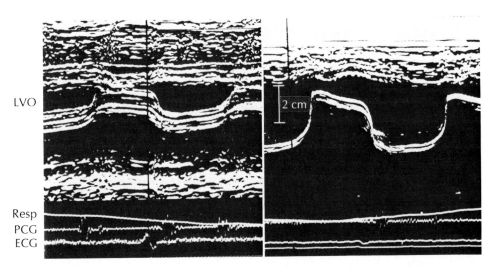

LVO

2 cm

Resp
PCG
ECG

Fig. 10-19. Mitral valve echocardiograms from two patients with mitral stenosis. The echogram on the left demonstrates a narrow left ventricular outflow tract (LVO); the one on the right illustrates a normal-sized outflow tract. Resp, respirations; PCG, phonocardiogram; ECG, electrocardiogram. (From Nanda, N. C., and others: Circulation **48:**1208, 1973.)

Fig. 10-20. Diagrammatic representation of a Starr-Edwards caged ball prosthesis. *1,* Length of the portion of the poppet expected to be projecting into the left ventricular outflow tract in the closed position (in systole) following prosthesis implantation. *2,* Height of cage. (From Nanda, N. C., and others: Circulation **48:**1208, 1973.)

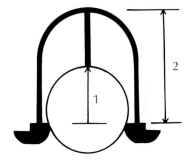

Table 9. Estimate of possible obstruction by caged ball prosthesis*

$\dfrac{\text{Poppet length (mm)}}{\text{LVO width (mm)}\dagger} \times 100$	Group 1 Normal LVO (12 pts.)	Group 2 Narrow LVO (7 pts.)
<50%	10	0
50%-59%	1	0
60%-69%	1	3
70%-80%	0	4

*From Nanda, N. C., Gramiak, R., Shah, P. M., and others: Echocardiographic assessment of left ventricular outflow width in the selection of mitral valve prosthesis, Circulation **48:**1208, 1973.
LVO, left ventricular outflow tract by echocardiography; poppet length, known length of the poppet expected to project into the LVO in systole following prosthesis implantation.

Table 10. Postoperative mortality*

Patient category	In-hospital mortality	Cause of death
Group 1 Normal LVO and caged ball prostheses (12 pts.)	8%	1 intra-operative
Group 2 Narrow LVO and caged ball prostheses (7 pts.)	71%	1 respiratory complications 4 low output state
Group 3 Narrow LVO and low profile prostheses (7 pts.)	14%	1 recent myocardial infarction

*From Nanda, N. C., Gramiak, R., Shah, P. M., and others: Echocardiographic assessment of left ventricular outflow width in the selection of mitral valve prosthesis, Circulation **48**:1208, 1973.
LVO, left ventricular outflow tract by echocardiography.

sition because it would not project far enough into the left ventricle to obstruct the outflow tract and produce a low cardiac output state or irritate the ventricular septum or free wall producing arrhythmias (Figs. 10-19 and 10-20). A study from our laboratory (Table 9) has shown the in-hospital mortality rate in patients with narrow left ventricular outflow and caged ball prosthesis to be 71% as compared with 8% when the left ventricular outflow was normal in width (Table 10).

• Surgical implantation of a prosthesis in a very small aortic root may also produce obstruction. The likelihood of this complication may increase when the width of the aortic root is less than 25 mm, although in our experience echocardiography generally overestimates the aortic lumen diameter when compared with surgery, probably because the wide ultrasonic beam passes partially through the sinuses of Valsalva.

• Associated cardiac diseases such as involvement of other valves and the presence of idiopathic hypertrophic subaortic stenosis may be recognized. Pericardial effusion developing after surgery may be detected and its size and distribution evaluated.

BIBLIOGRAPHY

Gimenez, J. L., Winters, W. L., Jr., Davila, J. C., Connell, J., and Klein, K. S.: Dynamics of the Starr-Edwards ball valve prosthesis; a cinefluorographic and ultrasonic study in humans, Am. J. Med. Sci. **250**:652, 1965.

Winters, W. L., Gimenez, J. L., and Soloff, L.: Clinical applications of ultrasound in the analysis of prosthetic ball valve function, Am. J. Cardiol. 19:97, 1967.

Mahringer, W., and Hausen, W. J.: The origin of the ultrasound echocardiogram in mitral stenosis; studies on prosthetic valves with the aid of roentgen cinematography, Z. Kreisl.-Forsch. 58:1193, 1969.

Johnson, M. L., Paton, B. C., and Holmes, J. H.: Ultrasonic evaluation of prosthetic valve motion, Circulation 41(suppl. 2):3, 1970.

Mahringer, W., and Hausen, W. J.: Ultrasound cardiogram in patients with mitral valve disc prostheses, Angiology **21**:336, 1970.

Popp, R. L., and Carmichael, B. M.: Cardiac echography in the diagnosis of prosthetic mitral valve malfunction, Circulation 44(suppl. 2): 33, 1971 (abstract).

Siggers, D. C., Srivongse, S. A., and Deuchar, D.: Analysis of dynamics of mitral Starr-Edwards valve prosthesis using reflected ultrasound, Br. Heart J. 33:401, 1971.

Pfeifer, J., Goldschlager, N., Sweatman, T., Gerbode, E., and Selzer, A.: Malfunction of mitral ball valve prosthesis due to thrombus, Am. J. Cardiol. **29**:95, 1972.

Belenkie, I., Carr, M., Schlant, R. C., Nutter, D. O., and Symbas, P. N.: Malfunction of a Cutter-Smeloff mitral ball valve prosthesis; diagnosis by phonocardiography and echocardiography, Am. Heart J. **86**: 339, 1973.

Johnson, M. L., Holmes, J. H., and Paton, B. C.: Echocardiographic determination of mitral disc valve excursion, Circulation **47**:1274, 1973.

Miller, H. C., Stephens, J. D., and Gibson, D. G.: Echocardiographic features of mitral Starr-Edwards paraprosthetic regurgitation, Br. Heart J. **35**: 560, 1973.

Miller, H. C., Gibson, D. G., and Stephens, J. D.: Role of echocardiography and phonocardiography in the diagnosis of mitral paraprosthetic regurgitation with Starr-Edwards prostheses, Br. Heart J. **35:**1217, 1973.

Nanda, N. C., Gramiak, R., Shah, P. M., DeWeese, J. A., and Mahoney, E. B.: Echocardiographic assessment of left ventricular outflow width in the selection of mitral valve prosthesis, Circulation **48:**1208, 1973.

Oliva, P. B., Johnson, M. L., Pomerantz, M., and Levine, A.: Dysfunction of the Beall mitral prosthesis and its detection by cinefluoroscopy and echocardiography, Am. J. Cardiol. **31:**393, 1973.

Yuste, P., Minguez, I., Aza, V., Asin, E., Castrillo, L. A., and Martinez-Bordiu, C.: Mitral valve prostheses, and left ventricular function; an echocardiographic study, J. Cardiovasc. Surg. (Torino) (special issue) pp. 421-424, 1973.

Assad-Morell, J. L., Tajik, A. J., Anderson, M. W., Tancredi, R. G., Wallace, R. B., and Giuliani, E. R.: Malfunctioning tricuspid valve prosthesis; clinical, phonocardiographic, echocardiographic and surgical findings, Mayo Clin. Proc. **42:**443, 1974.

Ben-Zvi, J., Hildner, F. J., Chandraratna, P. A., and Samet, P.: Thrombosis on Bjork-Shiley aortic valve prosthesis; clinical, arteriographic, echocardiographic and therapeutic observations in seven cases, Am. J. Cardiol. **34:**538, 1974.

Douglas, J. E., and Williams, G. D.: Echocardiographic evaluation of the Bjork-Shiley prosthetic valve, Circulation **50:**52, 1974.

Ellis, J., Phillips, B., Friedewald, V. E., Jr., and Diethrich, E. B.: The evaluation of the Bjork-Shiley prosthetic valve by echocardiography, J. Clin. Ultrasound **2:**228, 1974 (abstract).

Gibson, T. C., Starek, J. K., Moos, S., and Craige, E.: Echocardiographic and phonographic characteristics of the Lillehei-Kaster mitral valve prosthesis, Circulation **49:**434, 1974.

Horowitz, M. S., Goodman, D. J., and Popp, R. L.: Echocardiographic diagnosis of calcific stenosis of a stented aortic homograft in the mitral position, J. Clin. Ultrasound **2:**179, 1974.

Mary, D. A. S., Pakrashi, B. C., Catchpole, R. W., and Ionescu, M. L.: Echocardiographic studies of stented fascia lata grafts in the mitral position, Circulation **49:**237, 1974.

Escarous, A.: The Bjork-Shiley tilting disc valve prosthesis; echocardiographic findings, Scand. J. Thorac. Cardiovasc. Surg. **9:**192-196, 1975.

Kawai, N., Segal, B. L., and Linhart, J. W.: Delayed opening of Beall mitral prosthetic valve detected by echocardiography, Chest **67:**239-241, 1975.

Mcilmoyle, G., Robertson, D. A., McDicken, W. N., and Evans, D. H.: Ultrasonic measurement of prosthetic heart valve action, Cardiovasc. Res. **9:**554-560, 1975.

Schuchman, H., Feigenbaum, H., Dillon, J. C., and

Chang, S.: Intracavitary echoes in patients with mitral prosthetic valves, J. Clin. Ultrasound **3:**111, 1975.

Yuste, P., Aza, V., Minguez, I., Asin, E., and Martinez-Bordiu, C.: Echocardiographic evaluation of mitral valve prosthesis malfunction. In Kazner, E., and others, editors: Ultrasonics in medicine, Amsterdam, excerpta Medica, 1975, pp. 239-244.

Berndt, T. B., Goodman, D. J., and Popp, R. L.: Echocardiographic and phonocardiographic confirmation of suspected caged mitral valve malfunction, Chest **70:**221-230, 1976.

Bloch, W. N., Jr., Felner, J. M., Wickliffe, C., and Symbas, P. N.: Echocardiographic diagnosis of thrombus on a heterograft aortic valve in the mitral position. Chest. **70:**399-401, 1976.

Brodie, B. R., Grossman, W., McLaurin, L., Starek, P. J., and Craige, E.: Diagnosis of prosthetic mitral valve malfunction with combined echo-phonocardiography, Circulation **53:**93-100, 1976.

Chandraratna, P. A. N., Lopez, J. M., Hildner, F. J., Samet, P., Ben-Zvi, J., and Gindlesperger, D.: Diagnosis of Bjork-Shiley aortic valve dysfunction by echocardiography, Am. Heart J. **91:**318, 1976 (abstract).

Etzold, K. F., Kingsley, B., and Larach, S.: Echocardiography of prosthetic heart valves; the effect of poppet shapes and materials on the interpretation of recordings. In White, D. N., and Ross, A. E., editors: Ultrasound in medicine, vol. 3, New York, 1977, Plenum Publishing Corp., p. 27.

Horowitz, M. S., Tecklenberg, P. L., Goodman, D. J., Harrison, D. C., and Popp, P. L.: Echocardiographic evaluation of the stent mounted aortic bioprosthetic valve in the mitral position in vitro and in vivo studies, Circulation **54:**91-96, 1976.

Nanda, N. C., Thomson, K., and Gramiak, R.: Late diastolic motion of the mitral prosthesis; echocardiographic studies. In White, D. N., and Ross, A. E.: Ultrasound in medicine, vol. 3, New York, 1977, Plenum Publishing Corp., p. 109.

Popp, R. L.: Echocardiographic assessment of prosthetic mitral valves. In Kalmanson, D., editor: The mitral valve, Acton, Mass., 1976, Publishing Sciences Group, pp. 325-332.

Srivastava, T. N., Hussain, M., Gray, L. A., Jr., and Flowers, N. C.: Echocardiographic diagnosis of a stuck Bjork-Shiley aortic valve prosthesis, Chest **70:** 94-98, 1976.

Raizada, V., Desser, K. B., Benchimol, A., and Molthan, M. E.: Echocardiographic and phonocardiographic findings after Hancock procine pulmonary artery graft implantation, Clin. Res. **25:**246A, 1977.

Raizada, W., Benchimol, A., Desser, K. B., and Sheasby, C.: Echocardiographic features of normal functioning Hancock porcine heterograft valve in the aortic position, Clin. Res. **25:**246A, 1977.

11 Complex malformations

Complex malformations are the result of faulty development of the embryonic heart. An understanding of the various stages of embryologic development is useful for an appreciation of the defects encountered in echocardiography and the variations that produce related lesions.

EMBRYOLOGY

The earliest form of the heart is a primitive cardiac tube formed in the third week of intrauterine life. It grows rapidly, bending and twisting itself into a loop. The upper portion of the tube (called the conus arteriosus) connects the lower portion of the tube (primitive ventricles, atrioventricular canal) with the truncus arteriosus, which later divides into the aorta and pulmonary artery (Fig. 11-1). External bulges, the developing atria, are visible on either side of the conal truncus. The great veins develop at the inferior end of the cardiac tube to form a primitive collecting chamber, the sinus venosus. Internally, two masses of tissue (endocardial cushions) grow (one from the front and one from the back) into the common atrioventricular canal and represent an attempt to partition the heart into left and right sides (Fig. 11-2). Similar tissues also grow down from the top of the common atrium and upward from the bottom of the common ventricle to divide the chambers. The atrial septum (septum primum) grows downward but does not divide the atria completely, and the atrial communication at its lower end is called the ostium primum. Subsequently, a second atrial septum develops to the right of the septum primum and has a hole in its middle, the foramen ovale. Next, the upper portion of the septum primum is resorbed, leaving the lower portion to remain as a flap valve over the foramen ovale. This permits blood to flow only from right to left. (It is not until after birth, when blood returns to the left side of the heart from the newly expanded lungs, that the foramen ovale is finally closed.)

The ventricular septum grows from the apex of the common ventricle toward the growing endocardial cushions and the two ridges present on the conotruncus. It partitions the common chamber into right and left ventricles. One of the ridges of the conotruncus fuses with the tricuspid valve and an endocardial cushion, resulting in the formation of the crista that separates the pulmonary valve from the tricuspid valve. The other ridge fuses with the ventricular septum, leaving the aortic root in continuity with the mitral valve. The upper portion of the ventricular septum thins out (membranous portion).

The truncus arteriosus is partitioned by ridges that grow in a spiral manner so that the aorta receives flow from the left ventricle and the pulmonary artery connects to the right ventricular outflow. Three small swellings grow out from each of the truncal ridges and differentiate to form three cusps of the aortic and pulmonary valves (Fig. 11-3). The atrioventricular valves are formed by thin-

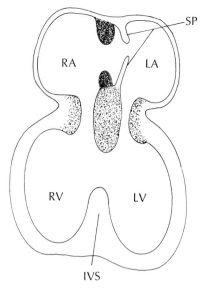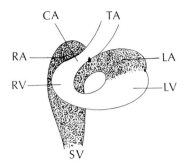

Fig. 11-1. Primitive cardiac tube. Elongation and twisting of the primitive cardiac tube has resulted in the establishment of the right-left relationships of the forerunners of future cardiac chambers. The truncus arteriosus (TA) will develop into the aorta and pulmonary arteries, and the conus arteriosus (CA) will become the ventricular outflow tracts. LA, primitive left atrium; LV, primitive left ventricle; RV, primitive right ventricle; RA, primitive right atrium; SV, sinus venosus.

ning and differentiation of masses of tissue that project from the endocardial cushions and from outer walls of the atrioventricular canal. The supporting apparatus (papillary muscles and chordae tendinae) arise by modification of the muscular tissues on the inner surfaces of the ventricles. Branches of the aorta and the pulmonary artery are then formed.

FETAL CIRCULATION

During fetal development, oxygenated blood derived from the maternal placenta enters the fetal heart via the inferior vena cava (Fig. 11-4). A prominent valve at the entrance of the inferior vena cava directs a major portion of this blood through the foramen ovale to the left side of the heart and thence to the systemic circuit. The unexpanded lungs have a high vascular resistance and hence a considerable proportion of the blood ejected from the right ventricle into the pulmonary artery is directed by the ductus arteriosus into the descending aorta, which at this time has a lower vascular resistance. At birth the breathing infant inflates his lungs, the pulmonary vascular resistance

Fig. 11-2. Atrial septal development. The septum primum (SP) and the contained ostium secundum are already developed, and the base of the septum primum is fused to the endocardial cushion *(light stippling)* closing the ostium primum. Failure of this fusion to take place results in formation of an ostium primum atrial septal defect. The septum secundum *(dark stippling)* is beginning to form and contains the foramen ovale. Incomplete development of the atrial septum in its upper part is the source of secundum atrial septal defects. The endocardial cushions also contribute to the development of the atrioventricular valves and to the upper portion of the interventricular septum. RA, right atrium; LA, left atrium; RV, right ventricle; LV, left ventricle; IVS, interventricular septum.

reduces considerably, and more blood flows into the pulmonary artery and the lungs. The increased volume of the blood returning from the pulmonary vascular bed raises the left atrial pressure above that in the right atrium and closes the atrial flap valve (formed from the septum primum), preventing left-to-right blood flow. Since more blood is now pumped by the left heart, the aortic pressure rises, and blood flow through the ductus arteriosus is no longer in the right-to-left direction. The ductus arteriosus is obliterated over the next several days, establishing the adult circulation pattern. Further decrease in the

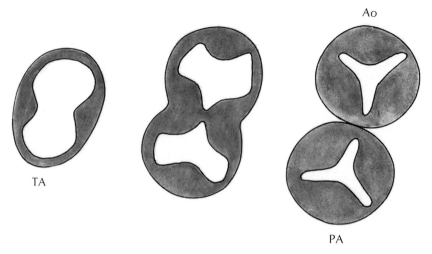

Fig. 11-3. Great vessel and semilunar valve formation. Connective tissue ridges form in the truncus arteriosus (TA) and grow to divide the truncus into two separate vessels. The valve cusps also originate from the connective tissue ridges. PA, pulmonary artery; Ao, aorta.

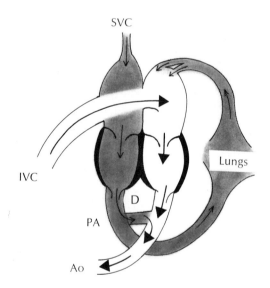

Fig. 11-4. Fetal circulation. The major flow pathways in the fetal heart bypass the right heart and the high resistance pulmonary circuit. Venous return streams mainly through the patent foramen ovale and is circulated by the left heart. The right heart pumps a reduced amount of blood, which is directed into the aorta and systemic circulation through the patent ductus arteriosus (D). Ao, aorta; PA, pulmonary artery; IVC, inferior vena cava; SVC, superior vena cava.

pulmonary vascular resistance occurs over the next six to eight weeks. For this reason the pulmonary artery remains larger than the aortic root during infancy.

ECHOCARDIOGRAPHIC EXAMINATION

Echocardiographic examination depends on a thorough knowledge of normal cardiac anatomy, since the ultrasonic findings represent departures from the patterns found in normal subjects. Experience in adult echocardiography, therefore, is a good foundation for the evaluation of these lesions. It should be noted that children may have heart disease seen in adults, and conditions such as mitral valve prolapse, IHSS, myxomas, congestive cardiomyopathies, vegetations, aneurysms, and pericardial effusions may be found in children. The echocardiographic features are the same when children are involved, and identical diagnostic criteria are utilized. It is also important to remember that adults may have a congenital heart lesion such as an atrial or ventricular septal defect, bicuspid aortic valve, Ebstein's anomaly, or tetralogy of Fallot that has not been previously diagnosed. Awareness of these possibilities leads to successful diagnosis.

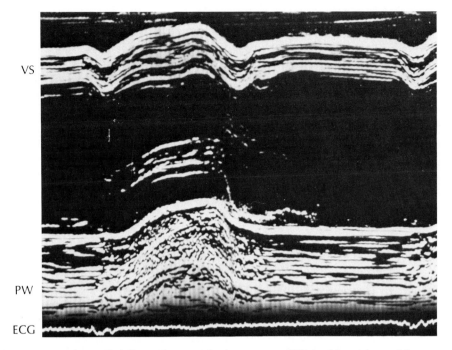

Fig. 11-5. Atrial septal defect. The ventricular septum (VS) in this patient with a secundum defect shows an abnormal anterior motion during systole. PW, left ventricular posterior wall; ECG, electrocardiogram.

Atrial septal defect

Anatomic and functional changes. Failure of the atrial septum to develop completely results in a communication between the right and left atrial cavities. The defect may be in the midportion of the septum (secundum type), low in the septum (primum type), or higher and more dorsal (sinus venosus type). There are ordinarily no associated anatomic defects with ostium secundum atrial septal defects. Ostium primum defects, on the other hand, are associated with clefts and deformities of the mitral valve and occasionally of the tricuspid valve and result in regurgitation as well. The anterior leaflet of the mitral valve may have abnormal chordae that attach to the ventricular septum. This narrows and elongates the left ventricular outflow tract. The posterior leaflet is normal in ostium primum defects. All defects result in a left-to-right shunt at the atrial level so that the entire right heart carries an increased volume of blood (volume overload). The right

ventricle and pulmonary artery become enlarged. The small vessels of the pulmonary vascular bed may become damaged as a late complication of the volume overload, resulting in the development of pulmonary hypertension. The elevated right heart pressures may reverse the atrial shunt so that cyanosis, which is not present in the uncomplicated cases, may follow. Heart failure can also result in shunt reversal.

Clinical summary. A systolic murmur due to increased flow through the pulmonic valve is usually present. For similar reasons a mid-diastolic murmur simulating tricuspid stenosis may be heard. The pulmonic component of the second heart sound is delayed from the overloaded right ventricle, and a widely split second heart sound results. Characteristically, the splitting is fixed, since the pulmonic component does not show normal respiratory variations because of the fixed volume overload of the shunt. A pansystolic murmur of mitral regurgitation is present in ostium primum defects. The ECG typically shows an incomplete right bundle branch block pattern. Ostium primum defects also show left axis deviation. The chest roentgenogram may show enlargement of the main pulmonary artery with engorgement of the pulmonary vessels. On fluoroscopy these vessels pulsate from the increased blood volume ejected through the pulmonary artery. The aorta is small and the right atrium large. Cardiac catheterization reveals an elevation of the oxygen content in the right atrium from left-to-right shunting through the defect, and the catheter may pass directly into the left atrium. The volume of blood flowing through the pulmonic (Qp) and systemic (Qs) circuits can be calculated. When Qp/Qs exceeds about 2.0, the functional burden from the right ventricular volume overload becomes significant. Slight gradients may be present across the tricuspid and pulmonic valves from the increased flow. Angiocardiog-

raphy reveals the shunt but is most useful to differentiate ostium primum from secundum defects. In ostium primum septal defects the left ventricular outflow tract is characteristically narrowed and appears as a "gooseneck" deformity. Mitral regurgitation is present when the anterior leaflet is cleft.

Echocardiographic features

• The right ventricle is enlarged.

• Ventricular septal motion is abnormal and is anterior in systole and posterior in diastole (Figs. 11-5 and 11-6).

• The left ventricular outflow tract is normal in secundum and sinus venosus defects but is narrowed in primum defects. (Outflow dimension less than 20 mm in adults; prolonged diastolic apposition of the mitral valve with the ventricular septum in children.) (Fig. 11-7.)

• A scan made from the mitral to the tricuspid valve will show a discontinuity between the mitral valve and the atrial sep-

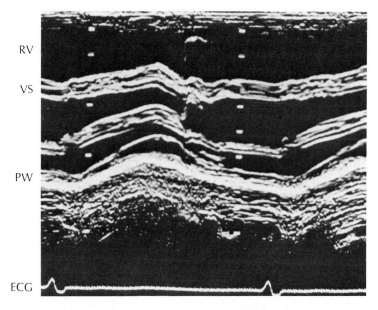

Fig. 11-6. Recording of the left ventricular cavity in a child with ostium primum atrial septal defect demonstrating an abnormal anterior movement of the ventricular septum (VS) during systole. Right ventricular cavity (RV) is enlarged, and its end-diastolic dimension approximates that of the left ventricle. Fragmentary recording of the mitral valve shows diastolic apposition with the ventricular septum. PW, left ventricular posterior wall; ECG, electrocardiogram.

tum in ostium primum defects. The atrial septum also appears to be more deeply placed than in normal subjects or may not be recorded. Ostium secundum and sinus venosus atrial septal defects occur higher in the atrial septum than primum defects so that mitral-to-tricuspid scans show continuity between the mitral valve and the atrial septum.

• The tricuspid valve may show diastolic fluttering (Table 8).

• The ventricular septum shows normal width unless severe pulmonary hypertension supervenes.

Comments

• Right ventricular enlargement is evaluated using a beam position that passes through the left ventricular cavity at a point just beyond the tips of the mitral leaflets. The width of the right ventricle is measured as the vertical distance from the endocardial surface of the anterior right ventricular wall to the right side of the septum at the R wave peak of the ECG and is corrected for body size using the determination of body surface area obtained from height-weight charts. The upper limit in normal adults is 1.2 cm/m^2

Table 8. Echocardiographic differentiation of ostium primum from ostium secundum atrial septal defects

Echo features	Ostium primum	Ostium secundum
LVO dimension	Narrow (under 20 mm)	Normal (20 mm or more)
Prolonged mitral-septal diastolic apposition	Present	Absent
Mitral valve-atrial septum continuity	Absent	Present
Tricuspid valve diastolic flutter	May be present (involvement of septal leaflet more common)	May be present
Multilayering of mitral/ tricuspid valves	May be present	Absent
Abnormal ventricular septal motion	Present	Present

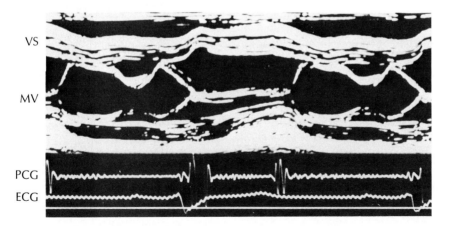

Fig. 11-7. Prolonged diastolic apposition of the mitral valve (MV) with the ventricular septum (VS) in a patient with an ostium primum atrial septal defect. The A wave is also seen to be in contact with the septum. PCG, phonocardiogram; ECG, electrocardiogram.

when the patient is examined in a supine position. The left decubitus position results in somewhat larger right ventricular dimensions. The size of the right ventricle can be estimated qualitatively during the examination by comparing the width of the right ventricle with that of the left ventricle. In normal subjects the right ventricular cavity measures about one fourth to one third as large as the left ventricle. Right ventricular enlargement, therefore, displaces the septum into a deeper position than in normal subjects. The degree of right ventricular enlargement roughly parallels the extent of shunting into the right heart.

• Ventricular septal motion recording should also be evaluated with the beam passing through the left ventricle just beyond the tips of the mitral leaflets. A beam position that is too high will show paradoxical motion of the septum in normal subjects, since the septum is attached to the anterior margin of the aortic root, which moves anteriorly in systole and posteriorly in diastole. Beam sweeping from the left ventricle into the aorta is a useful maneuver to show the entire spectrum of changes.

• The septum may also in some cases appear to be flat during systole, without clear anterior excursion. The presence of right ventricular enlargement identifies this finding as part of the atrial septal defect diagnostic picture.

• Abnormal septal motion plus right ventricular enlargement are not specific diagnostic signs of atrial septal defect but are indicators of right ventricular diastolic volume overload. These findings are also present in severe pulmonic and tricuspid regurgitation and in total anomalous pulmonary venous return (TAPVR). Additional findings in TAPVR are an abnormally small left atrial cavity and an echo-free space behind the left atrium or left ventricle arising in a common pulmonary venous trunk (Fig. 11-8). Scan this area carefully and look for a vessel that should be larger than a normal left pulmonic vein that can be seen behind the left ventricle or atrium.

Abnormal ventricular septal motion is also seen in left bundle branch block, coronary artery disease with lesions involving the left anterior descending vessel, after open heart surgery in which the pericardium is opened, and in congenital absence of the pericardium. However, in these conditions there is usually no indication of right ventricular enlargement.

• When shunts are small and the ratio of pulmonic to systemic blood flow is less than 2:1, the right ventricle may not be enlarged and septal motion appears normal.

• Pressure overload may increase the size of the right ventricle, but normal septal motion is retained.

• After successful surgical closure of an atrial septal defect the abnormal findings may persist for many months before the recordings return toward normal. Some may remain abnormal indefinitely.

• Ventricular septal motion may appear normal in ostium primum atrial septal defects. Mitral regurgitation from cleft leaflets produces volume overload of the left ventricle, which may balance the right ventric-

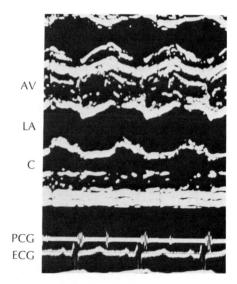

AV

LA

C

PCG
ECG

Fig. 11-8. Total anomalous pulmonary venous drainage. The left atrial wall is hyperactive and separates the left atrial cavity (LA) from a large common pulmonary venous chamber (C) located posteriorly. AV, aortic valve; PCG, phonocardiogram; ECG, electrocardiogram.

ular volume overload resulting from the atrial septal defect.

• In an adult, complete diastolic traces of the tricuspid valve are usually obtained when the right ventricle is enlarged.

• Diastolic fluttering of the tricuspid valve occurs as the result of turbulent flow produced by the shunt. It should not be regarded as primary evidence of pulmonic regurgitation. Diastolic fluttering may involve both anterior and septal leaflets and is generally observed in the presence of a large shunt (Qp/Qs > 2.3). The incidence of flutter is higher in ostium primum defects than in the secundum variety, probably because of the low position of the defect, which is located just above the tricuspid valve. For a similar reason, septal leaflet flutter is also more common in primum defects.

• The pulmonic valve should be examined carefully for the findings of pulmonary hypertension. A thick ventricular septum also suggests significant pulmonary hypertension.

• Pulmonic stenosis may coexist, but ultrasound findings may not be typical, as noted previously.

• Mitral valve prolapse is said to occur in about one third of cases with atrial septal defects. We have had difficulty recognizing coexisting mitral valve prolapse in proved cases for reasons not clear to us at the present time.

• The posterior left atrial wall may show a hyperdynamic motion pattern in the presence of a large atrial septal defect.

• When cleft mitral leaflets are present in ostium primum defects, the mitral valve may show a multilayered pattern. As mentioned earlier, this is a nonspecific finding. A more extensively deformed mitral valve may show a small excursion and delayed opening slopes. In our experience cleft tricuspid valves also demonstrate multilayering (Fig. 11-9).

• Postoperatively, the patch used in closing the defect can be identified by its thick or multilayered appearance behind the tricuspid valve. Contrast studies in the immediate postoperative period can be used to assess the effectiveness of surgical closure. An intraatrial conduit (pericardial or Teflon) surgically placed in the right atrium to redirect the blood from anomalous pulmonary veins opening in the right atrium to the left atrial

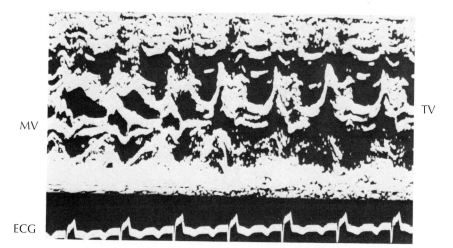

Fig. 11-9. Cleft tricuspid valve ostium primum atrial septal defect. A scan from the mitral valve (MV) to the tricuspid valve (TV) shows some diastolic mitral-septal apposition and discontinuity between the mitral valve and fragmentary echoes from the base of the atrial septum seen behind the tricuspid valve. The multilayering of the tricuspid valve results from a large cleft that involved the septal leaflet. The anterior mitral leaflet showed a smaller cleft not detected in this study. ECG, electrocardiogram.

cavity across the fossa ovalis may also be imaged as a prominent linear echo in the right atrial cavity.

Role of echocardiography

• Occasionally echocardiography demonstrates changes suggestive of atrial septal defect in adult patients when the clinical presentation is atypical. In clinically typical children and adults, a rough estimation of shunt size can be made from the size of the right ventricle and the presence of diastolic fluttering of the tricuspid valve. In addition, complicating conditions such as pulmonary hypertension can be recognized and evaluated. Ostium primum defects, which require a different surgical repair, can be specifically identified by the features of right ventricular volume overload plus narrowing of the left ventricular outflow tract. Secundum defects, on the other hand, cannot be diagnosed directly from the echocardiogram since other abnormalities, which produce right ventricular volume overload, result in the same echocardiographic pattern.

• The presence of normal ventricular septal motion on the echocardiogram cannot be used to exclude a significant secundum defect, since a few patients with large defects have not shown any motion abnormalities involving the septum.

Ventricular septal defects

Ventricular septal defects can occur as isolated holes in the septum or in combination with more complex developmental errors. Any portion of the ventricular septum may be involved and a left-to-right shunt at the ventricular level occurs. Since the shunt is into the right ventricle in systole, there is no diastolic volume overload in the right heart so that the picture of right ventricular volume overload is not produced. The major effect is seen on the left atrium and left ventricle, which become enlarged. The main pulmonary artery and the right ventricle may enlarge when pulmonary hypertension supervenes.

The size of isolated ventricular septal defects varies. They may occasionally be so large that normal continuity between the septum and aorta is lost in scans of the left heart. This is an unreliable finding since it

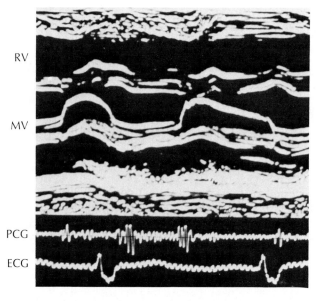

Fig. 11-10. Slow EF slopes of the mitral valve in a child with pulmonary hypertension complicating a ventricular septal defect. There was no evidence for mitral stenosis. RV, right ventricle; MV, mitral valve; PCG, phonocardiogram; ECG, electrocardiogram.

is also seen when the beam is not correctly aligned over a normal septum. Defects that are smaller than the width of the ultrasonic beam are not imaged, since an edge is always in the beam and is imaged as though it were centrally placed. Defects that pass through the septum at an angle are also not imaged. The echocardiographic findings, therefore, are usually not diagnostic of the ordinary isolated ventricular septal defect, and only secondary changes in the left atrial and left ventricular size may be apparent. Complications such as pulmonary hypertension occur, and should be looked for. The mitral valve may show a slow EF slope that mimics mitral stenosis as a result of pulmonary hypertension (Fig. 11-10). The tricuspid valve is normal in these cases.

Ventricular septal defects that involve the membranous portion of the septum can produce shunts that pass from the left ventricle into the right atrium. The tricuspid valve is often involved in the defect, and some local thickening of leaflet tissue occurs as the result of the defect and from the turbulent flow produced by the jet. In these cases, there is a high-frequency flutter of the tricuspid valve. (See p. 215 for a more complete description). In patients with small membranous septal defects, septal aneurysms have been demonstrated echocardiographically. Abnormal echoes having wide excursions protrude into the right ventricle and may be closely associated with the motion of the tricuspid valve (Figs. 11-11 and 11-12).

Patent ductus arteriosus

In some newborns the ductus fails to close and remains patent so that a shunt from the higher pressure aorta to the lower pressure pulmonary artery is established. The volume of the shunt is contained in the pulmonary circulation, the aorta, and the left heart chambers with the major functional load carried by the left heart and pulmonary circulation, so that respiratory distress is a common clinical finding in these newborns.

Cardiac auscultation demonstrates the

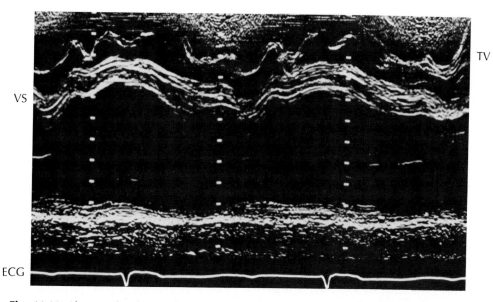

Fig. 11-11. Abnormal echoes in the right ventricular cavity in a patient with aneurysm of the membranous portion of the ventricular septum. An undulating linear echo is seen throughout the cardiac cycle merging with the anterior leaflet of the tricuspid valve (TV) on the right. The echo probably arises from the aneurysm itself as it bulges into the right ventricle. VS, ventricular septum; ECG, electrocardiogram.

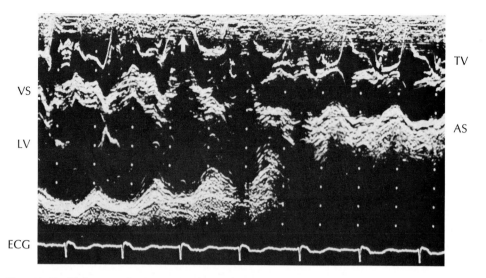

Fig. 11-12. Right ventricular cavity recordings in a patient with an aneurysm of the membranous portion of the ventricular septum. Abnormal echoes *(arrows)* from the aneurysm are superimposed on the tricuspid valve images. On the left the abnormal echo shows posterior displacement in systole mimicking tricuspid valve prolapse. It then merges with the opening segment of the tricuspid valve and may be mistaken for a late closing tricuspid valve commonly seen in Ebstein's anomaly. VS, ventricular septum; TV, tricuspid valve; LV, left ventricle; AS, atrial septum; ECG, electrocardiogram.

presence of a rough, machinerylike continuous murmur in systole and diastole over the pulmonic valve area. Cardiac catheterization reveals the presence of oxygenated blood in the pulmonary artery. Aortography may demonstrate the ductus directly and routinely shows radiopaque material flowing from the aorta to the pulmonary artery.

The ductus and pulmonary circulatory problems are not diagnosable by echocardiography, but the left atrium, whose size reflects the magnitude of the shunt, can be examined and followed. In normal newborns the ratio of left atrial to aortic diameter is about 0.75; that is, the aorta is slightly larger than the left atrium. In the presence of a large patent ductus the left atrium becomes larger than the aorta, and the ratio may exceed 1.19. Serial studies that chart left atrial size are most useful, and a rapid increase in left atrial size is one of the indications for immediate surgical closure of the patent ductus. Postoperatively, left atrial size returns to normal levels. A dramatic decrease in the size of

the left atrium has also been observed by us following administration of Indomethacin for closure of a patent ductus.

Coarctation of the aorta

Improper development of the aorta may result in coarctation, which is frequently preductal, but may be postductal or at the site of origin of the ductus arteriosus. Occasionally, the coarcted segment may be long and may involve other areas of the aorta. Clinically, the pulses in the lower limbs are diminished in volume and delayed as compared to the upper extremities. A systolic murmur may be audible in the upper back from the coarcted segment or from flow in the collateral vessels that develop to bypass the obstruction. Angiography demonstrates the site and extent of the coarcted segment.

The narrowed segment of the aorta is not available for direct ultrasonic examination since adjacent lung and bone block the passage of the ultrasonic beam. However, we have observed a high incidence of bicuspid

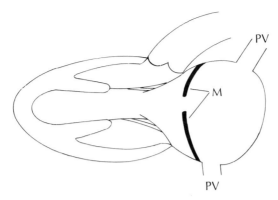

Fig. 11-13. Cor triatriatum. A fibromuscular membrane (M) partitions the left atrial cavity into two chambers. The pulmonary veins (PV) drain into the posterior chamber, which communicates with the distal chamber through one or more openings. The size of the communication determines the severity of obstruction.

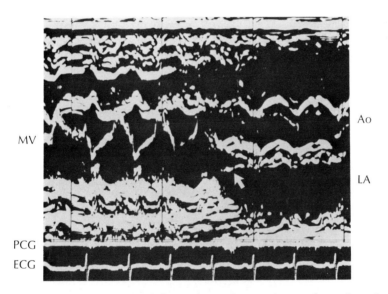

Fig. 11-14. Congenital obstructing left atrial membrane. A scan from the mitral valve (MV) to the aortic root (Ao) shows linear echoes at the outflow portion of the left atrium arising from a left atrial membrane *(arrow).* The left atrium (LA) is enlarged. The echoes seen deep to the aortic root also arise from the membrane and can represent diagnostic difficulties when the portion extending over the atrioventricular junction is not imaged. After surgery the obstructing portion of the membrane was absent, and the left atrium decreased in size, though the linear echoes immediately behind the posterior aortic wall persisted. PCG, phonocardiogram; ECG, electrocardiogram.

aortic valves detected ultrasonically, occasional aneurysms of the aorta at the level of the aortic valve, and mitral valve prolapse patterns. We have also observed, in some patients, echocardiographic findings indicating the presence of a functional left ventricular outflow tract obstruction identical to that found in patients with IHSS. The mitral valve and ventricular septum should be routinely studied with care, and provocative maneuvers such as amyl nitrite inhalation should be used in precatheterization studies to identify these patients preoperatively.

Cor triatriatum

The appearance of three atria is produced by a congenital fibromuscular membrane that divides the left atrial cavity into two chambers, the posterior containing the openings of the pulmonic veins (Fig. 11-13). An opening is present in the membrane; its size determines the degree of obstruction to the passage of blood before it reaches the mitral valve. Pulmonary hypertension is a common associated finding. This lesion is relatively rare, but echocardiography can show the presence of an additional structural echo in the left atrium and a normal mitral valve. Beam scanning in multiple positions is useful to show the position and extent of the membrane, but the diagnosis should be made with

caution since "lines" are commonly seen in the left atrium and probably arise from the normal orifices of the pulmonic veins. Echocardiographic or clinical evidence of pulmonary hypertension should be present before a diagnosis of cor triatriatum is made.

Membranes may also be present in a supravalvular position relative to the mitral valve. These produce similar clinical findings, and the echocardiogram will show the membrane echoes in the left atrium close to the mitral valve (Fig. 11-14). Scans from the mitral to the aortic valve may reveal an enlarged left atrial cavity and an obliquely situated linear echo pattern that crosses the left atrial cavity and bulges toward a normally moving mitral valve. The turbulent flow across the membrane may produce coarse undulations of the mitral valve. We have recently examined an infant who appeared to have a typical left atrial membrane (Fig.

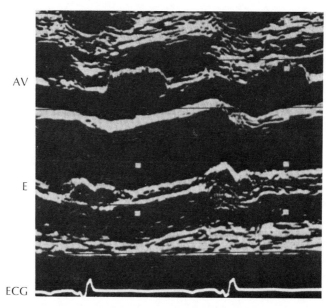

Fig. 11-15. Abnormal echoes in the left atrium mimicking cor triatriatum. The left atrial cavity recorded behind the aortic valve (AV) demonstrates moving echoes (E) reminiscent of cor triatriatum or supravalvular membrane. At surgery a small atrial septal defect was found with a small distorted left atrial cavity. The echo findings probably result from dilatation of the pulmonary veins but also resemble the findings of a common pulmonary venous chamber seen in total anomaly of the pulmonary venous return. A dilated coronary sinus may also present a similar echo pattern. This case illustrates the difficulty of separating these entities echocardiographically. ECG, electrocardiogram.

11-15). At surgery no membrane was found, but the left atrial cavity was small and distorted. We speculate that the echo findings resulted from dilatation of the pulmonary veins, whose lumen appeared to add depth to the left atrium while the edges of the orifice moved vigorously in the beam and created an echo source behind the aortic root.

Ebstein's anomaly

Anatomic and functional changes. This malformation chiefly affects the attachment of the tricuspid valve, which is displaced from its normal position at the atrioventricular ring into the right ventricular cavity (Fig. 11-16). All of the leaflets may not be displaced, and the anterior leaflet, which is the one most easily detected by echocardiog-

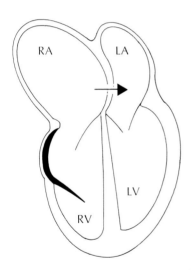

Fig. 11-16. Ebstein's anomaly. The attachment of one or more leaflets of the tricuspid valve is displaced downward into the right ventricular cavity (RV). This results in incorporation of a portion of the anatomic right ventricle into the functional right atrium (RA). Thinning of the walls of the "atrialized" right ventricle may be present. The right atrium is further dilated by functional tricuspid stenosis or incompetence and right-to-left shunting may occur across a foramen ovale or a secundum atrial septal defect, which is commonly present. The atrial septum may bulge into the left atrium (LA). LV, left ventricle.

raphy, may be very elongated and redundant. Other leaflets may be shortened. The right ventricular cavity is shortened as the result of tricuspid valve displacement, while the right atrium becomes markedly enlarged. The portion of the right ventricle that becomes part of the right atrium is said to be atrialized and may show thinning of its walls, including the ventricular septum. The tricuspid valve may show some functional stenosis or insufficiency, depending on the nature of the deformity. An atrial septal defect is commonly present with a right-to-left shunt so that some cyanosis occurs.

Clinical summary. Cyanosis is variable and may not appear until later in life. Variable murmurs occur, and the ECG shows right bundle branch block and prolonged P-R intervals, evidence of right atrial enlargement, but no evidence of right ventricular hypertrophy. Auscultatory findings may mimic mitral or tricuspid valve stenosis. The chest roentgenogram reveals an enormous right atrium and decreased filling of the pulmonary vessels. Cardiac catheterization shows the degree of right-to-left shunting, an elevated right atrial pressure, and a normal right ventricular pressure. Angiocardiography shows the tricuspid valve displacement characteristic of Ebstein's anomaly, right atrial enlargement, and the presence of the right-to-left atrial shunt.

Echocardiographic features
• The characteristic feature of Ebstein's anomaly is delayed closure of the tricuspid valve as compared to the mitral, probably related to atrialization and reduced pumping capacity of the right ventricle (Fig. 11-17). A difference of 40 msec or more is considered diagnostic, though this finding is not present in all cases.
• The tricuspid valve is detected considerably to the left of its usual position. The anterior leaflet may appear unusually large and tends to dominate the echocardiographic examination. Beam sweeping demonstrates that the tricuspid valve is present in the beam over wider angular displacement than the mitral valve. The tricuspid valve may be recorded simultaneously with the mitral

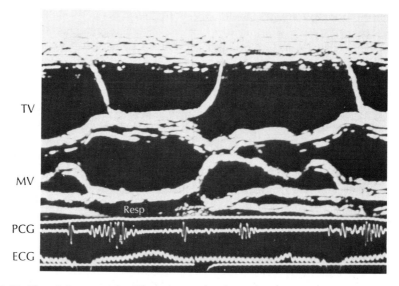

Fig. 11-17. Ebstein's anomaly. The tricuspid valve (TV) is prominently recorded and demonstrates markedly delayed closure as compared to the mitral valve (MV). Resp, respiration; PCG, phonocardiogram; ECG, electrocardiogram.

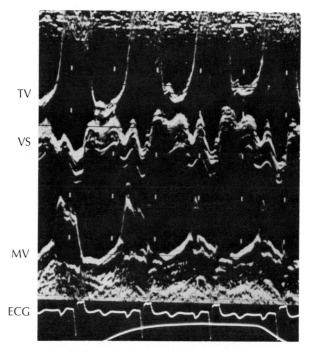

Fig. 11-18. Ventricular septum in Ebstein's anomaly. The ventricular septum (VS) is recorded in its usual position between the tricuspid valve (TV) and the mitral valve (MV). Normal septal motion has been replaced by a bizarre pattern that is primarily paradoxical in systole with a systolic dip and a sharp peak at the time of atrioventricular valve opening. This motion pattern probably arises from the effects of atrialization of the ventricular septum. Note that the closure of the tricuspid valve is significantly delayed as compared to the mitral. ECG, electrocardiogram.

valve and in front of the aortic root, even in adult patients.

• Septal motion may be paradoxical or bizarre. The atrialized portion of the septum appears thin, and its motion pattern is different from a normal septum (Fig. 11-18).

Comments

• It is useful to try to record the tricuspid valve and mitral valve together for comparison of the time of closure (C point) of both leaflets. The EF slope of the tricuspid valve may be flattened from associated functional stenosis or from reduced compliance of the right ventricle. An intracardiac conduction defect of the right bundle branch block type may also produce a late tricuspid valve closure of up to 30 msec. Uhl's anomaly (in which the right ventricle is papery thin) may also show delayed tricuspid valve closure of the type seen in Ebstein's anomaly.

• The pulmonary valve opening and closing movements may be markedly delayed as compared to the aortic valve due to the reduced pumping capacity of the right ventricle (Fig. 11-19).

• The mitral valve may be small and difficult to visualize. The left ventricular cavity is generally small, and in some patients the left ventricular posterior wall may show poor motion, representing true ventricular dysfunction or attenuated motion due to nonperpendicular relationship of the wall to the ultrasonic beam secondary to displacement of the left ventricle by the enlarged right atrium.

• Mitral and tricuspid valve prolapse as well as bicuspid aortic valves have been observed by us in association with this anomaly (Fig. 11-20).

• The right atrium may be so large that the atrial septum is displaced posteriorly and laterally into a position where it can be recorded behind the ventricular septum (Fig. 11-21).

Role of echocardiography. Marked delay in tricuspid valve closure is highly specific and can verify the clinical diagnosis and occasionally demonstrates an unsuspected case. Because of variability of anatomic findings, Ebstein's anomaly cannot be ruled out by ultrasonic examination.

Overriding tricuspid valve

This is a rare lesion in which the tricuspid valve ring is directed into the right and left ventricles. The tricuspid valve straddles the interventricular septum, and the right ventricle is underdeveloped. The septal leaflet of the tricuspid valve may have attachment to papillary muscles in the left ventricle, and the upper part of the ventricular septum is absent. Dextrotransposition of the

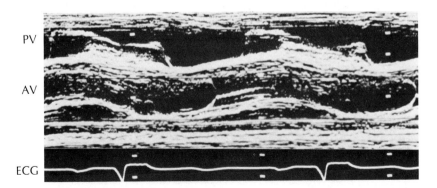

Fig. 11-19. Simultaneous recording of the pulmonic and aortic valves in Ebstein's anomaly. Pulmonic valve (PV) closure is markedly delayed as compared to the aortic valve (AV). The opening movement of the pulmonary valve is also delayed. Both findings probably result from inefficient pumping of the reduced right ventricular chamber. ECG, electrocardiogram.

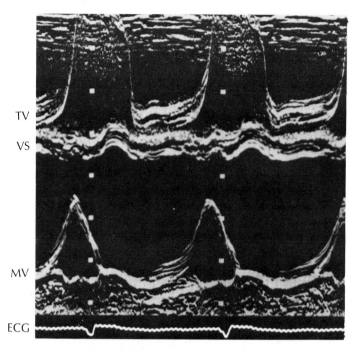

Fig. 11-20. Mitral valve prolapse in Ebstein's anomaly. The mitral valve shows a midsystolic step typical of mitral valve prolapse. The tricuspid valve shows a large amplitude of motion; its closure is markedly delayed as compared to the mitral valve. TV, tricuspid valve; VS, ventricular septum; MV, mitral valve; ECG, electrocardiogram.

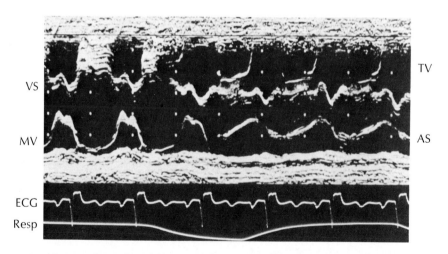

Fig. 11-21. Abnormal position of the atrial septum in Ebstein's anomaly. The beam has been angled from the mitral valve (MV) recording position medially into the usual tricuspid valve (TV) position. The atrial septum (AS) is identified by its continuity with the mitral valve. The ventricular septum (VS) shows an abnormal motion pattern from partial atrialization and can be seen lying between the tricuspid valve and the atrial septum. The displacement of the atrial septum posteriorly toward the outflow portion of the left atrium and mitral valve produced by a very large right atrium allows the beam to pass through the tricuspid valve, ventricular septum, and atrial septum in this unusual combination of anatomic findings. ECG, electrocardiogram; Resp, respirations.

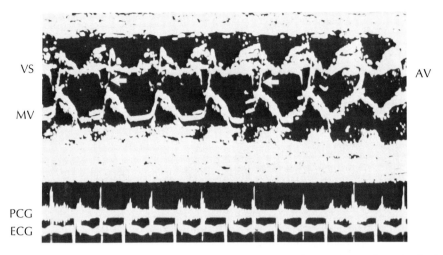

Fig. 11-22. Overriding tricuspid valve. The linear moving echo pattern *(arrow)* in the left ventricular outflow tract probably represents the septal leaflet of the tricuspid valve, which at autopsy was shown to have chordal attachments to the margins of a high ventricular septal defect of the type seen in atrioventricular canal defects. The motion pattern is bizarre, probably from the influence of the shunt, the abnormal position of the leaflet in both ventricular cavities, and from the anomalous attachment of chordae. The ventricular septal image (VS) is also abnormal and thin from tissue deficiency in this area. MV, mitral valve, AV, aortic valve; PCG, phonocardiogram; ECG, electrocardiogram.

great vessels is frequently present. Scans of the long axis of the left ventricle show the septum ending in the middle of the tricuspid valve, and tricuspid septal leaflet echoes are present below the level of the left side of the septum. They may also be seen in the left ventricular outflow tract in front of the mitral valve (Fig. 11-22). In extreme cases (double inlet left ventricle) both atrioventricular valves are demonstrated in the left ventricle. It is important to define the interventricular septum and to show that it does not separate the tricuspid valve and the mitral valve.

Complete atrioventricular canal defects

Anatomic and functional changes. Complete development of the endocardial cushions divides the primitive atrioventricular canal into right- and left-sided components. Abnormal development results in persistence of a portion of the embryonic atrioventricular canal so that the basal portion of the atrial septum and upper portion of the ventricular septum fail to meet and fuse

normally. A complex central defect results, which may allow mixing of blood from all four chambers. Since the cushions also contribute to the development of the atrioventricular valve leaflets and their rings, abnormalities of these structures are always present. A single large annulus is usually present to which the leaflets of a common atrioventricular valve are attached (Fig. 11-23). The common atrioventricular valve also may be divided into mitral and tricuspid components. Clefts in the tricuspid and mitral valves occur, and atrioventricular valve regurgitation is common.

Since blood flow can potentially occur between any of the four chambers of the heart, generalized cardiac enlargement and hypertrophy are common. Increased flow through the pulmonary vascular bed from the left-to-right shunting results in the early development of pulmonary hypertension. When severe, this results in right-to-left shunting and, therefore, cyanosis. This cardiac lesion is often seen in patients with Down's syndrome.

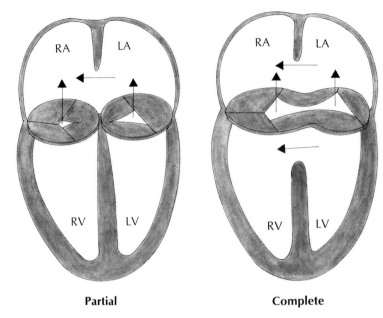

Partial   Complete

Fig. 11-23. Functional anatomy in atrioventricular canal defects. In partial canal defects a low atrial septal defect (ostium primum variety) allows shunting to occur at the atrial level. Clefts in the mitral and occasionally the tricuspid valve result in valvular regurgitation. The atrioventricular valves lie at the same level but are separate and the ventricular septum is intact. In the complete form of the defect, shunting also occurs at the ventricular level, since the upper portion of the ventricular septum is also defective. The atrioventricular valve rings are continuous and valve elements extend across the single ring, forming a common atrioventricular valve. RA, right atrium; LA, left atrium; RV, right ventricle; LV, left ventricle.

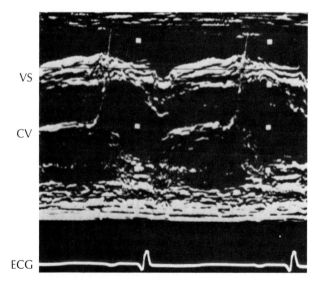

Fig. 11-24. Common atrioventricular canal defect. A common atrioventricular valve (CV) having a large amplitude of motion is recorded and appears to cross the ventricular septum as it opens in diastole. VS, ventricular septum; ECG, electrocardiogram.

Clinical summary. Growth and development are retarded, and heart failure occurs frequently. Murmurs may be absent when pressures are balanced, or murmurs of atrioventricular valve regurgitation, atrial septal defect, or ventricular septal defect may be present. The ECG may show combined ventricular and atrial hypertrophy. The chest roentgenogram reveals generalized enlargement of all chambers and pulmonary vas-

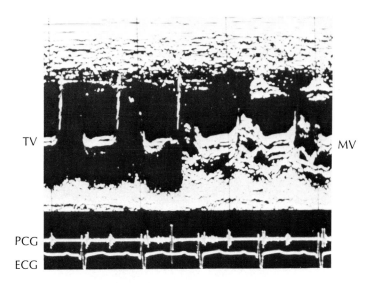

Fig. 11-25. Common atrioventricular canal defect. Demonstration of continuity between two components of the common atrioventricular valve showing systolic positions at identical depths from the chest wall. TV, tricuspid valve; MV, mitral valve; PCG, phonocardiogram; ECG, electrocardiogram. (From Nanda, N. C., and others: Ultrasound Med. **1:**19, 1975.)

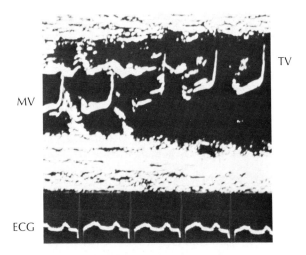

Fig. 11-26. Demonstration of a steplike continuity between the mitral and tricuspid valves in a patient with complete atrioventricular canal defect. MV, mitral valve; TV, tricuspid valve; ECG, electrocardiogram. (From Nanda, N. C., and others: Ultrasound Med. **1:**19, 1975.)

cular engorgement. Cardiac catheterization shows a free and bizarre passage of the catheter into all chambers, and angiocardiography demonstrates the anatomy of the defect as well as atrioventricular valve incompetence.

Echocardiographic features

• Separate tricuspid and mitral valves can be imaged in their expected anterior and posterior positions.

• A beam position closer to the aortic root may show that the mitral valve appears to pass through the ventricular septum as it opens in diastole (Fig. 11-24).

• A somewhat different beam position may demonstrate an apparent single leaflet that lies deep at the mitral level in systole but opens far anteriorly into the level of the tricuspid valve in diastole (Fig. 11-25). The septal image is absent in this region. Two large leaflets moving in opposite directions or two smaller leaflets moving parallel to each other have also been observed.

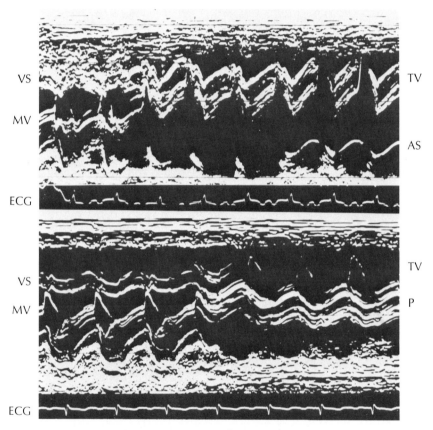

Fig. 11-27. Complete atrioventricular canal defect. A scan between the mitral (MV) and tricuspid (TV) components of a common atrioventricular valve depicts a staircase continuity of the valve leaflets attached to a common atrioventricular ring. The ventricular component of the septal defect is represented by an apparent thinning of the ventricular septum (VS), through which the valve appears to move. The atrial septal component is demonstrated by a lack of normal continuity between the mitral component and the atrial septal image (AS), which appears unattached and lies deep to the tricuspid component. After repair *(lower panel)* the surgically inserted patch (P) reestablishes continuity between the mitral valve and the atrial septum. ECG, electrocardiogram. (From Nanda, N. C., and others: Ultrasound Med. **2:**1, 1976.)

• Continuous scans from the mitral to tricuspid components of the abnormal atrioventricular valve complex show an abrupt termination of the interventricular septum and a staircase continuity of the position of the systolic segments of a common atrioventricular valve (Fig. 11-26).

• The atrial septal image appears to be unattached in these scans and to lose continuity with the mitral component of the common atrioventricular valve (Fig. 11-27). It also lies at a greater depth than seen in normal subjects or may be unrecordable. Occasionally, it may show high-frequency fluttering in systole and diastole, probably from complex shunting and turbulence at its lower, free edge (Fig. 11-28).

Comments

• Differentiation of the various forms of atrioventricular canal defects may be difficult or impossible. Separate mitral and tricuspid valves of a partial defect may appear like a common atrioventricular valve, probably because the wide beam fails to recognize the separation between them. Clefts in the atrioventricular valves may also escape detection, and double or multilayered atrioventricular valve images have proved unreliable in making this diagnosis. In two instances where the cleft mitral valve developed as a double orifice formed by a bridge of cusp tissue extending from the anterior segment of the anterior leaflet to the posterior leaflet, we observed a dense mass of linear echoes in the region of the mitral valve simulating a mass (Fig. 11-29).

• The finding of a mitral leaflet that appears to pass through the ventricular septum has been considered to be an important diagnostic point in identifying the ventricular septal defect that differentiates complete from partial (ostium primum ASD) canal defects. Recent work suggests that this may be a less reliable finding, since it has been seen occasionally in patients with a partial canal defect.

The staircase appearance is also less specific since we have encountered it in a patient with tricuspid atresia and in another with a partial canal defect.

• The abnormal attachment of the mitral valve results in a narrow left ventricular outflow tract with prolonged diastolic mitral-septal apposition also in patients who have

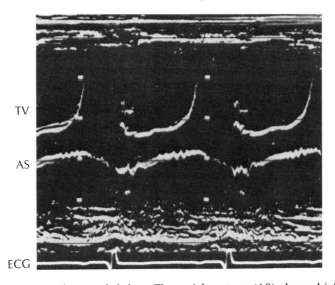

Fig. 11-28. Atrioventricular canal defect. The atrial septum (AS) shows high-frequency fluttering in systole and diastole, probably from complex shunting and turbulence present at its lower, free edge. TV, tricuspid valve; ECG, electrocardiogram.

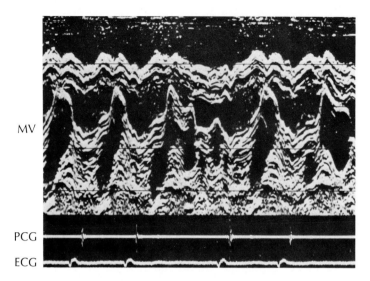

Fig. 11-29. Mitral valve recording in a patient with partial atrioventricular canal defect and "double" mitral orifice. Dense bands of echoes behind the mitral valve in both systole and diastole probably arise from tissue bridges connecting the two leaflets to form the double orifice. Absence of abnormal echoes in the left atrial cavity behind the aortic root excluded the presence of a mass lesion. MV, mitral valve; PCG, phonocardiogram; ECG, electrocardiogram.

complete defects. The abnormal ventricular septal motion is, in our experience, not a common feature with this entity.

Role of echocardiography. This defect can be recognized in patients whose clinical presentation may be atypical. In most instances, however, the echocardiographic examination confirms a clinical diagnosis. Usually, the separation of complete from partial canals can be made but may be difficult if the ventricular component of the defect is small or when a partial canal resembles a complete canal as judged by atrioventricular valve findings.

Tetralogy of Fallot

Anatomic and functional changes. Tetralogy of Fallot consists of four anatomic defects: infundibular stenosis, ventricular septal defect, right ventricular hypertrophy, and an abnormal anterior position of the aorta that overrides the defective interventricular septum (Fig. 11-30). The right ventricle and aorta become enlarged, whereas the main pulmonary artery and the pulmonary vessels in the lungs remain small. Valvular pulmo-

nary stenosis occurs commonly. In extreme cases, there may be atresia of the pulmonary artery.

When the degree of infundibular stenosis is severe, right heart pressures equal systemic, and shunting takes place from the right ventricle directly into the overriding aorta. Cyanosis is usually intense (as in the blue baby syndrome), but if the degree of infundibular stenosis is mild, the shunt may be small with little cyanosis (pink tetralogy).

Clinical summary. These patients may be intensely cyanotic and show clubbing of the tips of the fingers and toes. When they become fatigued, they frequently assume a squatting position, which probably decreases systemic venous return and increases peripheral resistance and therefore decreases the magnitude of the right-to-left shunt. Polycythemia is present, and cerebral thrombosis and abscess formation are commonly associated with tetralogy of Fallot. A systolic murmur is produced by the infundibular stenosis, and the pulmonic element of the second heart sound is soft or absent.

The chest roentgenogram shows a boot-

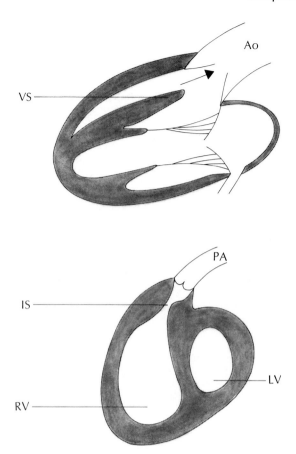

Fig. 11-30. Anatomic features of tetralogy of Fallot. A long-axis section of the left ventricle reveals a high ventricular septal defect and an enlarged aorta (Ao), which is anteriorly displaced so that it overrides the defective ventricular septum (VS) and receives blood from both ventricles. A sagittal section through the right heart *(below)* shows right ventricular hypertrophy and enlargement, an area of infundibular stenosis (IS) and a pulmonary artery (PA), which is small. LV, left ventricle.

shaped heart in which the apex appears elevated from the diaphragm, marked narrowing at the base of the heart from underdevelopment of the pulmonary artery, and reduction in the pulmonary vascular markings.

Cardiac catheterization reveals right ventricular pressures equal to left ventricular pressures and low pressures in the pulmonary artery. The oxygen saturation of blood in the left ventricle and aorta is reduced from right-to-left shunting. The catheter passes directly from the right ventricle into the aorta demonstrating the overriding. Angiocardiography shows the site and size of the ventricular septal defect, the degree of overrid-

ing, the location and nature of the infundibular stenosis, and the size and status of the pulmonary artery and valve.

Echocardiographic features

• Normal continuity between the interventricular septum and the anterior aortic root margin is disrupted, and the aorta is positioned more anteriorly so that it straddles or overrides the septum (Fig. 11-31).

• The aortic root is enlarged.

• The pulmonary valve is difficult to detect.

Comments

• The degree of aortic overriding may be difficult to judge. Very low beam positions tend to minimize the extent of overriding; very high positions tend to accentuate the separation between the interventricular septum and the anterior aortic margin. The best starting point for scans made into the aortic root is with transducer perpendicular to the chest wall over the mitral valve. With proper scanning procedure the degree of aortic overriding may be as accurately estimated as it can with angiocardiography.

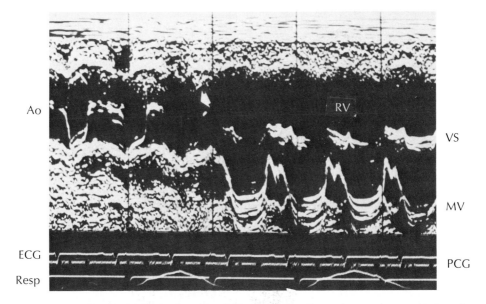

Fig. 11-31. Tetralogy of Fallot. Ultrasonic beam scanning from the aortic root (Ao) to the mitral valve (MV) shows loss of normal continuity between the anterior aortic margin and the ventricular septum (VS). The aortic root is dilated and overrides the ventricular septum. The arrow represents the subaortic ventricular septal defect. The mitral valve retains continuity with the posterior aortic margin. The mitral valve also shows pansystolic sagging, a relatively common finding in this entity. RV, right ventricle; PCG, phonocardiogram; ECG, electrocardiogram; Resp, respiration. (From Nanda, N. C.: Am. J. Med. **62:**836, 1977.)

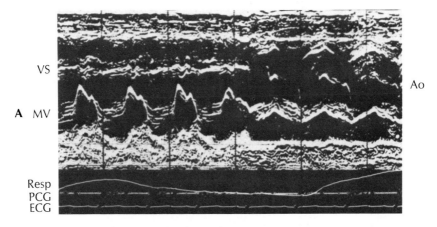

Fig. 11-32. For legend see opposite page.

• Surgical correction of this lesion involves closing the ventricular septal defect with a patch that can be demonstrated echocardiographically as a source of thick echoes between the ventricular septum and the anterior aortic margin. Alignment is restored to normal so that mitral-septal discontinuity is no longer present (Fig. 11-32). In some cases, we have seen early systolic preclosure of the aortic valve leaflets, which may be related to turbulent flow produced by the patch.

• Surgical patches may become partially detached and result in reestablishment of the ventricular septal defect. These usually can-

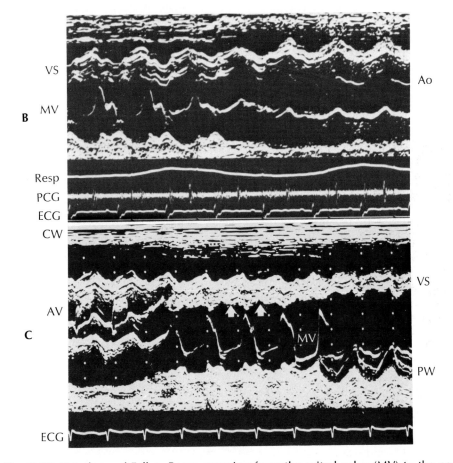

Fig. 11-32. Tetralogy of Fallot. Beam scanning from the mitral valve (MV) to the aorta (Ao) in a patient with tetralogy of Fallot **(A)** shows discontinuity between the ventricular septum (VS) and the anterior aortic margin with the aorta straddling the ventricular septum. **B** was obtained following surgical correction and demonstrates continuity between the septum and anterior aortic margin with restoration of alignment. The septal image appears thicker than the preoperative recording, probably as the result of the surgically inserted patch. Resp, respiratory excursion; PCG, phonocardiogram; ECG, electrocardiogram. **C,** The beam is swept from the aortic valve (AV) to the left ventricular cavity in a patient with tetralogy of Fallot following surgical repair. Dense echoes from the patch *(arrows)*, mimicking a thickened ventricular septum, are observed in front of the mitral valve (MV). A normal-appearing septum (VS) is delineated as the beam is angled further into the left ventricular cavity. The aortic valve shows early systolic preclosure of both right and noncoronary cusps, probably related to turbulence produced by the patch. There was no evidence for left ventricular outflow obstruction. CW, chest wall; PW, left ventricular posterior wall; ECG, electrocardiogram.

not be detected by echocardiography unless the degree of detachment is extreme.

• The mitral valve may close very deep to the aortic root and resemble the findings of a double outlet right ventricle. This can be a very difficult differential diagnosis. In older children with tetralogy of Fallot the mitral valve often sags posteriorly during systole in a pattern indistinguishable from mitral valve prolapse. There are usually no clinical findings to support this diagnosis, and caution in interpretation should be exercised.

• Pulmonary valve identification is important in differentiating tetralogy of Fallot from truncus arteriosus, which also shows overriding of the ventricular septum. This can be accomplished in about 50% to 60% of patients with tetralogy of Fallot and should be sought diligently in all patients.

• Isolated infundibular stenosis may produce coarse systolic fluttering of the pulmonary valve leaflet, but this has not been useful in our experience in tetralogy of Fallot. Direct ultrasonic visualization of the infundibular stenosis is not attainable by present M-mode techniques.

Role of echocardiography. Echocardiography can identify aortic overriding and es-timate its severity. Tetralogy of Fallot can be diagnosed if the pulmonary valve is identified in its usual position and differentiated from truncus arteriosus, which also demonstrates aortic overriding.

Truncus arteriosus

Anatomic and functional changes. In the embryo the great vessels are represented by a single common trunk, which later divides to form the pulmonary artery and aorta. If this division fails to take place, a single great vessel persists (truncus arteriosus, common trunk, truncal vessel). The main pulmonary artery may arise as a short stem from the truncus (Fig. 11-33) and then divide into right and left branches, or the two branches may arise separately from the posterior or lateral walls of the trunk. In one type, pulmonary arteries are absent, and the lungs are served by bronchial vessels arising from the descending aorta. A ventricular septal defect and overriding of the truncal vessel relative to the defective ventricular septum are always present. Both ventricular chambers, therefore, empty directly into the truncal vessel. The truncal valve is often abnormal and may be thickened and fleshy in charac-

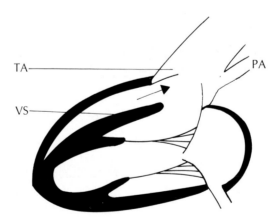

Fig. 11-33. Truncus arteriosus. The truncus arteriosus (TA) overrides a defective ventricular septum (VS) and serves as a single outflow vessel for both ventricles. In this illustration a small main pulmonary artery (PA) is shown arising from the truncus near its base. In other varieties of this anomaly, right and left pulmonary branches arise directly from the trunk, or the pulmonary arteries are absent and the blood supply to the lung is via bronchial arteries that arise from the descending aorta.

ter. Often there are more leaflets than in a normal semilunar valve, and truncal valve incompetence is relatively common. The right ventricular outflow tract is absent in this anomaly.

Blood flow to the lungs varies from in-creased to markedly diminished, depending on the size and number of vessels that arise from the truncal vessel to supply the lungs.

Clinical summary. The degree of cyanosis varies, depending on the blood supply to the lungs. The presence of a large dilated truncal

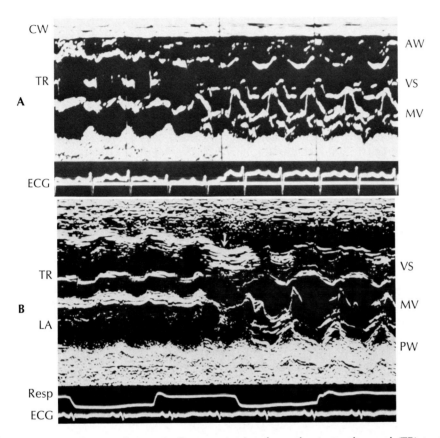

Fig. 11-34. Truncus arteriosus. **A,** Beam scanning from the truncal vessel (TR) to the mitral valve (MV) demonstrates marked overriding of the ventricular septum (VS). The anterior wall of the truncal vessel is continuous with the right ventricular anterior wall (AW), whereas the mitral valve is aligned with the posterior truncal wall. Mediastinal tissue separates the truncus from the chest wall (CW). The right ventricular outflow tract is absent. ECG, electrocardiogram. **B,** This echocardiogram was obtained in a patient with truncus arteriosus following surgery during which the ventricular septal defect was closed by a patch and the right ventricular blood directed to the main pulmonary artery by an extracardiac conduit containing a porcine prosthesis. The ultrasonic beam was swept from the truncus (TR) to the left ventricular cavity. Continuity between the anterior truncal wall and the ventricular septum (VS) has been restored by the patch *(arrow),* which presents as a thick, multilayered echo complex. The patch seems to protrude into the left ventricular outflow and resulted in obstruction to blood flow in this patient. Cardiac catheterization revealed a gradient of 55 mm Hg across the left ventricular outflow. PW, left ventricular posterior wall; MV, mitral valve; Resp, respiration; ECG, electrocardiogram.

vessel may be suspected because of the presence of an ejection click and a systolic murmur. At times, the murmur may be continuous in systole and diastole with the diastolic component related to blood flow to the lungs. The second heart sound contains only one component, since only a single semilunar valve is present.

The chest roentgenogram shows the mediastinum widened by the truncal vessel and ocassionally the abnormal pulmonary arteries which arise directly from the truncus. Cardiac catheterization reveals systemic pressures in the right ventricle, direct passage of the catheter into the truncal vessel, and absence of the pulmonary arteries in their usual site. Angiocardiography demonstrates the large truncal vessel straddling the interventricular septum and the pulmonary arteries that arise from the truncus.

Echocardiographic features

• The truncus overrides the ventricular septum (Fig. 11-34).

• The truncal vessel is usually somewhat larger than the aorta in tetralogy of Fallot.

• Truncal valve leaflets may appear abnormal or multiple.

• The mitral and tricuspid valves may flutter in diastole in the presence of truncal valve insufficiency.

Comments

• The echocardiographic diagnosis of truncus arteriosus may be difficult in certain forms of this anomaly. In those cases where the pulmonary artery arises from the base of the trunk, it may be possible to echo a smaller second vessel that does not contain valve leaflets and that lies at about the same depth as the trunk. In these cases, a false diagnosis of tetralogy of Fallot may be made. Demonstration of valve leaflets in two separate outflow vessels rules out truncus arteriosus.

• The right ventricular outflow tract is always absent in truncus arteriosus. Any space lying in front of the truncal vessel should be

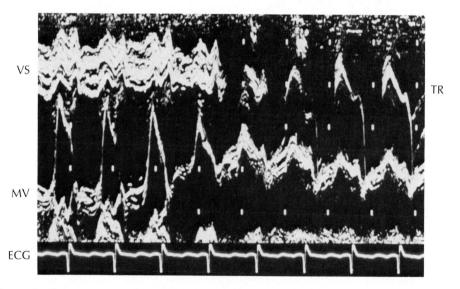

Fig. 11-35. Beam scanning from the mitral to the aortic valve in truncus arteriosus. The anterior truncal wall may be difficult to image since the right ventricular outflow tract is absent and the truncal wall lies in the near field of the transducer. In these instances the truncal valve (TR) may be mistaken for the anterior leaflet of the tricuspid valve unless careful attention is paid to beam direction during recording. When this question arises, immediate search for the tricuspid valve in the normal position will clarify the true anatomic findings. VS, ventricular septum; MV, mitral valve; ECG, electrocardiogram.

inspected carefully while searching for a moving anterior wall that will differentiate the right ventricular outflow tract from mediastinal tissue interposed between the trunk and chest wall (Fig. 11-34).

• Isolated images of the posterior cusp of the truncus may mimic a tricuspid valve recording especially when the anterior wall is not recorded or obscured by anterior reverberatory clutter (Fig. 11-35).

Role of echocardiography. Echocardiography may support the clinical diagnosis, but differentiation from tetralogy of Fallot is extremely difficult. Truncus arteriosus can be ruled out when a pulmonic valve is demonstrated.

Transposition complexes

Transposition of the great arteries

Anatomic and functional changes. When the fetus is approximately three weeks old, the primitive cardiac tube begins its earliest changes, which ultimately transform it into a four-chambered heart. As the tube grows, it folds or loops on itself with its convexity to the right (D-looping), and this results in the right ventricle being located anteriorly while the left ventricle is situated more posteriorly. The atrioventricular valves passively follow their respective ventricles so that the three-leaflet tricuspid valve fits between the right atrium and the right ventricle; the two-leaflet mitral valve is located between the left atrium and the left ventricle. The upper portion of this tube (common trunk or truncus arteriosus) divides into two portions, which ultimately form the aorta and the pulmonary artery. Ridges appear on the common trunk and grow spirally, resulting in twisting of the common trunk so that the origin of the aorta is posterior and leftward and the pulmonary root is located anteriorly and to the right.

The developmental error that results in dextrotransposition of the great vessels is incompletely understood. Current theories suggest that the division of the common trunk occurs in a different plane and that the normal spiraling of the great vessels is disrupted. As a result the aorta arises from the anterior or right ventricle while the pulmonary artery comes off from the posterior or left ventricle (Fig. 11-36). The root of the aorta is anterior, superior, and rightward in its location, whereas the pulmonary root is situated posteriorly, inferiorly, and to the left. The right ventricular outflow is situated immediately below the aortic root, and the normal continuity between the aortic root and the mitral valve is lost. On the other hand, continuity between the pulmonary valve and the mitral valve is present. The right ventricle pumps systemic venous blood into the aorta while the pulmonary artery carries pulmonary venous blood from the left ventricle back to the lungs. Thus the arterial and venous circuits are isolated, and shunting through septal defects or a patent ductus must be present to allow some systemic venous blood to reach the lungs and oxygenated blood to flow into the aorta. Coexisting lesions such as single ventricle and subpulmonic stenosis may occur.

If, during embryologic growth, the loop does not twist to the right but rather to the left (L-loop), the side-to-side relationship of the transposed vessels is reversed so that the pulmonary root is displaced more rightward as compared to the aortic root. The condition is called L-transposition. L-looping may also result in some cases in inversion of the ventricles so that the anatomic right ventricle is situated posteriorly and is connected to the pulmonary artery, while the anatomic left ventricle is displaced anteriorly and is continuous with the aorta. This form of L-transposition is commonly called corrected transposition of the great vessels, since the systemic venous blood from the right ventricle is pumped into the pulmonary circuit while the pulmonary venous blood is channeled into the aorta. Although the circulation is normal in an uncomplicated case, other intracardiac defects such as a ventricular septal defect with or without pulmonary hypertension or pulmonary stenosis frequently coexist with this entity.

Clinical summary. The diagnosis of dextrotransposition of the great vessels can be suspected in an infant who has minimal-to-mod-

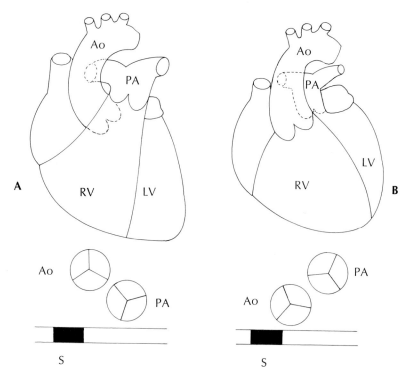

Fig. 11-36. Anatomy of dextrotransposition of the great vessels. In the normal heart **(A)**, the right ventricle (RV) is continuous with the pulmonary artery (PA), whereas the left ventricle (LV) and aorta (Ao) are in continuity. In dextrotransposition of the great vessels **(B)**, the aorta arises from the right ventricle and the pulmonary artery is connected to the left ventricle. Normally, the aortic valve (*dashed lines* in **A**) lies deep and medial to the pulmonary valve. This relationship is reversed in dextrotransposition of the great vessels so that the aorta is now anterior to the pulmonary artery (*dashed lines* in **B**). A schematic representation of the spatial position of the semilunar valves is shown below the anatomic sketches with the sternum (S) as a landmark.

erate cyanosis, no significant murmurs, and a single second sound (usually represents closure of the aortic valve close to the chest wall). The chest roentgenogram shows an enlarged heart. Cardiac catheterization demonstrates systemic pressures in the right ventricle, the aorta arising from the right ventricle, and the pulmonary artery arising from the left ventricle. Angiocardiography shows the altered great vessel relationship. The patient with corrected transposition of the great arteries without intracardiac defects has a normally functioning heart and may well go unrecognized as having congenital heart disease. However, the presence of associated intracardiac defects may bring him to the attention of the physician.

Echocardiographic detection techniques
• Normally, the anteriorly situated vessel (pulmonary root) is detected by lateral transducer angulation, whereas the posteriorly located vessel (aortic root) is identified by relatively medial transducer direction. In patients with dextrotransposition complex, this relationship is reversed. This results in the detection of the anteriorly placed aorta by medial beam angulation, while the posteriorly located pulmonary artery is identified more laterally (Fig. 11-37). This method depends on meticulous observation at the time of the examination of the transducer directions required to image the outflow vessels, and one may not be able to deduce the true identity of the vessel from mere inspection

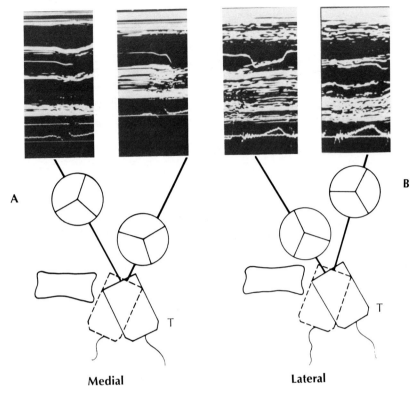

Fig. 11-37. Dextrotransposition of the great vessels. The spatial distribution of the great vessels is shown schematically in the normal **(A)** and in dextrotransposition of the great vessels **(B)** in relation to the sternum and to the transducer (T) angulation required for great vessel detection. In the normal the deep outflow vessel (aorta) is detected with medial beam angulation, whereas lateral angulation is required for the anteriorly situated pulmonary artery. In dextrotransposition of the great vessels, this relationship is reversed so that the anterior vessel (aorta) is found medially placed, whereas the deep vessel (pulmonary artery) requires lateral beam angulation. Representative ultrasonic traces show that the individual vessels cannot be recognized by their appearances, emphasizing the need for information concerning their spatial distribution.

of echocardiographic records. In levotransposition, two great vessels can be identified in the same positions seen in normal subjects, though the posterior vessel is the pulmonary artery and the anterior vessel is the aorta. For this reason, great vessel position detection is not adequate to diagnose levotransposition.

• Another useful method in the diagnosis of transposition is based on the fact that the pulmonary valve, which lies in a low resistance-low pressure circuit, closes later than the aortic valve. Comparison of the time intervals between the R wave of the electrocardiogram and the closure points of semilunar valves, therefore, can be used to determine whether they are part of a high (aorta) or low pressure system (pulmonary artery; Fig. 11-38). It is necessary to select cardiac cycles of equal length for this measurement technique. In this manner, levotransposition can be identified, since the vessel that lies in the anatomic position of the normal aorta can then be recognized as a transposed pulmonary artery. The valve closure timing technique can also be applied in dextrotransposition to determine if the posterior vessel is a pulmonary artery, but it does not aid in the

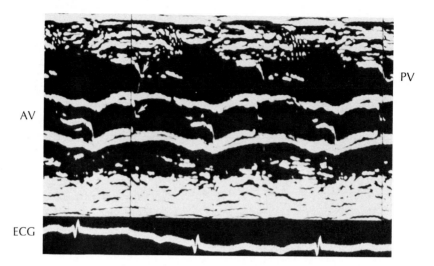

Fig. 11-38. Simultaneous recording of the pulmonary (PV) and aortic (AV) valves in a normal neonate. Delayed closure of the anterior semilunar valve as compared to the posterior *(arrow)* identifies it as the pulmonary valve and indicates normal spatial relationship of the great vessels. ECG, electrocardiogram.

separation of levotransposition and dextrotransposition. The method fails to recognize transposition in patients with equal resistances in the pulmonary and systemic circuits, since both semilunar valves will close simultaneously.

• In some cases the transposed pulmonary artery may lie directly behind the aorta so that the echocardiogram shows simultaneous recording of the two great vessels lying one in front of the other. A limitation of this techinque is the fact that both great vessels can occasionally be recorded simultaneously in infants with normally related great vessels (Fig. 11-38).

Comments

• The successful characterization of the transposition complex requires utilization of both the spatial orientation and valve closure timing methods, since both have their individual limitations. Dextrotransposition can be diagnosed by the spatial relationships alone; levotransposition requires spatial as well as valve closure timing information. The importance of intelligent observation of beam direction and the recording of valve leaflet motion in both outflow vessels cannot be overemphasized.

• We have studied over 50 patients with dextrotransposition complexes so far and have had few false diagnoses whenever the two vessels have been recorded. Difficulties arise when only one vessel is recorded. In these cases, a repeat echocardiographic examination, performed more diligently with the patient in the lateral decubitus position, may prove successful in recording both outflow vessels.

• Other congenital anomalies associated with transposition of the great arteries may be diagnosed by echocardiography. These include a single ventricle and mitral or tricuspid valve atresia. The presence of a large left atrial cavity suggests the presence of an incompetent mitral valve.

• In our experience, Ebstein's anomaly of the posteriorly located tricuspid valve commonly seen in patients with levotransposition and ventricular inversion may not result in delayed tricuspid valve closure when compared with the anteriorly placed mitral valve.

• In patients with transposition of the great vessels, effective palliation is provided by Rashkind's balloon septostomy in which an atrial septal defect is created using a special type of catheter. This results in a mixing

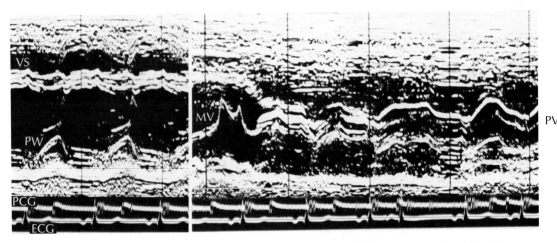

Fig. 11-39. Subvalvular narrowing in dextrotransposition of the great vessels with subpulmonic obstruction. A gradual transition of the ultrasonic beam through the mitral (MV) and pulmonary (PV) valves reveals a narrow subpulmonic segment. Echoes from the left ventricular cavity do not show evidence of asymmetric ventricular septal hypertrophy. VS, ventricular septum; PW, posterior left ventricular wall; PV, pulmonary valve; PCG, phonocardiogram; ECG, electrocardiogram. (From Nanda, N. C. and others: Circulation **51**:515, 1975. By permission of the American Heart Assn., Inc.)

of blood from the two circuits and permits survival of an infant suffering from this malformation until total physiologic correction, which entails the use of an intra-atrial baffle (Mustard's operation) is feasible. If balloon septostomy is ineffective, the atrial septum may have to be excised surgically (atrial septectomy, Blalock-Hanlon procedure).

• Diastolic fluttering of mitral and tricuspid valves is commonly seen following balloon septostomy or atrial septectomy in patients with transposition of the great vessels who have no evidence of semilunar valve insufficiency. The mechanism for this is not clear but may be related to abnormal direction of flow resulting from bidirectional shunting across the newly created atrial septal defect. Diastolic fluttering is uncommon before creation of the atrial septal defect.

Transposition of the great vessels associated with subpulmonic obstruction

Anatomic and functional changes. Obstruction in the subpulmonic area may be due to a discrete fibrous ring just below the pulmonary valve or to thickened, elongated muscle tissue. A ventricular septal defect may be associated. The left ventricle and the

ventricular septum may become hypertrophied. The pulmonary artery is usually small.

Clinical summary. The diagnosis can be suspected in an infant who has findings suggestive of transposition of the great vessels but who is more cyanotic from increased right-to-left shunting at the atrial level. The outflow obstruction may produce an ejection systolic murmur. The chest roentgenogram shows an enlarged heart with decreased pulmonary vascular markings suggestive of decreased pulmonary flow. Cardiac catheterization demonstrates a high pressure in the left ventricle and, if entered, a low pressure in the pulmonary artery. Angiocardiography identifies the type of subpulmonic stenosis and the altered great vessel relationship.

Echocardiographic features

• The majority of patients show significant apposition between the mitral valve and the ventricular septum in diastole. As mentioned previously, this is a useful echocardiographic indicator of a narrow left ventricular outflow tract.

• The width of the pulmonary artery is usually smaller than that of the aortic root. Ultrasonic demonstration of the pulmonary

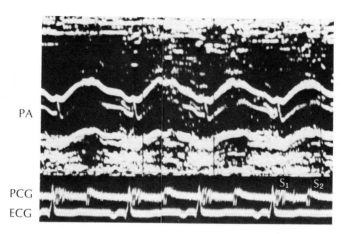

Fig. 11-40. Pulmonary valve recording in D-transposition of the great vessels associated with subpulmonic obstruction and ventricular septal defect. The pulmonary valve appears to close in early systole following brisk opening and remains closed till the next cardiac cycle. PA, pulmonary artery; PCG, phonocardiogram; S_1, first heart sound; S_2, second heart sound; ECG, electrocardiogram. (From Nanda, N. C., and others: Circulation **51**:515, 1975. By permission of the American Heart Assn., Inc.)

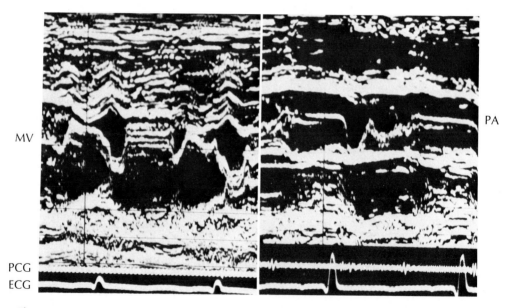

Fig. 11-41. Functional subpulmonic obstruction in dextrotransposition of the great vessels. The mitral valve (MV) shows a large abnormal systolic anterior movement (SAM) while the pulmonary valve demonstrates closure in early to mid systole with the onset of obstruction produced by the mitral SAM. PA, pulmonary artery; PCG, phonocardiogram; ECG, electrocardiogram. (From Nanda, N. C., and others: Circulation **51**:515, 1975. By permission of the American Heart Assn., Inc.)

artery larger than the aortic root is useful in excluding the presence of associated outflow obstruction in patients with transposition complexes.

• A localized area of narrowing may be delineated in the subpulmonic region by beam sweeping maneuvers from the mitral to the pulmonic valve. This is generally seen in patients with an elongated area of tunnellike obstruction (Fig. 11-39).

• A prominent movement of the pulmonary valve to its closure in early systole may be present. In some patients with associated ventricular septal defects the pulmonary valve may show no subsequent reopening until the next cardiac cycle, probably because of the runoff into the right ventricle (Fig. 11-40). Early systolic closure of the pulmonary valve may also be occasionally seen in patients with associated ventricular septal defects who have no evidence of subpulmonic stenosis.

• Abnormal systolic anterior movements of the mitral valve similar to those observed in patients with idiopathic hypertrophic subaortic stenosis may be seen occasionally (Fig. 11-41). They are often accompanied by a coarse systolic flutter or midsystolic closure of the pulmonary valve with opening later in systole, as well as by asymmetric ventricular septal hypertrophy. Additional work is required to elucidate the genesis of the observed mitral systolic abnormalities, since a recent report has indicated that they may be occasionally detected in patients with transposition who do not have outflow obstruction.

Intra-atrial baffle

Anatomic and functional changes. An intra-atrial baffle is often surgically inserted into the atrial chambers of patients with dextrotransposition of the great vessels (Mustard procedure) after excising the atrial septum (Fig. 11-42). The baffle or patch is usually constructed from the pericardium or a synthetic material (Teflon). Its atrial attachments are such that physiologic correction is achieved by directing pulmonary venous blood into the aorta through the tricuspid valve while the systemic venous return is

channeled into the pulmonary artery through the mitral orifice. This procedure has greatly improved the outlook of children with dextrotransposition of the great vessels. Complications can occur as a consequence of the use of intra-atrial baffles. These are systemic and pulmonary venous obstruction (since the baffle is attached near the insertion of these veins) and leaks in the patch resulting from shrinkage, calcification, or detachment.

Echocardiographic features

• Echoes from the intra-atrial baffle are most commonly identified behind the pulmonary root and in general consist of one or two linear signals resembling the motion pattern of an atrioventricular valve (Fig. 11-43). A sharp anterior movement occurs at the onset of diastole and is followed by flattening in mid and late diastole. In some instances a small anterior deflection may be observed during atrial systole. With the beginning of

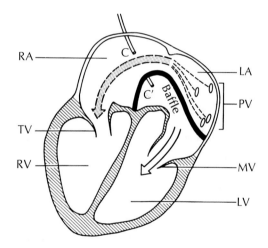

Fig. 11-42. Schematic representation of the intra-atrial baffle and its relation to various structures. The shaded arrow depicts blood flow from the pulmonary veins; the white arrow denotes systemic venous return. The atrial septum has been excised. LA, left atrium; PV, pulmonary veins; MV, mitral valve; LV, left ventricle; RV, right ventricle; TV, tricuspid valve; RA, right atrium; C and C′, catheters in front of and behind the intra-atrial baffle. (From Nanda, N. C., and others: Circulation **51:**1130, 1975. By permission of the American Heart Assn., Inc.)

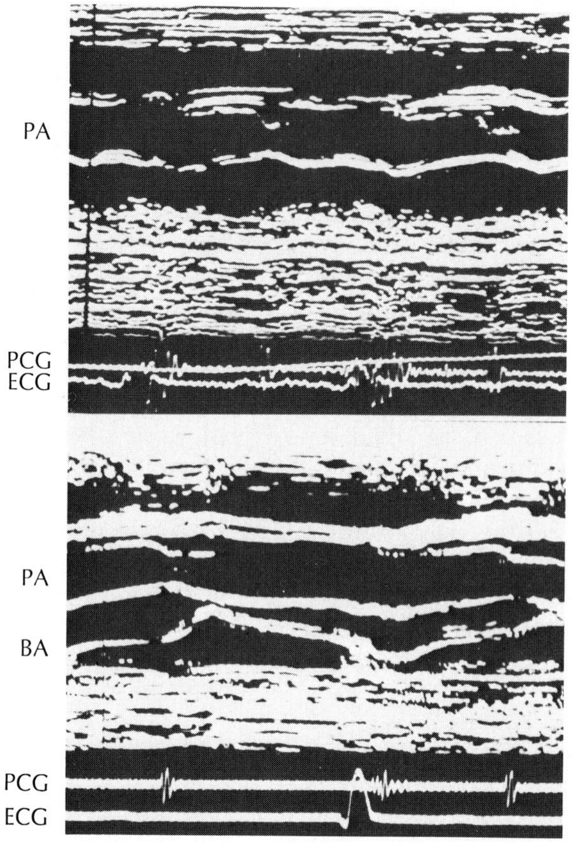

Fig. 11-43. Preoperative and postoperative pulmonary artery echocardiograms in dextrotransposition of the great vessels. *Upper panel,* Note absence of any abnormal echoes in the left atrium. *Lower panel,* Following Mustard's procedure, a linear echo having the motion pattern of a stenotic atrioventricular valve is now present in the atrial cavity behind the pulmonary artery and represents the intra-atrial baffle (BA). PA, pulmonary artery; PCG, phonocardiogram; ECG, electrocardiogram. (From Nanda, N. C., and others: Circulation **51:**1130, 1975. By permission of the American Heart Assn., Inc.)

ventricular systole, a rapid posterior movement is observed, and this is followed by no movement or very gradual anterior motion during the remainder of systole. The maximum excursion of the baffle in this region varies from 4 to 9 mm (average 6.6 mm). The space between the posterior wall of the pulmonary artery and the baffle echo represents a portion of the systemic venous atrium, whereas the echo-free zone posterior to the baffle echo is a segment of the pulmonary venous atrium. The intra-atrial baffle can also be observed as a single thick echo or a multi-layered complex with little detectable motion directly behind the tricuspid valve recording. Baffle images exhibiting larger amplitudes of motion and moving anteriorly in diastole and posteriorly in mid systole have also been recorded in the tricuspid valve region but are less common (Fig. 11-44). Occasionally, echoes from the intra-atrial baffle resembling those detected behind the pulmonary root may be seen behind the aorta or the mitral valve.

• Diastolic fluttering and undulations of both atrioventricular valves are observed in

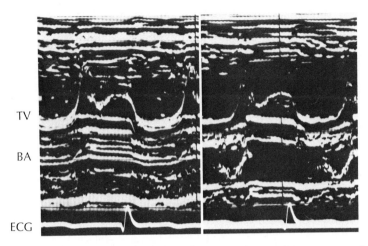

Fig. 11-44. Postoperative tricuspid valve echocardiograms in dextrotransposition of the great vessels. Multilayered images *(left)* as well as a large amplitude echo *(right)* from the intra-atrial baffle (BA) are observed behind the tricuspid valve (TV). ECG, electrocardiogram. (From Nanda, N. C., and others: Circulation **51:**1130, 1975. By permission of the American Heart Assn., Inc.)

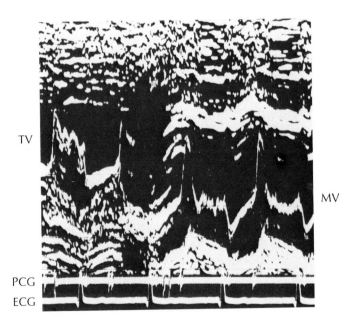

Fig. 11-45. Atrioventricular valve motion abnormalities in dextrotransposition of the great vessels following the Mustard procedure. The tricuspid valve (TV) shows undulating diastolic movements, whereas the mitral valve (MV) shows fine diastolic flutter. The thick linear echo observed behind the mitral valve originates in the intra-atrial baffle. PCG, phonocardiogram; ECG, electrocardiogram. (From Nanda, N. C., and others: Circulation **51:**1130, 1975. By permission of the American Heart Assn., Inc.)

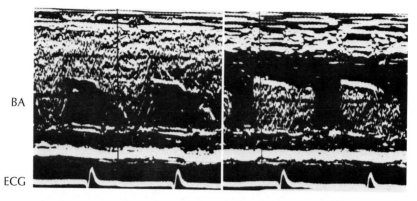

Fig. 11-46. Ultrasonic contrast studies. The intra-atrial baffle was initially imaged by a beam direction close to that used for tricuspid valve recording. Injection of indocyanine green into the pulmonary venous atrium produces echoes in front of the intra-atrial baffle (BA), which are limited by it posteriorly *(left)*, whereas injection into the systemic venous atrium results in opacification, which is confined behind the baffle *(right)*. ECG, electrocardiogram. (From Nanda, N. C., and others: Circulation **51**:1130, 1975. By permission of the American Heart Assn., Inc.)

almost all patients following the Mustard procedure (Fig. 11-45) in the absence of semilunar valve incompetence. The abnormal blood flow pathways and turbulence resulting from various insertions of the pericardial patch in the atrium may account for this finding.

• The appearance of abnormal ventricular septal motion in systole is also a common feature following the Mustard procedure. This may be a nonspecific response following open heart surgery, although tricuspid incompetence or significant shunting across a leaky baffle may be a contributory factor in some patients.

Comments

• Validation of the baffle echoes as well as of other anatomic landmarks in this area has been effected by the use of ultrasonic contrast agents through injections into catheters placed on either side of the baffle during the Mustard procedure (Fig. 11-46).

• Preliminary studies in our laboratory indicate that patients with significant baffle incompetence (from baffle detachment) show characteristic echocardiographic patterns. A prominent anterior deflection of the baffle echo recorded behind the pulmonary artery during atrial systole is the most prominent finding (Fig. 11-47). This large A-wave probably reflects increased mobility of a detached and incompetent baffle and is not observed with a competent patch. The large shunt may also produce dilatation of the pulmonary artery and enlargement of the systemic venous atrium recorded behind the pulmonary root. The unsupported baffle has also shown systolic oscillations. Normal motion patterns of the baffle return following placement of a new competent pericardial patch. Thus, serial studies of the size of the great vessels and of the newly constructed atrial chambers as well as observations of the motion pattern of the baffle echoes may provide indications of baffle dysfunction.

• We have used ultrasonic contrast injections through catheters surgically placed into the newly constructed atrial cavities to identify a leaking baffle in the immediate postoperative period (Fig. 11-48). One should be careful not to misidentify contrast reverberations (which occur posteriorly and are less dense) as evidence of leakage (Fig. 11-49).

• Baffle motion may be altered in the presence of pulmonary hypertension (Fig. 11-50).

• Resection of subpulmonic stenosis can be carried out concomitantly with the Mustard procedure but carries a high surgical mortality rate. This is mainly due to the incomplete relief of the subvalvular stenosis,

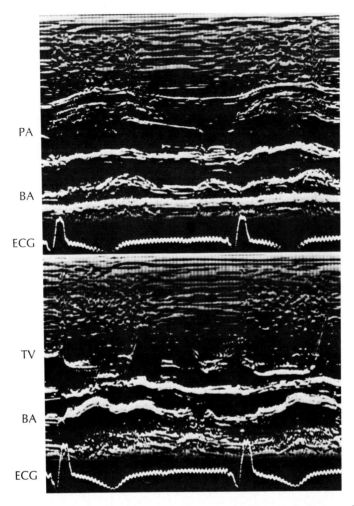

Fig. 11-47. Echocardiographic findings in baffle incompetence. *Upper panel,* a prominent deflection of the baffle recording (BA) behind the pulmonary artery (PA) is observed during atrial systole (A wave). The pulmonary artery as well as the systemic venous atrial chamber (represented by the space between the posterior pulmonary artery wall and the baffle echo) are both large in size. *Lower panel,* a prominent systolic anterior motion is seen in the baffle echo (BA) recorded behind the tricuspid valve (TV). ECG, electrocardiogram. (From Nanda, N. C., and others: Ultrasound Med. **2**:13, 1976.)

since surgical exposure of the posteriorly located left ventricle is difficult. Repair is particularly difficult in patients who have hypoplastic left ventricles and small pulmonary rings. An alternative technique that bypasses the pulmonary valve and the subvalvular region has been devised by Rastelli. In this procedure a porcine heterograft valve, which is mounted on a metallic stent, is inserted into an external conduit (made of Teflon) connecting the right ventricle to a distal portion of the pulmonary artery, which is divided proximally just above the pulmonary valve. The cardiac end of the transected pulmonary artery is oversewn. An intraventricular tunnel made with Teflon patch redirects left ventricular blood to the aorta through the ventricular septal defect.

• Lateral angulation of the transducer frequently detects strong echoes from the stent

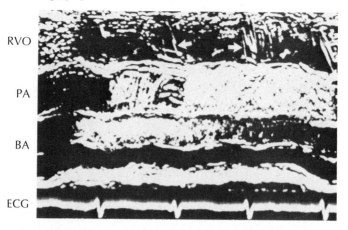

Fig. 11-48. Baffle incompetence. A contrast injection into the systemic venous atrial chamber is initially limited posteriorly by the baffle (BA) and anteriorly by the pulmonary artery (PA). The first systole fills the pulmonary artery as a consequence of corrected intracardiac flow. The presence of a leak in the baffle can be deduced from the appearance of contrast echoes *(arrows)* in the right ventricular outflow (RVO), which is part of the systemic circuit in dextrotransposition of the great vessels. Though the leaked involved the pulmonary venous atrial chamber seen below the baffle, it probably occurred away from the beam position used in this recording. ECG, electrocardiogram.

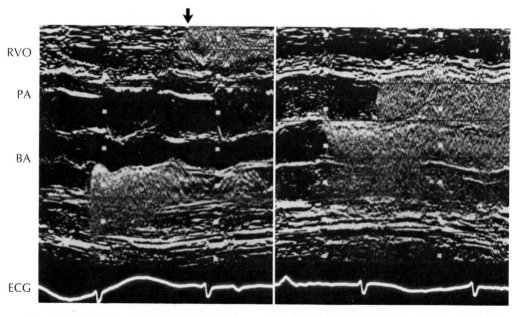

Fig. 11-49. Contrast studies in intra-atrial baffle. Injection of indocyanine green into the atrium receiving pulmonary venous blood *(left)* results in the appearance of contrast echoes posterior to the baffle image (BA) and in the right ventricular outflow tract (RVO) *(arrow)*. An injection was then made into the atrium receiving systemic venous blood *(right)* and reveals contrast echoes anterior to the baffle image and in the pulmonary artery. There is no evidence for baffle incompetence. Less dense echoes present behind the baffle in the pulmonary venous atrium represent contrast reverberations. The eccentric position of the pulmonary valve echo in diastole suggests that it may be bicuspid. PA, pulmonary artery; ECG, electrocardiogram.

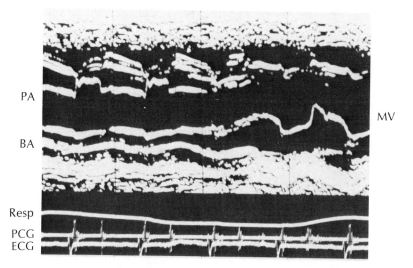

PA

BA

MV

Resp

PCG

ECG

Fig. 11-50. Pulmonary hypertension in dextrotransposition of the great vessels. The beam is swept from the pulmonary artery (PA) to the mitral valve (MV). The pulmonary artery is enlarged, and the pulmonary valve shows absence of the A dip and presence of systolic notching indicative of pulmonary hypertension. The baffle (BA) in this patient moves poorly and does not exhibit sharp anterior motion normally observed at the onset of diastole, probably related to the effects of pulmonary hypertension. Resp, respiration; PCG, phonocardiogram; ECG, electrocardiogram.

and by gentle scanning in that area, the leaflets of the porcine valve may be identified. Serial echocardiograms should prove useful in detecting prosthetic dysfunction by observing development of restricted cusp motion.

• Marked diastolic eccentricity of the pulmonary valve echo suggests the presence of a bicuspid valve in transposition complexes.

Role of echocardiography in transposition complexes

• Echocardiography offers a simple, non-invasive technique for the diagnosis of transposition of great vessels, which, if undiagnosed and untreated, has a high mortality rate. Careful observation of the beam direction used to locate the vessels as well as the closure characteristics of the semilunar valves are required for accurate categorization of transposition complexes into their dextro and levo forms. The great vessels are more difficult to find, in our experience, in levotransposition with ventricular inversion.

• Subpulmonic obstruction associated with transposition can be diagnosed and may be classified into anatomic types.

The following are echocardiographic fea-

tures of subpulmonic obstruction in transposition of great vessels:

1. Prolonged mitral-septal diastolic apposition
2. Pulmonary artery usually smaller than aortic root
3. Narrow subpulmonic segment (evident during beam sweeping from mitral to pulmonary valve)
4. IHSS type findings
   a. Abnormal mitral systolic anterior movement (SAM)
   b. Midsystolic closure of pulmonary valve
   c. Asymmetric ventricular septal hypertrophy (ASH)

• The intra-atrial baffle can be recognized and its motion pattern categorized. Various parts of the baffle can be examined using the valves as landmarks. Preliminary experience indicates that baffle detachment can be recognized.

Double outlet right ventricle

This is a relatively uncommon congenital defect in which both great vessels originate from the right ventricle. A ventricular septal

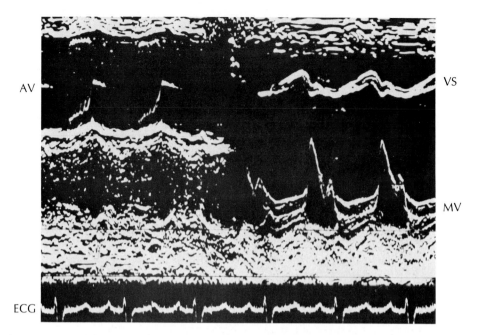

Fig. 11-51. Double outlet right ventricle. Beam sweeping from the aortic (AV) to the mitral valve (MV) shows the aorta overriding the ventricular septum (VS) as well as discontinuity between the posterior wall of the aorta and the mitral valve, which is recorded at a more posterior level. This combination of findings may also be seen in tetralogy of Fallot. ECG, electrocardiogram.

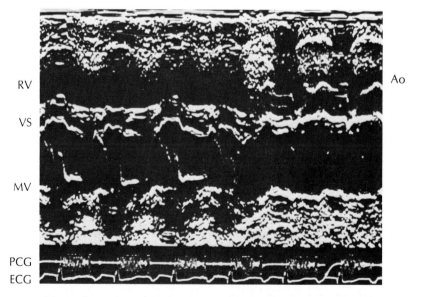

Fig. 11-52. Double outlet right ventricle. Beam angulation on the long axis of the left ventricle shows the aorta (Ao) arising totally from the right ventricle (RV). The pulmonary artery was identified by its typical appearance and in an anterior position adjacent to the aorta. The usual continuity between the mitral valve (MV) and the aorta could not be demonstrated. The ventricular septal defect through which the left ventricle empties could not be imaged. VS, ventricular septum; PCG, phonocardiogram; ECG, electrocardiogram.

defect is always present, and the mitral leaflet is displaced from its usual attachment to the posterior aortic wall by a ridge of conus tissue of variable size. Rarely, the mitral valve may be attached directly to the posterior aortic margin through the ventricular septal defect. In some instances the pulmonary artery may override the interventricular septum.

The echocardiographic findings are not specific, but mitral-aortic discontinuity has been emphasized, since the angiocardiogram shows separation of the mitral leaflet from the aorta by the muscular conus tissue. Echocardiographic discontinuity between the mitral and aortic valves has been described as a posterior position of the closed mitral valve related to the posterior wall of the aorta (Fig. 11-51). Unfortunately, this finding may also occur in tetralogy of Fallot and in patients with dilated left ventricles. Demonstration of mitral-aortic continuity, on the other hand, does not rule out double outlet right ventricle, since the conus tissue may be too small to produce separation, or the mitral valve may be attached directly to the aorta. Occa-

sionally, the aorta may be demonstrated arising entirely from the right ventricle with the posterior aortic margin imaged anterior and close to the ventricular septum during beam scanning (Fig. 11-52). We have seen this finding only in patients with double outlet right ventricles.

Some reports have appeared describing the specific echocardiographic appearance of conus tissue between the mitral valve and aorta. This finding should be of considerable importance in identifying patients with double outlet right ventricles.

Single ventricle

In this anomaly, there is a single ventricular chamber, which may contain two separate atrioventricular valves or a common atrioventricular valve. In the most common variety the single ventricle has the characteristics of a left ventricle, and there is a small, rudimentary outflow chamber from which a great vessel arises. Great vessel position is variable, and the two vessels may lie in normal, dextroposed, levoposed, or in side-by-side position.

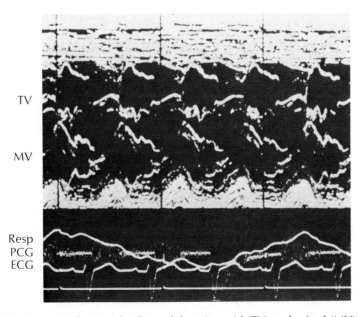

Fig. 11-53. Single ventricle. Two leaflets of the tricuspid (TV) and mitral (MV) valves are shown moving in a single ventricular cavity without an intervening septum. A septal image could not be obtained by scanning the beam throughout the ventricular cavity. Resp, respiratory excursions; PCG, phonocardiogram; ECG, electrocardiogram.

The identifying echocardiographic finding is the simultaneous visualization of two separate atrioventricular valves without an intervening septum (Fig. 11-53). A septal remnant and a small outflow chamber anterior to both atrioventricular valves are demonstrable in some patients. Echocardiographic continuity between the posterior semilunar valve and the posterior atrioventricular valve can be demonstrated. The posterior (mitral) atrioventricular valve should be evaluated carefully, since stenosis may involve this valve. Spatial orientation of the great vessels should be established by the techniques already described under transposition of the great vessels.

It is possible to mistake a muscle band for the interventricular septum and miss the diagnosis when a single A-V valve is present (Fig. 11-54).

Tricuspid atresia

Anatomic and functional changes. The tricuspid valve fails to develop in these patients, and there is no direct communication between the right atrium and right ventricle (Fig. 11-55). The foramen ovale remains patent or a secundum atrial septal defect is present, producing a right-to-left shunt and serving as the outlet for the systemic venous return. The right ventricle is small or markedly hypoplastic, and both atria become enlarged. A ventricular septal defect may be present to fill the hypoplastic chamber, or no communication may be present. There may be transposition of the great vessels and pulmonary atresia. Blood flow to the lungs may be through a ventricular septal defect into the underdeveloped right ventricle and thence into the pulmonary artery or, more commonly, through a patent ductus arteriosus.

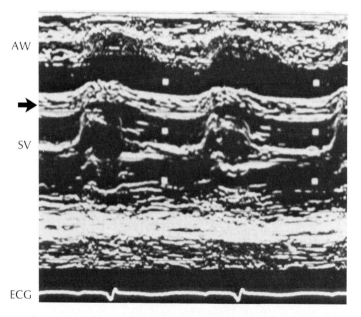

Fig. 11-54. Single ventricle with a single atrioventricular valve. The prominent linear echo complex *(arrow)* was believed to represent a ventricular septum lying in front of the mitral valve. At autopsy, this patient was found to have a single ventricle and mitral atresia. The septum-like echo was produced by a large papillary muscle, and the single atrioventricular valve (SV) was tricuspid. Retrospectively, difficulty in identifying this septum and its inconstant appearance represent clues to its true identity. Two-dimensional transverse scans of this area would probably have revealed the true nature of the anatomic findings. AW, anterior wall; ECG, electrocardiogram.

Clinical summary. The patients are usually intensely cyanotic, and the ECG shows predominance of left ventricular forces. This is an important finding, since cyanotic congenital heart disease usually involves the right ventricle and, therefore, right heart forces tend to predominate. Chest roentgenograms resemble tetralogy of Fallot. During cardiac catheterization, it is impossible to pass the catheter from the right atrium into the right ventricle, but the catheter will pass readily from the right atrium into the left atrium. Pressures in the atria are elevated, and the oxygen content of left atrial and ventricular blood is reduced. Angiocardiography shows the contrast agent flowing from the

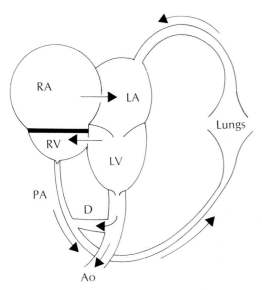

Fig. 11-55. Tricuspid atresia. The atretic tricuspid valve *(heavy line)* blocks flow in the right heart so that the right atrium (RA) becomes enlarged, whereas the right ventricle (RV) is small and underdeveloped. The right atrium empties into the left heart through an atrial septal defect, and blood flow to the lungs occurs primarily through a patent ductus (D). A ventricular septal defect is often present and allows some blood to flow through the small right ventricle and pulmonary artery (PA). In extreme cases, their contribution to the pulmonary blood flow may be insignificant, since the right ventricle and proximal pulmonary artery may be severely hypoplastic. LA, left atrium; LV, left ventricle; Ao, aorta.

right atrium to the left atrium, then into the left ventricle and aorta, and possibly into a small right ventricle through a ventricular septal defect. Often, a radiolucent defect is present in the cardiac image where the small underdeveloped ventricle is present. Pulmonary artery filling through a patent ductus arteriosus is evident.

Echocardiographic features (Figs. 11-56 and 11-57).

• The right ventricle is small or undetectable.

• A single atrioventricular valve is present and may have a large amplitude of motion.

• Scans made through the plane in which the normal mitral and tricuspid valves lie show that the atrioventricular valve that is imaged is continuous with the image of the atrial septum, thereby identifying it as the mitral valve. It may also be shown to be continuous with the posterior aortic margin.

• The left atrium is enlarged.

Comments

• The definitive diagnosis of tricuspid atresia may be difficult, since the single valve recorded could be either tricuspid or mitral. However, we have found that the atrioventricular valve–atrial septum relationship has been useful to identify the existing atrioventricular valve as the mitral. The position of the great vessels should be established by noting beam position and angle if possible.

• A rudimentary tricuspid valve may be detected when there is right heart hypoplasia without valve atresia.

• An estimation of the size of the right ventricle and right ventricular outflow tract should be attempted, since this is important in planning a corrective surgical procedure.

• The single AV valve may resemble a common atrioventricular valve seen in complete canal defects when scanned through the usual mitral-tricuspid plane. An erroneous diagnosis can be avoided by demonstrating an atrial septal relation that appears normal and by correlation with clinical findings.

• In the presence of a single atrioventricular valve, a confusing picture may sometimes be present, since the valve may appear to be located at different depth levels from

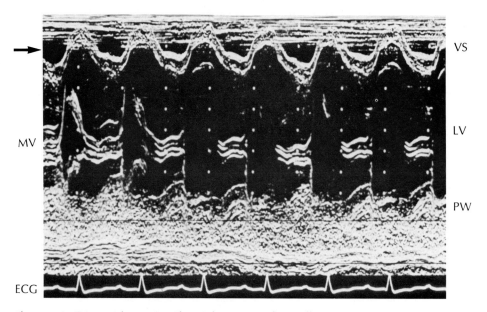

Fig. 11-56. Tricuspid atresia. The right ventricular wall moves poorly and is partially obscured by reverberations that extend into the small right ventricular cavity *(arrow)*. The left ventricle (LV) is markedly dilated, and the ventricular septum (VS) is hyperactive. The mitral valve (MV) demonstrates a large excursion. PW, posterior left ventricular wall; ECG, electrocardiogram.

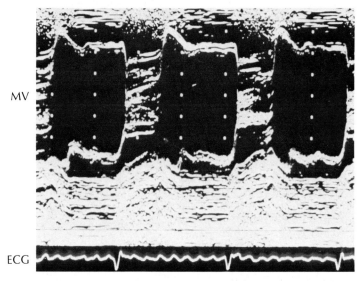

Fig. 11-57. Tricuspid atresia. The mitral valve is large and practically occupies the whole of the left ventricular cavity. Multilayered echoes in systole are consistent with valve redundancy or healed endocarditis. (This patient has been treated for endocarditis in the past.) MV, mitral valve; ECG, electrocardiogram.

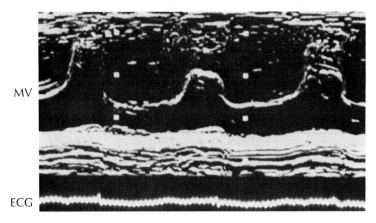

Fig. 11-58. Mitral valve recording in tricuspid atresia. Apparent changes in mitral valve (MV) amplitude are probably related to small variations in beam angulation. The dropouts that appear to separate the first cycle from the others should not be interpreted as evidence of two atrioventricular valves because of the amplitude difference. ECG, electrocardiogram.

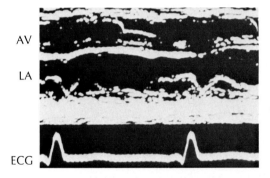

Fig. 11-59. Aortic root recording in a patient with tricuspid atresia. A prominent moving echo is seen in the middle of the left atrial cavity in late diastole and early systole, probably produced by bulging of the atrial septum into the left atrial cavity. AV, aortic valve; LA, left atrium; ECG, electrocardiogram.

the chest wall, depending on the transducer position and angulation. The valve amplitude may also vary, and thus it may appear that two valves are present. However, continuity between the apparent valve images as well as absence of ventricular septal recording between them helps resolve this problem (Fig. 11-58). These findings may also be seen in single ventricle when a single atrioventricular valve is present and in the hypoplastic

left heart syndrome with mitral atresia (see below).

• A prominently moving linear echo may be seen, apparently in the left atrial cavity recorded behind the aortic root in patients with tricuspid atresia (Fig. 11-59). This probably represents bulging of the atrial septum into the left atrium, which may occur in this condition.

Role of echocardiography. The clinical presentation is usually typical, and echocardiography confirms the clinical diagnosis. Associated abnormalities like transposition of the great vessels may be demonstrated.

Hypoplastic left heart syndrome

Anatomic and functional changes. This lesion involves various degrees of underdevelopment of the mitral valve, left ventricle, aortic valve, or ascending aorta. The mitral valve may be atretic or underdeveloped; the left ventricular cavity is always small and can be slitlike. The aortic root is often underdeveloped and may be only a few millimeters in size. The aortic valve may also be atretic or represented by a diaphragm with a central aperture or be bicuspid. The right atrium, right ventricle, and pulmonary artery are large and take over the additional burden of supplying the systemic circulation, usually through a patent foramen ovale and a patent ductus, which permit blood flow from the pulmonary artery into the aorta in its descending portion. Closure of the patent ductus arteriosus is a common cause of death in this uniformly fatal condition since there is no surgical corrective procedure available.

Clinical summary. These children may appear normal shortly after birth but soon go into shock with decreased blood pressure in the extremities and decreased volume of pulse in the peripheral arteries. The second heart sound may have only a single component generated by pulmonic valve closure, and murmurs may be absent. The ECG shows an absence of left ventricular forces and the chest roentgenogram demonstrates cardiomegaly. Cardiac catheterization and angiocardiography demonstrate the expected anatomic changes but are usually not performed when the echocardiographic findings are typical for hypoplastic left heart syndrome.

Echocardiographic features (Fig. 11-60)
• The left ventricular cavity may be small (less than 10 mm in end-diastole) or appear to be absent.
• The aortic root is unrecordable or small, and the contained cusps may show delayed systolic opening (Fig. 11-61).
• Mitral valve echoes may be impossible to detect or may reveal a markedly diminished amplitude of motion as compared to the tricuspid valve.
• Scans made through the mitral-tricuspid region show the single atrioventricular valve

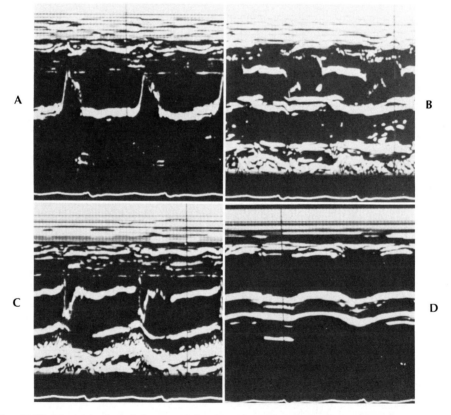

Fig. 11-60. Hypoplastic left heart syndrome. Normal-appearing tricuspid **(A)** and pulmonic valves **(B)** are shown. Exploration of the region of the mitral valve **(C)** demonstrated only the posterior leaflet of the tricuspid valve, and normal mitral leaflets were absent. The aortic root lumen **(D)** measured less than 5 mm in diameter and was about one-third the size of the pulmonary artery. At autopsy, there was mitral atresia and marked hypoplasia of the left ventricle and aorta.

to lie anterior to the position of the atrial septum, identifying it as the tricuspid valve.

Comments

• The right ventricle appears enlarged, and the pulmonary valve is much larger than the aortic valve and root. If the echocardiographic appearance is that of a single ventricular cavity, the scan that demonstrates the atrial septum is useful to identify a single atrioventricular valve as the tricuspid or to recognize a poorly moving echo complex as arising from an underdevleoped mitral valve.

• Tricuspid valve reverberation images occur occasionally and can be erroneously called a mitral valve (Fig. 11-62). They lie deep to the tricuspid and disappear if beam position and angle are changed.

• The tricuspid valve may show changes in amplitude of valve motion with minimal alterations in the transducer position (Fig. 11-63). These may be related to the ultrasonic beam striking different portions of the leaflet at different angles, which results in attenuated motion and image dropouts. In some

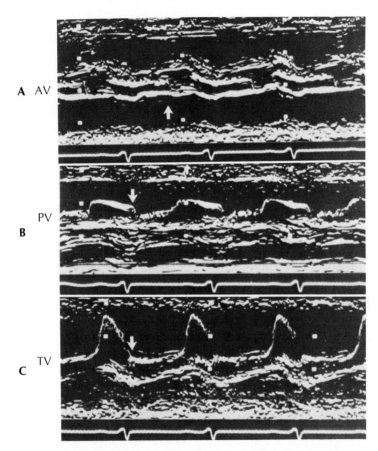

Fig. 11-61. Delayed aortic valve opening in hypoplastic left heart syndrome. There is a marked delay in aortic valve opening (**A,** *arrow*) as compared to pulmonary valve opening (**B,** *arrow*) and tricuspid valve closure (**C,** *arrow*). The valve, in fact, opens so late in systole that it just precedes pulmonary valve closure and tricuspid valve opening movement. Aortic valve stays open briefly, closes before the onset of the QRS complex, and remains closed for most of systole. These abnormal aortic valve findings are seen only when some left atrial-mitral-aortic continuity is retained in the presence of severe endocardial fibroelastosis involving a hypoplastic left ventricle. AV, aortic valve; PV, pulmonary valve; TV, tricuspid valve.

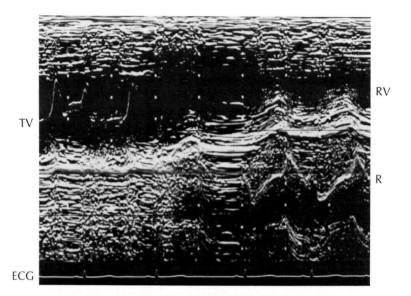

Fig. 11-62. Tricuspid valve reverberations in mitral valve atresia. Reverberatory echoes (R) from the tricuspid valve (TV), recorded posteriorly, resemble normal mitral valve recordings and may result in misdiagnosis. RV, right ventricle; ECG, electrocardiogram.

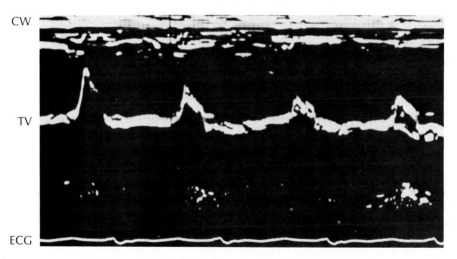

Fig. 11-63. Mitral atresia. The tricuspid valve (TV) demonstrates changes in the amplitude of valve motion with minimal alterations in the transducer position. These may be related to the ultrasonic beam striking different portions of the valve at different angles, resulting in apparently attenuated motion and image dropouts. In some instances the smaller amplitude echo may represent the movement of a smaller second (accessory) anterior tricuspid leaflet. CW, chest wall; ECG, electrocardiogram.

instances the smaller amplitude echo may represent the movement of a smaller accessory anterior tricuspid leaflet, a not uncommon anatomic finding.

• Aortic valve cusps may appear normal, even though the valve is deformed. Late opening of the aortic valve occurs (Fig. 11-61) when there is continuity of blood flow from the left atrium to the aorta in the absence of a ventricular septal defect. The function of the underdeveloped left ventricle is further compromised by the presence of endocardial fibroelastosis (see below).

• A bicuspid aortic valve may be detected by its eccentric diastolic position.

• The atretic aortic valve may be represented by a diaphragm or a small mass of undifferentiated endocardial tissue. This may dome in systole and mimic normal cusp opening. Observation of the aortic valve opening and closing motion on the echocardiogram thus does not necessarily imply the anatomic presence of a functioning valve.

• The pulmonary artery may be large and signs of pulmonary hypertension may be present.

• Certain newborns present with the clin-ical picture of left heart hypoplasia that is functional in origin, with no structural abnormality present. The echocardiogram in these infants appears normal and represents vital clinical information since these babies usually recover with supportive therapy.

• Examination of patients with hypoplastic left heart syndrome represents a trying experience for the echocardiographer, who must have confidence in his skills to detect the presence of normal structures and exercise diligence in the performance of the echocardiographic examination. An experienced echocardiographer can usually demonstrate the left heart structures in the normal newborn in a relatively short period of time. Prolonged examination and heroic devotion may lead to confusion and erroneous diagnoses. If normal left heart structures are not located in 20 to 30 minutes of effort, be confident that they are either absent or so deformed that recognition may not be possible.

Role of echocardiography. The echocardiographic examination is of critical importance in separating infants with functional left heart hypoplastic syndrome from those with structural abnormalities that are not

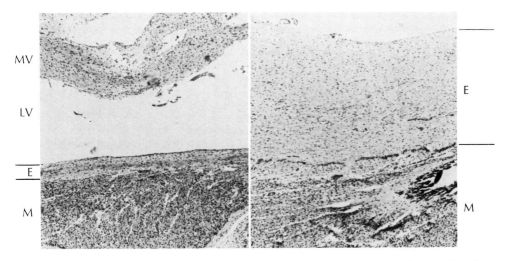

Fig. 11-64. Endocardial fibroelastosis. Two microscopic sections are shown. On the right, a section taken from a newborn with hypoplastic left heart syndrome shows a markedly thickened endocardium due to endocardial fibroelastosis. A normal endocardium in a newborn is shown on the left for comparison. MV, mitral valve; LV, left ventricle; E, endocardium; M, myocardium.

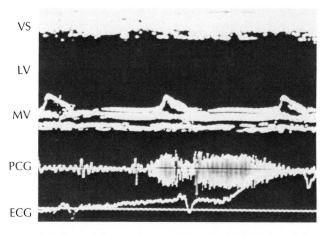

Fig. 11-65. Endocardial fibroelastosis in an infant. The left ventricular cavity (LV) is dilated, and the mitral valve (MV) appears to be diminutive with a low amplitude of motion. Late diastolic opening of the mitral valve is also evident. These findings are comparable to those seen with congestive cardiomyopathy. VS, ventricular septum; PCG, phonocardiogram; ECG, electrocardiogram.

curable and that regularly result in death. In addition, the echocardiographic examination obviates the need for further invasive diagnostic procedures in these critically ill newborns. Left heart hypoplasia represents one of the outstanding conditions in which the echocardiographic examination dominates the clinical management of the patient.

Endocardial fibroelastosis

There is marked thickening of the endocardial lining of the heart that may occur as an isolated abnormality or coexist with other lesions such as coarctation of the aorta, congenital aortic stenosis, and the hypoplastic left heart syndrome (Fig. 11-64). The endocardial thickening most often involves the left ventricle, left atrium, mitral valve, and chordae tendinae. The left ventricle cannot contract normally, and hypertrophy and dilatation occur. Mitral valve and chordae involvement and the ventricular dilatation result in mitral regurgitation with a sequel of pulmonary hypertension and right heart enlargement. In later stages, all four chambers of the heart are enlarged.

Endocardial fibroelastosis is suspected clinically in a child usually under 6 months of age who shows signs of cardiac enlargement, failure, and pulmonary hypertension in the absence of murmurs other than that of mitral regurgitation. The ECG shows left ventricular hypertrophy and cardiac catheterization demonstrates normal or elevated right heart pressure, elevated left ventricular end-diastolic pressure, and no evidence of intracardiac shunts. Angiocardiography demonstrates an enlarged left ventricle with poor wall motion and mitral regurgitation, if present.

The echocardiographic findings consist of left ventricular dilatation, poor wall motion, and decrease in the amplitude of aortic root excursion (Fig. 11-65). Mitral valve echoes are reduced in amplitude, but EF slopes are usually not abnormal. The echocardiograms resemble those seen in congestive cardiomyopathy in adults. Mild degrees of abnormality may not be detected echocardiographically.

If the lesion is sufficiently advanced, the ultrasonic examination is diagnostic. The elimination of pericardial effusion as a source of cardiac silhouette enlargement is an important function for echocardiography in these patients.

BIBLIOGRAPHY
Atrial septal defect

Diamond, M. A., Dillon, J. C., Haine, C. L., Chang, S., and Feigenbaum, H.: Echocardiographic features of atrial septal defect, Circulation **43:**129-135, 1971.

Glaser, J., Whitman, V., and Liebman, J.: The differential diagnosis of total anomalous pulmonary venous drainage in infancy by echocardiography, Circulation 46(suppl. 2):138, 1972. (abstract)

Gramiak, R., and Nanda, N. C.: Echocardiographic diagnosis of ostium primum septal defect, Circulation 45(suppl. 2):46, 1972 (abstract).

Tajik, A. J., Gau, G. T., Ritter, D. G., and Schattenberg, T.: Echocardiographic pattern of right ventricular diastolic volume overload in children, Circulation 46:36, 1972.

Tajik, A. J., Gau, G. T., and Schattenberg, T. T.: Echocardiogram in total anomalous pulmonary venous drainage; report of case, Mayo Clin. Proc. 47:247, 1972.

Chiotellis, P., Lees, R., Goldblatt, A., Liberthson, R., and Myers, G.: New criteria for echocardiographic diagnosis of atrial septal defect, Circulation 52(suppl. 2):134, 1975 (abstract).

Paquet, M., and Gutgesell, H.: Echocardiographic features of total anomalous pulmonary venous connection, Circulation 51:599-605, 1975.

Popio, K. A., Gorlin, R., Teichholz, L. E., Cohn, P. F., Bechtel, D., and Herman, M. V.: Abnormalities of left ventricular function and geometry in adults with an atrial septal defect; ventriculographic hemodynamic and echocardiographic studies, Am. J. Cardiol. 36:302, 1975.

Radtke, W. E., Tajik, A. J., Gau, G. T., Schattenberg, T. T., Giuliani, E. R., and Tancredi, R. G.: Atrial septal defect; echocardiographic observations; studies in 120 patients, Ann. Intern. Med. 84:246-253, 1976.

Ventricular septal defect

Carter, W. H., and Bowman, C. R.: Estimation of shunt flow in isolated ventricular septal defect by echocardiogram, Circulation 48(suppl. 4):64, 1973 (abstract).

King, D. L.: Visualization of ventricular septal defects by cardiac ultrasonography, Circulation 48:1215, 1973.

Oki, T., Sawada, S., Matsumura, K., and Mori, H.: Anterior mitral valve echo in patients with isolated ventricular septal defect and with tetralogy of Fallot, Jpn. Circ. J. 39:657-664, 1975.

Lewis, A. B., and Takahashi, M.: Echocardiographic assessment of left-to-right shunt volume in children with ventricular septal defect, Circulation 54:78, 1976.

Patent ductus arteriosus

Baylen, B., Meyer, R. A., and Kaplan, S.: Echocardiographic assessment of patent ductus arteriosus in prematures with respiratory distress, Circulation 50(suppl. 3):16, 1974 (abstract).

Laird, W. P., and Fixler, D. E.: Echocardiographic estimation of pulmonary-systemic flow in children with patent ductus arteriosus, Circulation 50(suppl. 3):184, 1974 (abstract).

Silverman, N. H., Lewis, A. B., Heymann, M. A., and Rudolph, A. M.: Echocardiographic assessment of ductus arteriosus in premature infants, Circulation 50:821, 1974.

Baylen, B. G., Meyer, R. A., Kaplan, S., Ringenburg, W. E., and Korfhagen, J.: The critically ill premature infant with patent ductus arteriosus and pulmonary disease—an echocardiographic assessment, J. Pediatr. 86:423-432, 1975.

Goldberg, S. J., Allen, H. D., Sahn, D. J., Friedman, W. F., and Harris, T.: A prospective 2½ year experience with echocardiographic evaluation of prematures with patent ductus arteriosus (PDA) and respiratory distress syndrome (RDS), Am. J. Cardiol. 35:139, 1975 (abstract).

Purohit, D. M., Caldwell, C. C., Webb, H. N., and Levkoff, A. H.: Effects of assisted ventilation on echocardiographic findings in two infants with patent ductus arteriosus, J. Thorac. Cardiovasc. Surg. 72:294-295, 1976.

Cor triatriatum

Matsumoto, M., Shimada, H., Hayashi, T., Nimura, Y., and Abe, H., Kitabatake, A., Matsuo, H., Kito, Y., and Nishizaki, H.: Ultrasound cardiogram and ultrasonocardiotomogram in a case of cor triatriatum, Med. Ultrason. 9:61, 1971.

Troy, B. L., Panepinto, M., Harp, R., Carvalho, A., Conn, R., and Smalley, P.: Diagnosis of cor-triatriatum by echocardiography, J. Clin. Ultrasound 1:257, 1973 (abstract).

Chung, K. J., Manning, J. A., Lipchik, E. O., Gramiak, R., and Mahoney, E. B.: Isolated supravalvular stenosing ring of left atrium; diagnosis before operation and successful surgical treatment, Chest 65:25, 1974.

Gibson, D. G., Honey, M., and Lennox, S. C.: Cor triatriatum; diagnosis by echocardiography, Br. Heart J. 36:835-838, 1974.

Nimura, Y., Matsumoto, M., Beppu, S., Matuso, H., and Sakakibara, H.: Noninvasive preoperative diagnosis of cor triatriatum with ultrasonocardiotomogram and conventional echocardiogram, Am. Heart J. 88:240-250, 1974.

Moodie, D. S., Hagler, D. J., and Ritter, D. G.: Cor triatriatum; echocardiographic findings, Mayo Clin. Proc. 51:289-295, 1976.

Ebstein's anomaly

Kotler, M. N., and Tabatznik, B.: Recognition of Ebstein's anomaly by ultrasound technique, Circulation 44(suppl. 2):34, 1971 (abstract).

Tajik, A. J., Gau, G. T., Giuliani, E. R., Ritter, D. G., and Schattenberg, T. T.: Echocardiogram in Ebstein's anomaly with Wolff-Parkinson-White pre-excitation syndrome, type B, Circulation 47:813, 1973.

Sahn, D. J., Hagan, A., and Friedman, W. F.: Cross-sectional echocardiographic features of Ebstein's malformation, J. Clin. Ultrasound 2:263, 1974 (abstract).

Yuste, P., Minguez, I., Aza, V., Senor, J., Asin, E., and Martinezaabordiu, C.: Echocardiography in the diagnosis of Ebstein's anomaly, Chest 66:273, 1974.

French, J. W., Baum, D., and Popp, R. L.: Echocardiographic findings in Uhl's anomaly, Am. J. Cardiol. 36:349, 1975.

Farooki, Z. Q., Henry, J. G., and Green, E. W.: Echocardiographic spectrum of Ebstein's anomaly of the tricuspid valve, Circulation 53:63-68, 1976.

Matsumoto, M., Matsuo, H., Nagata, S., Hamanaka, Y., and Fujita, T.: Visualization of Ebstein's anomaly of the tricuspid valve by two-dimensional and standard echocardiography, Circulation 53:59-79, 1976.

Milner, S., Meyer, R. A., Venables, A. W., Korfhagen, J., and Kaplan, S.: Mitral and tricuspid valve closure in congenital heart disease, Circulation 53:513, 1976.

Overriding tricuspid valve

Seward, J. B., Tajik, A. J., and Ritter, D. G.: Echocardiographic features of straddling tricuspid valve, Mayo Clin. Proc. 50:427-434, 1975.

LaCorte, M. A., Fellows, K. E., and Williams, R. G.: Overriding tricuspid valve; echocardiographic and angiocardiographic features, Am. J. Cardiol. 37:911, 1976.

Atrioventricular canal defect

Gramiak, R., and Nanda, N. C.: Echocardiographic diagnosis of ostium primum septal defect. Circulation 45(suppl. 2):46, 1972.

Williams, R. G., and Rudd, M.: Echocardiographic features of endocardial cushion defects. Circulation 49:418, 1974.

Sahn, D. J., Terry, R. W., O'Rourke, R., Leopold, G., and Friedman, W. F.: Multiple crystal echocardiographic evaluation of endocardial cushion defect, Circulation 50:25, 1974.

Eshaghpour, E., Turnoff, H. B., Kingsley, B., Kawai, N., and Linhart, J. W.: Echocardiography in endocardial cushion defects; a preoperative and postoperative study, Chest 68:172-177, 1975.

Nanda, N. C., Gramiak, R., and Manning, J. A.: Echocardiographic diagnosis of complete atrioventricular canal defect. In White, D. N., editor: Ultrasound in medicine, vol. 1, New York, 1975, Plenum Publishing Corp., p. 19.

Pieroni, D. R., Homcy, E., and Freedom, R. M.: Echocardiography in atrioventricular canal defect; a clinical spectrum, Am. J. Cardiol. 35:54-58, 1975.

Yoshikawa, J., Owaki, T., Kato, H., Tomita, Y., and Baba, K.: Echocardiographic diagnosis of endocardial cushion defects, Jpn. Heart J. 16:1, 1975.

Beppu, S., Nimura, Y., Nagata, S., Tamai, M., and Matsuo, H.: Diagnosis of endocardial cushion defect with cross-sectional and M-mode scanning echocardiography; differentiation from secundum atrial septal defect, Br. Heart J. 38:911-920, 1976.

Komatsu, Y., Nagai, Y., Shibuya, M., Takao, A., and Hirosawa, K.: Echocardiograhpic analysis of intracardiac anatomy in endocardial cushion defect, Am. Heart J. 91:210, 1976.

Tetralogy of Fallot

Chung, K. J., Nanda, N. C., Manning, J. A., and Gramiak, R.: Echocardiographic findings in tetralogy of Fallot, Am. J. Cardiol. 31:126, 1973.

Tajik. A. J., Gau, G. T., Ritter, D. G., and Schattenberg, T. T.: Echocardiogram in tetralogy of Fallot, Chest 64:107, 1973.

Morris, D. C., Felne, J. M., Schlant, R. C., and Franch, R. H.: Echocardiographic diagnosis of tetralogy of Fallot, Am. J. Cardiol. 36:908, 1975.

Truncus arteriosus

Chung, K. J., Alexson, C. G., Manning, J. A., and Gramiak, R.: Echocardiography in truncus arteriosus; the value of pulmonic valve detection, Circulation 48:281, 1973.

Chandraratna, P. A. N., Bhaduri, U., Littman, B. B., and Hildner, F. J.: Echocardiographic findings in persistent truncus arteriosus in a young adult, Br. Heart J. 36:732, 1974.

Transposition of great vessels

Gramiak, R., Chung, K. J., Nanda, N., and Manning, J.: Echocardiographic diagnosis of transposition of the great vessels, Radiology 106:187, 1973.

King, D. L., Steeg, C. N., and Ellis, K.: Demonstration of transposition of the great arteries by cardiac ultrasonography, Radiology 107:181, 1973.

Dillon, J. C., Feigenbaum, H., Konecke, L. L., Keutel, J., Hurwitz, R. A., Davis, R. H., and Chang, S.: Echocardiographic manifestations of d-transposition of the great vessels, Am. J. Cardiol. 32:74, 1973.

Henry, W. L., Maron, B. J., Griffith, J. M., and Epstein, S. E.: The differential diagnosis of anomalies of the great vessels by real-time, two-dimensional echocardiography, Am. J. Cardiol. 33:143, 1974.

Hagler, D. J., Tajik, A. J., and Ritter, D. G.: Fluttering of atrioventricular valves in patients with D-transposition of the great arteries after Mustard operation; echographic observation, Mayo Clin. Proc. 50:69-75, 1975.

Henry, W. L., Maron, B. J., Griffith, J. M., Redwood, D. R., and Epstein, S. E.: Differential diagnosis of anomalies of the great arteries by real-time, two-dimensional echocardiography, Circulation 51:283, 1975.

Maron, B. J., Henry, W. L., Griffith, J. M., Freedom, R. M., Kelly, D. T., and Epstein, S. E.: Identification of congenital malformations of the great arteries in infants by real-time two-dimensional echocardiography, Circulation 52:671-677, 1975.

Nanda, N. C., Gramiak, R., Manning, J. A., and Lipchik, E. O.: Echocardiographic features of subpulmonic obstruction in dextro-transposition of the great vessels, Circulation 51:515-521, 1975.

Nanda, N. C., Stewart, S., Gramiak, R., and Manning, J. A.: Echocardiography of the intra-atrial baffle in dextro-transposition of the great vessels, Circulation 51:1130-1135, 1975.

Aziz, K. U., Paul, M. H., and Muster, A. J.: Echocardiographic localization of interatrial baffle after Mustard operation for dextrotransposition of the great arteries, Am. J. Cardiol. 38:67-72, 1976.

Beardshaw, J. A., Gibson, D. G., Wright, J. S., Pearson, M. C., and Anderson, R. H.: Proceedings; echocardiographic diagnosis of corrected transposition, Br. Heart J. **38:**878, 1976.

Pennock, W., and Shelton, S. L.: Simultaneous echocardiographic recording of the semilunar valves in patients with normally related great arteries, Radiology **118:**397-399, 1976.

Double outlet right ventricle

Chesler, E., Jaffe, H. S., Beck, W., and Schrire, V.: Echocardiographic recognition of mitral-semilunar valve discontinuity; an aid to the diagnosis of origin of both great vessels from the right ventricle, Circulation **43:**725, 1971.

Strunk, B. L., Guss, S. B., Hicks, R. E., and Kotler, M. N.: Echocardiographic recognition of the mitral valve-posterior aortic wall relationship, Circulation **51:**594, 1975.

French, J. W., and Popp, R.: Variability of echocardiographic discontinuity in double outlet right ventricle and truncus arteriosus, Circulation **51:**848-854, 1975.

Henry, W. L., Maron, B. J., Griffith, J. M., Epstein, S. E.: Identification of double outlet right ventricle by two-dimensional echocardiography, Clin. Res. **24:**222A, 1976 (abstract).

Vaseenon, T., Zakheim, R. M., Park, M. K., Mattioli, L., and Diehl, A. M.: Echocardiographic diagnosis of double-outlet right ventricle, Chest **70:**362-366, 1976.

Single ventricle

Chesler, E., Jaffe, H. S., Vecht, R., Beck, W., and Schrire, V.: Ultrasound cardiography in single ventricle and the hypoplastic left and right heart syndromes, Circulation **42:**123, 1970.

Seward, J. B., Tajik, A. J., Hagler, D. J., and Ritter, D. G.: Preoperative and postoperative echocardiographic observations in common ventricle, Circulation **52**(suppl. 2):46, 1975. (abstract)

Felner, J. M., Brewer, D. B., and Franch, R. H.: Echocardiographic manifestations of single ventricle, Am. J. Cardiol. **38:**80-84, 1976.

Seward, J. B., Tajik, A. J., Hagler, D. J., Giuliani, E. R., Gau, G. T., and Ritter, D. G.: Echocardiogram in common (single) ventricle; angiographic-anatomic correlation, Am. J. Cardiol. **39:**217-225, 1977.

Tricuspid atresia

Chesler, E., Jaffe, S., Vecht, R., Beck, W., and Schrire, V.: Ultrasound cardiography in single ventricle and the hypoplastic left and right heart syndromes, Circulation **42:**123, 1970.

Meyer, R. A., and Kaplan, S.: Echocardiography in the diagnosis of hypoplasia of the left or right ventricle in the neonate, Circulation **46:**55, 1972.

LaCorte, M. A., Dick, M., Scheer, G., LaFarge, C. G., and Fyler, D. C.: Left ventricular function in tricuspid atresia, Circulation **52:**996, 1975.

Ferrer, P. L., Garcia, O. L., Hernandez, F., Jesse, M. J., and Castellanos, A.: Echocardiographic findings in isolated right ventricular hypoplasia, Clin. Res. **25:**221A, 1977.

Hypoplastic left heart syndrome

Chesler, E., Jaffe, H. S., Vecht, R., Beck, W., and Schrire, V.: Ultrasound cardiography in single ventricle and the hypoplastic left and right heart syndromes, Circulation **42:**123, 1970.

Lundstrom, N. R.: Ultrasoundcardiographic studies of the mitral valve region in young infants with mitral atresia, mitral stenosis, hypoplasia of the left ventricle and cor triatriatum, Circulation **45:**324, 1972.

Meyer, R. A., and Kaplan, S.: Echocardiography in the diagnosis of hypoplasia of the left or right ventricle in the neonate, Circulation **46:**55, 1972.

Farooki, Z. Q., Henry, J. G., and Green, E. W.: Echocardiographic spectrum of the hypoplastic left heart syndrome; a clinicopathologic correlation in 19 newborns, Am. J. Cardiol. **38:**337-343, 1976.

Ross, A., Nanda, N. C., Manning, J., and Gramiak, R.: Abnormal aortic valve movement in hypoplastic left heart syndrome associated with endocardial fibroelastosis (abstract). Submitted for publication.

Congenital heart disease (miscellaneous)

Keutel, J.: Echocardiographic examinations in children, Monatsschr. Kinderheilkd. **121:**520, 1973.

Machida, K., Yasukochi, H., Tada, S., Oshima, M., and Hackimori, K.: Ultrasonic measurements of left ventricular volume, mass and velocity of posterior wall movement in children, Nippon Acta Radiol. **33:**617, 1973.

Pieroni, D., Varghese, P. J., and Rowe, R. D.: Echocardiography to detect shunt and valvular incompetence in infants and children, Circulation **48**(suppl. 4):81, 1973 (abstract).

Kerber, R. E., Kioschos, J. M., and Lauer, R. M.: Use of an ultrasonic contrast method in the diagnosis of valvular regurgitation and intracardiac shunts, Am. J. Cardiol. **34:**722-727, 1974.

Lundstrom, N. R.: Clinical applications of echocardiography in infants and children. III. Estimation of left and right ventricular size; a comparison between echocardiography and angiocardiography, Acta Paediatr. Scand. **63:**257, 1974.

Meyer, R. A., Schwartz, D. C., Covitz, W., and Kaplan, S.: Echocardiographic assessment of cardiac malposition, Am. J. Cardiol. **33:**896, 1974.

Sahn, D. J., Deely, W. J., Hagan, A. D., and Friedman, W. F.: Echocardiographic assessment of left ventricular performance in normal newborns, Circulation **49:**232, 1974.

Godman, M. F., Fiddler, G. I., and Marquis, R. M.: Proceedings; echocardiography in evaluation of congenital mitral valve disease in infants and children, Br. Heart J. **37:**783, 1975.

Henry, W. L., Sahn, D. J., Griffith, J. M., Goldberg,

S. J., Maron, B. J., McAllister, H. A., Allen, H. D., and Epstein, S. E.: Evaluation of atrio-ventricular valve morphology in congenital heart disease by real-time cross-sectional echocardiography, Circulation 52(suppl. 2):120, 1975. (abstract)

Keutel, J.: Echocardiographic diagnosis and evaluation of rare congenital anomalies. In: Kazner, E., and others, editors: Ultrasonics in medicine, Amsterdam, 1975, Excerpta Medica, pp. 231-238.

Meyer, R. A., Stockert, J., and Kaplan, S.: Echographic determination of left ventricular volumes in pediatric patients, Circulation 51:297, 1975.

Nora, J. J., Lortscher, P. H., and Spangler, R. D.: Echocardiographic studies of left ventricular disease in Ullrich-Noonan syndrome, Am. J. Dis. Child. 129:1417-1420, 1975.

Seward, J. B., Tajik, A. J., Spangler, J. G., and Ritter, D. G.: Echocardiographic contrast studies; initial experience, Mayo Clin. Proc. 50:163, 1975.

Verani, M. S., and Lauer, R. M.: Echocardiographic findings in right coronary arterial-right ventricular fistula; report of a neonate with fatal congestive heart failure. Am. J. Cardiol. 35:444-447, 1975.

Assad-Morell, J. L., Seward, J. B., Tajik, A. J., Hagler, D. J., Giuliani, E. R., and Ritter, D. G.: Echophonocardiographic and contrast studies in conditions associated with systemic arterial trunk overriding the ventricular septum; truncus arteriosus, tetralogy of Fallot, and pulmonary atresia with ventricular septal defect, Circulation 53:663-673, 1976.

Cooperberg, P., Hazell, S., and Ashmore, P. G.: Parachute accessory anterior mitral valve leaflet causing left ventricular outflow tract obstruction; report of a case with emphasis on the echocardiographic findings, Circulation 53:908-911, 1976.

Duff, D. F., and Gutgesell, H. P.: The use of saline for ultrasonic detection of a right-to-left shunt in post operative period, Am. J. Cardiol. 37:132, 1976 (abstract).

LaCorte, M., Harada, K., and Williams, R. G.: Echocardiographic features of congenital left ventricular inflow obstruction, Circulation 54:562-566, 1976.

Seward, J. B., Tajik, A. J., Gutierrez, F., Hagler, D. J. Moodie, D. S., and Ritter, D. G.: Contrast echocardiography; peripheral vein injection of indocyanine green dye for detection and assessment of right-to-left intracardiac shunting, Am. J. Cardiol. 37:171, 1976.

Shub, C., Tajik, A. J., Seward, J. B., and Dines, D. E.: Detecting intrapulmonary right-to-left shunt with contrast echocardiography, Mayo Clin. Proc. 51:81, 1976.

Valdes-Cruz, L. M., Pieroni, D. R., Roland, J. M., and Varghese, P. J.: Echocardiographic detection of intracardiac right-to-left shunts following peripheral vein injections, Circulation 54:558-562, 1976.

Yabek, S. M., Isabel-Jones, J., Bhatt, D. R., Nakazawa, M., Marks, R. A., and Jarmakani, J. M.: Echocardiographic determination of left atrial volumes in children with congenital heart disease, Circulation 53:268, 1976.

Beardshaw, J. A., Gibson, D. G., Pearson, M. C., Upton, M. T., and Anderson, R. H.: Echocardiographic diagnosis of primitive ventricle with two atrioventricular valves, Br. Heart J. 39:266-275, 1977.

Seward, J. B., Tajik, A. J., Hagler, D. J., and Ritter, D. G.: Peripheral venous contrast echocardiography, Am. J. Cardiol. 39:202-212, 1977.

Sheikh, M., Kolia, G. M., Fox, L., Cevarrubias, E., and Ali, N.: Dilatation of aortic root producing pseudo overriding of aorta (ORA) pattern on echocardiography (ECH), Clin. Res. 25:254A, 1977.

Story, W. E., Felner, J. M., and Schlant, R. C.: Echocardiographic criteria for the diagnosis of mitral-semilunar valve continuity, Am. Heart J. 93:575-580, 1977.

Valdes-Cruz, L. M., Pieroni, D. R., Roland, J. M., and Shematek, J. P.: Recognition of residual postoperative shunts by contrast echocardiographic techniques, Circulation 55:148-152, 1977.

Congenital heart disease (review articles)

Chesler, E., Joffe, H. S., Beck, W., and Schrire, V.: Echocardiography in the diagnosis of congenital heart disease, Pediatr. Clin. North Am. 18:1163-1190, 1971.

Lundstrom, N. R., and Edler, I.: Ultrasoundcardiography in infants and children, Acta Paediatr. Scand. 60:117, 1971.

Winsberg, F.: Echocardiography of the fetal and newborn heart, Invest. Radiol. 7:152, 1972.

Meyer, R. A., and Kaplan, S.: Noninvasive techniques in pediatric cardiovascular disease, Prog. Cardiovasc. Dis. 15:341-367, 1973.

Lundstrom, N. R.: Clinical applications of echocardiography in infants and children, Acta Paediatr. Scand. 243(suppl.):1-38, 1974.

Meyer, R. A.: Echocardiography in congenital heart disease, Cardiovasc. Clin. 6:219-243, 1975.

Meyer, R. A.: Echocardiography in congenital heart disease, Semin. Roentgenol. 10:277-290, 1975.

Murphy, K. F., Kotler, M. N., Reichek, N., and Perloff, J. K.: Ultrasound in the diagnosis of congenital heart disease, Am. Heart J. 89:638-656, 1975.

Sahn, D. J., Allen, H. D., Goldberg, S. J., Solinger, R., and Meyer, R. A.: Pediatric echocardiography; a review of its clinical utility, J. Pediatr. 87:335-352, 1975.

Moss, A. J., Gussoni, C. C., Isabel-Jones, J.: Echocardiography in congenital heart disease, West. J. Med. 124:102-121, 1976.

Nanda, N. C.: Clinical applications of echocardiography. II. Mod. Conc. Cardiovasc. Dis. 45:139-142, 1976.

Silverman, N. H.: Newer noninvasive methods in pediatric cardiology; echocardiography, isotope angiography, Adv. Pediatr. 23:357-399, 1976.

Solinger, R., Elbl, F., and Minhas, K.: Echocardiography; its role in the severely ill infant, Pediatrics 57:543-563, 1976.

Friedman, W. F., Sahn, D. J., Hirschklau, M. J.: A review; newer noninvasive cardiac diagnostic methods, Pediatr. Res. 11(pt. 1):190-197, 1977.

12 Two-dimensional echocardiography

This chapter is included to provide some background information on two-dimensional cardiac imaging so that the reader may anticipate inclusion of this exciting new technique into clinical echocardiography when it becomes more widely utilized. Two-dimensional systems have been developed to provide better representation of structures than is available from the single line of information obtained during M-mode examination, which has been likened to an icepick, needle path, or flashlight view. In M-mode the position and motion of structures along a single line is recorded without information concerning adjacent structures (Fig. 12-1). Though M-mode scanning compensates for this defect somewhat, the records obtained by this technique do not contain precise information about structure size in the plane of the scan. For instance, the beam is recorded perpendicularly despite the fact that considerable angulation may have been used. As a result, a scanning maneuver that views a triangular or wedge-shaped portion of the heart is displayed as a rectangular record. This produces distortions at the extremes of angulation and tends to position structures in these areas deeper than they lie if measured from the nearest skin surface. Also, near structures that occupy the narrow portion of the wedge or triangle of tissue are stretched to accommodate the rectangular format of strip chart recorders. The rate at which the scan is made and the speed of the recording paper and not the anatomy determine the apparent spacing of structures. Slow scans and fast paper speeds produce abnormal elongations, whereas very slow paper speeds may shorten apparent relationships. An ideal M-mode scan, therefore, would require sliding a perfectly vertical beam (regardless of chest wall contour) at a rate that exactly matches the speed of the moving recording surface. This combination is virtually impossible to achieve in clinical settings.

There are other factors that also make M-mode scanning less than ideal in the anatomic presentation of echocardiographic findings. Not only does the anatomy of the heart change during an M-mode scan, but the motion of structures is also recorded. This results in a complex image that includes changing structure superimposed on intrinsic motion. Often, the records are confusing and difficult to interpret, especially when the examiner wishes to analyze the coordinated motion of a single structure such as a heart valve or wall. The analysis of ventricular septal motion or the appreciation of the entire motion pattern of a mitral valve with ruptured chordae are excellent examples of this difficulty.

Furthermore, movements that occur across the beam during a phase of the cardiac cycle may also produce confusing records. The apex of the heart, for instance, may

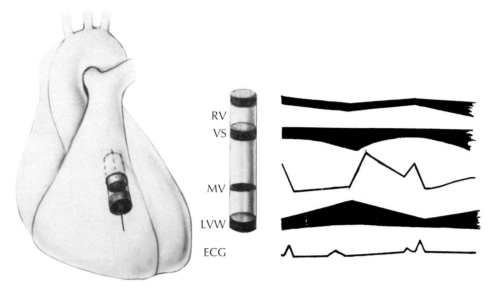

Fig. 12-1. One-dimensional echocardiography. The frontal projection of the heart demonstrates the concept that M-mode is equivalent to extraction of a plug of tissue that corresponds to the width of the beam passing through the heart. The removed plug is shown to the right and contains a portion of the right ventricle (RV), ventricular septum (VS), mitral valve (MV), and left ventricular posterior wall (LVW). A schematic of structure motion along with the ECG is included. ECG, electrocardiogram.

enter the beam only in systole during scanning of a large pericardial effusion and produce clumps of echoes that may appear to be separated from the heart in the pericardial effusion space. Though M-mode scanning is an integral and important part of echocardiographic examination, the limitations preclude the production of images that accurately duplicate the size and shape of heart cavities, valves, and lesions such as tumor masses, and the coordinated motion of the total structure cannot be appreciated.

STATUS OF TWO-DIMENSIONAL IMAGING

Two-dimensional cardiac imaging records structure distribution in motion in real-time and in planes equivalent to slices removed from the heart (Fig. 12-2). Early use of real-time devices has already demonstrated that M-mode information can vary considerably, depending on the portion of the valve leaflet under study, and that better M-modes are obtained when they are selected during a two-dimensional study.

Structure recognition in two dimensions is generally easier and more complete than with one dimension and does not depend so heavily on the demonstration of heart valves as landmarks. Heart valves themselves are generally easier to locate with the real-time systems, though we have occasionally required the more familiar M-mode to locate a heart valve, particularly when a complex anomaly is under study. Increased familiarity with two-dimensional imaging is expected to decrease the number of times this is necessary.

Certain cardiac motions are much easier to understand in two dimensions than in M-mode. The systolic displacement of the atrioventricular junction is readily appreciated in long axis views of the left ventricle but appears as a contractile pattern in M-mode. This is a reflection of the ability of two-dimensional systems to document motion of structures that move longitudinally in the plane of study but are across the beam in M-mode.

The ultrasonic plane under examination can be varied rapidly in real-time systems so that operator judgment can be exercised for

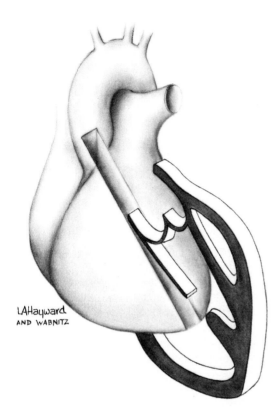

LAHayward
AND WABNITZ

Fig. 12-2. Two-dimensional scanning concept. Real-time, two-dimensional images are equivalent to slices of the heart that are removed and observed in motion. This illustration shows the cardiac cavities and valves viewed in the long axis of the left ventricle and the relationship of this plane to a frontal view of the heart.

ideal plane selection. Also, multiple parallel planes or the utilization of a sliding or tilting technique can be used to synthesize a three-dimensional concept of cardiac anatomy. Wild or erratic motions that occur in the presence of chordae rupture and with vegetations are much easier to understand and to characterize when viewed in two-dimensional motion.

The clinical role of two-dimensional imaging has not yet been defined, but there are early indications that its role in echocardiography will increase with usage. The more complete demonstration of structures such as heart valves has already provided some insight into the capabilities of two-dimensional imaging. The ability to view the leaflets of the aortic valve in longitudinal section has

demonstrated the position of the leaflets as the valve opens. This has permitted recognition of the congenitally stenotic valve, which domes on opening, and the size of the orifice has been estimated from these studies. In acquired mitral stenosis, short axis images of the mitral orifice have been obtained that accurately depict its width and compare well with measurements of the excised valve. Ultrasonic two-dimensional studies may prove to be more accurate in measuring orifice size than the traditional cardiac catheterization techniques, which are severely hampered by coexisting processes such as mitral regurgitation or aortic incompetence.

Vegetations on cardiac valves are generally easier to recognize in the two-dimensional format, especially when they are highly mobile and move some distance in the stream of blood flow. Associated destruction of tissues can be better appreciated. Other masses, such as myxomas, are much easier to recognize and their anatomic extent and motion more accurately characterized. In mitral valve prolapse, analysis of the extent of involvement of either leaflet may often be clearly delineated and abnormal motion patterns that are not recognizable on M-mode studies appear to be emerging.

Considerable promise exists that two-dimensional studies will play an important role in the evaluation of coronary artery disease. The origin of the left coronary artery has been demonstrated and an aneurysm shown. Ventricular aneurysms and abnormalities in segmental wall motion have been demonstrated. The potential exists, with the availability of devices that can encompass the entire left ventricle in its long axis, that left ventricular volumes and performance can be evaluated with ultrasonic techniques.

The supravalvular extension of aortic root dissection has been imaged in our laboratory and promises to improve the accuracy of the ultrasonic technique and, we hope, demonstrate the sources of false-positives seen in M-mode. Transverse studies of the aortic root add valuable diagnostic information by demonstrating portions of aortic walls not seen in M-mode.

Pericardial effusion is much easier to recognize in two dimensions, and sources of false-positives, such as pulmonic veins or subepicardial fat, cause much less confusion in diagnosis. The distribution of fluid toward the apex or behind other chambers such as the left atrium is usually obvious and makes recognition easier. In more complicated situations, such as in those patients who have had a left pneumonectomy and are examined for a question of pericardial effusion, the gross distortion of anatomy may make the M-mode examination very confusing while two-dimensional studies can demonstrate these effusions with clarity.

Complex cardiac malformations are conditions in which two-dimensional echocardiography should show its full potential in describing anatomic alterations. The spatial relationship of great vessels to each other, their relationship to cardiac chambers, and identification of the pulmonary artery and aorta by the direction taken after origin from the heart have been demonstrated. The displacement and abnormal attachment of the tricuspid valve in Ebstein's disease have been recorded. The tricuspid valve has also been differentiated from the mitral by noting the number of leaflets and the shape of the orifice when the valve is open. This finding is of use in identifying complexes that involve ventricular inversion. Obstructing membranes in the left ventricular outflow tract, as well as in the atrial cavities, can be imaged successfully.

There are certain drawbacks in two-dimensional cardiac imaging as it exists today. Anatomic analysis may be difficult or confusing, since the anatomic planes that are imaged are often nonstandard in the sense that there is not an abundance of cross-sectional anatomic information to be used for comparison with the ultrasonic images. Classic cross sections of the heart have been made mostly in planes that parallel or cross the major axes of the trunk and not in those that relate one intracardiac structure to another as required in two-dimensional echocardiography. Also, a variety of planes is needed to describe the anatomy as small changes in the scanning plane are made dur-

ing examination. This material should develop as clinical applications of two-dimensional imaging grow.

The resolution of motion with current scanners is limited by the frame repetition frequency, which is generally too low to record very rapid events like fine fluttering of heart valves or valve opening and closing rates. Here, M-mode has a distinct advantage and a firm position in diagnostic echocardiography. Structure boundaries are also more clearly defined in M-mode so that certain measurements may be made with greater precision.

Image recording in two-dimensional studies often utilizes a television camera chain to record the images on videotape. This introduces image-degrading features and is avoided in newer systems that record directly onto videotape without an intervening camera. However, videotape is a difficult format to use when it is necessary to present images to large groups and requires a compatible TV tape player. Single-frame exposures are generally made photographically with self-developing film but suffer in quality when viewed alone without the component of motion.

A wide variety of clinical conditions has not yet been studied so that the place of two-dimensional imaging in respect to M-mode has not yet been defined. Eventual utility depends on the demonstration of findings that are not seen on M-mode or that are shown with greater ease and clarity in two dimensions. Diagnostic accuracy, the incidence of false-positives and false-negatives, and clarification of some of the pitfalls of one-dimensional imaging remain to be fully defined. New functional information based on a comprehensive evaluation of structure size, character, and motion will be required to ensure a firm future for two-dimensional cardiac imaging in motion.

CURRENT SYSTEMS

Three basic systems are commercially available for the production of real-time two-dimensional images of the heart. They can be compared according to their operational features that influence the nature of the image and to certain advantages and disadvantages in their fundamental concepts. However, two-dimensional cardiac imaging is a rapidly changing field. New modifications are constantly emerging, and it is difficult to state a preference for one particular system when all factors are considered. The potential user must evaluate the applications in which two-dimensional imaging might be useful in practice and determine how a particular system meets his needs. The expense of some systems will also influence the decision.

Mechanical sector scanners

Basic concept. Mechanical sector scanners, as the name implies, mechanically angle a transducer through a sector repeatedly and at a rapid rate, thereby scanning a fan-shaped area with the point of the fan at the transducer surface (Fig. 12-3). Each angular excursion of the crystal results in the production of a frame with every beam sweep so that a full cycle of angulation produces two frames as the crystal is angled and then returns to the starting position. The number of lines contained in the image is determined by the pulse repetition frequency (PRF) and the number of frames required for a study. These devices usually operate at a PRF of about 4000/sec so that each frame contains about 133 lines when a frame rate of 30/sec is used. The image is most pleasing when the individual lines are closely spaced to produce good border continuity and a high density of information in the area under study. Very wide sectors and high frame rates may show spaces between the lines of information, since a fixed number of available pulses must be divided more often and spread over a wider area. In some systems the speed of crystal motion may be greatest at its midpoint, and the image will reveal less information density in the midportion of the sector as compared to the edges. The result is usually not objectionable.

System features. The transducer is mounted on the end of a housing that primarily contains a motor and a drive assembly that oscillate the crystal (Fig. 12-4). The housing is much larger than the transducer used in M-mode operation but is relatively easy to hold and to maneuver. Some vibration is experienced by the operator, but this is not an objectionable feature. The crystal is about the same diameter as conventional transducers and operates at about 2.0 MHz. Some devices permit crystal changing to obtain higher frequencies when desirable. The usual sector angle is 30 degrees with a frame rate of 30/sec, but wider sectors up to 60 degrees and frame rates of 30 to 60/sec can be selected by the operator. The ultrasonic system is identical to that used in M-mode, and in some cases the two-dimensional imager can be added to an already available ultrasonoscope by the addition of a module containing system controls, a display oscilloscope, and a camera that can be programmed to obtain still-frame photographs. The display oscilloscope has television type controls for adjustment of brightness and contrast for optimal display of the gray scale image. An ECG is displayed along with the sector scan image. A TV tape recorder and a strip chart recorder are also included, and the entire unit is packaged so that it is mobile and can be used for bedside examination.

In operation, a liberal quantity of coupling gel is applied to the chest wall and the oscillating crystal is positioned much as it is in M-mode examinations. The examiner directs a sector plane into the heart while observing the moving image on the oscilloscope. TV tape recording is accomplished with a foot switch. The crystal produces a vibrating sensation on the chest wall that is not unpleasant but that may become painful with prolonged examination. Coupling the transducer to the chest wall may be more difficult than with conventional transducers, especially when the chest wall is very thin or when large sector angles are employed. The coupling gel may require frequent renewal, since the motion of the crystal displaces the gel or may whip air in, reducing its transmission efficiency. The images obtained are of high quality, and all structures that can be detected by M-mode can be studied by sector scanning.

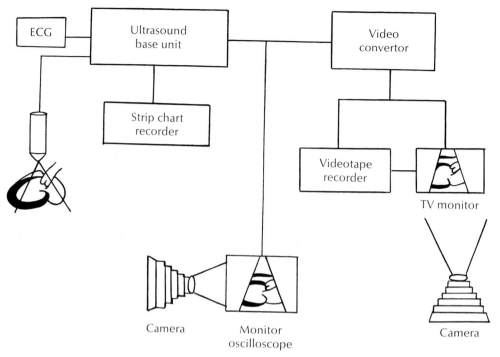

Fig. 12-3. Mechanical scanning system. This block diagram demonstrates components of a typical mechanical sector scanner. The ultrasound base unit generates the ultrasonic pulses and receives echoes from the sector scanner along with the patient's ECG. The signal may be sent to a strip chart recorded to obtain M-mode traces with a stationary crystal. For two-dimensional motion display the ultrasound output may be directed to a monitor oscilloscope, which can be photographed during the examination using an ECG trigger to obtain stationary images at a point in the cardiac cycle. For motion display, the ultrasound signal is converted to a video format (a TV camera is used in some systems) for storage in a tape recorded with simultaneous display on a TV monitor. The images may be photographed directly, but better results are obtained from the videotape operated in stop frame mode.

M-modes can be obtained but require that the crystal be stopped after the desired target is located and positioned in the center of the sector scan field.

Some foreign manufacturers have placed a crystal internally in the housing so that there are no vibrations transmitted directly to the patient. A major disadvantage of sector scanners is the fact that structures that are anteriorly located are incompletely demonstrated in the narrow portion of the field.

The cost of these systems is relatively low when compared to other, more complex, sector scanners, which deflect the beam electronically without crystal vibration. However, an add-on device costs about as much as a complete M-mode system with a strip chart recorder, so that a complete mechanical sector scanner is about twice as expensive.

Electronic sector scanners (phased array)

Basic concept. Electronic sector scanners provide an image similar to that obtained from mechanical scanners but differ in the manner in which beam scanning is accomplished. The applicator is small, about the same size as a conventional transducer, but the crystal is composed of small elements arranged linearly in an array. There are generally about 30 individual elements spaced over a total distance of around 15 mm. In

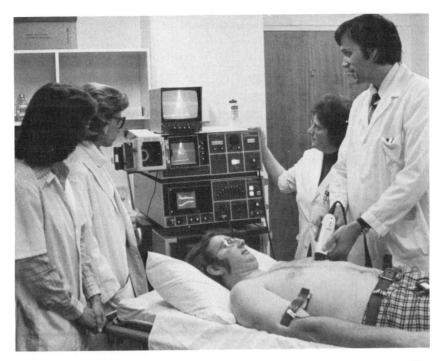

Fig. 12-4. Patient examination with a mechanical sector scanner. A commercially available sector scanner is shown during a routine two-dimensional real-time study. The examiner holds the transducer assembly with two hands and requires an assistant to adjust instrument gain controls. The image is displayed on a larger viewing monitor as well as on a smaller oscilloscope from which still photographs may be obtained by the attached camera. A television tape recorder is operated by a foot switch for motion recording along with the comments of the examiner.

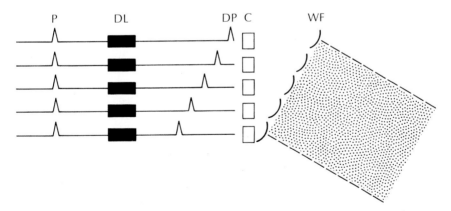

Fig. 12-5. Phased-array principle. Pulses of electrical energy (P) are simultaneously generated in leads supplying individual crystals (C) in a linear array. Delay lines (DL) slow the passage of each pulse so that the delayed pulses (DP) arrive at the crystals in a staggered linear sequence. The wavelets generated by each crystal summate into a wavefront (WF), which is angled in respect to the face of the array. The resultant beam is therefore propagated at an angle. By varying the magnitude and the sequence of the delays, the beam can be made to scan in a sector.

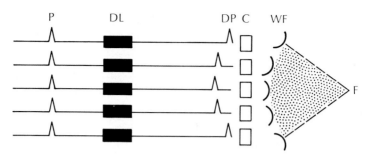

Fig. 12-6. Phased-array focusing. Focusing can be effected by programming the delays so that the delayed pulses arrive at the crystals (C) in a spherical sequence and therefore produce a summated wavefront (WF) that is convex and results in a beam that focuses to a narrow point (F). By altering the curvature of the relationship of the delayed pulses (DP), the examiner can alter the point of focus, but this point is fixed for any individual pulse emission, which is necessarily brief. The same principle can be applied in the receive phase to narrow the field from which echoes are accepted. More time is available so that the focus of the receiving system can be changed to correspond to the depth of tissues returning echoes. In this manner, a narrow tissue path equivalent to a narrow sending beam can be utilized along the entire range for each returning pulse. P, pulses of electrical energy; DL, delay lines.

operation the individual elements are excited sequentially with a small delay interposed in the activation of individual crystals. This results in a wavefront generated at an angle to the face of the transducer (Fig. 12-5). Variations in the degree of delay can be used to swing the beam rapidly in a sector format. The phased-array principle can also be used to focus the beam. If the magnitude of the delays between elements is changed so that the wavefronts emerging from the crystals located at the edge of the array are deflected toward the central portion of the beam, a focusing effect can be produced that narrows the beam (like an acoustic lens) (Fig. 12-6). By proper programming of delays the point of focus can also be altered during the receive phase so that it is possible to zoom the zone of best focus. This dynamic focusing, therefore, can result in a marked improvement in the width of the beam throughout the range of observation, which is typically 15 cm in sector scanners. This dynamic beam narrowing improves lateral resolution throughout the area of interest. These devices are considerably more complex than mechanical sector scanners and require some form of computer to program the delays.

System features. The transducer is small, about the same size as a conventional transducer. Obviously, a motor housing is not required, and there is no vibratory sensation for the operator or patient (Fig. 12-7). Free mobility and angulation of the transducer are possible. The scanning angle is adjustable and may be extended up to about 90 degrees for wide-angle viewing of a large portion of the heart. Frame rates up to 30/sec are utilized, and the same constraints between scanning angle, frame rate, and line density as described for mechanical scanners pertain to phased arrays. Focusing may be selectable at a given depth or dynamic to achieve a greater depth of field. The images are also presented in gray scale, and the quality may be similar to mechanical scanners or better. An ECG display is included.

The systems may be rather large so that all may not be transportable to the bedside. The electronics are sufficiently different from conventional M-mode machines so that an add-on device is not available today.

High quality M-modes can be obtained from any angle in the sector by positioning a bright line on the sector scan image to indicate the portion of the heart from which

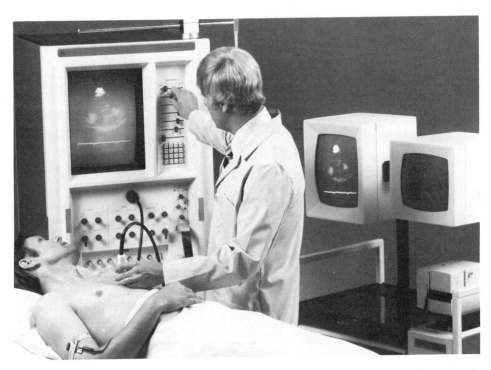

Fig. 12-7. Phased-array sector scanner. The transducer in this commercial system is small and can be held with one hand. The display oscilloscope shows the real-time 80-degree sector along with the ECG and patient identification. Still photography is carried out from an independent oscilloscope. The system contains a video recorder for motion recording.

the tracing is recorded. This line can be moved while observing the sector scan so that well directed M-mode sweeps can be made simultaneously with motion recording.

Phased-array systems are generally similar to mechanical scanners in all other features except cost. At the present time, these devices cost about two to four times as much as complete mechanical sector scanners, depending on the sophistication of the beam-forming system. It is anticipated, however, that cost will decrease as less expensive methods for producing delays are generated and as the price of the computational systems required for beam steering diminishes.

Fixed-beam, linear arrays

Basic concept. Fixed-beam linear arrays are the first system developed to produce real-time, two-dimensional images of the heart in motion. A multielement array usu-

ally 6 to 8 cm in length and containing 20 to 60 individual elements is used to form an ultrasonic beam that is electronically swept along the length of the array and in a direction perpendicular to the line of crystals. The beam is formed by exciting several adjacent elements so that the resultant beam has the same width as that obtained from a standard transducer. The excitation sequence is advanced by adding an element or a small group of elements in the advancing direction while subtracting a similar contribution from the trailing portion of the beam. In this manner, a well-collimated beam is made to sequence rapidly, up to 60 times per second, along the length of the array. Phasing is not employed to angle the beam, but some systems use phasing to obtain focus at a prescribed depth.

Display is in a raster format with the echo returns shown on an oscilloscope as lines

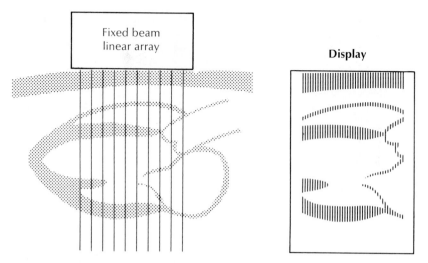

Fig. 12-8. Fixed beam linear array principle. A fixed beam linear array is shown with ten representative beams that are produced individually and in a rapid sequence. The echo returns from each individual beam are displayed along lines that lie adjacent to each other and in correct anatomic relationship to the echoing structures. The display is presented as if formed from more beams than shown in the schematic for better border continuity.

that correspond to the beam position from which the echoes are recorded. Rapid sequencing results in a real-time motion image (Fig. 12-8).

System features. Linear multielement arrays generate large rectangular images so that structures lying near the chest wall are displayed more completely than is possible with sector scanners. This is particularly advantageous in congenital heart disease, in which right heart distortions are common. The relatively large transducer may also represent a disadvantage and create a coupling problem in individuals with thin, irregular chest walls. The plane of the scan may be changed readily by sliding the transducer or tilting it medially or laterally in respect to its long axis. Angulation along the long axis of the transducer is not possible, since contact with the chest wall must be maintained. The obligatory perpendicular relationship between the beam and the chest wall images the structures around the base of the heart well so that high-quality images of the aortic root, left atrium, mitral valve, and proximal left ventricle can be obtained. The sloping

posterior left ventricular wall, as it inclines toward the apex, is not seen as well as with sector scanners.

These units are sufficiently small to allow portability to the bedside (Fig. 12-9). Display and hard copy features are similar to those described under sector scanners. M-mode recordings can be readily obtained from a single line of the image or, if desired, two M-modes can be recorded from two different lines to observe and compare the simultaneous motion patterns of two different structures, such as the aortic and mitral valves. These devices are also not unduly expensive and fall in the general range of mechanical sector scanners.

CARDIAC EVALUATION BY PLANES

The examination technique is quite similar to that used in M-mode echocardiography, but the fact that the beam is two dimensional in real-time cardiac imaging requires new terminology to describe the maneuvers we have found successful in patient examination.

Sliding describes a searching technique in which the transducer is moved over the pre-

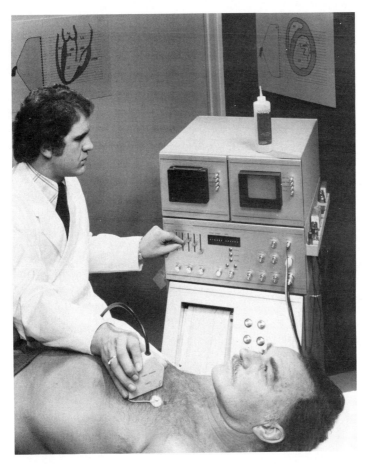

Fig. 12-9. Fixed beam multielement array. The equipment used for multibeam imaging of cardiac cross-sectional anatomy is shown. The examiner has placed the transducer over the patient's heart and is adjusting sensitivity controls. The strip chart recorder is producing a simultaneous M-mode from a portion of the array.

cordium, passing the sector into various portions of the heart. It is most useful for evaluation of the size of the cardiac window and determination of the size and shape of the heart for preliminary estimation of the general direction of specific planes within the heart. Sliding can also impart three-dimensional information by demonstrating successive adjacent planes that can be visually added by the examiner into a composite multisectional view (Fig. 12-10).

Angulation extends the view of the heart obtained by a particular sector and involves scanning the fan-shaped examination plane along its arc or width, thereby adding ana-tomic information by sequentially increasing the longitudinal extent of the area under study (Fig. 12-11). The effect is equivalent to increasing the size of the sector beyond that directly available from the instrument.

Tilting displaces the sector in a direction perpendicular to its width and is useful for changing the plane of study and for the development of three-dimensional spatial orientation of structures in a particular scanning plane (Fig. 12-12).

Pivoting is a rotational motion that changes the direction of the axis of the sector scan in relation to intracardiac structures. It is accomplished by rotating the transducer on its

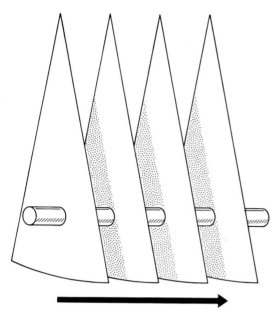

Fig. 12-10. Sector sliding. A series of sectors is shown as the transducer slides along a linear structure. Each sector displays a cross section, and continuity is evident since the structure image persists though the transducer is moved.

longitudinal axis while retaining a known target in the sector. Pivoting aligns the sector for ideal demonstration of intracardiac planes to include more than one target or to view more completely linear structures such as papillary muscles or a great vessel. In its extreme form, pivoting can provide two views of the same area obtained at 90 degrees to each other (Fig. 12-13). Though angulation, tilting, and pivoting imply a fixed reference point on the chest wall, they are often used in combination with sliding at the discretion of the examiner.

The landmarks used in two-dimensional echocardiography are essentially the same as those employed in one-dimensional studies. However, the recognition patterns are different in two-dimensional studies, and it is necessary to become familiar with a new image presentation to recognize structures. Reference to anatomic sketches and representative sector scans included in this chapter allow an echocardiographer entering the field of two-dimensional imaging to speed up the orientation process.

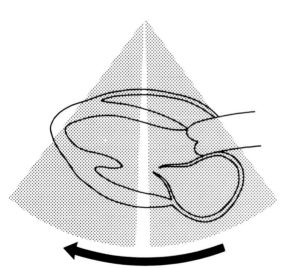

Fig. 12-11. Sector angulation. The limited fields of view obtained by a sector scanner can be increased by angling the sector in a straight line to include other structures lying in the same plane. Adjacent images can be summated into a broad impression of anatomy.

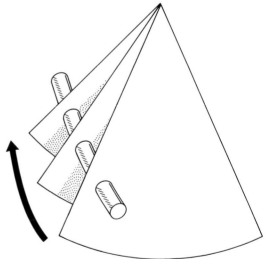

Fig. 12-12. Sector tilting. The sector may be tilted from a fixed point on the chest wall to pass the examining plane laterally through adjacent areas of interest. Tilting is useful to adjust the sector to a target of clinical interest or to obtain a more complete spatial orientation of structures.

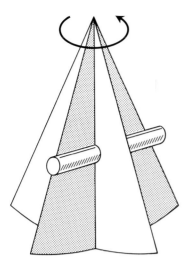

Fig. 12-13. Sector pivoting. A fixed reference point is employed, and the sector is rotated over a target of interest. Pivoting provides ideal alignment of the examining plane to a region or structure, or two views may be obtained to show longitudinal and cross-sectional features.

Our exposure to real-time echocardiography has been with a mechanical sector scanner, and we are confident that landmark recognition can be transferred directly to phased-array examinations and to studies carried out with fixed beam multielement arrays. The known landmarks, such as heart valves, cavities, and great vessels, can be used to describe various planes in the heart for maximal extraction of structural and functional information. Some planes are identified by the inclusion of two valves at the extremes of the sector image, whereas others require added landmarks located anteriorly and posteriorly for proper plane description. In transverse sections of the left ventricle and great vessels, ideal circular configurations are sought. Based on this approach, our experience has shown seven major planes of clinical interest and promise to extend the diagnostic capabilities of echocardiography.

A landmark that has not been recognized in M-mode echocardiography is the central fibrous junction that lies in the region where the ventricular and atrial septa join between the rings of the atrioventricular valves and just under the aortic root. It is composed of fibrous tissues that support valve rings and join centrally to constitute a mass of connective tissue. The central fibrous junction is recognized as a roughly circular area of high reflectance between the septa and the atrioventricular valves and should not be confused with an abnormal process such as calcification or tumor mass. Frequently, it can be seen more readily than the valves or septa and forms a valuable landmark for pivoting or tilting of the examination plane to bring adjacent structures into view. This landmark is altered in atrioventricular canal defects that involve disruption of this portion of the heart. Also, alterations in the attachment of the atrioventricular valves, as occurs in Ebstein's malformation, can be recognized by observing the relationship of the attachment site to the central fibrous junction.

Image presentation in two-dimensional echocardiography has varied, with some authors displaying the heart in an upright or apex-down position, with anterior structures on the left, while others have used the M-mode convention placing anterior structures at the top of the image. In 1976, the Standards Committee of the American Institute of Ultrasound in Medicine (AIUM) adopted an interim standard to introduce uniformity in publications and public presentations. Their recommendations in two-dimensional imaging of the heart may be summarized as follows:

• Transverse scans should be displayed as if viewed from the patient's feet so that right heart structures are present in the left side of the image and vice versa. Anterior structures are therefore at the top of the image.

• Longitudinal images should be displayed as if viewed from the patient's left side. Structures at the base of heart, for example, the aorta, will appear on the right side of the image while the cardiac apex is shown on the left. Anterior structures, as in transverse sections, remain at the top.

• Coronal or horizontal images that pass from the apex to the base of the heart are recommended for display as if viewed from the front of the patient so that the apex is oriented downward while the base of the heart is at the top of the image. Right-sided structures are to be shown on the left and left-sided structures on the right.

The images included in this chapter comply with the AIUM Interim Standard in the presentation of long- and short-axis views. However, we have elected to depart from the standard when coronal images are shown. It is our view that coronal planes should be displayed in the format present when they are acquired, namely, with the apex of the heart at the top of the image and the base at the bottom. This relationship corresponds to the image displayed on the oscilloscope during examination, so that it is easier to retain anatomic orientation while the examination is in progress.

Anatomic reference drawings, made in a frontal view, are presented to show the position and inclination of the major transverse examining planes with an insert to demonstrate their anteroposterior direction. Longitudinal plane reference drawings are similar but the insert reveals the orientation of the plane relative to the right and left sides.

Schematic anatomic expansions of sector images are included to show the position of the sector in the anatomic plane. Structure labeling is on the schematic to spare the sector image from conflicting lettering and arrows. Each schematic contains a pair of crossed lines that indicate anterior (A), posterior (P), right (R), left (L), superior or cephalic (S), and inferior or caudal (I) directions in the image. The reader should be aware that coronal sections may have only minimal anteroposterior inclination within the heart; however the base usually lies deeper than the apex relative to the chest wall, and this justifies our use of anterior and posterior designations on these anatomic planes.

Left ventricular long axis

This plane is an excellent starting point in real-time imaging of the heart, since most echocardiographers already appreciate the

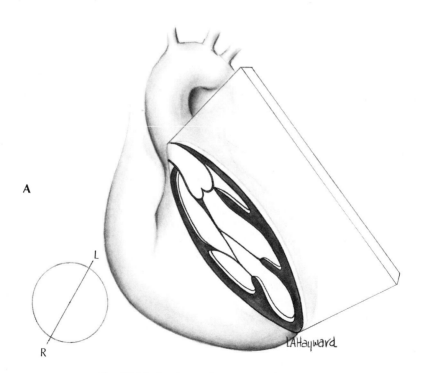

Fig. 12-14. For legend see opposite page.

anatomy and motion of structures in this plane (Fig. 12-14). Imaging of the long axis begins with the scanner placed in the precordial position, in which the mitral valve can usually be detected, and sliding it until the mitral valve is recognized by its position and motion pattern. Tilting medially or laterally identifies the beam orientation in which the mitral valve shows the greatest motion amplitude. If the aortic root is not clearly seen,

pivoting of the transducer to direct the superior portion of the sector medially in respect to the mitral valve aligns the scanning plane along the long axis of the left ventricle. Angulation caudally brings the papillary muscles, the left ventricular cavity, and finally the cardiac apex into view. The posterior left ventricular wall is seen as it slopes anteriorly toward the cardiac apex, which is located near the chest wall. Angulation toward

Text continued on p. 389.

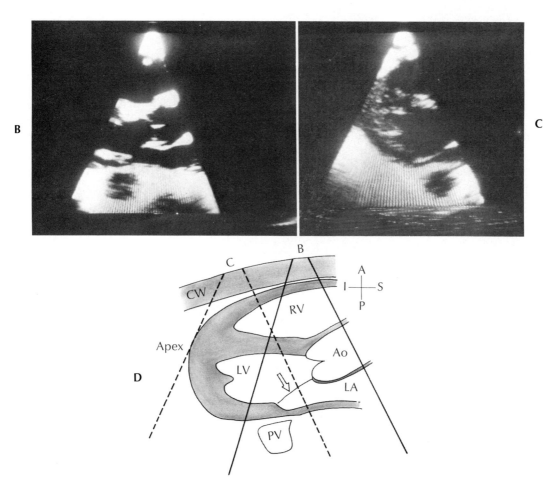

Fig. 12-14. Left ventricular long axis anatomy. The position and angulation of the anatomic plane for long axis study are shown in **A.** The small insert is an end-on view of the heart to demonstrate the medial orientation of the plane. Two-sector scans (**B** and **C**) were obtained in a patient with right ventricular (RV) enlargement and show the structures commonly imaged in this plane **(D).** The closed mitral valve is indicated by an arrow. The leaflets of the aortic valve are also closed in this frame obtained during isovolumic contraction. The base of a papillary muscle is imaged, as is an enlarged pulmonary vein (PV) behind the heart. CW, chest wall; LV, left ventricular cavity; Ao, aortic root; LA, left atrium.

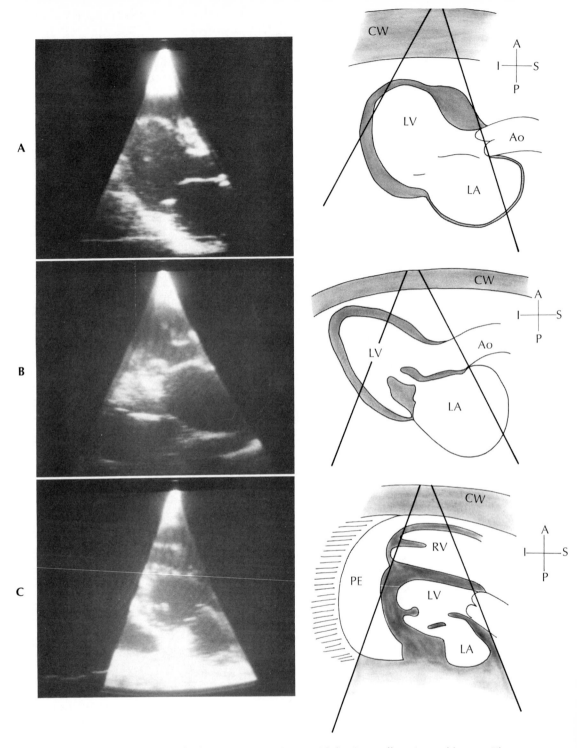

Fig. 12-15. Left ventricular long axis in patients with horizontally oriented hearts. These projections of the left ventricular long axis are obtained in a beam direction that more or less looks along the axis of the left ventricle and shows the cardiac chambers and valves from a viewpoint at or near the apex. The cardiac tilt allows inclusion of more of the left heart in the sector than is possible with vertically oriented hearts. In **A** there is asymmetric hypertrophy of the ventricular septum. **B** is from a patient with mitral stenosis and shows heavily calcified cusps and an enlarged left atrium (LA). Pericardial effusion (PE) and an enlarged right ventricle (RV) are demonstrated in **C.** Note the papillary muscle images in the right and left (LV) ventricles. CW, chest wall; Ao, aortic root.

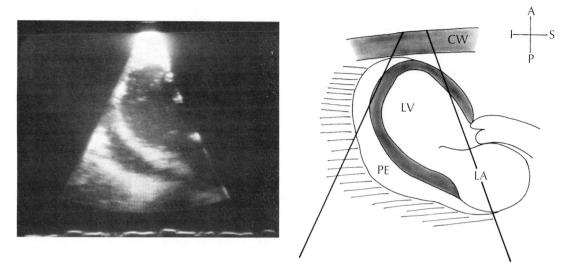

Fig. 12-16. Apical long axis view of the left ventricle. A pericardial effusion space (PE) hugs the posterior left ventricular wall and extends somewhat behind the left atrial cavity. It thins dramatically at the ventricular apex. LV, left ventricle; LA, left atrium; CW, chest wall.

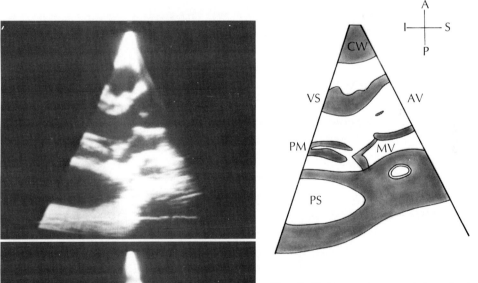

Fig. 12-17. Long axis scan of the mitral and aortic valves following left pneumonectomy. The excursion of the mitral valve (MV) is evident between early systole **(A)** and diastole **(B).** The pneumonectomy space (PS) lies behind the left ventricle and is difficult to differentiate from pericardial fluid. Narrowing of the left atrial cavity seen behind the aortic valve (AV) probably results from postoperative distortion. VS, ventricular septum; PM, papillary muscles.

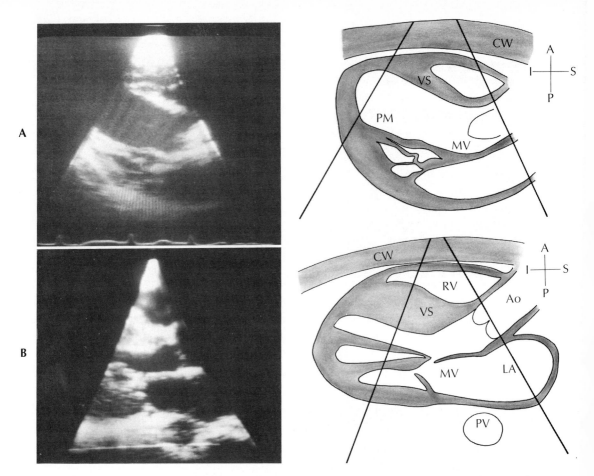

Fig. 12-18. Long axis scans. A patient with mitral stenosis is shown in **A.** The mitral apparatus between the papillary muscles (PM) and mitral valve (MV) is thickened and distorted by the rheumatic process. The aortic root is poorly seen because the plane is tilted for optimal demonstration of the papillary muscles. **B** shows asymmetric hypertrophy of the ventricular septum (VS). CW, chest wall; RV, right ventricular cavity; Ao, aortic root; LA, left atrium; PV, pulmonary vein.

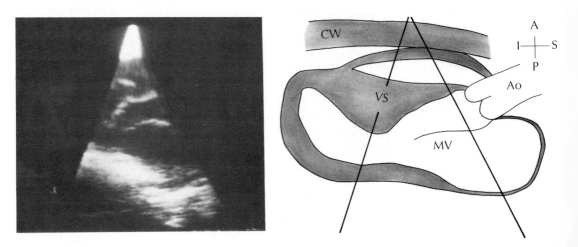

Fig. 12-19. Midventricular outflow obstruction from asymmetric septal hypertrophy. This long-axis sector of the mitral valve (MV) and aortic root (Ao) shows the ventricular septum (VS) to thicken dramatically in the left ventricular cavity beyond the tip of the mitral valve. In systole, midventricular cavity obstruction was produced, which differs from the outflow tract obstruction seen in IHSS. CW, chest wall.

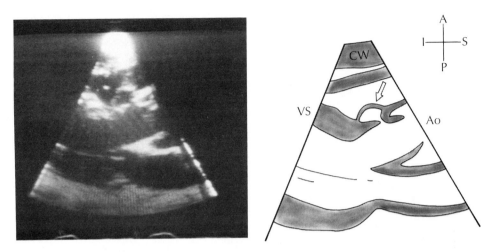

Fig. 12-20. Aneurysm formation involving the membranous septum. The aneurysmal bulge *(arrow)* is demonstrated in a long-axis plane of the left ventricle and aortic root (Ao) obtained during ventricular systole. In diastole the aneurysm collapsed, which suggests a ventricular origin rather than one from the sinus of Valsalva. At cardiac catheterization there was evidence of a ventricular septal defect. The plane that demonstrated the aneurysm best failed to image the mitral valve, though chordae can be seen in the left ventricular cavity. VS, ventricular septum; CW, chest wall.

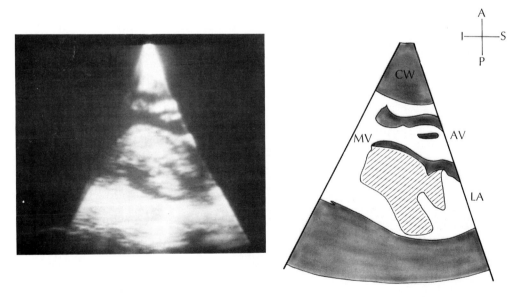

Fig. 12-21. Left atrial myxoma. The long axis sector of the mitral (MV) and aortic (AV) valves shows a dense mass of abnormal echoes *(cross-hatched)* in the enlarged left atrial cavity and extending behind the mitral valve. A large myxoma was removed at surgery. CW, chest wall; LA, left atrium.

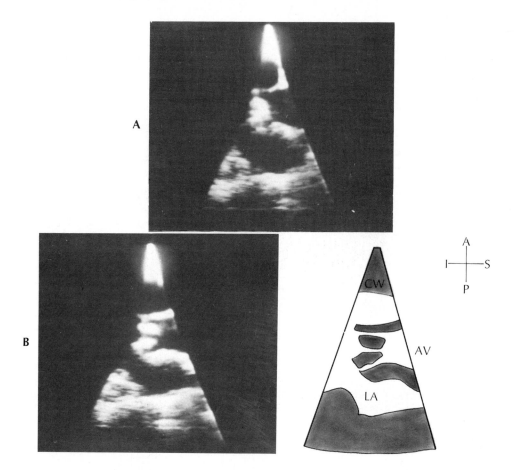

Fig. 12-22. Calcific aortic valve disease. This long axis sector demonstrates a calcified aortic valve (**A,** diastolic frame) with restricted motion of the leaflets in systole (**B).** CW, chest wall; AV, aortic valve; LA, left atrium.

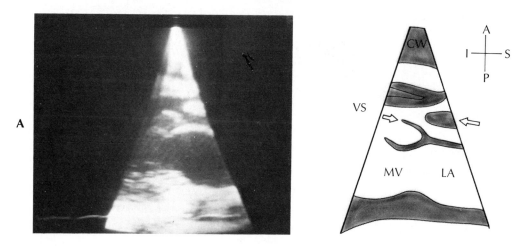

Fig. 12-23. For legend see opposite page.

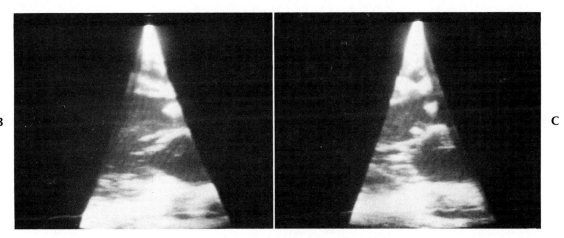

Fig. 12-23. Bacterial endocarditis (left ventricular long axis planes). Vegetations *(arrows)* are present on the mitral (MV) and aortic valves. This series, made in diastole **(A)** and early systole **(B and C)** shows a striking change in the mitral vegetation as the valve moves toward closure. VS, ventricular septum; LA, left atrium; CW, chest wall.

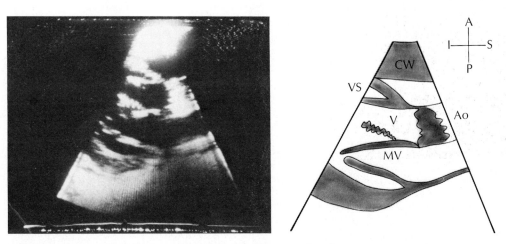

Fig. 12-24. Nonbacterial endocarditis of the mitral valve in systemic lupus ery-thematosis. This long axis plane shows the mitral valve (MV) in a semiclosed position and the vegetation (V) attached to the anterior leaflet. The serrated appearance of the margins of the vegetation (verruca) arise in a rapid flutter of about 600 cycles/sec, which is recorded as an M-mode in this single-beam sweep. The apparent filling of the aortic root (Ao) with echoes is an artifact produced by an oblique plane selected for optimal demonstration of the vegetation. VS, ventricular septum; CW, chest wall.

the head may also be used to demonstrate the base of the ascending aorta in the supra-valvular area as it arches anteriorly. A complete long-axis view of the left ventricle usually cannot be obtained in a single transducer position in patients with vertically situated hearts because of the limited sector angle and the narrow representation of anterior structures. However, when the heart assumes a more horizontal position, an apically placed sector may scan along the entire long axis, aortic origin, mitral valve, and left atrium (Figs. 12-15 and 12-16). Pivoting of the transducer in an apical position alters the long

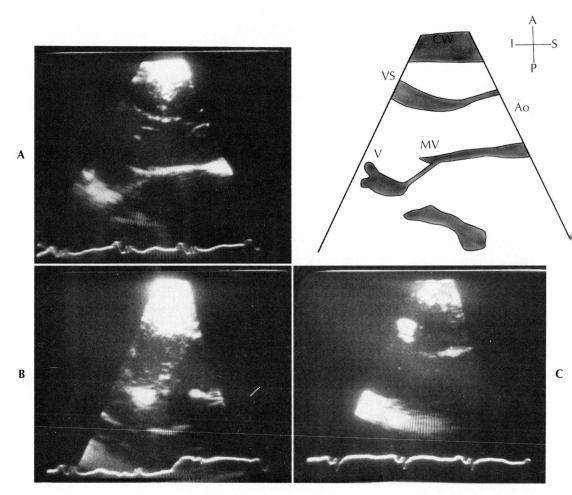

Fig. 12-25. Mitral valve vegetation and chordae rupture. A large vegetation (V) is seen attached to the distal portion of a ruptured chord, which has retained its mitral valve (MV) attachment **(A).** During the cardiac cycle, this mass could be seen flinging wildly in the left ventricular cavity **(B** and **C)** around its mitral valve attachment. VS, ventricular septum; Ao, aortic root.

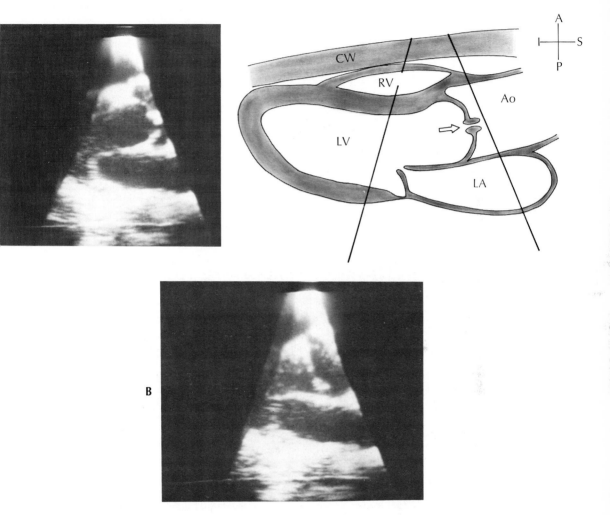

Fig. 12-26. Congenital aortic stenosis. The systolic image **(A)** shows the leaflets of a congenital bicuspid valve doming upward with the orifice *(arrow)* delineated by thickened cusp margins. In diastole **(B)** the dome has collapsed and forms an oblique line across the aortic root (Ao). CW, chest wall; RV, right ventricle; LV, left ventricle; LA, left atrium.

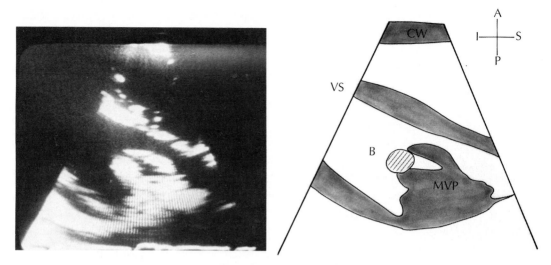

Fig. 12-27. Caged ball prosthesis. The ball *(cross-hatched)* is seen as a roughly circular image that appears smaller than its true size and is probably a tangential section. The cage of this mitral valve prosthesis (MVP) is partially seen, and the sewing ring is obscured in the heavy echoes at the base. VS, ventricular septum; CW, chest wall.

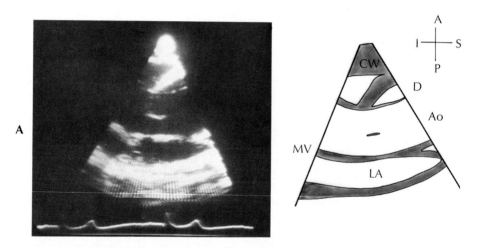

Fig. 12-28. Supravalvular aorta (long axis scans). A dissection space (D) is shown involving the anterior aortic (Ao) wall and extending into the supravalvular portion, which is dilated **(A).** In **B,** there is dilatation of the aorta in its supravalvular portion as a consequence of congenital aortic valve stenosis. MV, mitral valve; LA, left atrium; CW, chest wall.

axis view so that various portions of the left ventricular wall and right ventricular cavity can be examined.

Long axis scans have been clinically the most rewarding and have been useful in assessing normal mitral valve motion (Fig. 12-17), asymmetric septal hypertrophy (Figs. 12-18, 12-19, 12-15), septal aneurysms (Fig. 12-20), tumors (Fig. 12-21), and valvular abnormalities (Figs. 12-22 to 12-26 and 12-15). Papillary muscles and chordae can be evaluated for structural changes (Fig. 12-18), pericardial effusion and other fluid collections identified (Figs. 12-15 to 12-17), pros-

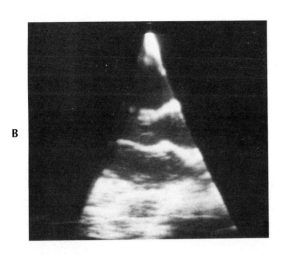

B

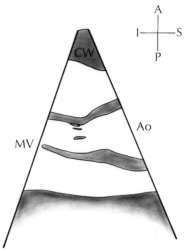

Fig. 12-28, cont'd. For legend see opposite page.

thetic valve motion studied (Fig. 12-27), and the supravalvular aorta examined for enlargement and wall abnormalities (Fig. 12-28).

Left ventricular short axis

The left ventricular short axis can be examined by pivoting the sector plane at an angle of 90 degrees from the long axis position (Fig. 12-29). Tilting is usually required to transect the left ventricular cavity perpendicular to the long axis so that the left ventricle is represented as a circular configuration with both short axes of equal dimension. Sector angulation is required to center the left ventricle in the beam for more complete visualization of the entire circumference. Sliding of the transducer permits alterations of the level of cross section and may be extended cephalically to the subaortic area through various portions of the mitral valve and more distally through the body of the left ventricle and the apex.

The mitral orifice can be examined and requires careful positioning of the sector plane at the tips of the leaflets to locate the minimal size of the orifice. A position located too far cephalically passes through the bodies of the leaflets and demonstrates an apparent orifice that is larger than the true size in the presence of mitral stenosis.

Left ventricular cross sections have shown systole-diastole variations in chamber size

Text continued on p. 399.

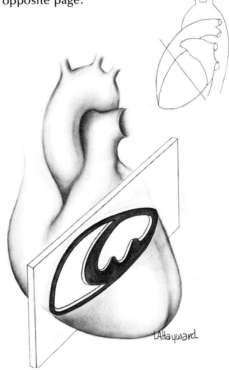

Fig. 12-29. Anatomy of the left ventricular short axis plane. A frontal sketch of the heart shows the spatial orientation of the plane for imaging the short axis of the left ventricle. The foreshortened anatomic image shows the left ventricle as an oval with papillary muscles on the posterior aspect, whereas the right ventricle is crescentic in cross section. The small insert is a lateral projection demonstrating the anteroposterior disposition of the plane.

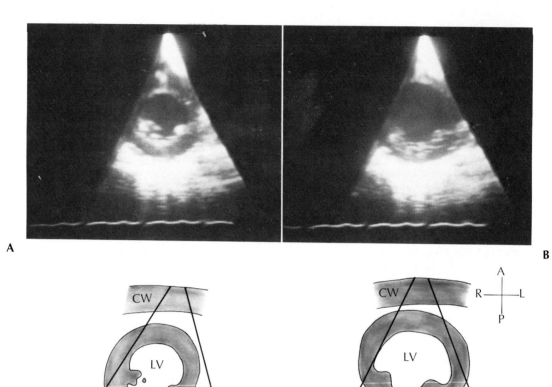

A

B

Fig. 12-30. Transverse scans of the left ventricular cavity. These sections were obtained just beyond the tips of the mitral leaflets and show the papillary muscles projecting into the left ventricular (LV) cavity. The endocardial echo is best seen in the systolic image **(A)**; the diastolic image **(B)** shows enlargement of the cavity. CW, chest wall.

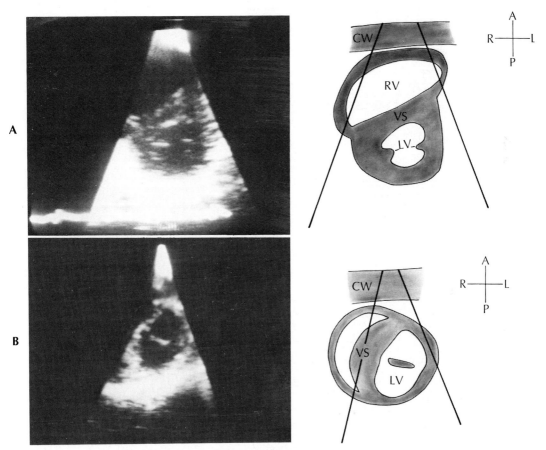

Fig. 12-31. Abnormalities of left ventricular cavity shape. Pulmonary hypertension **(A)** has enlarged the right ventricle (RV) and flattened the ventricular septum (VS). An asymmetrically thickened ventricular septum **(B)** flattens the contour of the left ventricular cavity (LV), where a portion of the mitral valve is seen. CW, chest wall.

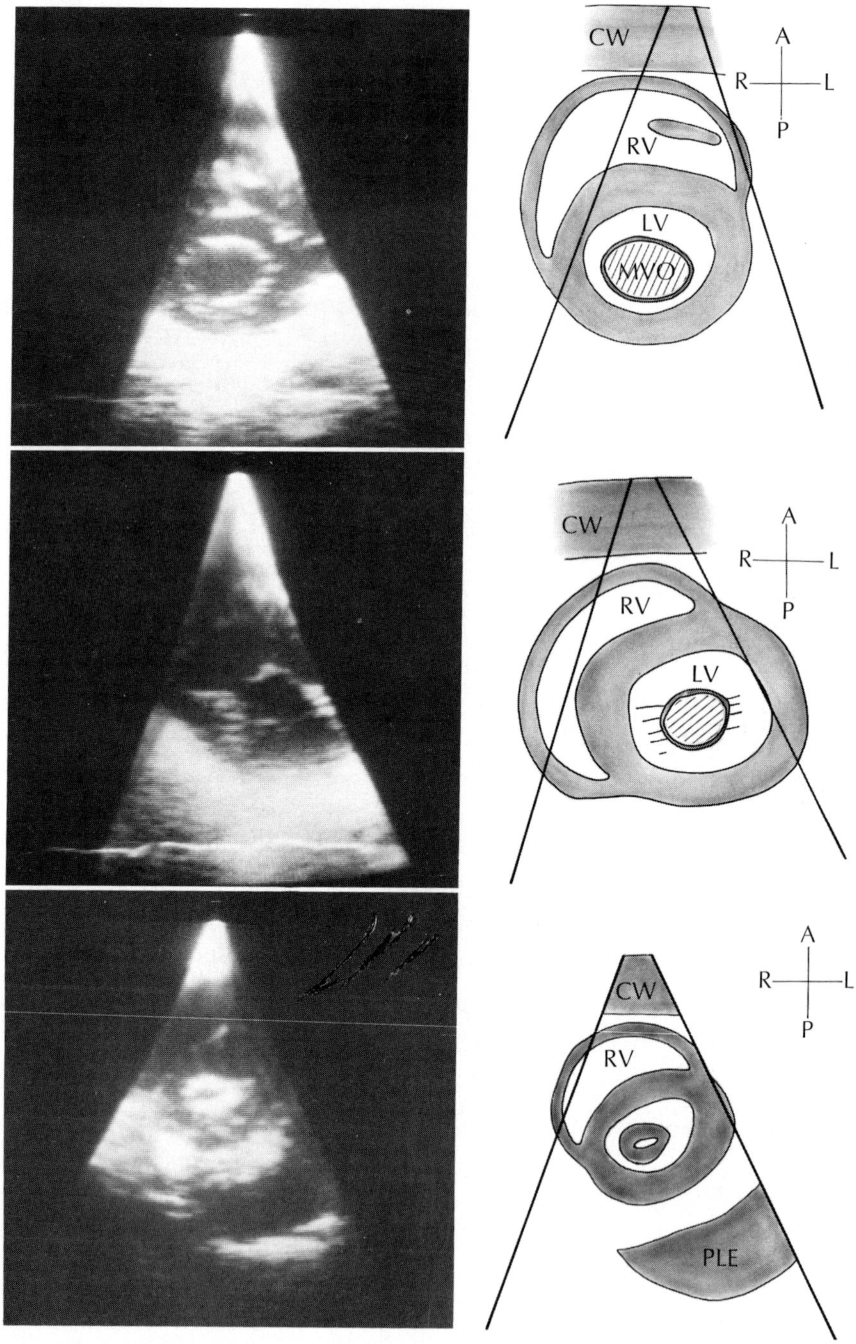

Fig. 12-32. Mitral valve orifices. A normal mitral valve orifice (*cross-hatched,* MVO) is demonstrated in a left ventricular (LV) cross section **(A).** Mild reduction of orifice size is present in a patient **(B)** with mild congenital mitral stenosis. Severe, rheumatic mitral stenosis **(C)** reveals a thickened and calcified valve with a markedly reduced, slitlike orifice. Incidental findings are a right ventricular papillary muscle in **A** and a pleural effusion (PLE) located behind the heart in **C.** CW, chest wall; RV, right ventricle.

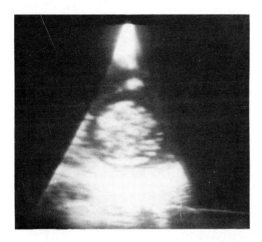

Fig. 12-33. Mitral orifice in left atrial myxoma. This short axis scan of the left ventricle was obtained at the level of the mitral valve and shows complete filling of the mitral orifice in diastole by tumor tissue, which prolapses into the left ventricular inflow.

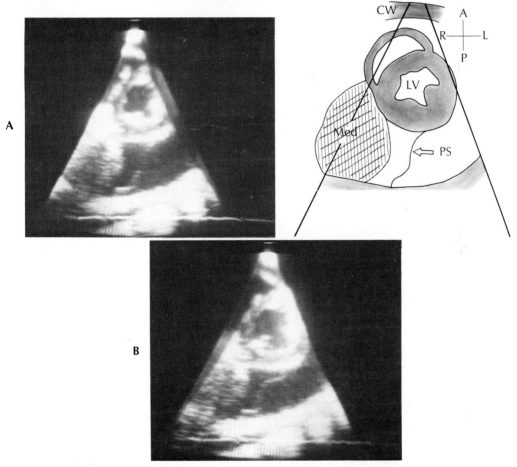

Fig. 12-34. Left ventricular short axis scan following pneumonectomy. The large sonolucent pneumonectomy space (PS) behind the left ventricle (LV) represents fluid that accumulates after lung removal. A fibrinous strand *(arrow)* extends posteriorly from the left ventricle to the posterior chest wall. In systole **(A)** it is pulled to a straight line and buckles in diastole **(B).** The displaced mediastinum (Med) produces a mass of echoes seen medially adjacent to the pneumonectomy space. CW, chest wall.

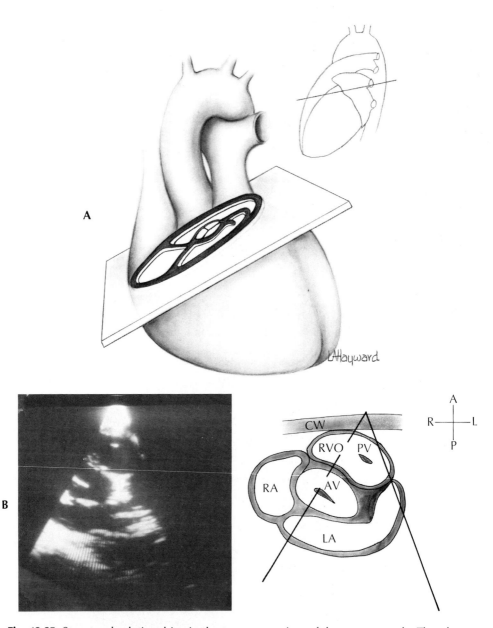

Fig. 12-35. Structural relationships in the transverse view of the great vessels. The plane that passes through the valves of the great vessels is shown in frontal and lateral views in **A.** A sector scan obtained in this plane **(B)** demonstrates the relationship of the aortic (AV) and pulmonic (PV) valves and continuity between the right ventricular outflow tract (RVO) and pulmonary artery, which lies to the left of the pulmonary valve. The left atrium (LA) lies posteriorly, and the position of the right atrium (RA) relative to the aorta is shown in the sketch. CW, chest wall.

and can be useful to show segmental abnormalities of wall motion. Papillary muscles can be imaged and their contractility pattern evaluated (Fig. 12-30). Flattening of the left ventricle has been demonstrated in the presence of pulmonary hypertension and asymmetric septal hypertrophy (Fig. 12-31). Normal and abnormal mitral orifice can be imaged and valve area measured (Figs. 12-32 and 12-33). A fibrinous adhesion following left pneumonectomy is shown in Fig. 12-34.

Transverse views of the great vessels

Transverse views of the great vessels are made by placing the transducer at the level of the aortic valve and rotating the sector plane transversely to the long axis of the aorta. With proper tilt the aortic root is seen as a circular image containing the leaflets of the aortic valve and origins of the coronary arteries. Inclusion of the pulmonary valve in the examining plane may require some pivoting toward the left shoulder so that the aortic root may appear oval in shape (Figs. 12-35 and 12-36).

We have found the transverse aortic plane to be ideal for the evaluation of bicuspid aortic valves which can show the distribution of valve tissue and the variable and irregular line of closure (Fig. 12-37). Other disease processes involving the aortic valve and left atrium may also be recognized (Figs. 12-38 and 12-39). This plane has also been used to diagnose dextrotransposition of the great vessels by showing parallelism and abnormal relationship of the outflow vessels instead of the normal curved course of the right ventricular outflow tract and pulmonary artery as they wrap around the aortic root.

Aortic-tricuspid plane

Identification of this plane may begin with a transverse orientation of the transducer to the aortic root. This is followed by rotation of the inferior portion of the sector rightward, accompanied by tilting of the plane under the sternum until the tricuspid valve and aortic root are imaged together. Minor adjustments of beam direction demonstrate the atrial septum extending posteriorly in an

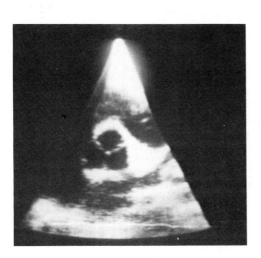 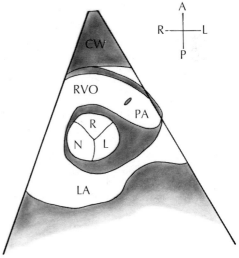

Fig. 12-36. Transverse section of the aortic root. This plane is less oblique than the aortic-pulmonary plane and images the aorta as a circular cross section. The diastolic image shows three cusps of the aortic valve in their closed position. The right coronary cusp (R) is anteriorly placed, whereas the noncoronary (N) and left (L) cusps are posteriorly situated. In this section the right ventricular outflow tract (RVO) and pulmonary artery (PA) are shown as they wrap around the aortic root. LA, left atrium; CW, chest wall.

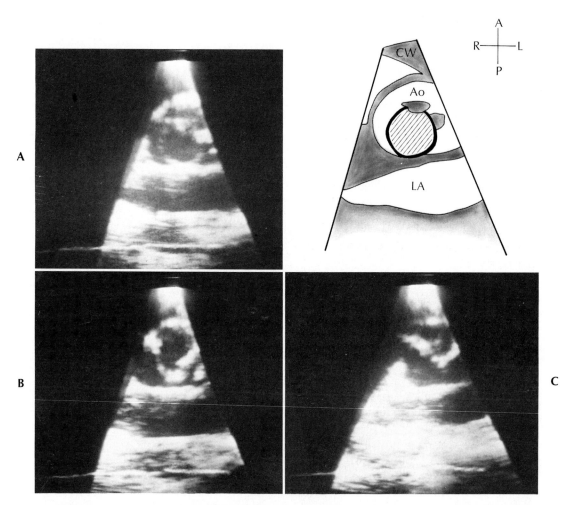

Fig. 12-37. Short axis cross section of a congenitally bicuspid aortic valve. The systolic frame **(A)** was made through the base of the doming valve *(cross-hatched)* and reveals two areas of cusp thickening. In **B,** obtained in early diastole, the dome is beginning to collapse and closes **(C)** in a curvilinear, approximately transverse, position. The line of closure is irregular and shows serrations produced by folding of redundant valvular tissue. Ao, aortic root; LA, left atrium; CW, chest wall.

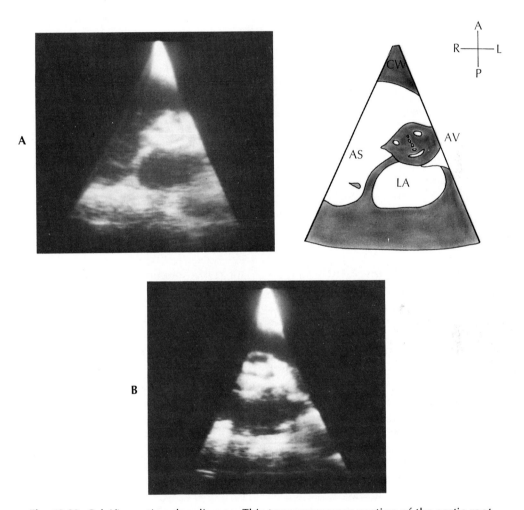

Fig. 12-38. Calcific aortic valve disease. This transverse cross section of the aortic root demonstrates a heavily calcified aortic valve with minimal cusp separation during systole. **A,** Diastolic frame. **B,** Systolic frame. CW, chest wall; AV, aortic valve; AS, atrial septum; LA, left atrium.

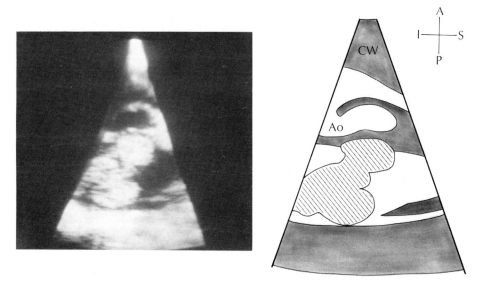

Fig. 12-39. Left atrial myxoma. The short axis cross section of the aortic root (Ao) demonstrates a lobulated tumor *(cross-hatched)* in the left atrium, which is enlarged. At surgery a multilobed myxoma was removed. CW, chest wall.

oblique line from the aortic root behind the tricuspid valve (Fig. 12-40). This plane offers the potential to examine the atrial septum for defects and right heart structures, especially the right ventricular outflow tract.

Mitral-tricuspid plane

The plane between the mitral and tricuspid valves is easiest to image by first obtaining a cross-sectional view of the left ventricular cavity and mitral valve and then angling the sector to the right to view right heart cavities. Pivoting of the plane is required to include the tricuspid valve in the image, and tilting provides optimal visualization of tricuspid valve leaflets (Fig. 12-41). This plane demonstrates the body and inflow portion of the right ventricle as well as the attachment site of tricuspid leaflets (Fig. 12-42). We have found it particularly useful in the study of Ebstein's malformation (Fig. 12-43) in viewing an abnormal attachment of the septal leaflet and to demonstrate elongation of the anterior leaflet. In this view the posteriorly located central fibrous junction serves as a reference point in evaluating displacement of the origin of the septal leaflet, which should

normally be at the level of the central fibrous junction. Variations that pass this plane somewhat low in the right atrial cavity may demonstrate the eustachian valve of the inferior vena cava as a linear structure whose medial extent is directed toward the central fibrous junction. Minor tilts of the plane show the space behind the eustachian valve as an oval configuration where the inferior vena cava enters the right atrium.

Mitral-pulmonic plane

The mitral-pulmonic plane requires placement of the sector in a sagittal orientation over the mitral valve with some medial tilting for optimal mitral imaging. This is followed by pivoting of the plane toward the left shoulder until the pulmonic leaflets are visible in the superior portion of the sector (Fig. 12-44). Angulation and tilting can be used to follow the course of the main pulmonary artery and of the right and left main branches. The posterior arching of the pulmonary artery becomes evident and can be utilized to distinguish the pulmonary artery from the aorta in conditions where their origins at the base of the heart are altered. Pulmonary

Fig. 12-40. Aortic-tricuspid plane anatomy. The orientation of this plane to a frontal view of the heart and to an end-on view is illustrated in **A.** Both sector scans were obtained from a patient with a bicuspid aortic valve (AV) in whom the diastolic image **(B)** reveals a folded line of closure extending in an anteroposterior direction. In **C,** the origin of the left coronary artery (LCA) is shown as it courses over the musculature of the left ventricle *(crosshatched).* The atrial septum *(arrow)* lies between the left (LA) and right (RA) atria. CW, chest wall; RV, right ventricle; TV, tricuspid valve.

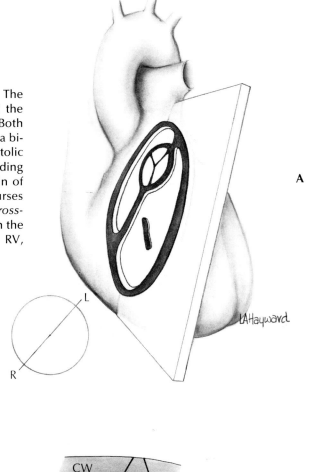

A

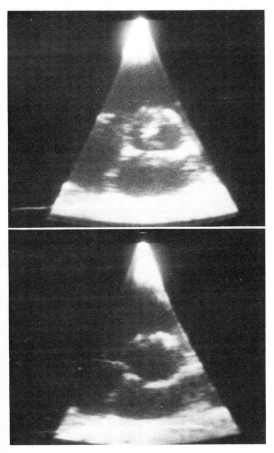

B

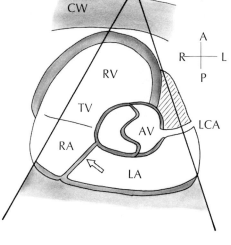

C

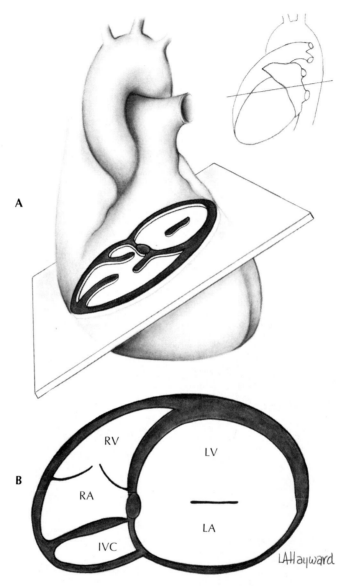

Fig. 12-41. Mitral-tricuspid plane. The normal relationship of heart cavities, the frontal position of the plane and its anteroposterior orientation are shown in **A.** In **B,** the structures encountered in this plane are shown schematically. The anterior mitral valve leaflet lies between the left ventricle (LV) and left atrium (LA), the central fibrous junction is located at the site of attachment of the septal leaflet of the tricuspid valve between the right ventricle (RV) and right atrium (RA), and the eustachian valve forms the anterior border of the entrance of the inferior vena cava (IVC) into the right atrium.

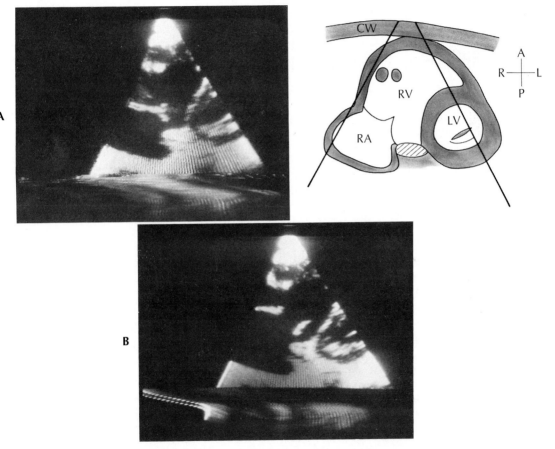

Fig. 12-42. Mitral-tricuspid plane in right ventricular enlargement. The right heart cavities are markedly enlarged and seen in "long axis" view. A more vertical plane than usual could be utilized so that the left ventricle (LV) is viewed across its short axis. The right ventricular cavity (RV) contains two papillary muscles, and the central fibrous junction (cross-hatched) appears elongated and forms part of the boundary between the right atrium (RA) and the right ventricle. **A** was recorded during isovolumic contraction as the tricuspid valve first closes. In early diastole (**B**) the tricuspid leaflets open as the distended right atrium begins to empty. CW, chest wall.

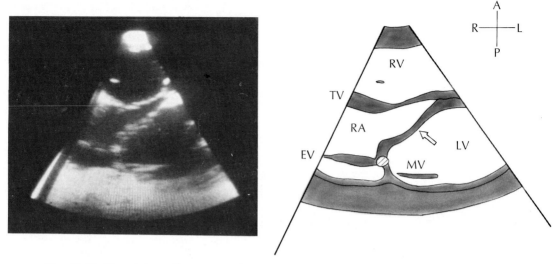

Fig. 12-43. Ebstein's malformation. A transverse plane between the mitral (MV) and tricuspid (TV) valves in a patient with Ebstein's malformation shows a large anterior leaflet of the tricuspid valve, which closes more anteriorly in the right ventricle (RV) than normal. The portion of the ventricular septum that is incorporated into the right atrium as the result of anterior tricuspid valve displacement is thin *(arrow)* and bulges toward the left ventricle (LV) in diastole. The eustachian valve (EV) is seen in the posterior portion of the right atrial cavity (RA) and extends to the central fibrous junction *(cross-hatched).*

valve doming, poststenotic dilatation, and branch stenoses of the left pulmonary artery may be demonstrable in this plane. This plane approximates the long axis of the right ventricular outflow tract. Caudal plane angulation or sliding is valuable in assessing its status and demonstrating a cross-sectional image of the body of the right ventricle.

Apical four-chamber view

In some patients, especially those in whom the heart is more horizontally situated, the transducer may be placed over the apex of the heart and the examining plane directed to include both ventricular cavities and the intervening ventricular septum (Fig. 12-45). The decubitus position is especially useful in obtaining this view as it often displaces the apex toward the anterior axillary line. The first landmark usually is the central fibrous junction recognized by its high intensity echoes and mid or posterior position in the sector. The septa can usually be seen extend-

ing vertically from the central fibrous junction. Sliding of the transducer is then employed to obtain an optimal presentation of the cardiac apex. Pivoting of the horizontally oriented examination plane is required to elevate the portion of the sector demonstrating right heart cavities to obtain the best visualization of their extent. The atrioventricular valve leaflets that are transversely oriented in the sector are demonstrated as they open toward the transducer into the ventricular cavities. Angulation may be required to emphasize structures of clinical interest, since the sector may not be wide enough to demonstrate the whole lateral extent of both the right and left heart, especially the ventricular cavities. Tilting of the plane anteriorly from the ideal will show the base of the aorta, while posterior tilting will show the posterior portions of the AV rings.

An equivalent horizontal view of the structures of the base of the heart may also be recorded in patients with more vertically placed hearts when the apex is not directly

Fig. 12-44. Anatomy of the mitral-pulmonic plane. The position and angulation of this plane are shown in **A** with a representation of the degree of medial orientation shown in an end-on view of the heart. **B** demonstrates the appearance of the right ventricular outflow tract (RVO), pulmonary artery (PA) and valve, mitral valve (MV), and left atrium (LA). The distal course of the main pulmonary artery and a portion of its left branch are illustrated in **C**, obtained in a different patient. The dense echo pattern adjacent to the pulmonary artery probably arises in the wall of the left atrial appendage. CW, chest wall; LV, left ventricle.

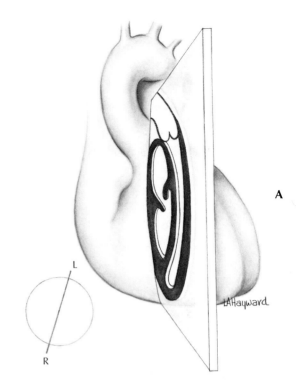

A

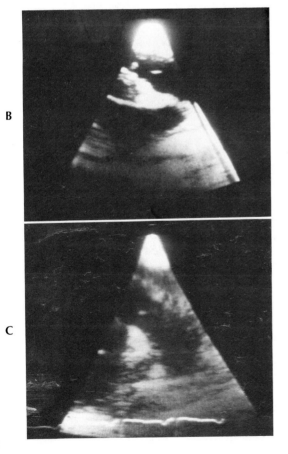

B

C

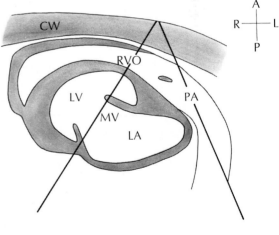

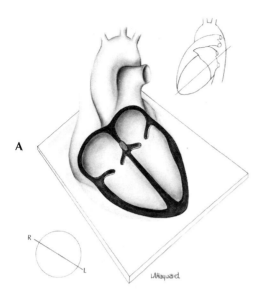

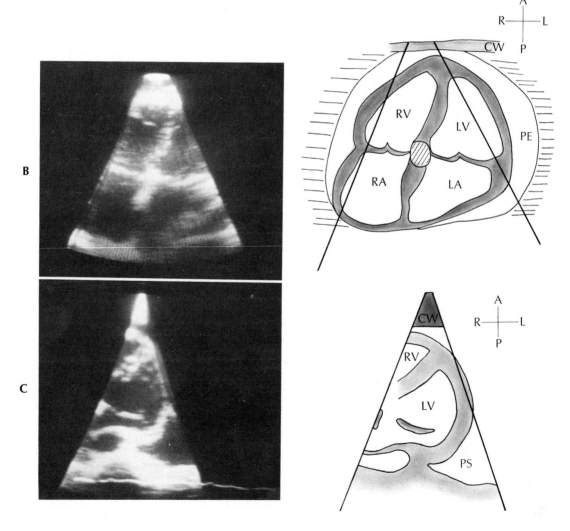

Fig. 12-45. Apical view of four cardiac chambers. A frontal projection of the heart (**A**) shows the horizontal plane, which contains the four cardiac chambers, septa, and AV valves. This plane is somewhat higher on the right (end-on view) and is directed posteriorly and upward (lateral view). A sector scan is shown in **B** and demonstrates a pericardial effusion (PE) and a strong echo from the central fibrous junction *(cross-hatched)*. **C** and the accompanying sketch are from a patient with a left pneumonectomy, which accounts for the fluid seen adjacent to the heart. The apex of both ventricular cavities and the ventricular septum are clearly shown. The left atrium appears distorted, probably from extrinsic pressure related to cardiac displacement. RV, right ventricle; RA, right atrium; PS, pneumonectomy space; LV, left ventricle; LA, left atrium; CW, chest wall.

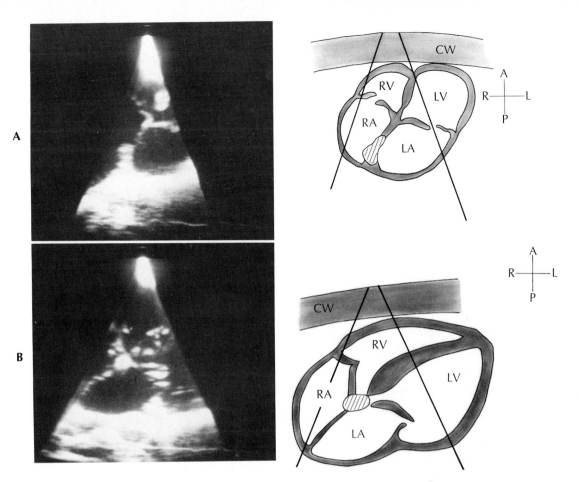

Fig. 12-46. Apical four-chamber view of the atrial cavities. The AV valves and atrial septum are illustrated in **A.** The thickening of the posterior portion of the atrial septum *(cross-hatched)* corresponds to the site of a surgically inserted patch for the closure of an atrial septal defect. In **B,** the central fibrous junction *(cross-hatched)*, seen where the ventricular and atrial septa join between the AV valves is represented as a bright echo source in the sector image. CW, chest wall; RV, right ventricle; LV, left ventricle; RA, right atrium; LA, left atrium.

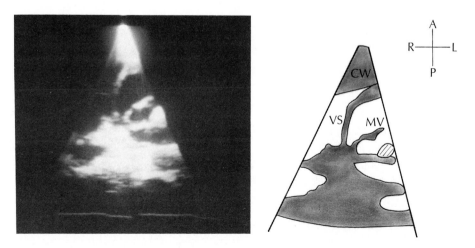

Fig. 12-47. Mitral annular calcification. This plane is somewhat more oblique than the standard four-chamber view. Calcification *(cross-hatched)* is present in the mitral annulus. The mitral valve (MV) showed normal motion pattern. CW, chest wall; VS, ventricular septum.

available (Fig. 12-46) because of overlying lung. The transducer is placed as close to the apex as possible and directed at the central fibrous junction as described.

Apical four-chamber views are useful to study the atrial and ventricular septa, mitral or tricuspid annulus, and abnormal attachment of tricuspid leaflets and to visualize masses in the atrial cavities (Figs. 12-46 to 12-50). These are the best projections for depiction of the apex of the left ventricle, where aneurysms and clots commonly occur. Pericardial effusion displaces lung from the apex and tilts the heart so that excellent apical views may be obtained showing the distribution of pericardial effusions.

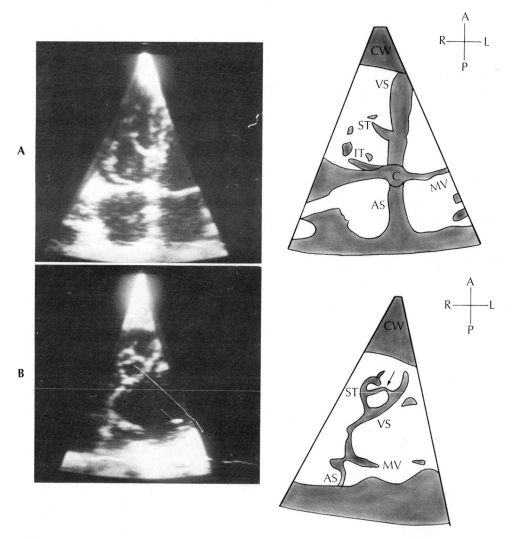

Fig. 12-48. Ebstein's malformation. **A,** An apical four-chamber view shows displacement of the septal leaflet (ST) of the tricuspid valve into the right ventricle. The inferior leaflet (IT) is seen near the tricuspid annulus. A large segment of the right ventricular cavity from the central fibrous junction (C) to the origin of the tricuspid septal leaflet functions like the right atrium (atrialization of right ventricle). **B** is a somewhat more oblique plane which shows an abnormal chordae tendinae *(arrow)* attaching the septal leaflet (ST) of the tricuspid valve to the upper portion of the ventricular septum (VS). CW, chest wall; MV, mitral valve; AS, atrial septum.

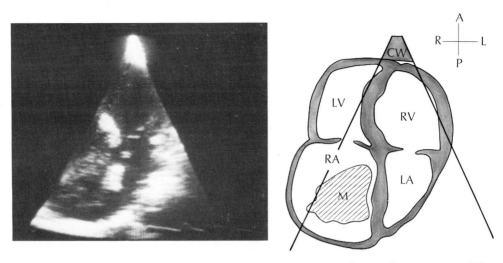

Fig. 12-49. Right atrial myxoma. An apical four-chamber view shows a large myxoma (M) in the right atrial cavity (RA). Atrial and ventricular septa are incompletely seen because of dropouts. RV, right ventricle; LV, left ventricle; LA, left atrium; CW, chest wall.

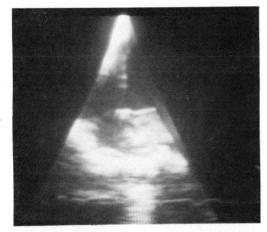

A

Fig. 12-50. Left atrial myxoma. In **A** (systolic frame) an apical four-chamber view shows a tumor in the left atrial cavity. During diastole **(B),** a large segment of the tumor (cross-hatched) prolapses into the left ventricular cavity beyond the central fibrous junction (C). There is, however, no appreciable clearing of the left atrial cavity, suggesting that the mass is enormous in size. Multiple, translucent areas within the tumor may represent areas of hemorrhage. A very large lobulated myxoma, which almost completely filled the left atrial cavity, was found at surgery. Multiple areas of hemorrhage were present within the tumor. CW, chest wall; VS, ventricular septum; C, central fibrous junction.

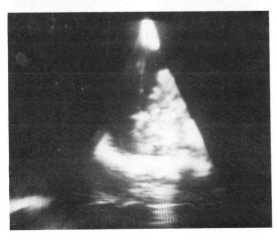

B

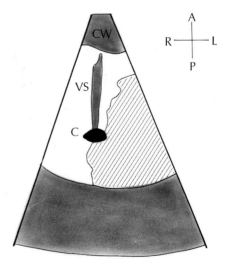

REGIONAL CARDIAC EVALUATION

The discussion in this chapter has been principally focused on the identification of individual cardiac planes and the structures contained in them. However, each examiner must be prepared to carry out regional cardiac evaluation and to obtain the maximum information available by employing a variety of approaches to visualize the area where the disease process may be located. This requires a multiplanar approach as well as the use of observation and recording as the examining planes are shifted through several landmark planes to view an area in continuity. This approach demonstrates a region completely as well as its relationship to other structures of interest. It is convenient for the purposes of this presentation to describe individual chambers and to consider the related valves as separate entities.

Structures not readily detected by today's systems are mentioned in the descriptions; however their presence in the anatomic planes suggests that they are available for imaging and that improved instrumentation with a broader field of view and better resolution should result in their recognition and lead to improved diagnosis.

Right atrium

Exploration of the right atrial cavity can begin with the transverse plane of the great vessels, which passes through the upper portion of the right atrial cavity transversely (Fig. 12-51). Tilting or sliding this plane cephalically directs the examination toward the superior vena cava and the right atrial appendage. The atrial septum is seen in its superior portion. The lower portion of the right atrium is examined in the mitral-tricuspid plane, roughly parallel to the transverse great vessel plane. Scanning between them surveys the atrial septum through the region of the fossa ovalis. The eustachian valve, inferior vena cava, central fibrous junction, opening of the coronary sinus, and inferior aspect of the AV ring are all located in this general region, low in the right atrium. The aortic-tricuspid plane is an oblique longitudinal section of the right atrium immediately

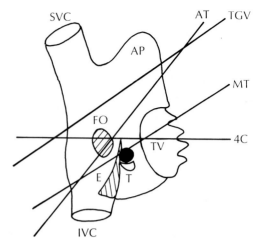

Fig. 12-51. Examining planes and right atrial anatomy. The examining planes that traverse the right atrial cavity are shown as lines that indicate the region where a portion of the plane passes through the right atrium. The relationship of structures to individual planes and extension of examining capability by plane displacement can be inferred. SVC, superior vena cava; AP, right atrial appendage; FO, fossa ovalis (cross-hatched); E, eustachian valve (cross-hatched); T, thebesian valve and adjacent orifice of the coronary sinus (black); TV, tricuspid valve; IVC, inferior vena cava; AT, aortic-tricuspid plane; TGV, transverse plane of the great vessels; MT, mitral-tricuspid plane; 4C, apical four-chamber view.

behind the tricuspid valve and passes through the atrial septum vertically at the fossa ovalis. A horizontal view of the anteroposterior plane of the right atrium is obtained in the apical four-chamber view. It is possible to obtain the area of the right atrium; tilting of the plane cephalically and caudally allows scanning of the entire extent of the right atrial cavity. The tricuspid ring could be evaluated by this same maneuver. The atrial septum is seen along its axis and the central fibrous junction identified.

Tricuspid valve

The tricuspid valve is visible in several of these standard views. In the mitral-tricuspid plane the anterior and septal leaflets are well seen, including the attachment of

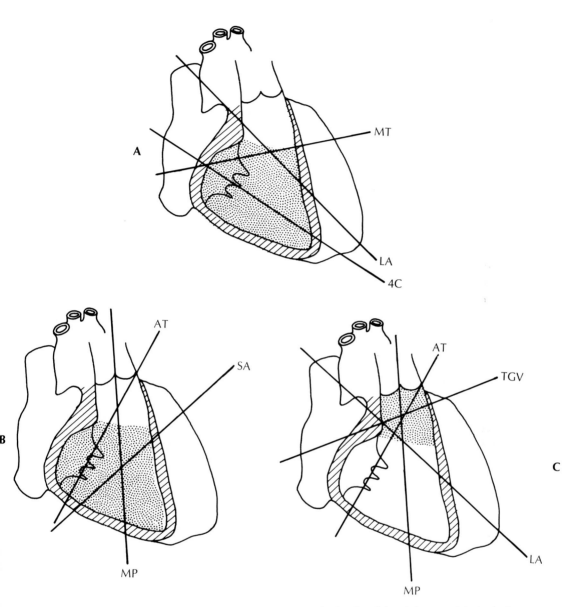

Fig. 12-52. Right ventricular regional examination. The body of the right ventricle including the inflow portion is stippled in **A** and **B;** examining planes are shown as lines. The "long axis" representations are demonstrated in **A. B** denotes the "short axis" views. In **C** the right ventricular outflow is stippled, and planes passing through the region are identified. Note that the transverse plane of the great vessels (TGV) has been pivoted to include only the aorta. MT, mitral-tricuspid plane; LA, long axis of the left ventricle; 4C, apical four-chamber view; AT, aortic-tricuspid plane; SA, short axis of the left ventricle; MT, mitral-tricuspid plane; MP, mitral-pulmonic plane.

the septal leaflet at the central fibrous junction. Medial angulation of the plane should demonstrate the attachment of the anterior leaflet while downward tilting should encompass the posterior leaflet and its attachment. The apical four-chamber view also allows visualization of all three tricuspid leaflets and represents an axial presentation of their motion pattern. The aortic-tricuspid plane demonstrates mostly the anterior leaflet, and portions of the tricuspid valve may be seen in the short axis views of the left ventricle. The valve apparatus can be imaged in those views that show the right ventricular cavity.

Right ventricle

The complex configuration of the right ventricular cavity results in representation of portions in all seven standard planes. By considering the body and inflow portion as an entity separate from the right ventricular outflow tract, the discussion of regional anatomy can be simplified somewhat (Fig. 12-52).

Inflow and body of the right ventricle are seen most completely in four-chamber views that demonstrate this region from the apex to the tricuspid valve and may include long axis views of the papillary muscles, the anterior right ventricular wall, and the ventricular septum. The long axis plane of the left ventricle passes obliquely through the right ventricular cavity as compared to the four-chamber representation and lies higher and closer to the base of the right ventricular outflow tract. The view of the right ventricle obtained in the mitral-tricuspid plane initially passes through the superior portion of the body of the right ventricle, just below the right ventricular outflow tract and traverses the cavity to exit through the superior aspect of the inflow portion. These planes can be considered to represent "long axis" views of the region, though they obviously are not strictly parallel to each other.

Approximate "short axis" planes are obtained in other sections that view the right ventricular body. The aortic-tricuspid plane includes the proximal or inflow portion of the cavity, while the short axis view of the left ventricle made through the mitral valve images the midportion of the body of the ventricle and demonstrates its crescentric shape. The mitral-pulmonic plane passes vertically through the body of the right ventricle in continuity with the right ventricular outflow tract.

The outflow portion of the right ventricle is demonstrated longitudinally in the mitral-pulmonic plane, while the transverse representation of the great vessels shows a short axis cross section of the right ventricular outflow tract. These planes are virtually perpendicular to each other. The aortic-tricuspid plane passes through the right ventricular outflow tract obliquely, while the long axis section of the left ventricle demonstrates the base of the right ventricular outflow tract obliquely.

Pulmonary artery

The pulmonary artery is shown partially in the oblique transverse plane of the great vessels as a space distal to the pulmonary valve leaflets. In infants and children, it is possible to adjust the orientation of this plane so that the pulmonary artery is viewed transversely as a circular cross section. The mitral-pulmonic plane offers the best opportunity to examine the long axis of the pulmonary artery as it arches posteriorly. It is also possible to include portions of the left branch by appropriate tilting toward the left. Tilting of the plane to the right passes it through the pulmonary artery bifurcation, and further tilting or sliding brings the right pulmonary artery into view as it lies behind the aorta and superior to the left atrium.

Pulmonic valve

The pulmonic valve is demonstrable in the planes that image the pulmonary artery to determine the number of cusps present and to evaluate leaflet doming in systole.

Left atrium

The left atrial cavity is transected by six of the seven planes used in two-dimensional cardiac imaging (Fig. 12-53). Those which pass through the left atrium transversely are

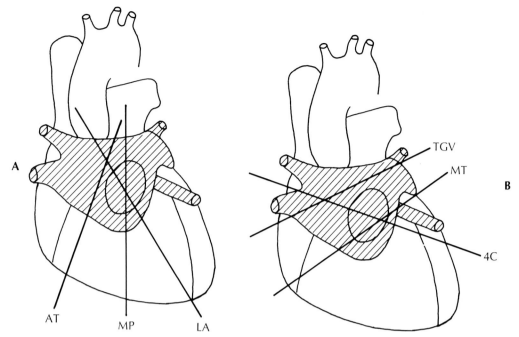

Fig. 12-53. Planes passing through the left atrium. The left atrium is shaded, and the mitral ring is shown as an oval. Longitudinally oriented planes are shown in **A** and transverse planes in **B**. The inclination of individual planes is not evident, and the lines represent a midpoint of the passage of the planes through the left atrial cavity. AT, aortic-tricuspid plane; MP, mitral-pulmonic plane; LA, long axis of the left ventricle; TGV, transverse view of the great vessels; MT, mitral-tricuspid plane; 4C, apical four-chamber view.

the transverse view of the great vessels and the mitral-tricuspid plane. The transverse view of the great vessels examines the upper portion of the left atrial cavity and may include the left atrial appendage. Superior tilting of this plane should scan the uppermost portion of the left atrium and the transverse sinus of the pericardium can be demonstrated between the left atrium and the aortic root. The superior pulmonic veins and the inferior right pulmonic vein lie within this anatomic area. The mitral-tricuspid plane examines a small portion of the lower extent of the left atrium and its outflow portion. Tilting of this plane upward permits examination of the midportion of the left atrium and portions of the mitral ring. Inferior scanning shows the atrioventricular junction where the coronary sinus passes transversely in the A-V groove. The left inferior pulmonic vein

can be imaged in cross sections at the extreme leftward portion of this plane.

The atrial septum is imaged in these transverse planes and has been described in the right atrial section.

The three longitudinal axes that pass through the left atrial cavity are the long axis of the left ventricle, the mitral-pulmonic plane, and the aortic-tricuspid view. The long axis passes somewhat obliquely through the midportion of the left atrium, including portions of the mitral ring. The inferior left pulmonic vein and coronary sinus are demonstrable in relation to the left atrial cavity. The mitral-pulmonic section passes through the same area in the left atrium, though it is more vertically placed and most closely approximates the longitudinal axis. Lateral tilting or sliding of this plane images the left atrial appendage. The aortic-tricuspid plane passes through the middle of the outflow portion of the left atrium. The left coronary artery is included in this anatomic cross section between the left atrium and the right heart outflow.

The apical four-chamber view transects the left atrium horizontally and shows its depth and lateral extent. As in right atrial examination, tilting of this plane can view the A-V ring and give estimates of left atrial volume.

The planes that image the left atrial cavity also demonstrate the oblique sinus of the pericardium.

Mitral valve

Three examination planes provide the bulk of diagnostic information concerning the mitral valve. The left ventricular long axis shows the lengths of both leaflets and their attachments to the posterior aortic margin and at the atrioventricular junction. The plane of systolic coaptation is well demonstrated. The subvalvular apparatus is best evaluated in this anatomic plane. Short axis views of the left ventricle permit evaluation of the leaflets in transverse section, and this plane can be modified by sliding from the subaortic area to the tips of the leaflets where the orifice is demonstrated. Further extension to the left ventricular cavity shows the chordae and papillary muscles in transverse orientation. The apical four-chamber view provides a horizontal cross section of the leaflets and offers a clear view of the plane of coaptation of the mitral valve for assessment of conditions that alter the systolic stability of the valve. The origin of the anterior leaflet relative to the central fibrous junction can be seen. The subvalvular apparatus is demonstrated in a long axis view. The mitral valve is also included in the mitral-tricuspid plane in which an oblique transverse image of the anterior leaflet is obtained. The mitral-pulmonic plane is similar to the left ventricular long axis presentation, though it is somewhat obliqued.

Left ventricle

The entire length of the left ventricular cavity can be examined in the long axis plane

to show the ventricular septum and its attachment to the aortic root, the left ventricular outflow tract, the body of the cavity, and the apex (Fig. 12-54). Sliding the transducer leftward brings the anterior free wall of the left ventricle into view. Medial tilting of the plane from a leftward origin permits scanning of the ventricular septum in its antero-posterior dimension. The posterior wall may be surveyed by similar tilting of the plane from the standard long axis transducer position. Portions of the lateral wall may also be included with this maneuver. The short axis plane offers the potential to examine the entire circumference of the left ventricular cavity from the outflow portion to the apex by sliding the plane longitudinally in relation

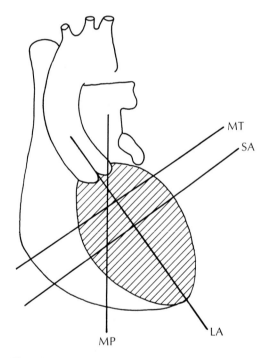

Fig. 12-54. Left ventricular regional examination. The shaded left ventricle is shown in relationship to the aortic root in a frontal image of the heart. The long axis (LA) and short axis (SA) planes lie perpendicular to each other and represent standard left ventricular views. The mitral-pulmonic (MP) and mitral-tricuspid (MT) planes provide skewed or tangential cross sections of a portion of the left ventricular cavity.

to the long axis. The apical 4-chamber view is best suited for examination of the apex and the walls of the left ventricle. A pivoting motion at the apex should also provide circumferential information concerning the entire left ventricular cavity. The mitral-pulmonic plane shows the inflow portion of the left ventricle in oblique cross section while the mitral-tricuspid plane inspects the left ventricular outflow tract in an oblique short axis that passes through the ventricular septum in its upper half.

Proximal aorta

The long axis plane includes a longitudinal representation of the proximal aorta in which the right sinus of Valsalva forms the anterior aortic boundary at its base. The proximal aorta arches anteriorly, and the right pulmonary artery lies behind the aorta above the left atrial cavity. The transverse views of the great vessels at the level of the aortic valve include the origins of the coronary arteries from the sinuses of Valsalva. A cross section of the aorta may be obtained in the supravalvular portion by sliding the plane cephalically. The right pulmonary artery is shown longitudinally, and the superior vena cava lies to the right and slightly posterior. Downward displacement of the plane demonstrates the relationship of the ventricular septum, left ventricular outflow tract, and mitral valve to the aortic root. The aortic-tricuspid plane ordinarily images an oblique plane passing through the aortic root. In those instances in which the aortic origin from the left ventricle may be tilted, a true cross section may be obtained in this plane.

Aortic valve

Those short axis views that represent the aorta as a circular configuration are best suited for simultaneous imaging of all valve cusps for evaluation of the number present and for estimation of orifice size by shifting the plane upward to the level of the tips of the cusps. In long axis the right coronary and noncoronary cusps can be imaged as they open and close, and valve doming can be demonstrated in cases of aortic stenosis.

ADDITIONAL EXAMINATION TECHNIQUES

So far, the discussion in this chapter has emphasized precordial access to the heart. When additional or more specific cardiac or great vessel information is required, it is feasible to perform two-dimensional, real-time imaging from suprasternal or subxiphoid transducer positions as has been described under M-mode techniques. However, the information obtained in two-dimensional scanning is far superior to that obtained in M-mode, since structures that lie parallel to the ultrasonic beam may be imaged and recognized more definitively. In some patients, especially those in whom the cardiac window is small or the chest wall is deformed, too thin, or too irregular for easy transducer seating and angulation, valuable information can be obtained concerning cardiac chamber and valvular anatomy and function, especially from a subxiphoid position.

Subxiphoid technique and anatomy

An easy starting point in subxiphoid examination is the identification of the inferior vena cava with the sector plane oriented sagitally or vertically and the transducer placed just below the xiphoid process and about 2 to 3 cm to the right of midline. The inferior vena cava is recognized as a linear sonolucent space lying at a depth of about 10 cm and bounded anteriorly by the liver, which contains a characteristic speckled pattern (Fig. 12-55). Minor tilting of the examination plane will identify branches of major hepatic veins within the substance of the liver, and as they terminate in the inferior vena cava. Cephalic sliding and tilting of the examination plane will show the dome of the liver lying under the right leaf of the diaphragm, recognized by its upward convex margin and disappearance of typical liver parenchymal texture. The inferior vena cava enters the right atrial cavity from its inferior aspect and the eustachian valve is seen as a linear echo source arising anteriorly at the junction of the inferior vena cava and right atrium.

The cardiac cavities displayed in this sag-

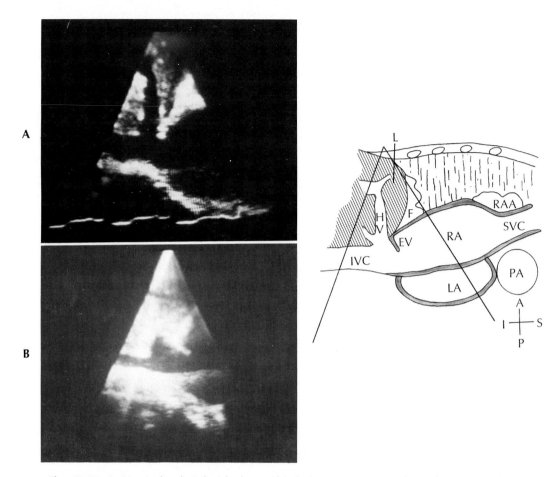

Fig. 12-55. A, Vertical subxiphoid plane of inferior vena cava and atrial cavities. The anteriorly situated liver (L), hepatic vein branches (HV) and inferior vena cava (IVC) are shown below the diaphragm. The eustachian valve (EV) marks the junction of the inferior vena cava and right atrium (RA). The left atrium (LA) is separated from the right atrium by the atrial septum. A variable sized fat pad (F) is often interposed between the diaphragm and right atrium. Other structures that could possibly be detected from this position are a portion of the right atrial appendage (RAA), the superior vena cava (SVC), and the right pulmonary artery (PA) seen in cross section. Two-dimensional sector scan **A** was obtained from the region enclosed in the straight lines and shows hepatic veins entering the inferior vena cava. **B** illustrates the eustachian valve and atrial septum more clearly.

ittal, right subxiphoid view are the anteriorly situated right atrium and the posteriorly placed left atrium with the interatrial septum demonstrated as a longitudinal, linear echo source. Theoretically, additional cephalic angulation should image the entrance of the superior vena cava, though we have not accomplished this to date.

Variations of this sagittal examination plane include placement of the transducer to the left of the xiphoid process with medial tilting of the plane, at which time a portion of the right ventricular cavity, the anterior tricuspid leaflet, the right atrium, the interatrial septum, and the left atrial cavity are imaged in sequence as depth increases (Fig. 12-56). It is interesting to speculate at this point that a plane intermediate between

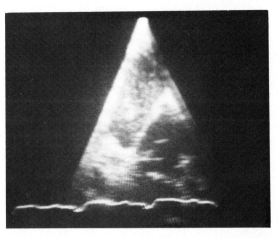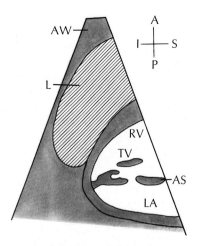

Fig. 12-56. Vertical subxiphoid plane just to left of midline. Some tilting of the plane to the right will pass it through a portion of the right ventricle (RV) and will include echoes from the tricuspid valve (TV). The atrial septum (AS) appears fragmented, probably from dropouts. LA, left atrium; L, liver; AW, abdominal wall.

those described could be selected to demonstrate the right coronary artery, which lies longitudinally in the atrioventricular groove. Tilting of the plane to the left from a close left paraxiphoid position passes it through the same plane previously described for imaging of the short axis of the left ventricle (Fig. 12-29). The information obtained from the subxiphoid approach, however, differs from that acquired precordially, since it is now possible to image the tricuspid valve leaflets in the anterior portion of the sector (Fig. 12-57). We have been able to show the position and motion of all three leaflets of the tricuspid valve and to record an oval cross-sectional image of the orifice of the tricuspid valve.

Orientation of the examining plane transversely to parallel the left costal margin provides images equivalent to the horizontal four-chamber view obtained from the cardiac apex (Fig. 12-45) but directed more ideally at the atrial and ventricular septa, especially their junction (Fig. 12-58). The atrioventricular valves, chordae, and papillary muscles may be more clearly imaged since they lie perpendicular to the beam. Cephalic tilting of the plane detects the aortic valve in cross section.

Clinical applications. The vertical view of

the inferior vena cava is useful to recognize a distended inferior vena cava in conditions such as tricuspid regurgitation, congestive heart failure, or any other process that increases right atrial pressure or volume. The normal inferior vena cava will show a cyclic change in its diameter, which is larger on inspiration, breath-holding, or during the Valsalva maneuver. Distension by elevated right atrial pressure dampens or obliterates these cyclic changes.

This plane has found outstanding clinical application in the evaluation of pericardial effusion. Since the pericardium attaches to the heart at the junction of the inferior vena cava and the right atrium, pericardial fluid can be recognized as a sonolucent space between the diaphragm and the right atrial wall. The special utility of this examination plane is in those cases in which left pleural effusion complicates the ultrasonic diagnosis when viewing the heart from standard precordial examination positions. The inferior vena cava plane is to the right of midline and, therefore, away from the left pleural space. If the pleural effusion also involves the right side, careful evaluation of the echo patterns can be used to differentiate right pleural effusion from pericardial fluid since the pleural

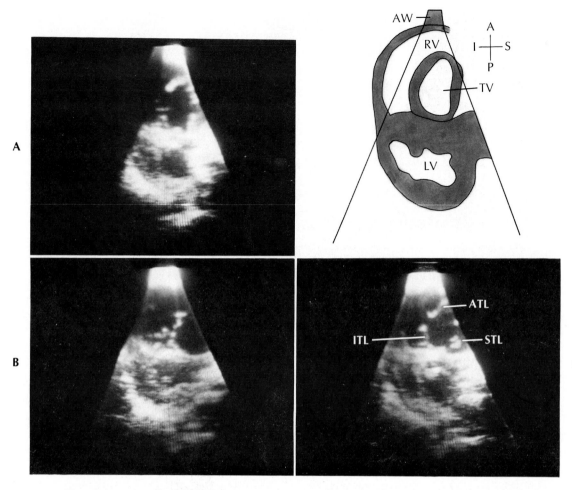

Fig. 12-57. Vertical subxiphoid short axis view of the right and left ventricular cavities. This view is particularly useful to image the orifice of the tricuspid valve (TV) in diastole in the right ventricular cavity (RV). In addition, in **A** and **C** all three leaflets of the tricuspid valve can be seen. The systolic image is shown in **B**. AW, abdominal wall; LV, left ventricle; ATL, anterior leaflet of the tricuspid valve; STL, septal leaflet of the tricuspid valve; ITL, inferior leaflet of the tricuspid valve.

space does not extend into this region; therefore a sonolucent space adjacent to the right atrial wall near the junction with the inferior vena cava indicates the presence of pericardial fluid. This relatively easy examination technique has also been useful in our experience in ruling out the presence of pericardial effusion.

In rare instances, examination of this region will indicate the presence of a thrombus or tumor masses that encroach on the right atrial cavity. This may be a useful observation in the differential diagnosis of a right atrial mass since right atrial myxomas do not usually extend into the inferior vena cava. The finding of inferior vena cava involvement indicates an abdominal origin of the disease process.

The vertically oriented planes obtained from a subxiphoid position, especially when tilted toward the left heart, provide a unique opportunity to study the structure and mo-

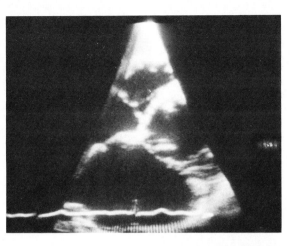
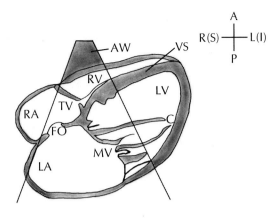
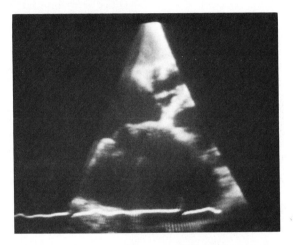

Fig. 12-58. Horizontal four-chamber view obtained from a subxiphoid position. This study was obtained from a patient with mitral stenosis and shows an enlarged left atrial cavity (LA) and an atrial septum that bulges into the right atrium (RA). The localized, thin bulge in the atrial septum probably represents the fossa ovalis (FO). Angulation of the sector to the left was successful in imaging the length of both ventricular cavities including papillary muscles and chordae (C) as they attached to the atrioventricular valves. RV, right ventricle; LV, left ventricle; VS, ventricular septum; AW, abdominal wall; MV, mitral valve; TV, tricuspid valve.

tion of the tricuspid valve. Since it is possible to image all three leaflets as they form the tricuspid funnel, the shape and size of the orifice is obtainable from this vantage point to evaluate tricuspid stenosis or the presence of vegetations attached to any of the valve leaflets. Also, when the precordial approach is limited by a very small cardiac window, this view could provide the only available information about the mitral valve and the left ventricular cavity. We have used the horizontal subxiphoid four-chamber view to study the length of the atrial septum and to identify the fossa ovalis as well as to demonstrate atrial septal defects and an aneurysm of the atrial septum. In a patient with mitral stenosis the atrial septum could be seen bulging into the right atrium and an additional localized bulge in a thinner area of the septum was identified in the anatomic location of the fossa ovalis (Fig. 12-58). In another patient with a secundum atrial septal defect demonstrated at cardiac catheterization, an extensive localized protrusion of the atrial septum into the right atrial cavity was detected in this view. The atrial septum appeared extremely thin and fragmentary in outline. In motion viewing the septal bulge tended to undulate, and the diagnosis of an atrial septal aneurysm was suggested. At surgery a fenestrated aneurysm with an extremely thin wall was excised, and the defect was patched.

A complete canal defect demonstrates the utility of this examination plane to examine structures at the base of the heart (Fig. 12-59). The normal continuity of the atrial and ventricular septa and the central fibrous junction was absent, producing atrial and ventricular septal defects. The common atrioventricular valve could be seen passing through the central defect and extending into both ventricular cavities. Papillary muscles in both ventricular cavities and chordae inserting into the tricuspid valve could be readily seen. In addition, abnormal chordal insertion into the crest of the defective ventricular septum was demonstrated.

In partial canal defects the ventricular septum extends to the level of the atrioventricular rings without demonstration of a ventricular septal defect. The atrial septum, on the other hand, shows a typical defect at its base.

We have been impressed by the clarity and detail observed in studies of the subvalvular apparatus of the mitral valve obtained from the horizontal plane subxiphoid view as compared to studies obtained from precordial projections. This may be related to the improved coupling of our mechanical sector scanner to the softer tissues of the abdominal wall.

The horizontal subxiphoid view has the potential to provide additional supportive findings in other conditions or to identify specific anatomic structures. Left atrial membranes and intra-atrial baffles can be examined, the insertion of pulmonary veins and their anomalies evaluated, and valvular abnormalities such as Ebstein's anomaly or tricuspid atresia studied. Since we have demonstrated the aortic valve in this examination plane, the full length and width of the right

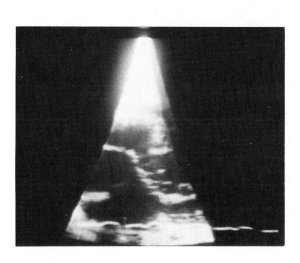
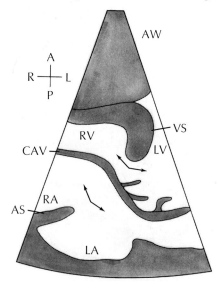

Fig. 12-59. Horizontal subxiphoid four-chamber view in complete atrioventricular canal defect. The deficient ventricular (VS) and atrial (AS) septa are shown with a common atrioventricular valve (CAV) passing through a large central defect. The arrows indicate the pathways of atrial and ventricular shunting, of which the right-to-left atrial component was demonstrated using peripheral contrast injections. RA, right atrium; LA, left atrium; LV, left ventricle; RV, right ventricle; AW, abdominal wall.

ventricular outflow tract can be imaged when additional anterior tilting of the plane is employed.

Since the subxiphoid views provide images of the atrial cavities and the atrial septum, they should be attempted in all patients suspected of harboring an intra-atrial mass, particularly to demonstrate its size and extent and possible site of attachment.

Suprasternal technique and anatomy

As in M-mode examinations, the transducer may be placed in the suprasternal notch or in the supraclavicular fossae to obtain clinically useful information. We have found that a mechanical sector scanner is easiest to apply in the right supraclavicular fossa, since soft tissues are more abundant here than in the suprasternal notch. The pa-

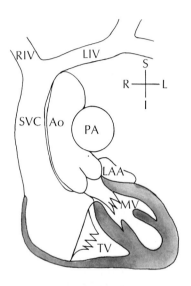

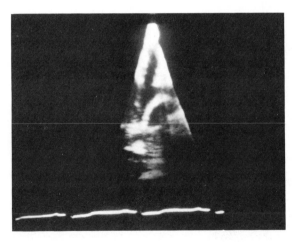

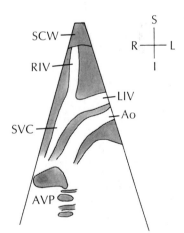

Fig. 12-60. Suprasternal demonstration of great vessel anatomy. The sketch of the heart in a coronal plane demonstrates the anatomic structures encountered in suprasternal or right supraclavicular examination of the great vessels. The corresponding clinical image is from a patient with an aortic valve prosthesis (AVP) in which poppet motion could be clearly seen. SCW, right supraclavicular wall; RIV, right innominate vein; LIV, left innominate vein; SVC, superior vena cava; Ao, ascending aorta and portion of arch; PA, pulmonary artery; TV, tricuspid valve; MV, mitral valve; LAA, left atrial appendage.

tient is positioned with a pillow under the shoulders to allow increased extension of the head and neck. In children, it may be necessary to administer mild sedation to assure cooperation.

A horizontal plane that produces a coronal section of the upper mediastinum can be employed to demonstrate the great veins as they merge to form the superior vena cava, which is seen in its full extent as it enters the right heart (Fig. 12-60). Beneath the left innominate vein, a portion of the aortic arch is demonstrated along with the ascending aorta, lying to the left of the superior vena cava and terminating at the level of the aortic valve. The right pulmonary artery may be seen just to the left of the ascending aorta. Deeper cardiac structures have been difficult to image because of the long sound paths required.

More complete visualization of the arch of the aorta requires that the left side of the examining plane be pivoted posteriorly until the image of the aortic arch is obtained. The

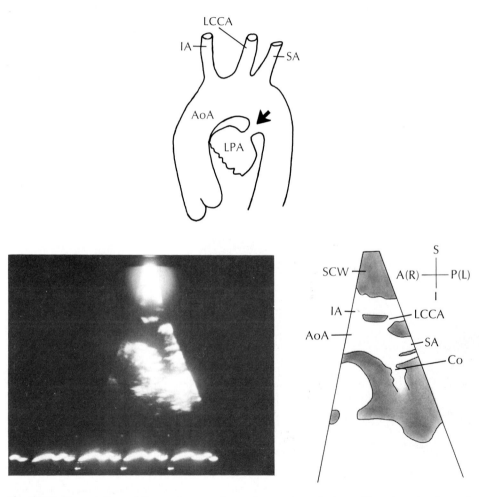

Fig. 12-61. Coarctation of the aorta seen from a suprasternal plane. The plane is pivoted from the coronal plane to demonstrate the aortic arch (AoA) and the great arteries originating from the aorta. The aortic arch narrows abruptly just beyond the origin of the subclavian artery (SA) and the region of coarctation (Co) is imaged. The arrow shows the position of ductus arteriosus. SCW, right supraclavicular wall; IA, innominate artery; LCCA, left common carotid artery; LPA, left pulmonary artery.

origin of the major aortic branches and the proximal descending aorta are usually demonstrable (Fig. 12-61).

Clinical applications. The suprasternal horizontal plane is ideally suited to study the motion of aortic valve prostheses, since the poppet moves along the line of sight and is therefore recorded more accurately than is possible from a precordial position. Aortic aneurysms and their superior extent can also be delineated. Mediastinal masses, which may mimic aortic aneurysms, may lend themselves to easy identification by this method.

The plane that images the aortic arch has been used to evaluate the presence and extent of aortic coarctation by demonstrating the area of narrowing and relating it to the origin of the left subclavian artery. The potential exists for direct imaging of the ductus arteriosus as it courses from the inner aspect of the aortic arch to the origin of the left pulmonary artery.

Two-dimensional contrast echocardiography

The techniques and agents described earlier for M-mode contrast echocardiography can be used in conjunction with real-time, two-dimensional scanning to demonstrate blood flow patterns in the heart and great vessels. Peripheral venous injections of contrast agents fill right heart cavities and show right-to-left passage of contrast medium. A left-to-right shunt may be demonstrated as a negative jet of noncontrast blood as it shunts into the right heart (Fig. 12-62). For example, in tetralogy of Fallot, contrast injections have been used to identify the site of the ventricular septal defect and show shunting into the overriding aorta. The complex intracardiac shunting seen in patients with tricuspid atresia has been revealed as contrast passes from the right to the left atrium and then to the mitral valve. Filling of the small right ventricular cavity occurs from the left ventricle.

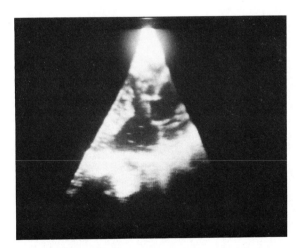 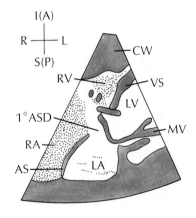

Fig. 12-62. Contrast demonstration of a left-to-right atrial shunt. This image was recorded with an apical four-chamber view in a patient with an ostium primum atrial septal defect. A negative jet effect is present in the contrast-filled right atrial cavity (RA) near the base of the intact ventricular septum (VS). The defect in the base of the atrial septum (AS) is also shown. A few contrast echoes in the left atrial cavity (LA) indicates the presence of a small right-to-left component of the shunt. In this type of defect the central fibrous junction loses its prominence or is absent, and this feature serves to distinguish it from a very large secundum atrial septal defect in our experience. 1° ASD, primum defect in atrial septum; RV, right ventricle; LV, left ventricle; MV, mitral valve apparatus; CW, chest wall.

Two-dimensional echocardiography is distinctly superior to M-mode in studying contrast agent flow patterns. The reverberations that occur with dense contrast filling are more easily recognized in two dimensions because of their broad, unstructured appearance. Jets, on the other hand, tend to be confined and localized so that it may be pos-sible to estimate the size of the defect in a semiquantitative manner by observing the flow of contrast. The quantity of contrast crossing a septal defect has been an unreliable indicator of shunt size, since precise control over the intensity of the contrast effect is difficult to standardize.

In patients who have had surgical repair

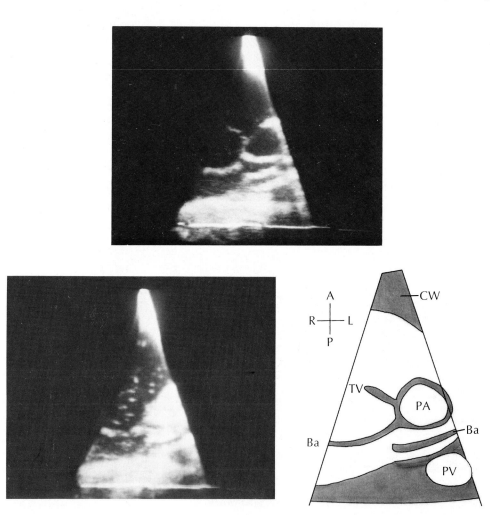

Fig. 12-63. Baffle incompetence. The examining plane in this child with dextrotransposition of the great vessels and Mustard procedure corresponds to the aortic-tricuspid plane previously described and images the transposed pulmonary artery (PA) (in the normal position of the aorta), tricuspid valve (TV), and limbs of the surgically inserted baffle (Ba). Following intravenous contrast injection, the pulmonary artery and systemic venous portion of the atrium (behind the pulmonary artery) filled first and contained dense contrast echoes. There was also immediate appearance of scattered contrast echoes in the pulmonary venous portion of the reconstructed atrial cavities as well as in the right ventricular cavity indicative of baffle incompetence. CW, chest wall; PV, pulmonic vein.

of septal defects, the competence of the patch may be tested with contrast material delivered to the left heart through catheters placed to monitor cardiac output and pressure in the postoperative period. These studies are best carried out a few days postoperatively to allow time for the patch and suture material to become sealed as the result of the healing process.

Baffles inserted into the atrial cavities for physiologic correction of dextrotransposition of the great vessels have been studied to detect evidence of incompetence (Fig. 12-63). Contrast injections into peripheral veins first opacify the systemic portion of the reconstructed atrial cavities with subsequent filling of the pulmonary artery. We have seen small shunts passing into the pulmonary venous portion of the atrium that have not been obvious on dye curve or saturation studies obtained during cardiac catheterization. The clinical significance of these small shunts is not clear, but the findings emphasize the sensitivity of the real-time, two-dimensional

contrast study in demonstrating baffle incompetence. This increased sensitivity over M-mode techniques is probably a function of the wide field of view of the two-dimensional system, which offers a greater opportunity to detect evidence of leakage.

The microbubbles responsible for the ultrasonic contrast effect represent individual echo sources that withstand dilution and retain their echogenicity even when small quantities of gas are injected. In addition, their particulate nature allows observation of flow direction, especially when relatively small numbers of microbubbles are injected. In the presence of tricuspid regurgitation, the recirculation of contrast echoes from the right ventricle to the right atrium is easily seen as individual echo sources flow through the tricuspid valve bidirectionally. In one patient with tricuspid regurgitation the leaflets of the valve appeared to be held open during systole, as though ventricular dilatation resulted in a relative shortening of the chordae as well as enlargement of the tricuspid an-

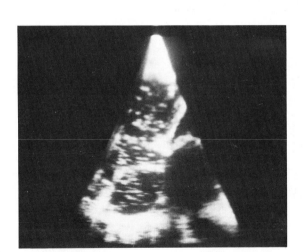
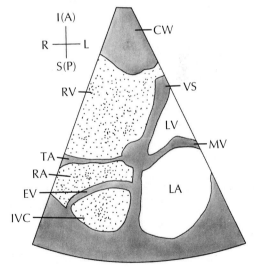

Fig. 12-64. Contrast validation of the eustachian valve. The plane of this apical four-chamber view was pivoted to image the tricuspid annulus (TA), the eustachian valve (EV), and the entrance of the inferior vena cava (IVC). The prominent anterior position of the eustachian valve and filling of the inferior vena cava following an arm vein injection probably result from right heart enlargement and tricuspid regurgitation in this patient with mitral stenosis. CW, chest wall; RV, right ventricle; RA, right atrium; VS, ventricular septum; LV, left ventricle; MV, thickened mitral valve; LA, left atrium.

nulus. Using an apical four-chamber view, the contrast echoes could be seen flowing back from the right ventricle into the right atrium through the gaping tricuspid valve.

Reflux of contrast material into the inferior vena cava following arm vein injection in our experience reinforces the diagnosis of tricuspid regurgitation.

We have used contrast techniques to validate the echo pattern arising from the eustachian valve and entrance of the inferior vena cava in apical and subxiphoid four-chamber views as well as in the mitral-tricuspid plane. This has been particularly useful when the inferior vena cava is enlarged and the eustachian valve becomes prominent and is displaced toward the tricuspid ring, raising the possibility of an abnormal structure or process in the right atrial cavity (Fig. 12-64). The posterior, medial location, the

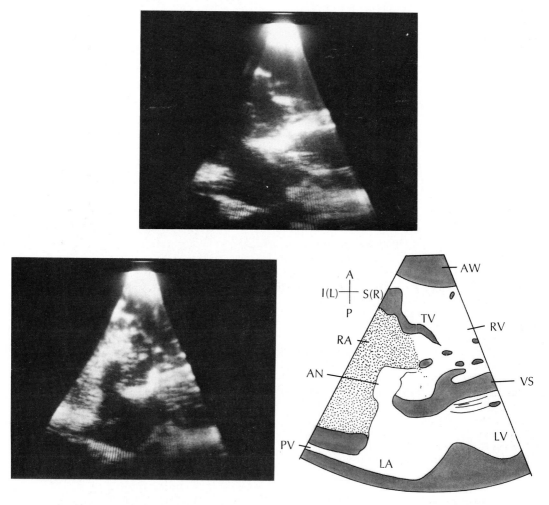

Fig. 12-65. Contrast validation of atrial septal aneurysm. The bulging, thin-walled atrial septal aneurysm (AN) is partially seen from a subxiphoid horizontal plane as it extends into the right atrial cavity (RA). Following intravenous contrast administration, the extent of the aneurysmal sac is clearly outlined. AW, abdominal wall; TV, tricuspid valve; VS, ventricular septum; LA, left atrium; PV, entrance of pulmonic vein into left atrium; RV, right ventricle; LV, left ventricle.

linear nature of the echo pattern, the gentle anterior convexity, the sonolucency behind it, and its relative lack of motion serve to identify the eustachian valve complex and to differentiate it from localized disease processes in the right atrium. For example, the aneurysm of the atrial septum, which we have described earlier, was seen in the right atrial cavity in a position that might confuse it with a normal eustachian valve. However, its convexity projected laterally, the margins were less distinct and thinner than those of the eustachian valve, and there was considerable variation in its size and contour during the cardiac cycle. Also, right atrial contrast filling failed to flood both sides of the aneurysm with contrast echoes (Fig. 12-65).

BIBLIOGRAPHY

Asberg, A.: Ultrasonic cinematography of the living heart, Ultrasonics 6:113, 1967.

Bom, N., Lancee, C. T., Honkoop, J., and Hugenholtz, P. C.: Ultrasonic viewer for cross-sectional analyses of moving cardiac structures, Biomed. Eng. 6:500, 1971.

Hertz, C. H., and Lundstrom, K.: A fast ultrasonic scanning for heart investigation, 3rd international conference on medical physics, Gotenburg, Sweden, Aug., 1972.

Bom, N., Lancee, C. T., VanZwieten, G., Kloster, F. E., and Roelandt, J.: Multiscan echocardiography, I. Technical description, Circulation 48:1066, 1973.

Gramiak, R., Waag, R., and Simon, W.: Cine ultrasound cardiography, Radiology 107:175, 1973.

Griffith, J. M., Henry, W. L., and Epstein, S. E.: Real time two-dimensional echocardiography, Circulation 48(suppl. 4):124, 1973 (abstract).

King, D. L.: Cardiac ultrasonography: cross-sectional ultrasonic imaging of the heart, Circulation 47:843, 1973.

Kloster, E. E., Roelandt, J., TenCate, F. J., Bom, N., and Hugenholtz, P. G.: Multiscan echocardiography. II. Technique and initial clinical results, Circulation 48:1075, 1973.

Bom, N., Hugenholtz, P. G., Kloster, F. E., Roelandt, J., Popp, R. L., Pridie, R. B., and Sahn, D. J.: Evaluation of structure recognition with the multiscan echocardiograph; a cooperative study in 580 patients, Ultrasound Med. Biol. 1:243, 1974.

Eggleton, R. C., and Johnston, K. W.: Real-time mechanical scanning system compared with array techniques, Institute of Electrical and Electronic Engineers, Proceedings in Sonics and Ultrasonics, 1974.

Griffith, J. M., and Henry, W. L.: A sector scanner for real time two-dimensional echocardiography, Circulation 49:1147, 1974.

Kisslo, J., vonRamm, O. T., and Thurstone, E. L.: Thaumascan; clinical cardiac imaging, J. Clin. Ultrasound 2:237, 1974 (abstract).

Kratochwil, A., Jantsch, C., Mosslacher, H., Slany, J., and Wenger, R.: Ultrasonic tomography of the heart, Ultrasound Med. Biol. 1:275, 1974.

McDicken, W. N., Bruff, K., and Paton, J.: An ultrasonic instrument for rapid B-scanning of the heart, Ultrasonics 12:269-272, 1974.

Roelandt, J., Kloster, F. E., TenCate, F. J., Van Dorp, W. G., Honkoop, J., Bom, N., and Hugenholtz, P. G.: Multidimensional echocardiography; an appraisal of its clinical usefulness, Br. Heart J. 36:29, 1974.

Sahn, D. J., Terry, R., O'Rourke, R., Leopold, G., and Friedman, W. F.: Multiple crystal echocardiographic evaluation of endocardial cushion defect, Circulation 50:25-32, 1974.

Sahn, D. J., Terry, R., O'Rourke, R., Leopold, G., and Friedman, W. F.: Multiple crystal and cross-sectional echocardiography in the diagnosis of cyanotic congenital heart disease, Circulation 50:230-238, 1974.

Sahn, D. J., Williams, D. E., Shackelton, S., and Friedman, W. F.: The validity of structure identification for cross-sectional echocardiography, J. Clin. Ultrasound 2:201, 1974.

Teichholz, L. E., Cohen, M. V., Sonnenblick, E. H., and Gorlin, R.: Study of left ventricular geometry and function by B-scan ultrasonography in patients with and without asynergy, N. Engl. J. Med. 291:1220, 1974.

vonRamm, O., Kisslo, J., Thurstone, F. L., Johnson, M. L., and Behar, V. S.: A new high resolution, real-time, two-dimensional ultrasound sector scanner, Circulation 50(suppl. 3):27, 1974 (abstract).

Eggleton, R. C., Feigenbaum, H., Johnston, K. W., Weyman, A. E., Dillon, J. C., and Chang, S.: Visualization of cardiac dynamics with real-time B-mode ultrasonic scanner. In White, D., editor: Ultrasound in medicine, vol. 1, New York, 1975, Plenum Publishing Corp., p. 385.

Henry, W. L., Griffith, J. M., Michaelis, L. L., McIntosh, C. L., Morrow, A. G., and Epstein, S. E.: Measurement of mitral orifice area in patients with mitral valve disease by real time, two-dimensional echocardiography, Circulation 51:829, 1975.

Henry, W. L., Maron, B. J., Griffith, J. M., Redwood, D. R., and Epstein, S. E.: Differential diagnosis of anomalies of the great arteries by real-time, two-dimensional echocardiography, Circulation 51:283, 1975.

Henry, W. L., Sahn, D. J., Griffith, J. M., Goldberg, S. J., Maron, B. J., McCallister, H. A., Allen, H. D., and Ebstein, S. E.: Evaluation of atrioventricular valve morphology in congenital heart disease by real-time cross sectional echocardiography, Circulation 52(suppl. 2):120, 1975.

Kisslo, J., Griedman, G., Johnson, M., and VonRamm, O.: Two dimensional echocardiographic assessment of normal mitral leaflet motion. Circulation **52**(suppl. 2): 32, 1975 (abstract).

Kisslo, J., vonRamm, O. T., and Thurstone, F. L.: Thaumascan; clinical cardiac imaging. In White, D., editor: Ultrasound in medicine, vol. 1, New York, 1975, Plenum Publishing Corp., pp. 379-383.

Popp, R. L., Brown, O. R., and Harrison, D. C.: Diagnostic accuracy of an ultrasonic multiple transducer cardiac imaging system, Am. Heart J. **90**:329-334, 1975.

vonRamm, O. T., and Thurstone, F. L.: Thaumascan; design considerations and performance characteristics. In White, D., editor: Ultrasound in medicine, vol. 1, New York, 1975, Plenum Publishing Corp., p. 373.

Weitzel, D., Stopfkuchen, H., and Jungst, B. K.: Ultrasonic cross-sectional investigation of the heart in children by the rapid image rate method. In: Kazner, E., and others, editors: Ultrasonics in medicine, Amsterdam, 1975, Excerpta Medica, pp. 245-250.

Weyman, A., Feigenbaum, H., Dillon, J., and Chang, S.: Evaluation of left ventricular apical aneurysms by real-time cross sectional echocardiography, Circulation **52**(suppl. 2):33, 1975.

Williams, D. E., Sahn, D. J., and Friedman, W. F.: Cross-sectional echocardiography in assessing the severity of valvular aortic stenosis, Circulation **52**: 828-834, 1975.

French, J. W., Silverman, N. H., Martin, R. P., Schiller, N. B., and Popp, R. L.: Examination of operative patients with conotruncal abnormalities using an ultrasonic wide-angle scanner, Circulation **54**(suppl. 2):45, 1976.

Friedman, W. F.: Radioisotopes and cross-sectional ultrasound in congenital heart disease, Adv. Cardiol. **17**:32-39, 1976.

Gilbert, B. W., Schatz, R., Behar, V. S., and Kisslo, J. A.: Two-dimensional echocardiographic and angiographic correlations of mitral valve prolapse, Circulation **53-54**(suppl. 2):234, 1976.

Gramiak, R., and Waag, R. C.: Cardiac reconstruction imaging in relation to other ultrasound systems and computed tomography, Am. J. Roentgenol. **127**:91-99, 1976.

Kisslo, J., vonRamm, O. T., Haney, R., Jones, R., Juk, S. S., and Behar, V.: Echocardiographic evaluation of tricuspid valve endocarditis, Am. J. Cardiol. **38**: 502-507, 1976.

Kisslo, J., von Ramm, O. T., and Thurstone, F.: Cardiac imaging using a phased array ultrasound system. II. Clinical technique and application, Circulation **53**:262, 1976.

Martin, R. P., French, J. W., Pittman, M. M., and Popp, R. L.: Analysis of idiopathic hypertrophic subaortic stenosis by wide-angle phased array echocardiography, Circulation **54**(suppl. 2):190, 1976.

Mathews, E., Jr., Henry, W. L., Ronan, J. A., and Griffith, J. M.: Two-dimensional echocardiographic evaluation of mitral valve prolapse—an explanation of the patterns seen with M-mode echocardiograms, Circulation **54**(suppl. 2):235, 1976.

Nishimura, K., Hibi, N., Kato, T., Fukui, Y., and Arakawa, T.: Real-time observation of cardiac movement and structures in congenital and acquired heart diseases employing high-speed ultrasonocardiotomography, Am. Heart J. **92**:340-350, 1976.

Nishimura, K., Hibi, N., Kato, T., Fukui, Y., Arakawa, T., Tatematsu, H., Miwa, A., Tada, H., Kambe, T., and Sakamoto, N.: Real-time observation of ruptured right sinus of Valsalva aneurysm by high-speed ultrasono-cardiotomography, Circulation **53**:732, 1976.

Popp, R. L., Martin, R. P., French, J. W., and Pittman, M. M.: Positional distribution of pericardial effusion by real-time two-dimensional echocardiography, Circulation **53-54**(suppl. 2):234, 1976.

Schiller, N., Drew, D., Acquatella, H., Boswell, R., Botvinick, E., Greenberg, B., and Carlsson, E.: Noninvasive biplane quantitation of left ventricular volume and ejection fraction with a real-time two-dimensional echocardiography system, Circulation **53-54**(suppl. 2):234, 1976.

vonRamm, O. T., and Thurstone, F. L.: Cardiac imaging using a phased array ultrasound system, I. system design, Circulation **53**:258, 1976.

Weyman, A. E., and Feigenbaum, H.: Echocardiography—where are we now and where are we going? Am. J. Med. **60**:315, 1976.

Weyman, A. E., Feigenbaum, K., Dillon, J. C., Johnston, K. W., and Eggelton, R. C.: Noninvasive visualization of the left main coronary artery by cross-sectional echocardiography, Circulation **54**:169-173, 1976.

Weyman, A. E., Feigenbaum, H., Hurwitz, R. A., Girod, D. A., Dillon, J. C., and Chang, G.: Cross-sectional echocardiography in evaluating patients with discrete subaortic stenosis, Am. J. Cardiol. **37**:358, 1976.

Weyman, A. E., Feigenbaum, H., Hurwitz, R. A., Girod, D. A., Dillon, J. C., and Chang, S.: Localization of left ventricular outflow obstruction by cross-sectional echocardiography, Am. J. Med. **60**:33, 1976.

Weyman, A. E., Wann, S., Feigenbaum, H., and Dillon, J. C.: Mechanism of abnormal septal motion in patients with right ventricular volume overload; a cross sectional study, Circulation **54**:179-186, 1976.

Williams, D. E., Sahn, D. J., and Friedman, W. F.: Cross-sectional echocardiographic localization of sites of left ventricular outflow tract obstruction, Am. J. Cardiol. **37**:250-255, 1976.

Anderson, W. A., Arnold, J. T., Clark, D., Davids, W. T., Hillard, W. J., Lehr, W. J., and Zitelli, L. T.: A new real-time phased array sector scanner for imaging the entire adult human heart. In White, D. N., and Brown, D. E.: Ultrasound in medicine, vol. 3, New York, 1977, Plenum Publishing Corp., p. 1547.

Dillon, J. C., Weyman, A. E., Feigenbaum, H., Eggelton, R. C., and Johnston, K. W.: Cross-sectional echocardiographic examination of the interatrial septum, Circulation **55**:115, 1977.

Gilbert, B. W., Haney, R. S., Crawford, F., McClelan, J., Gallis, H. A., Jouhson, M. L., and Kisslo,

J. A.: Two-dimensional echocardiographic assessment of vegetative endocarditis, Circulation **55:**346-353, 1977.

Gilbert, B. W., Schatz, R. A., von Ramm, O. T., Behar, V. S., and Kisslo, J. A.: Two-dimensional echocardiographic definition of mitral valve prolapse. In White, D. N., and Brown, R. E., editors: Ultrasound in medicine, vol. 3, New York, 1977, Plenum Publishing Corp., p. 87.

Henry, W. L., Maron, B. J., and Griffith, J. M.: Cross-sectional echocardiography in the diagnosis of congenital heart disease; identification of the relation of the ventricles and great arteries, Circulation **56:**267, 1977.

Hibi, N., Kato, T., Fukui, Y., Arakawa, T., Nishimura, K., Tatematsu, H., Miwa, A., Tada, H., Kambe, T., and Sakamoto, N.: Ultrasono-cardiographic study on tetralogy of Fallot by means of high speed mechanical sector scanning system. In White, D. N., Brown, R. E., editors: Ultrasound in medicine, vol. 3, New York, 1977, Plenum Publishing Corp. p. 149.

Kambe, T., Kato, T., Hibi, N., Fukui, Y., and Arakawa, T., Nishimura, K., Tatematsu, H., Miwa, A., Tada, H., Sakamoto, N.: Real-time observation of mitral valve movements in mitral stenosis by means of high speed ultrasono-cardiography. White, D. N., and Brown, R. E., editors: Ultrasound in medicine, vol. 3, New York, 1977, Plenum Publishing Corp., p. 71.

Kisslo, J. A., Robertson, D., Gilbert, B. W., vonRamm, O., and Behar, V. S.: A comparison of real-time two-dimensional echocardiography and cineangiography in detecting left ventricular asynergy, Circulation **55:** 134, 1977.

Kisslo, J. A., Robertson, D., von Ramm, O. T., Gilbert, B. W., and Behar, V. S.: Assessment of ventricular wall motion by two dimensional echocardiography. White, D. N., and Brown, R. E., editors: Ultrasound in medicine, vol. 3, New York, 1977, Plenum Publishing Corp., p. 5.

Kisslo, J. A., von Ramm, O. T., and Thurstone, F. L.: Dynamic cardiac imaging using a focused, phased-array ultrasound system, Am. J. Med. **63:**61, 1977.

Martin, R. P., French, J. W., Pittman, M. M., and

Popp, R. L.: Identification and localization of pericardial effusion by real-time two-dimensional echocardiography. In White, D. N., and Brown, R. E., editors: Ultrasound in medicine, vol. 3, New York, 1977, Plenum Publishing Corp.

Matsumoto, M., Matsuo, H., Inoue, M., Kitabatake, A., Nimura, Y., Tamura, S., Tanaka, K., and Abe, H.: Three dimensional echocardiographic images and two-dimensional echocardiograms in desired planes by a computerized system. In White, D. N., and Brown, R. E., editors: Ultrasound in medicine, vol. 3, New York, 1977, Plenum Publishing Corp., p. 1.

Nichol, P. M., Gilbert, B. W., and Kisslo, J. A.: Evaluation of mitral stenosis by two-dimensional echocardiography. In White, D. N., and Brown, R. E., editors: Ultrasound in medicine, vol. 3, New York, 1977, Plenum Publishing Corp., p. 99.

Nichol, P. M., Gilbert, B. W., and Kisslo, J. A.: Two-dimensional echocardiographic assessment of mitral stenosis, Circulation **55:**120, 1977.

Roelandt, J., Tencate, F. J., Bom, N., and Lancee, C. T.: Opportunities of two-dimensional ultrasonic cardiac imaging. In White, D. N., and Brown, R. E. editors: Ultrasound in medicine, vol. 3, New York, 1977, Plenum Publishing Corp., p. 177.

Sahn, D. J., Henry, W. L., Allen, H. D., Griffith, J. M., and Goldberg, S. J.: The comparative utilities of real-time cross-sectional echocardiographic imaging systems for the diagnosis of complex congenital heart disease, Am. J. Med. **63:**50, 1977.

Schiller, N. B., and Silverman, N.: Clinical experience with cardiac imaging using a new phased-array 80 degree sector-scanner. In White, D. N., and Brown, R. E., editors: Ultrasound in medicine, vol. 3, New York, 1977, Plenum Publishing Corp., p. 179.

Weyman, A. E., Feigenbaum, H., Hurwitz, R. A., Girod, D. A., and Dillon, J. C.: Cross-sectional echocardiographic assessment of the severity of aortic stenosis in children, Circulation **55:**773, 1977.

Nanda, N. C., and Gramiak, R.: Evaluation of bicuspid valves by two-dimensional echocardiography, Am. J. Cardiol. **41:**372, 1978.

Appendix

Normal measurements in adults*

RV dimension, supine (R)	0.7-2.3 cm
RV dimension, left lateral (R)	0.9-2.6 cm
LV dimension, supine (R)	3.7-5.6 cm
LV dimension, left lateral (R)	3.5-5.7 cm
LV posterior wall thickness (R)	0.6-1.1 cm
LV posterior wall excursion	0.7-1.7 cm
Ventricular septal thickness (R)	0.6-1.1 cm
Ventricular septal excursion	0.3-0.8 cm
LV fractional shortening or ΔD	0.25-0.42
LV ejection fraction	45%-84%
Mean V_{cf} (LV)	1.02-1.94 circ/sec
Ventricular septal thickening	0.30-0.65
Ventricular septal velocity (S)	3.3-7.0 cm/sec
LV posterior wall thickening	0.36-0.95
Mean LV posterior wall velocity (S)	3.0-7.1 cm/sec
Max LV posterior wall velocity (S)	3.0-8.3 cm/sec
Max LV posterior wall velocity (D)	9.1-28 cm/sec
LV outflow tract dimension (beginning S)	2.0-3.5 cm
Left atrial dimension (end-S)	1.9-4.0
Aortic root diameter (R)	2.0-3.7
Aortic cusp separation (early S)	1.5-2.6

*Data from Feigenbaum, H.: Echocardiography, ed. 2, Philadelphia, 1976, Lea & Febiger, and Felner, J. M., and Schlant, R. C.: Echocardiography; a teaching atlas, New York, 1976, Grune & Stratton, Inc.
R, measurement taken at the R wave of ECG; RV, right ventricle; LV, left ventricle; S, ventricular systole; D, ventricular diastole; V_{cf}, velocity of circumferential fiber shortening; circ, circumferences.

Normal measurements (cm) in children*

Weight (lbs)	RV (R) dimension	LVO dimension (beginning systole)†	LV (R) dimension	RVO (R) dimension†	LV posterior wall and VS thickness (R)	LA dimension (end-systole)	Aortic root diameter (R)
0-25	0.3-1.5	0.9-1.7	1.3-3.2	1.1-2.0	0.4-0.6	0.7-2.3	0.7-1.7
26-50	0.4-1.5	1.8-2.3	2.4-3.8	1.5-2.3	0.5-0.7	1.7-2.7	1.3-2.2
51-75	0.7-1.8	2.0-2.8	3.3-4.5	1.9-2.2	0.6-0.7	1.9-2.8	1.7-2.3
76-100	0.7-1.6	2.4-3.4	3.5-4.7	2.0-2.7	0.7-0.8	2.0-3.0	1.9-2.7
101-125	0.8-1.7	2.5-3.5	3.7-4.9	2.0-2.6	0.7-0.8	2.1-3.0	1.7-2.7
126-200	1.2-1.7	2.0-3.3	4.4-5.2	2.4-3.1	0.7-0.8	2.1-3.7	2.2-2.8

*Data from Feigenbaum, H.: Echocardiography, ed. 2, Philadelphia, 1976, Lea & Febiger.
†Obtained from our laboratory (James Powers).
R, measurements taken at the R wave of the ECG; RV, right ventricle; LV, left ventricle; VS, ventricular septum; LA, left atrium; LVO, left ventricular outflow tract; RVO, right ventricular outflow tract.

Measurements in normal newborns*

	Range (mm)
Mitral valve excursion	6-12
Tricuspid valve excursion	7-14
Aortic root diameter (S)	7-13.6
Pulmonary root diameter (S)	10.7-15.8
Left atrial dimension (S)	4-13.5
Ventricular septal thickness (D)	2.1-4.5
LV posterior wall thickness (D)	1.6-4.6
LV cavity diameter (short-axis) (D)	12-24.1
LV cavity diameter (short-axis) (S)	8-18.6
LV outflow dimension (beginning systole)†	9-15
RV anterior wall thickness (D)	1.1-4.7
RV dimension (D)	6.1-17.7
RV outflow dimension†	11-19
Mean V_{CF} (LV)	0.92-2.2 circ/sec

*Data from Feigenbaum, H.: Echocardiography, ed. 2, Philadelphia, 1976, Lea & Febiger.
†Data from our laboratory (James Powers)
D, diastole; S, systole; LV, left ventricle; RV, right ventricle; circ, circumferences.

Normal measurements from the suprasternal transducer position*

Aortic arch lumen diameter	24 ± 1.1 mm
Right pulmonary artery lumen diameter	20 ± 1.2 mm
Left atrial cephalocaudad diameter	52 ± 12.7 mm
Left atrial anteroposterior diameter	42 ± 7.3 mm

*From Goldberg, B. B.: Ultrasonic measurement of the aortic arch, right pulmonary artery and left atrium, Radiology 101:383-390, 1971.

Mitral valve diastolic flutter

Condition	Type	Etiology
Normal infants	High frequency	Thin, small leaflets
Aortic valve incompetence	High frequency	Regurgitant jet striking the open leaflets
Truncal insufficiency	High frequency	Regurgitant jet striking the open leaflets
Dextrotransposition of great vessels following balloon septostomy	High frequency	Bidirectional shunting at atrial level
Dextrotransposition of great vessels following Mustard procedure	High and low frequency	Abnormal blood flow pathways and turbulence produced by the intra-atrial baffle
Chordae-papillary muscle rupture	High and low frequency	Unsupported leaflets
Congenital mitral incompetence	High frequency	Small, thickened leaflets and deformed subvalvular apparatus
Cor triatriatum	High and low frequency	Turbulence produced by supravalvar membrane
Atrial flutter/fibrillation	Coarse undulations; not true flutter	

Decreased mitral valve EF slopes

1. Mitral orifice obstruction
   a. Mitral stenosis
   b. Left atrial tumor
   c. Large vegetation
2. Decreased left ventricular compliance
   a. Asymmetric ventricular septal hypertrophy
   b. Aortic valve disease
   c. Systemic hypertension
3. Pulmonary hypertension (related to secondary changes in left ventricular compliance)
4. Incomplete examination of the mitral valve

Posterior displacement of the mitral systolic segment

1. Mitral valve prolapse
2. Enlargement of the left ventricle
3. Large pericardial effusion
4. Prolonged P-R interval resulting in mitral valve preclosure (apparent displacement only)
5. Tetralogy of Fallot
6. High chest wall transducer placement
7. Papillary muscle dysfunction
8. Congenitally cleft mitral valve

Abnormal systolic anterior movements of the mitral valve

1. Idiopathic hypertrophic subaortic stenosis
2. Mitral valve prolapse
3. Aortic incompetence (usually severe or acute)
4. Myocardial infarction
5. Left ventricular aneurysm
6. Severe pulmonary hypertension
7. Atrial septal defect
8. Parachute mitral valve
9. Dextrotransposition of the great vessels with or without subpulmonic obstruction
10. Discrete subaortic membranous stenosis
11. Systemic hypertension associated with concentric left ventricular hypertrophy.
12. Shock syndrome (hypovolemia; inotropic agents)
13. ? Normal volunteers in standing position
14. ? Simultaneous contractions of the atrium and the ventricle in complete heart block

Paradoxical ventricular septal motion

1. Right-sided volume overload–atrial septal defect, severe pulmonary or tricuspid valve incompetence, total anomalous pulmonary venous drainage
2. Left bundle branch block; right ventricular pacing; right ventricular premature beats; Wolff-Parkinson-White syndrome

3. Coronary artery disease, especially lesions involving the proximal left anterior descending vessel
4. Cardiac surgery (may be related to incision of the pericardium and formation of adhesions)
5. ? Congenital absence of the pericardium
6. ? Constrictive pericarditis

Discontinuity between anterior aortic wall and ventricular septum

1. Tetralogy of Fallot
2. Double-outlet right ventricle
3. Truncus arteriosus
4. Dilated aortic root (apparent discontinuity)
5. High transducer position (apparent discontinuity)

Systolic preclosure of aortic valve

1. Early systolic (type 1; preclosure completed in the first third of left ventricular ejection)

   Prominent
   a. Discrete subaortic membranous stenosis
   b. Aortic root dilatation (nondissecting and dissecting aortic aneurysms, sinus of Valsalva aneurysms)
   c. Tetralogy of Fallot (especially post repair)
   d. Truncus arteriosus (especially post repair)
   Small
   Nonspecific (coronary artery disease with left ventricular aneurysms, acquired mitral or aortic valve disease, atrial septal defects, pulmonary valve stenosis, coarctation of aorta, ? normal subjects)
2. Midsystolic (type 2)
   IHSS

3. Gradual systolic collapse of aortic valve (type 3)

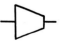

   a. Left ventricular systolic leaks—mitral regurgitation, ventricular septal defect, left ventricular aneurysm
   b. Low cardiac output

Usefulness of echocardiography in the detection of left ventricular outflow obstruction

Lesion	M-mode echo	Two-dimensional echo
Supravalvular aortic stenosis	Useful but can be missed	Useful; may be better than M-mode
Aortic valve stenosis		
Congenital	Almost always missed in the absence of valve calcification Poststenotic dilatation of aorta may serve as a clue to diagnosis	Useful; better than M-mode
Acquired (calcific)	Useful in diagnosis; less valuable in estimating severity	Better localization of small calcifications
Subaortic membranous or tunnel stenosis	Generally better than 2-D	No significant advantage over M-mode
IHSS, mid LV cavity obstruction	Generally better than 2-D	SAMs difficult to appreciate; useful for detecting site of septal hypertrophy
Large mitral prosthesis	Useful as a predictor before insertion	Not known

Echocardiography in infective endocarditis

Criteria for diagnosis
1. Aortic valve
   a. Shaggy, nonuniform thickening in systole and/or diastole with unrestricted leaflet motion
   b. Dense, shaggy echoes moving longitudinally across the aortic valve and into LVO
   c. Diastolic oscillations of the aortic valve, which appears thickened
2. Mitral valve
   a. Thick, shaggy echoes attached to or moving behind the leaflets that show unrestricted motion
   b. Systolic flutter of the prolapsing segments of the mitral valve
   c. Presence of fuzzy leaflet echoes in the left atrial cavity during systole
3. Tricuspid and pulmonary valves
   a. Shaggy thickening of the leaflet(s), which show unrestricted motion
   b. Mass of echoes moving with the leaflets

Associated abnormalities developing during course of disease
1. Diastolic flutter of mitral valve
2. Mitral valve preclosure
3. Flail mitral leaflets; chordae rupture
4. Coarse systolic flutter of aortic valve leaflets
5. Localized thickening of aortic wall (abscess formation)

Differential diagnosis
1. Fibrotic and/or calcified mitral and aortic valves
2. Flail mitral valve—cusp redundancy
3. Iatrogenic structures—catheters
4. Myxomatous degeneration of a valve
5. Cardiac tumors

M-Mode echo findings in transposition of great vessels

	Deduced great vessel spatial orientation		Timing of semilunar valve closure
	Anterior	**Posterior**	
Normal	Lateral	Medial	Anterior after posterior
DTGV	Medial	Lateral	Posterior after anterior
LTGV	Lateral	Medial	Posterior after anterior

DTGV, dextrotransposition of great vessels; LTGV, levotransposition of great vessels.

Two-dimensional echocardiographic findings in transposition of great vessels

Med, medial; Lat, lateral; Ant, anterior; Post, posterior, Ao, aorta, PA, pulmonary artery; RVO, right ventricular outflow tract; N, normal; DTGV, dextrotransposition of great vessels; LTGV, levotransposition of great vessels.

General review articles

Edler, I.: Diagnostic use of ultrasound in heart disease, Acta Med. Scand. **308**:32, 1955.

Wild, J. J., and Reid, J. M.: Diagnostic use of ultrasound, Br. J. Phys. Med. **19**:248, 1956.

Effert, S., Erkens, H., and Grossebrockhoff, F.: Ultrasonic echo method in cardiological diagnosis, Germ. Med. Mth. **2**:325, 1957.

Edler, I., Gustafson, A., Karlefors, T., and Christensson, B.: Ultrasound cardiography, Acta Med. Scand. **370**(suppl.):68, 1961.

Joyner, C. R., and Reid, J. M.: Application of ultrasound in cardiology and cardiovascular physiology, Progr. Cardiovasc. Dis. **5**:482, 1963.

Feigenbaum, H., and Zaky, A.: Use of diagnostic ultrasound in clinical cardiology, J. Indiana State Med. Assoc. **59**:140, 1966.

Kossoff, G.: Diagnostic applications of ultrasound in cardiology, Australas. Radiol. **10**:101, 1966.

Reid, J.: A review of some basic limitations in ultrasonic diagnosis. In Grossman, C. C., Holmes, J. H., Joyner, C., and Purnell, E. W., editors: Diagnostic ultrasound, Proceedings of the First International Conference, University of Pittsburgh, 1965, New York, 1966, Plenum Publishing Corp., p. 1.

Segal, B. L.: Echocardiography, Cardiology **50**:160-180, 1967.

Gramiak, R., and Shah, P. M.: Cardiac ultrasonography; a review of current applications; Radiol. Clin. North Am. **9**:469-490, 1971.

Feigenbaum, H.: Clinical applications of echocardiography, Prog. Cardiovasc. Dis. **14**:531-558, 1972.

Pridie, R. B., Behnam, R., and Wild, J.: Ultrasound in cardiac diagnosis, Clin. Radiol. **23**:160-173, 1972.

Chesler, E.: Ultrasound in cardiology, S. Arf. Med. J. **47**:1625-1637, 1973.

Feigenbaum, H.: Newer aspects of echocardiography, Circulation **47**:833, 1973.

Smith, W. K., Jr., and Frankl, W. S.: Ultrasound cardiography in clinical practice, Med. Clin. North Am. **57**:959-974, 1973.

Gramiak R.: Echocardiography, J.A.M.A. **229**:1099, 1974.

Abbasi, A. S.: Current application of echocardiography, Angiology **26**:303-316, 1975.

Chandraratna, P. A.: Clinical applications of echocardiography, Ceylon Med. J. **20**:185-191, 1975.

Feigenbaum, H.: The value of echocardiography in older patients, Geriatrics **30**:106-108, 110-111, 1975.

Ferrer, P. L., Gottlieb, S., Kallos, N., Wexler, H., and Miale, A., Jr.: Applications of diagnostic ultrasound and radionuclides to cardiovascular diagnosis. II. Cardiovascular disease in the young, Semin. Nucl. Med. **5**:387-418, 1975.

Gottlieb, S., Sheps, D., Myerburg, R. J., and Miale, A. J.: Applications of diagnostic ultrasound and radionuclides to cardiovascular diagnosis. I. Acquired cardiovascular disease in the adult, Semin. Nucl. Med. **5**:353-386, 1975.

Gramiak, R., Nanda, N. C., and Gross, C. M.: Echocardiography in acquired cardiac and pericardial disease, Semin. Roentgenol. **10**:291-297, 1975.

Morganroth, J.: Clinical echocardiography, Compr. Ther. **1**:61-68, 1975.

Popp, R. L., and Lopes, M.G.: Echocardiography in cardiac diagnosis, Cardiovasc. Clin. **6**:199-218, 1975.

Johnson, M. L., and Kisslo, J. A.: Basic diagnostic echocardiography, DM **23**:1-58, 1976.

Naggar, C. Z.: Ultrasound in medical diagnosis. I. Applications in cardiology, Heart Lung **5**:895-907, 1976.

Nanda, N. C.: Clinical applications of echocardiography, I. Mod. Concepts Cardiovasc. Dis. **45**:135-138, 1976.

Nanda, N. C.: Clinical applications of echocardiography. II. Mod. Concepts Cardiovasc. Dis. **45**:139-142, 1976.

Parisi, A. F., Tow, D. E., and Sasahara, A. A.: Clinical appraisal of current nuclear and other noninvasive cardiac diagnostic techniques, Am. J. Cardiol. **38**:722-730, 1976.

Popp, R. L.: Echocardiographic assessment of cardiac disease, Circulation **54**:538-552, 1976.

Gramiak, R., and Nanda, N. C.: Ultrasound in the evaluation of patients for cardiac surgery; Int. Surg., in press.

Parisi, A. F., Tow, D. E., Felix, W. R., Jr., and Sasahara, A. A.: Noninvasive cardiac diagnosis. II. N. Engl. J. Med. **296**:368-374, 1977.

Parisi, A. F., Tow, D. E., Felix, W. R., Jr., and Sasahara, A. A.: Noninvasive cardiac diagnosis. III. N. Engl. J. Med. **296**:427-432, 1977.

Index

A

A dip
  and diastolic pressure gradient across pulmonary
    valve, 229
  and pulmonary artery pressure, 227
Adriamycin causing left ventricular dysfunction, 256
A-mode displays of signal processing in ultrasound, 49
Anatomy
  echocardiographic; *see* Echocardiography, anatomy
  heart; *see* Heart, anatomy
  ultrasound; *see* Ultrasound, anatomy
Aneurysms
  aortic, 177-184
    aortic valve preclosure in, 140
  atrial septal, two-dimensional contrast echocardiog-
    raphy of, 428
  of interatrial septum, 204
  of sinus of Valsalva, 184
    right, 184
  ventricular, left, 13
  of ventricular septum
    of right ventricular cavity, abnormal echoes in, 321-
     322
    two-dimensional echocardiography of, 387
Angiocardiography of heart, 23-27
Angulation in two-dimensional echocardiography, 379,
  380
Anomalies
  complex, 312-368
  Ebstein's; *see* Ebstein's anomaly
  pulmonary venous drainage, total anomalous, 318
Aorta; *see also* Aortic root
  coarctation of; *see* Coarctation of aorta
  proximal, two-dimensional echocardiography of, 417
  supravalvular
    in aortic root dissection, 180
    poststenotic dilatation of, 172
    two-dimensional echocardiography of, 392-393
Aortic
  aneurysms, 177-184
  echocardiography, normal, 22
  heterograft, porcine, in mitral position, 300
  incompetence
    auscultatory findings in, 21
    phonocardiography of, 21
  root; *see also* Aorta
    motion of aortic cusp systolic preclosure, 140

Aortic—cont'd
  root—cont'd
    recording
     in newborn, 224
     in tricuspid atresia, 359
     transverse section of, in two-dimensional echocar-
      diography, 399
    stenosis; *see* Stenosis, aortic
    valve; *see* Aortic valve
    and discontinuity of wall with ventricular septum, 434
Aortic valve
  aneurysm, aortic valve preclosure in, 140
  beam scanning
    from left ventricular cavity to, in pericardial and
     pleural effusions, 278
    to left ventricular cavity after left pneumonectomy,
     278
    to mitral valve in mediastinal tumor, 288
    to mitral valve in pericardial effusion, 287
    to pulmonary valve, 225
    to tricuspid valve, 194
    from tricuspid valve to, in right heart enlargement,
     74
    in truncus arteriosus, 340
  bicuspid, 169-177
    anatomic and functional changes, 169-172
    clinical summary, 172
    demonstrating reversal of eccentricity, 174
    eccentricity index in, 171
    echocardiographic features, 172-173
    echocardiography, role of, 177
    two-dimensional echocardiography of, 400
    with unequal cusps, 175
  calcification
    calcific disease, 166, 182, 388, 401
    in stenosis, 165
    surgically resected, 165
  cusps
    right coronary, flutter of, 187
    systolic preclosure of, aortic root motion in, 140
    ultrasonic anatomy of, 70
  delayed opening of, in hypoplastic left heart syn-
    drome, 361
  disease, 164
    calcific, 166, 182
     two-dimensional echocardiography of, 388,
     401

Aortic valve—cont'd
disease—cont'd
findings in, 164-185
eccentricity index in, 171
calculation of, 171
in endocarditis, bacterial, 185, 187
flutter
from bacterial endocarditis, 187
of right coronary cusp, 187
functional changes, 185-190
incompetence, 143, 144
Austin-Flint murmur in, 145
mitral valve flutter in, 143
SAMs in, 123
leaflets, unsupported, 185
in mitral incompetence, 188
motion and premature ventricular contraction, 189
movement toward closure in pericardial effusion, 285
normal, tracing, 160
after pneumonectomy, two-dimensional echocardiography of, 385
preclosure in aortic aneurysm, 140
prosthesis; *see* Prosthetic valves, aortic
recording
in Ebstein's anomaly, 327
in newborn, 344
with simultaneous recording of heart sounds, 189
technique, 162
ultrasonic anatomy during, 71
variations in, anatomic and functional, 163
regurgitation, 142-146, 164-169
anatomic changes, 142-143, 164
clinical summary, 143-144, 164-165
congenital, 169-177
anatomic and functional changes, 169-172
clinical summary, 172
echocardiographic features, 172-173
echocardiography, role of, 177
echocardiographic features, 144-146, 165-166
echocardiography, role of, 146, 169
functional changes, 142-143, 164
relationship to pulmonary valve, 78
root
echocardiography, 178
motion abnormality in pericardial effusion, 286
motion in mitral regurgitation, 168
normal, 161, 167
in pericardial effusion, 289
in right ventricular enlargement, 169
root dissection, 177-183
anatomic and clinical summary, 177-179
atypical echocardiographic findings in, 181
echocardiographic features, 178, 179
echocardiography, role of, 183-184
root size variations in, 179
supravalvular aorta in, 180
stenosis; *see* Stenosis, aortic
structures in beam, 160
subaortic stenosis and
idiopathic hypertrophic, 119
membranous, 139
systolic preclosure of, 434
technical considerations, 160-164
tricuspid, ultrasonic beam passing through, 173
two-dimensional echocardiography of, 417
unicuspid, 174
vegetations, 184-185, 186

Arrhythmia, cardiac, pulmonary valve in, 242
Arteries
coronary; *see* Coronary artery disease
great; *see* Transposition of great arteries
pulmonary; *see* Pulmonary artery
Artifacts
beam width, 34
from mitral prosthesis, 304
reverberation, 305
mechanism of, 39
of time-varied gain, 60
Atresia
mitral valve, 362
tricuspid valve reverberations in, 362
tricuspid, 356-359
anatomic changes, 356
aortic root recording in, 359
clinical summary, 357
echocardiographic features, 357
echocardiography, role of, 359
functional changes, 356
mitral valve recording in, 359
Atrioventricular
canal defects
anatomy, functional, 330
common, 330-331
clinical summary, 331-332
complete, 329-334
anatomic changes, 329
echocardiographic features, 332-333
echocardiography, role of, 334
functional changes, 329
steplike continuity between mitral and tricuspid valves in, 331
two-dimensional echocardiography by subxiphoid technique of, 422
partial
cleft tricuspid valve in, 319
mitral valve recording in, 334
valve
motion abnormalities in dextrotransposition of great vessels after Mustard procedure, 349
single, and single ventricle, 356
Atrium
abnormal echoes in, mimicking cor triatriatum, 324
cavities of, two-dimensional echocardiography of
apical four-chamber view, 409
subxiphoid technique, 418
fibrillation of, 218, 219
mitral valve in, 147
pulmonary valve in, 241
tricuspid valve in, 219
flutter of, 218
mitral valve in, 147
pulmonary valve in, 241
left
pericardial effusion behind, 272
planes passing through, 415
reverberations in, 162
two-dimensional echocardiography of, 414-416
membrane of, left, congenital obstruction, 323
myxoma of; *see* Myxoma, atrial
right
anatomy, and two-dimensional echocardiography examining planes, 412
membrane in, tricuspid valve of, in infant, 204

Atrium—cont'd
  right—cont'd
    in shunt; *see* Shunt, congenital left ventricular–right atrial
    tricuspid valve recording with ultrasonic beam passing through, 198
    two-dimensional echocardiography of, 412
  septum of
    abnormal position in Ebstein's anomaly, 328
    aneurysm, two-dimensional contrast echocardiography of, 428
    defect; *see* Septal defect, atrial
    development of, 313
    identification, 193
      using contrast injections, 194
    recording, ultrasonic anatomy during, 79
    reverberations behind, 197
    shunt, left-to-right, two-dimensional contrast echocardiography of, 425
Auscultatory findings in clinical disease, 21
Austin-Flint murmur in aortic incompetence, 145
Axial resolution, 33

B
Bacterial endocarditis; *see* Endocarditis, bacterial
Baffle
  incompetence of, 352
    echocardiographic findings in, 351
    two-dimensional echocardiography of, 426
  intra-atrial; *see* Intra-atrial baffle
Ball valve; *see* Prosthetic valves, ball
Beall valve, 294
Beam
  angulation, 38
    with artifact from mitral prosthesis, 304
  pathway in right ventricular outflow–pulmonary artery area, 75
  pattern, 32
    returning, 38
  position, 38
  scanning
    from aortic to mitral valve
      in mediastinal tumor, 288
      in pericardial effusion, 287
    from aortic valve to left ventricular cavity after left pneumonectomy, 278
    in left ventricle long axis, 67
    from left ventricular cavity
      to aortic valve in pericardial and pleural effusions, 278
      to mitral valve in pericardial effusion, 279
    of left ventricular cavity in pericardial effusion, 282
    technique in pericardial effusion, 271
    from tricuspid to aortic valve in right heart enlargement, 74
    from tricuspid valve to left ventricle, 74
  shape, 32
  structure size, 38
  ultrasound; *see* Ultrasound, beam
  width, 35
    artifacts, 34
Bioprostheses; *see* Prosthetic valves, bioprostheses
Bjork-Shiley valve, 294
Block, heart
  complete, 18
    pulmonary valve in, 241
    with ventricular pacemaker, 209

Block, heart—cont'd
  first-degree, mitral valve in, 147
Blood pressure
  normal, 24
  overload, effects on ventricle
Blood supply of heart, 7

C
Calcification
  of aortic valve; *see* Aortic valve, calcification
  of mitral valve; *see* Mitral valve, calcification
Cardiology, clinical, 3-27
Cardiomyopathy
  congestive, 129, 130-133
    anatomic changes, 130
    in child, 132
    clinical summary, 131
    echocardiographic features, 131-133
    functional changes, 130
    mitral valve in, 148
    tricuspid valve, late opening in, 218
  manifestations of, 14
  ventricular hypertrophy in, concentric left, 132
Carotid pulse tracing, normal, 22
Catheter(s)
  heart; *see* Heart catheters, right
  pacing; *see* Pacing catheter
  ventricular, right
    outflow, 210
    reverberations, 211
Catheterization of hearts, 23-27
Chambers; *see* Heart chambers
Chest
  fluoroscopy, 23
  radiography, 23
Children, congestive cardiomyopathy of, 132
Chordae
  of mitral valve; *see* Mitral valve, chordae
  rupture of, two-dimensional echocardiography of, 390
Circulation
  coronary, 7
  fetal, 313-314
  normal, 5
Cleft tricuspid valve in atrioventricular canal defect, 319
Coarctation of aorta, 322-324
  two-dimensional echocardiography of, by suprasternal technique, 424
Complex malformations, 312-368
Conduction; *see* Heart conduction
Contrast
  identification of structures during pulmonary valve recording, 76
  injections
    in atrial septum identification, 194
    of indocyanine green in ultrasound, 216
    in left ventricle, 63
  studies of ventricular septal defect, 64
    after surgical closure, 64
Cor triatriatum, 323, 324-325
  left atrium, abnormal echoes mimicking, 324
Coronary
  artery disease, 257-259
    anatomic and functional changes, 257-258
    clinical summary, 258
    echocardiographic features, 258-259
    echocardiography, role of, 259
    left ventricular cavity in, 258

Coronary—cont'd
  circulation, 7
  sinus
    pacing catheter, 211
    ultrasonic identification, 280
Crystal size, 32

D

Dextrotransposition of great vessels, 343
  anatomy, 342
  atrioventricular valve motion abnormalities in, after
      Mustard procedure, 349
  pulmonary artery echocardiograms in, 348
  pulmonary hypertension in, 353
  subvalvular narrowing in, with subpulmonic obstruc-
      tion, 345
  tricuspid valve echocardiograms in, 349
Disc valve; see Prosthetic valves, disc
D-transposition; see Dextrotransposition of great vessels

E

Ebstein's anomaly, 325-327
  anatomic changes, 325
  atrial septum, abnormal position in, 328
  clinical summary, 325
  echocardiographic features, 325-327
  echocardiography, role of, 327
  functional changes, 325
  mitral valve prolapse in, 328
  simultaneous recording of pulmonary and aortic valves
      in, 327
  two-dimensional echocardiography in, 406, 410
  ventricular septum in, 326
Eccentricity index in aortic valve, 171
  calculation of, 171
Echo imaging, effect of instrument controls on, 47
Echocardiography
  anatomy, 66-81
    of aortic valve cusps, 70
    during aortic valve recording, 71
    during atrial septal recording, 79
    of mitral valve, normal, 68
    of tricuspid valve, 72
  aortic, normal, 22
  of aortic valve
    bicuspid, 172-173, 177
    regurgitation, 142-146, 165-166, 169
      congenital, 172-173, 177
    root, 178
    root dissection, 178, 179, 183
      atypical findings, 181
    stenosis, 169
      acquired, 165-166
      congenital, 172-173, 177
  of cardiomyopathy, congestive, 131-133
  in coronary artery disease, 258-259
  electrocardiographic leads used in, 16
  with electrocardiography, 55
  examination in complex malformations, 314-364
  fundamentals of, 1-84
  of heart catheters, right, 209-210, 213
  heart target characteristics in, 65-66
  in infundibular stenosis, 236
  interventions during, 83-84
  of mitral valve
    calcification, 94
    in cardiomyopathy, congestive, 131

Echocardiography—cont'd
  of mitral valve—cont'd
    findings in disease, 91-159
    in mitral stenosis, 103
    normal, 89
    prolapse, 105-107, 111-112
    regurgitation, rheumatic, 100-103
    in rupture of mitral apparatus, 113-115
    technique, 62
    useful measurements, 90
    vegetations, 115-116
  in myxoma, 127
    atrial, right, 202, 205
    ventricular outflow, right, 236-239
  one-dimensional, 370
  of pericardial effusion, 273-274, 291
  of prosthetic valve, 296, 305-310
  of pulmonary valve
    hypertension, 227-230, 232
    stenosis, 234, 235-236
  recording philosophy in, 81-83
  reverberations in, 41
  of shunt, congenital left ventricular–right atrial, 217
  Starr-Edwards prosthesis, 302
  of subaortic obstruction, 138-139, 141-142
  of subaortic stenosis, idiopathic hypertrophic, 119-
      120, 126-127
  of subxiphoid, 80, 417-423
  targets in, position of, 66
  technique of, 54-84
    general considerations, 54-65
    suprasternal, 81
    transducer-holding, two-handed, 56
  of tricuspid valve
    echocardiographic relationships, 73
    endocarditis, 205, 207
    prolapse, 200, 201
    stenosis, 199, 200
  two-dimensional; see Two-dimensional echocardiog-
      raphy
Echo-free spaces
  around heart, 275
  in pericardial effusion; see Pericardium, effusion,
      echo-free spaces
  from pneumonectomy, left, 277
Electrical alternans and pericardial effusion, 283
Electrocardiography, 16-18
  in conduction disturbances, 17
  with echocardiography, 55
  leads used in echocardiography, 16
  in rhythm disturbances, 17
Embryology, 312-313
Endocardial
  fibroelastosis, 363, 364
  pacing catheter, right ventricular, 212
Endocarditis
  aortic prosthesis, left ventricular outflow in, 308
  bacterial
    aortic valve in, 185
    aortic valve flutter from, 187
    mitral valve in, 116
    subacute, healed, mitral chordae rupture and,
        112
    systolic flutter in, and mitral valve prolapse, 110
    two-dimensional echocardiography of, 388-389
  infective, echocardiography in, 435
  mitral chordae rupture secondary to, 110

Endocarditis—cont'd
  nonbacterial, of mitral valve in lupus erythematosus, two-dimensional echocardiography of, 389
  tricuspid, 205-207
    anatomic and functional changes, 205
    clinical summary, 205
    echocardiographic features, 205
    echocardiography, role of, 207
Eustachian valve, two-dimensional contrast echocardiography of, 427

F

Fetal circulation, 313-314
Fibrillation; *see* Atrium, fibrillation of
Fibroelastosis, endocardial, 363, 364
Fibroma, ventricular, 257
Fluoroscopy of chest, 23
Flutter
  of aortic valve
    from bacterial endocarditis, 187
    of right coronary cusp, 187
  atrial; *see* Atrium, flutter
  of mitral valve
    in aortic incompetence, 143
    diastolic, 433
    systolic, in prolapse and bacterial endocarditis, 110
  of pulmonary valve, diastolic, 240
  tricuspid; *see* Tricuspid valve, flutter
Frequency, 32

G

Gain
  control, segmental, 48
  near-gain suppression, 61
  settings, 58
    around heart, 275
  time-varied
    artifact of, 60
    effects of, 59
"Ghost" echoes, mitral, 114

H

Heart
  anatomic relationships of, normal, 4
  anatomy
    abnormal, 7-16
    normal, 3-7
    right, 198
  angiocardiography and, 23-27
  apex of
    examination of, 245
    in pericardial effusion, 271, 276, 282
  arrhythmia in, pulmonary valve in, 242
  block; *see* Block, heart
  blood supply of, 7
  catheterization, 23-27
  catheters, right, 208-213
    clinical summary, 208-209
    echocardiographic features, 209-210
    echocardiography, role of, 213
  chambers
    enlargement due to intracardiac shunting, 11
    function, 5-7
    position, 5-7
  clinical investigations of, 16-27
  conduction
    disturbances, electrocardiography in, 17

Heart—cont'd
  conduction—cont'd
    system, 6
  disease, congenital, 133-137
  echo-free spaces around, 275
  enlargement, right
    beam scanning from tricuspid to aortic valve in, 74
    right ventricular scan in, 78
  failure, 15
    right, and pulmonary hypertension, 229
  function
    abnormal, 7-16
    normal, 3-7
  gain settings around, 275
  graphic recordings of, 18-23
  horizontally oriented, two-dimensional echocardiography of, 384
  hypoplastic left heart syndrome; *see* Hypoplastic left heart syndrome
  intracardiac reverberations, 251
  lining abnormalities, 12-13
  murmurs; *see* Murmurs
  obstructions, left, mechanisms that produce, 8
  orientation and ultrasound recording, 82
  output, low, with prosthetic valves, 295
  pathologic examinations of, 27
  relationships, 3-4
  retrocardiac spaces, false, 281
  shunting causing chamber enlargement, 11
  sounds; *see* Sounds
  structures
    abnormalities of, 7-12
    underdevelopment of, shunting as compensatory mechanism, 12
  swinging, 283-288
  tamponade, 288
  target characteristics in echocardiography, 65-66
  tube, primitive, 313
  window, 4
    location of, 57
Heart-lung interface reverberations, 281
Hemolysis and prosthetic valve, 295
Heterograft, porcine aortic, in mitral position, 300
Hypertension, pulmonary, 223, 226-232
  anatomic and functional changes, 226-227
  clinical summary, 227
  complicating ventricular septal defect, 320
  in dextrotransposition of great vessels, 353
  echocardiographic features, 227-230
  echocardiographic findings in, 227
  heart failure and, right, 229
  mitral valve in, 95
  pulmonary valve in, 228, 233
  two-dimensional echocardiography in, 395
Hypertrophic subaortic stenosis; *see* Stenosis, subaortic, idiopathic hypertrophic
Hypertrophy
  of ventricle
    left, concentric, in cardiomyopathy, 132
    right, tricuspid valve in, 200
  of ventricular septum
    asymmetric, 117
    outflow obstruction from, two-dimensional echocardiography of, 386
    two-dimensional echocardiography of, 386
Hypoplastic left heart syndrome, 359-364
  anatomic changes, 359-360

Hypoplastic left heart syndrome—cont'd
  aortic valve, delayed opening in, 361
  clinical summary, 360
  echocardiographic features, 360-361
  echocardiography, role in, 363-364
  functional changes, 359-360

I

IHSS; *see* Stenosis, subaortic, idiopathic hypertrophic
Image loss, lung-induced, 42
Imaging
  echo, effect of instrument controls on, 47
  modes in ultrasound, 30
  sound speed and, 42
Indocyanine green for ultrasonic contrast injections, 216
Infant
  with membrane in right atrium, tricuspid valve in, 204
  pulmonary artery recording in, 77
Instruments in ultrasound, 43-44
  controls, 44-48
    effect on echo imaging, 47
Intensity ratios, 45
Interatrial septum
  aneurysm of, 204
  in biatrial myxoma, 206
Interventions during echocardiography, 83-84
Intra-atrial baffle, 347-353; *see also* Baffle, incompetence of
  anatomic changes, 347
  contrast studies in, 352
  echocardiographic features, 347-350
  functional changes, 347
  schematic representation, 347
  ultrasonic contrast studies in, 350
Intracardiac reverberations, 251

L

Lateral resolution, 34
Left ventricle; *see* Ventricle, left
Lung-heart interface reverberations, 281
Lung-induced image loss, 42
Lupus erythematosus, endocarditis of mitral valve in, two-dimensional echocardiography of, 389

M

Malformations; *see* Anomalies
Measurements, normal
  in adults, 432
  in children, 432
  in newborn, 433
  from suprasternal transducer position, 433
Mediastinal tumor, 288
Mitral
  apparatus, 6
  insufficiency
    auscultatory findings in, 21
    phonocardiography of, 21
Mitral valve, 87-159
  atresia, 362
    tricuspid valve reverberations in, 362
  in atrial flutter-fibrillation, 147
  in atrial septal defect, ostium primum, 135
  in atrioventricular canal defect, 331
  in bacterial endocarditis, 116

Mitral valve—cont'd
  beam scanning
    from aortic valve to
      in mediastinal tumor, 288
      in pericardial effusion, 287
    from left ventricular cavity to, in pericardial effusion, 279
  calcification
    annular, 96
      two-dimensional echocardiography of, 409
    echocardiography of, 94
    effect of instrument sensitivity in evaluation of, 96
    of leaflets, 92
    in mitral stenosis, 93
    of posterior cusp in stenosis, 97
    in vitro studies of, 98
  in cardiomyopathy, congestive, 148
  chordae
    motion mimicking SAM, 121
    rupture, 111, 113
      and endocarditis, 110, 112
    thickening in mitral stenosis, 92
  "double" orifice, 334
  echocardiographic anatomy, normal, 68
  echocardiographic measurements of, useful, 90
  echocardiography of
    in cardiomyopathy, congestive, 131
    findings in disease, 91-159
  EF slopes
    decreased, 434
    relationship to mitral stenosis severity, 100
    in rheumatic mitral regurgitation, 101
    slow, in pulmonary hypertension complicating ventricular septal defect, 320
  endocarditis in lupus erythematosus, two-dimensional echocardiography of, 389
  flutter
    in aortic incompetence, 143
    diastolic, 433
  functional observations of, 146-152
  "ghost" echoes in, 114
  in heart block, first-degree, 147
  incompetence
    aortic valve in, 188
    congenital, mitral valve recording in, 134
  leaflets
    calcification, 92
    systolic separation of, 130
    thickening in mitral stenosis, 92
    ulceration, 92
  in myxoma, biatrial, 128
  myxomatous degeneration of, 104
  normal
    echocardiogram, schematic representation, 89
    measurement technique, 88
    tracing, 87-91
  orifice
    in left atrial myxoma, two-dimensional echocardiography of, 397
    two-dimensional echocardiography of, 396
  parachute, 133
    mitral valve recording in, 134
  in pericardial effusion, 286
  after pneumonectomy, two-dimensional echocardiography of, 385
  prolapse, 103-112

Mitral valve—cont'd
prolapse—cont'd
anatomic changes, 103-105
auscultatory findings in, 21
clinical summary, 103-105
in Ebstein's anomaly, 328
echocardiographic features, 105-107
echocardiography, role of, 111-112
findings in evaluation of, schematic representation, 108
with pericardial effusion, 150, 284
phonocardiography of, 21
potential error source in, 109
SAM in, 106
systolic flutter in, and bacterial endocarditis, 110
typical, 105
prosthesis; *see* Prosthetic valves, mitral
in pulmonary hypertension, 95
recording
in mitral incompetence, congenital, 134
in parachute mitral valve, 134
in partial atrioventricular canal defect and "double" mitral orifice, 334
technique, 62, 89
in tricuspid atresia, 359
regurgitation
aortic root motion in, 168
mechanisms of, 9
rheumatic, 100-103
anatomic changes, 100
clinical summary, 100
echocardiographic features, 100-102
echocardiography, role of, 102-103
functional changes, 100
mitral EF slopes in, 101
relationship to pulmonary valve, 78
rupture of apparatus, 112-115
anatomic changes, 112-113
clinical summary, 113
echocardiographic features, 113-114
echocardiography, role of, 115
functional changes, 112-113
simultaneous echocardiography and phonocardiography of, 151
stenosis; *see* Stenosis, mitral
structures in beam, 87
in subaortic stenosis
discrete, 137
discrete membranous, 142
membranous, 138
surgically resected, 92
systolic abnormalities, 118
of anterior movements, 434
in pericardial effusion, 122
systolic segment, posterior displacement of, 434
technical considerations of, 91
two-dimensional echocardiography of, 409, 416
ultrasound of, 101
vegetations, 115-116
anatomic changes, 115
clinical summary, 115
echocardiographic features, 115
echocardiography, role of, 115-116
functional changes, 115
two-dimensional echocardiography of, 390
in ventricular end-diastolic pressure elevation, left, 149

M-mode
echo findings, in transposition of great vessels, 435
recording, transducer motion during, 36
Mortality, postoperative, with prosthetic valves, 310
Murmurs, 18-23
Austin-Flint, in aortic incompetence, 145
extra, phonocardiography of, 20
Muscle band in right ventricular cavity, 247
Mustard procedure in dextrotransposition of great vessels, 349
Myocardial
contraction, 253
ejection fraction, 253
fractional shortening, 253
mean velocity of circumferential fiber shortening, 253
dysfunction, 13-15
Myxoma, 127-130
anatomic changes, 127
atrial, 128
echocardiographic features, 202
left
mitral orifice in, two-dimensional echocardiography of, 397
mitral stenosis simulating, 93
recorded at insufficient instrument insensitivity, 90
two-dimensional echocardiography of, 387, 402, 411
right, 202-205
anatomic and functional changes, 202
clinical summary, 202
echocardiography, role of, 205
two-dimensional echocardiography of, 411
biatrial, 129
interatrial septum in, 206
mitral valve in, 128
clinical summary, 127
echocardiographic features, 127
functional changes, 127
ventricular outflow, right, 236-239
anatomic and functional changes, 236
clinical summary, 236
echocardiographic features, 236-239
echocardiography, role of, 239
pulmonary valve in, 237
Myxomatous degeneration of mitral valve, 104

N

Newborn
normal measurements in, 433
pulmonary and aortic root recordings in, 224
simultaneous recording of pulmonary and aortic valves in, 344

P

Pacemaker, transvenous right ventricular, and complete heart block, 209
Pacing catheter
coronary sinus, 211
ventricular, right, 208
endocardial, 212
demonstration of, 208
Pacing wires; *see* Heart catheters, right
Parachute mitral valve, 133
mitral valve recording in, 134

Patent ductus arteriosus, 321-322
  auscultatory findings in, 21
  phonocardiography of, 21
Pathologic examinations, 27
Pericarditis, constrictive, 235, 290
  left ventricular wall motion in, 290
Pericardium
  absence of, surgical or congenital, 290
  effusion in, 15, 268-292
    anatomic summary, 268-270
    anterior wall motion in, 270
    aortic root in, 289
    aortic root motion abnormality in, 286
    aortic valve movement toward closure in, 285
    behind atrium, left, 272
    beam scanning
      from aortic to mitral valve in, 287
      from left ventricular cavity to aortic valve in, 278
      from left ventricular cavity to mitral valve in, 279
      technique, 271
    cardiac apex in, 271, 276, 282
    clinical summary, 270
    echocardiographic findings, 273-274
    echocardiography, role of, 291
    echo-free spaces
      anterior, 275-277
      posterior, 277-283
    electrical alternans and, 283
    examination technique, 270-273
    mitral valve in, 286
    mitral valve abnormal systolic anterior movement in, 122
    mitral valve prolapse and, 150, 284
    posterior wall motion in, 270
    pulmonary valve systolic notching in, 285
    schematic representation, 269
    tricuspid valve prolapse and, 284
    ventricular cavity in, left, beam scanning of, 282
    ventricular outflow tract in, right, 289
    ventricular wall in, left, 280
    ventricular wall motion alteration in, right, 287
  sinus of
    oblique, 269
    transverse, 268, 273
  thickening, 290
Phonocardiography
  in clinical disease entities, 21
  of mitral valve, with simultaneous echocardiography, 151
  of murmurs, extra, 20
  of sounds, extra, 20
Piezoelectric effect, 28
Pivoting in two-dimensional echocardiography, 379-381
Planes; see Two-dimensional echocardiography, planes in
Pleural effusion, 15
  beam scanning from left ventricular cavity to aortic valve in, 278
  left, demonstration of, 276
Pneumonectomy
  left
    beam scanning from aortic valve to left ventricular cavity after, 278
    echo-free spaces from, 277
    mitral and aortic valves after, two-dimensional echocardiography of, 385

Pneumonectomy—cont'd
  two-dimensional left ventricular short axis scan after, 397
Porcine aortic heterograft in mitral valve position, 300
Postoperative mortality with prosthetic valves, 310
Poststenotic dilatation of supravalvular aorta, 172
Premature contraction, ventricular, and aortic valve motion, 189
Pressure
  blood; see Blood pressure
  pulmonary artery; see Pulmonary artery pressure
Prosthetic valves, 293-311
  aortic
    dysfunction of, echocardiographic findings, 307
    endocarditis due to, left ventricular outflow in, 308
    imaged from parasternal transducer position, 301
    imaged from suprasternal transducer position, 298
    structures in beam, 296
  ball, 293, 294
    caged
      advantages, 293
      disadvantages, 293-294
      estimate of possible obstruction by, 309
      mitral, 297
      Starr-Edwards; see Starr-Edwards prosthesis
      two-dimensional echocardiography of, 392
    variance, 295
  bioprostheses, 293
    advantages, 294
    disadvantages, 294
  complications of, 295
  disc
    advantages, 294
    central, 293, 294
    disadvantages, 294
    eccentric, 293, 294
    variance, 295
  echocardiographic examination, 296
  echocardiographic findings, 305-307
  echocardiography, role of, 307-310
  function of, clinical assessment, 295
  hemolysis and, 295
  leak, perivalvular, 295
  low cardiac output with, 295
  measurement technique, 301-304
  mitral
    beam with artifact from, 304
    caged ball, 297
    dysfunction of
      echocardiographic findings, 305-307
      spontaneous contrast effects in, 307
    examination technique, 296
    low-gain recordings, 302, 303
    porcine heterograft, 300
    Silastic, 299
    structures in beam, 295-296
  mortality with, postoperative, 310
  normal tracings, 296-301
  selection of, 293-294
  Starr-Edwards; see Starr-Edwards prosthesis
  suture ring dehiscence, 295
  thrombosis complicating, 295
  tricuspid
    Starr-Edwards prosthesis, 298
    structures in beam, 296

Prosthetic valves—cont'd
   types of, 293
   vegetations complicating, 295
Pulmonary
   artery
      area, ultrasonic beam traversing, 226
      beam pathway in area of, 75
      echocardiograms in dextrotransposition of great
         vessels, 348
      pressure
         mean, relationship to pulmonary valve opening
            slope, 228
         relation to A dip, 227
      recording, in infant, 77
      in transposition of great arteries, 231, 232
      two-dimensional echocardiography of, 414
   hypertension; *see* Hypertension, pulmonary
   insufficiency
      auscultatory findings in, 21
      phonocardiography of, 21
   stenosis; *see* Stenosis, pulmonary
   valve, 222-243
      in arrhythmia, cardiac, 242
      in atrial flutter-fibrillation, 241
      beam scanning from aortic to, 225
      contour variations, 226
      detection, 75
      diastolic pressure gradient across, relationship to A
         dip, 229
      findings in disease, 226-239
      flutter, diastolic, 240
      in heart block, complete, 241
      hemodynamic correlations, 222-224
      hypertension; *see* Hypertension, pulmonary
      measurement technique, 223
      in myxoma, right ventricular outflow, 237
      normal, 75, 223
         tracing, 222-224
      opening
         with atrial systole, 233
         slope, relationship to mean pulmonary artery
            pressure, 228
      recording
         contrast identification of structures during, 76
         demonstrating anterior and posterior cusps, 224
         in Ebstein's anomaly, 327
         in newborn, 224, 344
         in transposition of great vessels with subpulmonic
            obstruction, 346
      relationship of aortic and mitral valve to, 78
      stenosis; *see* Stenosis, pulmonary
      structures in beam, 222
      systolic notching in pericardial effusion, 285
      technical considerations, 224-226
      two-dimensional echocardiography of, 414
   venous drainage, total anomalous, 318
Pulmonic; *see* Pulmonary

R

Radiography of chest, 23
Recorder paper types, strip chart of, 53
Recording(s)
   made with direct print paper, 52
   techniques in ultrasound, 51-53
Reflection(s)
   complex, 40
   principles of, 37

Reflector
   characteristics, 36
   shape, 38
Refraction, principles of, 37
Regurgitation
   aortic; *see* Aortic valve regurgitation
   mitral; *see* Mitral valve regurgitation
Resolution
   axial, 33
   lateral, 34
Retrocardiac spaces, false, 281
Reverberation(s)
   artifact, 305
      mechanism of, 39
   in echocardiography, 41
Rheumatic; *see* Mitral valve regurgitation, rheumatic
Rhythm disorders, 15-16
   electrocardiography in, 17
Right ventricle; *see* Ventricle, right
Rupture
   chordae, two-dimensional echocardiography of, 390
   mitral
      apparatus; *see* Mitral valve, rupture of apparatus
      chordae; *see* Mitral valve chordae, rupture

S

SAMs
   in aortic incompetence, 123
   mitral chordae motion mimicking, 121
   in mitral valve prolapse, 106
   partial, in IHSS, 120
Scanners; *see* Two-dimensional echocardiography,
      scanners
Scanning
   beam; *see* Beam scanning
   ventricle, left, in IHSS, 120
Semilunar valve formation, 314
Septal defect
   atrial, 315-320
      anatomic changes, 315
      auscultatory findings in, 21
      clinical summary, 315-316
      echocardiographic features, 316-317
      echocardiography, role of, 320
      functional changes, 315
      ostium primum
         echocardiographic differentiation from ostium
            secundum, 317
         left ventricular cavity recording in, 316
         mitral valve in, 135
         tricuspid valve in, 215
      phonocardiography of, 21
      secundum type, tricuspid flutter in, 214
   ventricular, 320-321
      auscultatory findings in, 21
      contrast study in, 64
      phonocardiography of, 21
      pulmonary hypertension complicating, 320
      surgical closure of, contrast studies after, 64
Septal dropouts and left ventricular dimensions, 250
Shunt
   atrial, left-to-right, two-dimensional contrast echo-
      cardiography of, 425
   congenital left ventricular–right atrial, 215-217
      anatomy and functional changes, 215
      clinical summary, 215-217
      echocardiographic features, 217

Shunt—cont'd
  congenital left ventricular–right atrial—cont'd
    echocardiography, role of, 217
    tricuspid systolic flutter in, 217
Shunting
  intracardiac, chamber enlargement due to, 11
  in underdevelopment of cardiac structures as compensatory mechanism, 12
Silastic mitral prosthesis, 299
Sinus
  coronary; see Coronary sinus
  of pericardium; see Pericardium, sinus of
  of Valsalva, aneurysm of, 184
    right, 184
Sliding in two-dimensional echocardiography, 378-379, 380
Sounds, 18-23
  extra, phonocardiography of, 20
  origin of, 19
  simultaneous recording of aortic valve, 189
Starr-Edwards prosthesis, 294
  diagrammatic representation, 309
  echocardiogram from, 302
  tricuspid, 298
Stenosis
  aortic
    acquired, 164-169
      anatomic changes, 164
      clinical summary, 164-165
      echocardiographic features, 165-166
      echocardiography, role of, 169
      functional changes, 164
    auscultatory findings in, 21
    calcific, 165
    congenital, 169-177
      anatomic and functional changes, 169-172
      clinical summary, 172
      echocardiographic features, 172-173
      echocardiography, role of, 177
    with IHSS, 124
    phonocardiography of, 21
    supravalvular, 176
    two-dimensional echocardiography of, 391
  infundibular, 236
    anatomic and functional changes, 236
    clinical summary, 236
    echocardiographic features, 236
    echocardiography, role of, 236
  mitral, 91-100
    anatomic changes, 91-92
    auscultatory findings in, 21
    calcific, simulating left atrial myxoma, 93
    calcified posterior cusp in, 97
    clinical summary, 92-95
    echo features in, 95
    functional changes, 91-92
    mitral echocardiography in, 103- 309
    narrow ventricular outflow tract in, left, 99
    phonocardiography in, 21
    severity of, relationship of mitral EF slope to, 100
    thickening of both leaflets and chordae in, 92
    two-dimensional echocardiography of, 386
    typical, 93
    ventricular outflow dimension in, left, 99
  pulmonary, 232-236
    anatomic and functional changes, 232-234
    auscultatory findings in, 21

Stenosis—cont'd
  pulmonary—cont'd
    clinical summary, 234
    echocardiographic features, 234
    echocardiography, role of, 235-236
    phonocardiography of, 21
    severe, 234
  subaortic
    discrete
      membranous, 136
      mitral valve in, 137, 142
    idiopathic hypertrophic, 116-127
      anatomic changes, 116-118
      with aortic stenosis, 124
      aortic valve movements in, 119
      auscultatory findings in, 21
      clinical summary, 118-119
      echocardiographic features, 119-121
      echocardiography, role of, 126-127
      functional changes, 116-118
      phonocardiography of, 21
      SAMs in, partial, 120
      with subaortic obstruction, discrete membranous, 141
    membranous
      aortic valve in, 139
      mitral valve in, 138
  tricuspid, 199-200
    anatomic and functional changes, 199
    auscultatory findings in, 21
    clinical summary, 199
    echocardiographic features, 199
    echocardiography, role of, 200
    phonocardiography of, 21
Subaortic; see also Aortic
  obstruction, 137-142
    anatomic changes, 137-138
    echocardiographic features, 138-139
    echocardiography, role of, 141
    functional changes, 137-138
    with IHSS, 141
    tunnel narrowing in, 142
  stenosis; see Stenosis, subaortic
Subpulmonic obstruction
  with dextrotransposition of great vessels, 345
  transposition of great vessels and; see Transposition of great vessels and subpulmonic obstruction
Subxiphoid echocardiogram, 80
  two-dimensional; see Two-dimensional echocardiography, subxiphoid technique
Suppression
  control errors, 62
  near-gain, 61
Systolic anterior motion; see SAMs

T

Tamponade, cardiac, 288
Tetralogy of Fallot, 334-338
  anatomic changes, 334
  anatomic features, 335
  clinical summary, 334-335
  echocardiographic features, 335
  echocardiography, role of, 338
  functional changes, 334
Thrombosis complicating prosthetic valve, 295
Tilting in two-dimensional echocardiography, 379, 380

Time-varied gain
  artifact of, 60
  effects of, 59
Transducer
  construction, 44
  motion during M-mode recording, 36
Transducer-holding technique, two-handed, 56
Transposition, 341-353
  complexes, 341-353
    role of echocardiography in, 353
  dextrotransposition; *see* Dextrotransposition of great
    vessels
  of great arteries, 341-345
    anatomic changes, 341
    clinical summary, 341-342
    echocardiographic detection techniques, 342-344
    functional changes, 341
    pulmonary artery in, 231, 232
  of great vessels
    M-mode echo findings in, 435
    and subpulmonic obstruction, 345-347
      anatomic changes, 345
      clinical summary, 345
      echocardiographic features, 345-347
      functional changes, 345
      pulmonary valve recording in, 346
    two-dimensional echocardiography of, 436
Tricuspid aortic valve, ultrasonic beam passing through,
  173
Tricuspid valve, 192-221
  atresia; *see* Atresia, tricuspid
  in atrial fibrillation, 219
  in atrial septal defect, ostium primum, 215
  in atrioventricular canal defect, 331
  beam scanning
    from aortic valve to, 194
    to aortic valve in right heart enlargement, 74
    to left ventricle, 74
    to right ventricular cavity, 195
  cleft, in atrioventricular canal defect, 319
  in double outlet right ventricle after surgery, 212
  echocardiograms in dextrotransposition of great ves-
    sels, 349
  echocardiographic anatomy, 72
  echocardiographic relationships of, 73
  endocarditis; *see* Endocarditis, tricuspid
  findings in disease, 199-219
  flutter
    diastolic, 213-215
      in atrial septal defect of secundum type, 214
    systolic, in left ventricular–right atrial shunt,
      217
  functional observations, 219-220
  insufficiency
    auscultatory findings in, 21
    phonocardiography of, 21
  in large right ventricle, 197
  late opening in congestive cardiomyopathy, 218
  leaflets
    posterior, 196
    septal, 196
      identification of, 196
  in membrane in right atrium in infant, 204
  normal, 192
    tracing, 194-196
  overriding, 327-329
  prolapse, 200-201

Tricuspid valve—cont'd
  prolapse—cont'd
    anatomic and functional changes, 200
    clinical summary, 200
    echocardiographic features, 200
    echocardiography, role of, 201
    pericardial effusion and, 284
  prosthesis; *see* Prosthetic valves, tricuspid
  recording
    complete, 193
    ultrasonic beam exiting through right atrium, 198
  reverberations in mitral valve atresia, 362
  septal leaflet, imaging of, 247
  stenosis; *see* Stenosis, tricuspid
  structures in beam, 192-193
  systolic abnormalities, 201
  systolic anterior movements abnormality, 217-219
    in heart block with ventricular pacemaker, 209
  technical considerations, 196-199
  two-dimensional echocardiography of, 412-414
  vegetation, 207
  in ventricular hypertrophy, right, 200
Truncus arteriosus, 338-341
  anatomic changes, 338-339
  aortic valve beam scanning in, 340
  clinical summary, 339-340
  echocardiographic features, 340
  echocardiography, role of, 341
  functional changes, 338-339
Tumor, mediastinal, 288
Two-dimensional echocardiography, 369-431
  angulation, 379, 380
  of aorta, proximal, 417
  of aortic valve, 417
  of atrium
    left, 414-416
    right, 412
  concepts of, 371
  contrast, 425-429
  fixed-beam, linear arrays, 377-378, 379
    basic concept, 377-378
    system features, 378
  four-chamber view, apical, 406-411
  of mitral valve, 416
  pivoting, 379-381
  planes in, 378-417
    aortic-tricuspid, 399-401
      anatomy, 403
    left ventricular long axis, 382-393
      anatomy, 383
    left ventricular short axis, 393-399
      anatomy, 393
    mitral-pulmonic, 402-406
      anatomy, 407
    mitral-tricuspid, 402, 404
  of pulmonary artery, 414
  of pulmonary valve, 414
  regional evaluation with, 412-417
  scanners
    electronic sector, 374-377
      basic concept, 374-376
      system features, 376-377
    mechanical sector, 373-374, 375
      basic concept, 373
      system features, 373-374
    phased array; *see* Two-dimensional echocardiog-
      raphy, scanners, electronic sector

Two-dimensional echocardiography—cont'd
sliding, 378-379, 380
status of, 370-372
subxiphoid anatomy, 417-423
subxiphoid technique, 417-423
horizontal four-chamber view obtained by, 421
suprasternal anatomy, 423-425
suprasternal technique, 423-425
clinical applications, 425
systems of, current, 372-378
tilting, 379, 380
in transposition of great vessels, 436
transverse views of great vessels, 398, 399
of tricuspid valve, 412-414
of ventricle
left, 416-417
right, 413, 414

U

Ulceration of mitral valve, 92
Ultrasound, 28-53
A-mode displays of signal processing in, 49
anatomy
of aortic valve cusps, 70
during aortic valve recording, 71
during atrial septal recording, 79
basic principles of, 28-53
beam; *see also* Beam
effects of tissues in, 29
passing through tricuspid aortic valve, 173
traversing pulmonary artery area, 226
traversing right ventricular outflow area, 226
biologic effects, 50-51
contract studies in intra-atrial baffle, 350
in coronary sinus identification, 280
imaging modes in, 30
indocyanine green contrast injections in, 216
instruments, 43-44
controls, 44-48
effect on echo imaging, 47
of mitral valve, 101
M-mode recording, transducer motion during, 36
physical principles of, 28-43
pulse-echo system, basic, 43
recording
and heart orientation, 82
techniques, 51-53
signal processing, 48-50
structure motion, 35

V

Valve
aortic; *see* Aortic valve
atrioventricular, single, and single ventricle, 356
eustachian, two-dimensional contrast echocardiography of, 427
mitral; *see* Mitral valve
prosthetic; *see* Prosthetic valves
pulmonary; *see* Pulmonary valve
semilunar, formation of, 314
tricuspid; *see* Tricuspid valve
Veins, pulmonary, total anomalous drainage, 318
Vena cava, persistent left superior, 280
and two-dimensional echocardiography by subxiphoid technique, 418
Ventricle
fibromas of, 257

Ventricle—cont'd
left, 244-267
aneurysm of, 13, 250
beam scanning from tricuspid valve to, 74
cavity of
beam scanning from aortic valve to, after left pneumonectomy, 278
beam scanning from, to aortic valve in pericardial and pleural effusions, 278
beam scanning from, to mitral valve in pericardial effusion, 279
beam scanning in pericardial effusion, 282
in coronary artery disease, 258
echo in volume overload, 145
echocardiogram of, 244
recording in ostium primum atrial septal defect, 316
shape abnormalities, two-dimensional echocardiography of, 395
transverse scans in two-dimensional echocardiography, 394
and two-dimensional echocardiography by subxiphoid technique, 420
contrast injection into, 63
dimensions of
septal dropouts and, 250
variations in, 249
dysfunction of, due to adriamycin, 256
echocardiography, role of, 255-257
end-diastolic pressure elevation, mitral valve in, 149
function determination, 251-255
echocardiographic measurement technique, 251-252
estimation of parameters, 252-254
hypertrophy of, concentric, in cardiomyopathy, 132
long axis of, beam scanning in, 67
mass of, 254
normal tracing of, 245-256
outflow
in aortic prosthesis endocarditis, 308
dimension of, in mitral stenosis, 99
narrow tract in mitral stenosis, 99
obstruction of, usefulness as echocardiography in, 435
performance of, 25
scan of, in idiopathic subaortic stenosis, 120
in shunt; *see* Shunt, congenital left ventricular–right atrial
structures in beam, 244-245
technical considerations, 246-251
two-dimensional echocardiography of, 385, 416-417
volume of, 252-253
overload, cavity echo in, 145
wall of
high speed recording of, 248
motion of, in constrictive pericarditis, 290
in pericardial effusion, 280
recording of, 246
thickness of, 253-254
obstruction, of mid-left cavity, 125-126
premature contraction and aortic valve motion of, 189
pressure overload of, effects of, 11
right
catheter reverberations, 211